CANCER   2

A COMPREHENSIVE TREATISE

ETIOLOGY: Viral Carcinogenesis

Therapies will be covered in subsequent volumes.

CANCER 2

A COMPREHENSIVE TREATISE

ETIOLOGY: Viral Carcinogenesis

FREDERICK F. BECKER, EDITOR
New York University School of Medicine

PLENUM PRESS • NEW YORK AND LONDON

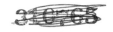

Library of Congress Cataloging in Publication Data

Becker, Frederick F
   Etiology—viral carcinogenesis.

   (His *Cancer, a comprehensive treatise*; v. 2)
   Includes bibliographies and index.
   1. Viral carcinogenesis.   I. Title.   [DNLM: 1. Neoplasms.
QZ200 B397c]
RC261.B42 vol. 2 [RC268.57] 616.9'94'008s [616.9'94'071]
ISBN 0-306-35202-8 (v. 2)   75-11770

© 1975 Plenum Press, New York
A Division of Plenum Publishing Corporation
227 West 17th Street, New York, N.Y. 10011

United Kingdom edition published by Plenum Press, London
A Division of Plenum Publishing Company, Ltd.
Davis House (4th Floor), 8 Scrubs Lane, Harlesden, London, NW10 6SE, England

Printed in the United States of America

Contributors

to Volume 2

J. Michael Bishop, Department of Microbiology, University of California, San Francisco, California

Hidesaburo Hanafusa, The Rockefeller University, New York, New York

Yohei Ito, Department of Microbiology, Faculty of Medicine, University of Kyoto, Kyoto, Japan

M. A. Jerkofsky, Department of Microbiology, College of Medicine, The Milton S. Hershey Medical Center of The Pennsylvania State University, Hershey, Pennsylvania

George Khoury, Laboratory of Biology of Viruses, National Institutes of Allergy and Infectious Diseases, National Institutes of Health, Bethesda, Maryland

Elliott D. Kieff, Division of Biological Sciences, The University of Chicago, Chicago, Illinois

Michael M. Lieber, Viral Leukemia and Lymphoma Branch, National Cancer Institute, National Institutes of Health, Bethesda, Maryland

Dan H. Moore, Institute for Medical Research, Camden, New Jersey

F. Rapp, Department of Microbiology, College of Medicine, The Milton S. Hershey Medical Center of The Pennsylvania State University, Hershey, Pennsylvania

Bernard Roizman, Division of Biological Sciences, The University of Chicago, Chicago, Illinois

Norman P. Salzman, Laboratory of Biology of Viruses, National Institutes of Allergy and Infectious Diseases, National Institutes of Health, Bethesda, Maryland

Gordon H. Theilen, Department of Surgery, School of Veterinary Medicine, University of California at Davis, Davis, California vi

CONTRIBUTORS

GEORGE J. TODARO, Viral Leukemia and Lymphoma Branch, National Cancer Institute, National Institutes of Health, Bethesda, Maryland

HAROLD E. VARMUS, Department of Microbiology, University of California, San Francisco, California

Preface

The impact of basic research on oncology has been particularly impressive in the recent search for the cause of malignancy. Equally impressive is our appreciation of the cause of tumors based on observation. Even in the earliest era of the study of infectious diseases, it was proposed that tumorous growth in animals and birds resulted from "minute" infectious particles. Experiments then supported the hypothesis that the etiologic agent in many animal tumors was viral.

The development of molecular biology, supported by technical advances and conceptual understanding of macromolecular action, led to an explosive increase in studies of animal oncogenic viruses. For a decade, new findings emerged from research laboratories revealing the enormous variety of such agents, the complexity of their interactions with cells, and the tantalizingly possible mechanisms by which they might cause malignant transformation of the cell. Repeatedly, clues emerged which suggested the intervention of viral agents in human tumors. A breathless excitement pervaded both the scientific and public communities as highly publicized findings rapidly followed one another. The excitement was no less scientific than it was practical, for implicit in the concept of the viral oncogen is the possibility of specific virostatic or virotoxic agents or of immunization.

Yet, despite the incredible facility of our laboratories and the advances in technique as this volume goes to press, crucial questions remain unanswered: Have we created a "race" of laboratory, viral oncogens, unrelated to wild types? Are there human viral-induced tumors? If so, which are they and how many are there? By what means does the virus integrate into the apparatus of the host cell and later its normal control, resulting in malignancy? Once altered, is that cell capable of directed reversion?

This book presents progress which has been made in the search for the viral etiology of tumors and delineates the vast landscape of future research.

New York   Frederick F. Becker

Contents

RNA Viruses

The Molecular Biology of RNA Tumor Viruses   1

J. Michael Bishop and Harold E. Varmus

Avian RNA Tumor Viruses 2

HIDESABURO HANAFUSA

Mammalian Type C RNA Viruses   3

~ MICHAEL M. LIEBER AND GEORGE J. TODARO

Mammary Tumor Virus 4

Dan H. Moore

Feline Leukemia–Sarcoma Complex: A Model for RNA Viral Tumorigenesis 5

Gordon H. Theilen

DNA Viruses

DNA Viruses: Molecular Biology   6

F. RAPP AND M. A. JERKOFSKY

Herpes Simplex and Epstein–Barr Viruses in Human Cells and Tissues: A Study in Contrasts 7

BERNARD ROIZMAN AND ELLIOTT D. KIEFF

Papilloma–Myxoma Viruses 8

YOHEI ITO

Replication and Transformation by Papovaviruses   9

GEORGE KHOURY AND NORMAN P. SALZMAN

RNA
Viruses

The Molecular Biology of RNA Tumor Viruses

J. MICHAEL BISHOP AND HAROLD E. VARMUS

1. Introduction

RNA tumor viruses are useful tools for the study of oncogenesis because they rapidly induce tumors in animals and efficiently transform cells in culture. These viruses are distinguished by certain morphological features (Bernhard, 1960; Sarker *et al.*, 1971*a*), an exceptionally large single-stranded RNA genome (about 30,000 nucleotides, Duesberg, 1970) and an RNA-directed DNA polymerase which transcribes the viral genome into single- and double-stranded DNA (Baltimore, 1970; Temin and Mizutani, 1970; Temin and Baltimore, 1972). This transcription, the mechanism by which it occurs, the fate of its products in the infected cell, and the role of the products in both the viral life cycle and virus-induced transformation of the host cell are the principal subjects of our discussion.

The following chapter is not a comprehensive introduction to RNA tumor viruses, but a treatise on the mechanisms which mediate the reproduction and cellular effects of these viruses. Our objective is to prepare the reader to understand the detailed discussions of specific classes of viruses in the subsequent chapters of this volume. We have identified and discussed aspects of viral structure and physiology which appear to be shared by most if not all RNA tumor viruses. The literature citations are not comprehensive and are designed to provide an overview of the major investigative trends in the contemporary study of the molecular biology of RNA tumor viruses.

J. MICHAEL BISHOP and HAROLD E. VARMUS ● Department of Microbiology, University of California, San Francisco, California.

J. M. BISHOP
AND
H. E. VARMUS

RNA tumor viruses are ubiquitous in nature and are associated with a large variety of neoplasms in their natural hosts (Huebner and Gilden, 1971). Consequently, these viruses have become favorite subjects for investigators who are seeking evidence that viruses are involved in the etiology of human tumors. The study of RNA tumor viruses began with the discoveries that avian leukemia (Ellerman and Bang, 1909) and sarcomas (Rous, 1911) can be transmitted horizontally by cell-free infectious agents. However, many viruses which possess both 70S RNA and RNA-directed DNA polymerase are not oncogenic. Some are cytopathic, others are symbiotic with their hosts. Virtually all such viruses, whether oncogenic or not, conform to one of two architectural forms defined by electron microscopy, *viz.*, type B and type C virus particles (Bernhard, 1960; Sarker *et al.*, 1971*a*). These two forms are distinguished by certain features of their morphological maturation and differences in their mature structure (Sarkar *et al.*, 1971*a*), but the outlines of their architectures are quite similar (Fig. 1). A third class of particle—type A—is an intracellular form which appears in two locations: (1) within the cytoplasm, where it is probably a precursor to mature type B particles (Sarkar *et al.*, 1971*a*; Tanaka *et al.*, 1972; for a dissenting opinion, see Smith and Wivel, 1973), and (2) within cisternae, where its nature and function are enigmatic (Wivel and Smith, 1971; Wivel *et al.*, 1973).

There is no universally accepted taxonomic designation for viruses with 70S RNA and RNA-directed DNA polymerase. Since many of these viruses are not oncogenic, we will use the structural designations of B- and C-type particles to denote a single taxonomic class.

For convenience, we can divide the oncogenicity of RNA tumor viruses into three general classes: induction of sarcomas (sarcoma viruses), induction of leukemias and related disorders (leukemia or leukosis viruses), and induction of carcinoma of the breast (mammary tumor viruses, rigorously identified only in mice to date). These categories are outlined here because they have useful

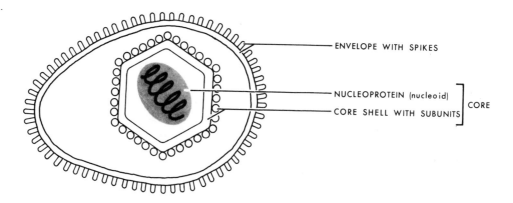

FIGURE 1. The virion of RNA tumor viruses.

correlates in cell culture. *Sarcoma viruses* transform cultured fibroblasts to a neoplastic state and are known as *transforming viruses* in laboratory parlance. *Leukosis viruses* cannot transform cultured fibroblasts (although certain strains of virus can cause cytopathic effects in cultured fibroblasts under special circumstances, Kawai and Hanafusa, 1972a; Graf, 1972) and are known as *nontransforming viruses*. However, there are also "nontransforming" (or *transformation-defective*) variants of sarcoma viruses; these are laboratory rather than natural isolates, but at least some of them are leukemogenic (Biggs *et al.*, 1973). Last, there are C-type viruses which are *not oncogenic* under any circumstances and are likewise *nontransforming*. We exclude mammary tumor virus from this nomenclature for the present because it cannot reproducibly infect cells in culture.

3. Architecture and Antigens of Virions

We describe here only the outlines of virion architecture (Fig. 1). The details vary from one virus to another and many are presently controversial. The virion is enclosed by an envelope which is derived from the plasma membrane of the host cell and retains the basic structure of that organelle (de Thé *et al.*, 1964; Ishizaki *et al.*, 1973). The external surface of the virion envelope contains protruding spikes (or knobs) which are more prominent on B-type than on C-type particles (Nowinski *et al.*, 1970). These spikes are composed of glycoproteins and have multiple functional roles, including the sites responsible for adsorption of the virion to a host cell, type-specific viral antigen(s), and, in at least some cases, hemagglutinin (Bolognesi *et al.*, 1972a; Rifkin and Compans, 1971; Robinson *et al.*, 1970; Duesberg *et al.*, 1970; Witter *et al.*, 1973). Within the envelope is a "core shell." Some investigators have been able to demonstrate geometrical symmetry and subunits in this structure (Nermut *et al.*, 1972). The shell in turn encloses a ribonucleoprotein complex (or "nucleoid") which contains the viral genome and, possibly, low molecular weight RNAs separate from the genome (Davis and Rueckert, 1972). The shell and ribonucleoprotein comprise a unit known as the "core." This can be isolated on the basis of its increased density, and there is provisional evidence that it is infectious (Bolognesi *et al.*, 1972b). It contains RNA-directed DNA polymerase as well as several other enzymes often found in these viruses (Mizutani and Temin, 1971).

The generally recognized protein constituents of virions include either four (mammalian viruses) or five (avian viruses) polypeptides and two glycoproteins (Nowinski *et al.*, 1972a; Fleissner, 1971). [This accounting omits the polypeptide(s) of RNA-directed DNA polymerase, which are not usually detected by compositional analysis of virions.] A variable number of other proteins have also been described, usually in relatively small amounts (Bolognesi and Bauer, 1970; Cheung *et al.*, 1972). There is no conclusive evidence that any of these "minor" proteins is a *bona fide* viral component. Genetic analysis of avian viruses has demonstrated that type-specific antigens (Vogt, 1971b; Kawai and Hanafusa, 1972b) and RNA-directed DNA polymerase (Hanafusa *et al.*, 1972b; May *et al.*,

1972; Linial and Mason, 1973) are encoded in the viral genome. It is possible that some of the other virion proteins may be derived from the host cell, as has been described for polyoma virus (Frearson and Crawford, 1972).

Three classes of viral antigens have been identified and their determinants provisionally localized on structural proteins of the virion: (1) Group-specific antigens, shared by all related viruses derived from a single host species (e.g., avian leukemia–sarcoma viruses, murine leukemia–sarcoma viruses); determinants are located on at least two polypeptides in the core of the virion. (2) Type-specific antigens, which define the most specific serological subgroups presently identified and which elicit neutralizing antibodies; the major determinants are located on glycoprotein(s) in the spikes (knobs) of the virion. (3) Interspecies ("interspec") antigens, which are shared by viruses derived from different host species and which, to date, have been found only in mammalian viruses (Geering et al., 1970; Gilden et al., 1971; Schafer et al., 1973); three distinct "interspec" determinants have been described, two located on a core protein which also has group-specific antigenicity (Gilden et al., 1971; Strand and August, 1974; Parks and Scolnick, 1972), the third located on a glycoprotein of the envelope spikes (Strand and August, 1974). Application of highly sensitive immunological techniques indicates that both group- and type-specific antigenic determinants can be found on most if not all viral proteins (Strand and August, 1974).

4. Nucleic Acids

Purified preparations of B- and C-type viruses contain a variety of nucleic acids (Table 1), some of which are also constituents of the uninfected host cell (Wollmann and Kirsten, 1968; Obara et al., 1971; Faras et al., 1973a; Erikson et al.,

TABLE 1

The Nucleic Acids of an RNA Tumor Virus[a]

Nucleic acid	Amount (%)	Sources
70S RNA	70	Virus
Aggregate of		
20–35S "subunits"	(95)	Virus
5S	(1)	Cell
4S	(4)	Cell
28S rRNA	2	Cell
18S rRNA	1	Cell
7S	5	Cell
5S	2	Cell
4S	20	Cell
dsDNA[b]	0.5	Cell

[a] These data are derived from analyses of Rous sarcoma virus (Faras et al., 1973a).
[b] Double-stranded DNA.

1973). The pattern of these latter nucleic acids in the virus varies from one species of host to another. At present, the only reasonable generalization is that all infectious virus particles probably contain at least two types of RNA: the high molecular weight RNA (50–70S) which typifies this entire class of viruses, and a set of low molecular weight RNAs which generally includes 4S RNAs (Bonar *et al.*, 1967; Erikson, 1969; Bishop *et al.*, 1970*a*; Emanoil-Ravicovitch *et al.*, 1973). None of the remaining RNAs listed in Table 1 has been established as an inevitable constituent of RNA tumor viruses. Some preparations of virus also contain miniscule amounts of DNA (Levinson *et al.*, 1970; Biswal *et al.*, 1971), which is probably a contaminant derived from host cells (Levinson *et al.*, 1972).

4.1. The Viral Genome

Optimally, a viral genome is identified by the isolation of an infectious nucleic acid. This has not been reproducibly achieved for RNA tumor viruses and is theoretically unlikely if a virion-contained function (i.e., RNA-directed DNA polymerase) is essential for the initiation of infection. However, 50–70S RNA is the only universal constituent of RNA tumor viruses large enough to accommodate multiple viral genes and is considered to be the viral genome. The relatively large size and extensive secondary structure of this RNA have impeded analysis of its molecular weight and structural conformation. Data from several conventional procedures set the mass of the native molecule at $9–12 \times 10^6$ daltons; the three or four major subunits observed following denaturation have molecular weights of $2.5–3.5 \times 10^6$ (Erikson, 1969; Duesberg, 1968; Maisel *et al.*, 1973). The precise values vary considerably from one strain of virus to another, although the different members of a particular class of virus (e.g., all helper-independent avian sarcoma viruses) generally have genomes of identical molecular weight. Measurement of the length of 50–70S RNA by electron microscopy is extremely difficult, since the RNA must be denatured to facilitate visualization: this usually precludes examination of the intact 50–70S structure. However, recent work has set a minimum size of 6×10^6 daltons for the ostensibly undissociated genome of Rous sarcoma virus (W. Mangel, H. Delius, and P. Duesberg, personal communication), and an earlier report contained micrographs of molecules long enough to have a mass of $10–12 \times 10^6$ daltons (Granboulan *et al.*, 1966). In our view, these data do not establish a reliable molecular weight for the viral genome, but they do substantiate the view that each genome contains more than one high molecular weight subunit (Duesberg, 1970; also, see below).

The 50–70S RNA is an aggregate which dissociates when treated with heat or a denaturing solvent (Erikson, 1969: Duesberg, 1968). The principal constituents of this aggregate are high molecular weight "subunits" (about 3×10^6 daltons) and 4S RNA (Erikson and Erikson, 1971), but small amounts of other low molecular weight RNAs (e.g., 5S and 7S) have also been identified (Faras *et al.*, 1973*a*; Canaani and Duesberg, 1972; Nichols and Waddell, 1973; Sawyer and Dahlberg, 1973). The high molecular weight subunits of both avian and murine viruses are single-stranded RNAs with poly(A) at the 3'-termini (Stephenson *et al.*, 1973; personal communications from R. Perry and R. Erikson). (Previous reports that the subunits have pU at the 3'-ends were erroneous—probably because of a technical artifact.) The 5'-terminus of the subunits from one avian sarcoma virus is Ap (Silber *et al.*, 1973); no data for other viruses are presently available.

The subunits from any clone of avian virus all have the same length, but the subunits from infectious avian sarcoma virus (class "a" subunits) are approximately 10% larger than the subunits from either transformation-defective variants of the sarcoma virus or avian leukemia virus (class "b" subunits) (Duesberg and Vogt, 1970; Martin and Duesberg, 1972; Vogt, 1971*a*; Duesberg *et al.*, 1973*b*; Duesberg and Vogt, 1973*a, b*; Maisel *et al.*, 1973). These differences between the masses of subunits are probably generated by deletions from the genomes of sarcoma viruses during passages at high multiplicities (Vogt, 1971*a*; Duesberg *et al.*, 1973*b*; Duesberg and Vogt, 1973*b*; Lai *et al.*, 1973).

Another form of deletion generates transforming viruses which are replication defective; that is, they cannot produce infectious particles unless replication occurs in the presence of a helper virus (generally a related leukemia virus) (Hanafusa, 1965; Hartley and Rowe, 1966; Kawai and Hanafusa, 1973). The genomes of helper-dependent avian sarcoma (transforming) viruses have subunits which are approximately the same size as class "b" subunits of avian nontransforming viruses (Duesberg *et al.*, 1973*a, b*). Although different regions must be deleted to generate avian *helper-dependent transforming* and *helper-independent nontransforming* viruses, the deletions are of approximately the same size. This description assumes that the starting point in both instances is the RNA of the helper-independent sarcoma (transforming) virus containing genes for replication, transformation, and leukemogenesis; there is biological evidence that avian sarcoma viruses do contain genes for leukemogenesis which become manifest after deletion of transforming (sarcomagenic) genes (Biggs *et al.*, 1973). The genomes of helper-dependent murine sarcoma (transforming) viruses are considerably *smaller* than the genomes of helper-independent murine leukemia viruses (Maisel *et al.*, 1973) and may be more defective than their avian counterparts. In addition, tests by molecular hybridization indicate that the genomes of murine leukemia and sarcoma viruses are less closely related than are the genomes of avian leukemia and sarcoma viruses (Stephenson and Aaronson, 1971). Any effort to explain the genetic relationships between the leukemia and sarcoma viruses of mice would be speculative and premature.

The presence of several high molecular weight subunits in each 50–70S structure (three or four per genome) introduces the possibility that the viral genome is polyploid, i.e., that the subunits contain identical genetic information (Vogt, 1973). If true, this would limit the genome to approximately 10–20 cistrons, which is barely sufficient to account for the identified structural proteins of the virion, the RNA-directed DNA polymerase, and gene product(s) responsible for cellular transformation. The complexities of the genomes of Rous sarcoma virus and murine leukemia virus have also been estimated by molecular hybridization (Taylor *et al.*, 1974; Fan and Paskind, 1974); the data indicate that the mass of unique nucleotide sequences in both viral genomes exceeds 9×10^6 daltons. These results are inconsistent with the hypothesis that the genomes are polyploid, although small amounts of genetic reiteration cannot be excluded. The nonidentity of the subunits would indicate that the high rate of genetic recombination seen with these viruses is due to reassortment of subunits. By contrast, the segregation of deletion mutants (Duesberg,. 1968), the frequent formation of heterozygotes (Weiss *et al.*, 1973), and biochemical evidence for genetic crossing over in recombination (Vogt and Duesberg, 1973) are more readily explained if the genome is polyploid (see Vogt, 1973, and Duesberg and Vogt, 1973*a*, for details of this argument). Results from chemical analyses of viral RNA indicate that the molecular weight of unique nucleotide sequences in the viral genome is approximately 3×10^6 (Billeter *et al.*, 1974; Beeman *et al.*, 1974). We consider this to be the most reliable of available evidence and conclude that the genome is probably polyploid.

4.2. Virions Without Genomes

Virus particles which contain no 70S have been isolated (Phillips *et al.*, 1973). These particles generally contain some of the other forms of RNA noted in Table 1 (particularly 4S, 18S, and 28S RNAs), but they are not infectious and it is not certain that they contain viral genes. The genesis of these particles is unexplained.

4.3. Genetic Interactions Among Viral Genomes

Two forms of genetic deficiency are prominent among RNA tumor viruses: an inability to produce infectious virus and a failure to convert cultured fibroblasts to a neoplastic state. Both deficiencies can be attributed to deletions from the viral genome (see above). However, the molecular consequences of these deletions are known in only one instance, *viz.*, the helper-dependent (replication-defective) strains of avian sarcoma viruses, which cannot direct the synthesis of glycoprotein(s) found in the viral envelope and essential for the infectivity of the virion (Scheele and Hanafusa, 1971; Kawai and Hanafusa, 1973). A helper virus can provide the missing structural protein(s) by phenotypic mixing.

Spontaneously occurring variants of RNA tumor viruses which are deficient in RNA-directed DNA polymerase may also be deletion mutants (Hanafusa and Hanafusa, 1971; Peebles *et al.*, 1972). In the case of RSVα, the mutant virions lack any protein capable of cross-reacting with polymerase in an immunological test (Hanafusa *et al.*, 1972*b*). Virions of these defective strains can acquire polymerase by phenotypic mixing during virus maturation (Hanafusa and Hanafusa, 1971), and the genome can readily acquire polymerase gene(s) by recombination with another strain of virus (Hanafusa and Hanafusa, 1971). (See the chapter by Hanafusa in this volume for a more extensive treatment of RSVα.)

Genetically different strains of RNA tumor viruses recombine at an exceptionally high frequency (Vogt, 1971*b*; Kawai and Hanafusa, 1972*b*). This could most easily be ascribed to reassortment of subunits from haploid genomes. However, Vogt and Duesberg (1973) have analyzed recombined genomes with physical techniques and have concluded that the recombination event involves crossing over between genomes rather than genetic reassortment among subunits. This conclusion, of course, is consistent with the thesis that the genome is polyploid.

4.4. Low Molecular Weight RNAs

Most available evidence indicates that the low molecular weight RNAs in RNA tumor viruses are derived from the host cell during assembly of the virus (see above); some investigators have considered these RNAs to be trivial contaminants (Bader and Steck, 1969). The 4S RNAs found free in virions (*free 4S RNAs*) and those associated with the 50–70S aggregate (*70S-a 4S RNAs*) possess structural features of tRNA (Faras *et al.*, 1973*a*; Bishop *et al.*, 1970*a*; Erikson and Erikson, 1971; Sawyer and Dahlberg, 1973; Rosenthal and Zamecnik, 1973*a*) and can be acylated with amino acids (Travnicek, 1968; Rosenthal and Zamecnik, 1973*b*; Erikson and Erikson, 1970; Wang *et al.*, 1973). The 70S-a 4S RNAs are a partial sample of the population of tRNAs represented in free 4S RNAs (Erikson and Erikson, 1971; Sawyer and Dahlberg, 1973; Faras *et al.*, 1973*a*; Rosenthal and Zamecnik, 1973*b*). One of the 4S RNAs, found in both the free and 70S-a fractions, is a primer for the initiation of DNA synthesis when 70S RNA serves as template for RNA-directed DNA synthesis *in vitro* (Canaani and Duesberg, 1972; Faras *et al.*, 1973*b*, 1974; Dahlberg *et al.*, 1974). There is no evidence that any of the other 4S RNAs have functions in the life cycle of the virus.

Although probably derived from the host cell, the tRNAs found in virus are not a random assortment of cellular tRNAs (Travnicek and Riman, 1970; Rosenthal and Zamecnik, 1973*b*; Erikson and Erikson, 1970; Wang *et al.*, 1973) and may be distinctive for specific strains of virus (Wang *et al.*, 1973). Generally, the same isoaccepting species of tRNA for a particular amino acid are present in the same relative amounts in virus and host cell, but there are exceptions to this rule. Avian myeloblastosis virus contains species of arginine and histidine tRNAs which are chromatographically distinct from the corresponding tRNAs of the cell (Gallagher and Gallo, 1973); this virus may also lack one of several species of lysyl-tRNA (Travnicek and Riman, 1970). A single species of met-tRNA (not an initiator tRNA) predominates among the *free* met-tRNAs of avian sarcoma and leukosis viruses (Elder and Smith, 1973; unpublished data of B. Cordell-Stewart and the authors), whereas appreciable amounts of all four of the known avian met-tRNAs are included in the 70S-a 4S RNAs and the initiator met-tRNA is particularly abundant (Elder and Smith, 1974; unpublished data of B. Cordell-Stewart and the authors). The significance of these observations is not known, but speculations that the 70S-a initiator tRNA is a primer for DNA synthesis (Elder and Smith, 1974) are probably not correct (see below).

Transforming avian viruses alter the proportion of various tRNAs in the host cell, and the sample of tRNAs included in viruses produced by transformed cells is different from the sample in the same virus produced by nontransformed cells (Wang *et al.*, 1973). These observations are thought to implicate viral genes in both the regulation of cellular synthesis of tRNAs and the packaging of tRNAs into virions.

The 5S and 7S RNAs found in some viruses (both separate from and associated with the viral genome) are identical to RNAs found in uninfected host cells. The 5S RNA is a constituent of normal ribosomes (Faras *et al.*, 1973*a*) and is probably essential for cellular protein synthesis. The 7S RNA (Bishop *et al.*, 1970*b*; Erikson *et al.*, 1973; Nichols and Waddell, 1973; Sawyer and Dahlberg, 1973) is associated with polyribosomes (Walker *et al.*, 1974), but its function is unknown. To date, neither of these RNAs has been implicated in either viral structure or replication.

5. RNA-Directed DNA Polymerase

5.1. Definition

RNA-directed DNA synthesis may not be unique to B- and C-type viruses (Temin and Baltimore, 1972), but it is nevertheless a universal element in the replication of these viruses (Temin, 1971, 1972). The responsible enzyme is a constituent of virions, encoded in the viral genome (Linial and Mason, 1973; Wyke and Linial, 1973). The best evidence for the last statement comes from experiments with two strains of conditional mutants of Rous sarcoma virus (Linial and Mason, 1973). These mutants possess temperature-sensitive RNA-directed DNA polymerase and are unable to either replicate or transform cells at the restrictive temperature (Linian and Mason, 1973; Baltimore *et al.*, 1974; Wyke and Linial, 1973). There are corresponding deficits in the synthesis of proviral DNA and viral RNA in cells infected at the restrictive temperature (see below).

The definition of RNA-directed DNA polymerase is a somewhat arbitrary exercise based on the enzyme's capacity to transcribe certain template-primers into DNA. Present practice considers the response to two such complexes as specific for RNA-directed DNA polymerase: (1) $poly(rC) \cdot oligo(dG)$; the oligomer serves as primer for the initiation of DNA synthesis (Baltimore and Smoler, 1971; McCaffrey *et al.*, 1973); and (2) 70S RNA from and B- or C-type virus; one or more RNA primer(s) (apparently a 70S-a 4S RNA) is intrinsic to this molecule (Verma *et al.*, 1971; Leis and Hurwitz, 1972; Faras *et al.*, 1973*b*, 1974; Dahlberg *et al.*, 1974). The widely used $poly(rA) \cdot oligo(dT)$ has only limited diagnostic value because it will serve as template-primer for several cellular DNA polymerases which cannot respond to either $poly(rC) \cdot oligo(dG)$ or 70S RNA. All viral RNA-directed DNA polymerases tested to date respond to appropriate synthetic template-primers [such as $poly(rA) \cdot oligo(dT)$ and $poly(rC) \cdot oligo (dG)$]. However, polymerases purified from several classes of C-type viruses transcribe viral 70S RNA either poorly or not at all *in vitro* (Wang and Duesberg, 1973; Verma *et al.*, 1974; Kang and Temin, 1973), and there is a corresponding deficiency in the amount of

RNA-directed DNA synthesis *in vitro* by virions of these viruses (Wang and Duesberg, 1973; Verma *et al.*, 1974; Kang and Temin, 1973). The reason for this is not known, but the defect is probably in the enzyme because the 50–70S RNA from these viruses is an effective template for RNA-directed DNA polymerase from other sources (Wang and Duesberg, 1973; Kang and Temin, 1973). These are paradoxical observations because the allegedly defective polymerases come from viruses which clearly replicate through the agency of RNA-directed DNA synthesis.

5.2. RNase H

RNase H has been described in RNA tumor viruses (Molling *et al.*, 1971; Baltimore and Smoler, 1972; Grandgenett *et al.*, 1972), normal eukaryotic cells (Hausen and Stein, 1970; Keller and Crouch, 1972), and bacteria (Berkower *et al.*, 1973). The nucleases from all three sources specifically hydrolyze the RNA constituent of a DNA · RNA hybrid; single-stranded RNA is not a substrate. The nuclease from RNA tumor viruses is a processive exonuclease; hydrolysis proceeds from either 3′- or 5′-termini of the substrate, and these termini must be in duplex hybrid (Leis *et al.*, 1973). The RNase H activity in avian tumor viruses resides on the same protein as RNA-directed DNA polymerase; nuclease and polymerase are inseparable by physical techniques (Baltimore and Smoler, 1972; Keller and Crouch, 1972; Grandgenett *et al.*, 1973), and both are affected by single conditional mutations in the viral genome (Baltimore *et al.*, 1974).

The RNase H of cells may participate in the replication of DNA by removing RNA primers from template subsequent to the initiation of DNA synthesis (Keller and Crouch, 1972; Berkower *et al.*, 1973). The RNase H of avian sarcoma viruses presumably has a function in the life cycle of the virus, because the enzyme is encoded in the viral genome (Baltimore *et al.*, 1974). The nature of that function is presently unknown. The viral nuclease has been implicated in the initiation of duplex DNA synthesis by RNA-directed DNA polymerase (Molling *et al.*, 1971), but this view is challenged by the observation that the polymerase of mammalian viruses is capable of duplex DNA synthesis, yet lacks RNase H activity as an intrinsic property of the enzyme molecule (Wang and Duesberg, 1973; Verma *et al.*, 1974).

5.3. Composition and Antigenicity

The RNA-directed DNA polymerase of avian sarcoma–leukemia viruses has a molecular weight of approximately 160,000 and is composed of two subunits, α (mol wt 65,000–70,000) and β (mol wt 105,000–110,000) (Grandgenett *et al.*, 1973; Kacian *et al.*, 1971). By contrast, the polymerases from mammalian viruses have a molecular weight of approximately 70,000 and are presumably composed of polypeptides analogous to the α subunit of the avian polymerases (Tronick *et al.*, 1972). (There is at least one exception to this statement: the purified DNA polymerase of hamster leukemia virus has a molecular weight of 120,000 and is composed of two subunits of molecular weight 68,000 and 53,000, Verma *et al.*, 1974). The enzymes from mammalian viruses transcribe 70S RNA poorly (if at all) and are probably devoid of RNase H activity (but there is controversy on the latter point; for example, see Wang and Duesberg, 1973; Grandgenett *et al.*, 1972). These deficiencies cannot presently be ascribed to the absence of β subunits, because the α subunit of avian polymerases allegedly possesses the entire functional capacity of the enzyme molecule, *viz.*, RNA-directed and DNA-directed DNA synthesis and RNase H activity (Grandgenett *et al.*, 1973). The function of the β subunit is not known.

Antibodies against a number of representative RNA-directed DNA polymerases are now available and have been used in efforts to define the extent of serological relatedness among polymerases from various viruses. Three conclusions seem safe: (1) there is no serological cross-section between the polymerases of avian viruses and those of mammalian viruses (Nowinski *et al.*, 1972*b*; Parks *et al.*, 1972); (2) there is similarity but not identity among the antigenic determinants of polymerases from various mammalian C-type viruses (Parks *et al.*, 1972; Scolnick *et al.*, 1972*a, c*; Todaro and Gallo, 1973; Oroszlan *et al.*, 1971); and (3) the polymerase of B-type mouse mammary tumor virus is antigenically distinct from the polymerases of mammalian C-type viruses (Parks *et al.*, 1972; Oroszlan *et al.*, 1971). Otherwise, the available data are too fragmentary and uncertain to merit discussion here. Previously unidentified cross-reactions are being recognized as the potency of antibody preparations improves and the sensitivity of test procedures increases.

5.4. Enzymatic Properties of RNA-Directed DNA Polymerase

The properties of RNA-directed DNA polymerases have been extensively reviewed elsewhere (Temin and Baltimore, 1972; Sarin and Gallo, 1973). We will discuss a few features which bear on the structure and replication of RNA tumor viruses.

All DNA polymerases require a 3′-hydroxyl terminus (or "primer") for the initiation of polymerization. RNA-directed DNA polymerase conforms to this rule (Baltimore and Smoler, 1971; Smoler *et al.*, 1971; Leis and Hurwitz, 1972; Hurwitz and Leis, 1972). The primer can be the 3′-terminus either of the template itself (Leis and Hurwitz, 1972) or of a separate polynucleotide held to the template by hydrogen bonds (Baltimore and Smoler, 1971; Smoler *et al.*, 1971; Canaani and Duesberg, 1972; Faras *et al.*, 1973*b*). In either event, DNA is synthesized in the 5′ to 3′ direction (Smoler *et al.*, 1971).

RNA-directed DNA polymerases can utilize either DNA or RNA as template. The efficiency of DNA synthesis is a function of individual combinations of template and primer; the enzymes have no general preference for either DNA or RNA as template. The efficiency with which RNA-directed DNA polymerase can transcribe DNA from naturally occurring RNAs (i.e., heteropolymers as opposed to synthetic homopolymers or copolymers) is unique among the known DNA polymerases, but DNA polymerase I from *Escherichia coli* has been used to transcribe ribosomal RNA and tobacco mosaic virus RNA without additional primers (presumably by initiating on the 3′-terminus of the template) (Loeb *et al.*, 1973) and globin messenger RNA with oligo(dT) as primer (Modak *et al.*, 1973; Proudfoot and Brownlee, 1974).

Representative classes of template–primers for the RNA-directed DNA polymerases of B- and C-type viruses are shown in Fig. 2. The principal primer on viral 70S RNA (for avian viruses, at least) is a unique species of 4S RNA which is found both separate from and attached to the viral genome (Dahlberg *et al.*, 1974; Faras *et al.*, 1974). At least 90% of DNA synthesis *in vitro* is initiated on this RNA (Dahlberg *et al.*, 1974). There is presently no information concerning the initiation of viral DNA synthesis in the infected cell.

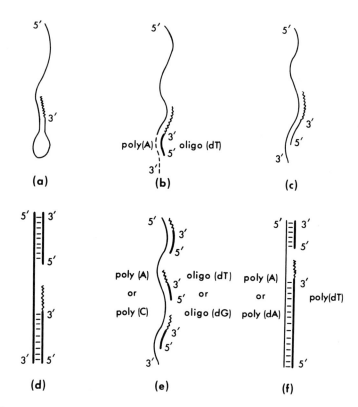

FIGURE 2. Template–primers for RNA-directed polymerase of RNA tumor viruses. Symbols used are as follows: ——, RNA chains; ——, DNA chains; – – –, poly(A); ᨓ, nascent DNA. (a) Single-stranded RNA devoid of poly(A), such as the genome of f2 bacteriophage; DNA synthesis initiates on the looped-back 3′-terminus of the template. (b) Single-stranded RNA with 3′-terminal poly(A) (such as globin messenger RNA or poliovirus RNA), primed by oligo(dT) added to the enzyme reaction. (c) Single-stranded RNA template with a discrete RNA primer, such as the 70S RNA of Rous sarcoma virus. (d) Duplex DNA, with a gap in one strand providing template and primer for DNA synthesis. (e, f) Template–primer complexes of synthetic homopolymers.

The 4S primer associated with the 70S RNA of Rous sarcoma virus has many structural features of tRNA (Faras *et al.*, 1974), although it lacks the characteristic nucleotide ribothymidine (Faras *et al.*, 1974). An identical 4S RNA has been isolated from normal avian cells (Sawyer and Dahlberg, 1974), but its function there is not known. There is presently no evidence that this 4S RNA can transfer an amino acid to polypeptide synthesis. The primer can be aminoacylated with either methionine or tryptophan; its chromatographic behavior and its nucleotide sequence indicate that it is a tryptophan tRNA (Faras *et al.*, 1974; personal communication from J. E. Dahlberg, and unpublished data of B. Cordell-Stewart and the authors).

Viral 70S RNA is a better template (about five- to fiftyfold) for RNA-directed DNA polymerase than any other naturally occurring RNA heteropolymer tested to date (Faras *et al.*, 1972; Duesberg *et al.*, 1971). We and others have attributed this fact to the presence of a distinct primer molecule associated with the template. This view is substantiated by several observations: (1) Denaturation of 70S RNA (and release of 4S RNAs) eliminates its advantage over other RNAs as template (Duesberg *et al.*, 1971; Faras *et al.*, 1972); the residual DNA synthesis probably initiates on the 3'-termini of genome subunits. (2) The initial level of template activity of 70S RNA can be partially restored (about 70% of maximum) by annealing subunits with either 4S RNA previously isolated from 70S RNA (Canaani and Duesberg, 1972) or purified 4S primer (unpublished data of B. Cordell-Stewart). (3) The template activity of other RNAs can be made equal to or better than that of 70S RNA by attachment of a low molecular weight primer; this is usually accomplished by annealing oligo(dT) to the 3'-terminal poly(A) of messenger or viral RNA (Duesberg *et al.*, 1971).

Transcription of viral 70S RNA by RNA-directed DNA polymerase *in vitro* fails to reconstruct the synthesis of provirus as it occurs *in vivo* (Table 2). The enzymatic product consists of relatively short chains of DNA (about 100–1000

TABLE 2

Transcription of RSV 70S RNA in Vitro and in Vivo[a]

	in vitro	*in vivo*
Template	70S RNA	70S RNA
Enzyme	RSV DNA polymerase	RSV DNA polymerase
Primer(s)	4S RNA	?
Products	H	(H)
	ssDNA	(ssDNA)
	dsDNA	dsDNA
Chain length (nucleotides)	100–1000	(~7500)
Fraction of template transcribed	10–100%	(100%)

[a] Items in parentheses represent provisional conclusions. The table is derived from published and unpublished data of the authors. Abbreviations: ssDNA, single-stranded DNA; dsDNA, double-stranded DNA; H, DNA–RNA hybrid.

nucleotides) transcribed in large measure from a very limited portion of the template molecule (Gelb *et al.*, 1971; Varmus *et al.*, 1971; Garapin *et al.*, 1973). These deficiencies pertain to DNA synthesis by either holoenzyme (i.e., virions activated to synthesize DNA by treatment with nonionic detergent) or purified enzyme with viral 70S RNA as template. The most widely proffered explanation of these observations is that the host cell provides an essential factor or factors which facilitate comprehensive transcription from the incoming viral genome. To date, this view has not been directly substantiated by experimental data, although proviral DNA isolated from acutely infected cells is considerably larger than the DNA transcribed from 70S RNA *in vitro* (Table 2 and below).

The widespread use of highly labeled products of viral polymerase in nucleic acid hybridization experiments is one of the significant consequences of the discovery of this enzyme. However, the size and sequence heterogeneity of the products synthesized *in vitro* has limited interpretation of the results of these experiments (Varmus *et al.*, 1972*b*, 1973*b*).

6. The Viral Life Cycle

6.1. Specificity of Virus–Cell Interactions

Permissive cells support the replication of virus and are converted to a neoplastic state by transforming viruses, whereas *nonpermissive* cells may be transformed at a low frequency (about 10^{-4} to 10^{-6}) but cannot support viral replication (Temin, 1971; Altaner and Temin, 1970). There is evidence that the frequency with which a restricted virus penetrates a nonpermissive host cell and initiates an incomplete infectious cycle is much greater than the frequency of transformation (Kotler, 1971; Varmus *et al.*, 1973*c*), but the mechanisms that restrict transformation and production of virus are not known. In general, avian viruses replicate only in avian cells and mammalian viruses in mammalian cells, but the host range varies greatly among known viruses (Termin, 1971).

The susceptibility of a permissive cell to infection by various strains of virus is a stable genetic property of the cell. This property has facilitated the classification of viruses from several species (e.g., chickens, mice, cats) into subgroups according to their capacity to infect genetically defined sets of permissive cells (see other chapters in this volume). The host range of chicken viruses is determined by one or more glycoproteins in the envelope of virus particles; consequently, viruses of the same antigenic type usually share host range. Chicken cells resistant to infection by particular subgroups of avian viruses probably do not permit virus penetration (Piraino, 1967; Crittenden, 1968; Love and Weiss, 1974). By contrast, host range and antigenic type of murine viruses are genetically independent properties. Restricted murine virus probably penetrates the resistant mouse cell only to have its life cycle interrupted at some subsequent point (Huang *et al.*, 1973; Krontiris *et al.*, 1973).

The description of host range for avian and murine viruses and the analysis of the cellular genetic determinants of this phenomenon represent milestones in the study of RNA tumor viruses. Host range provides one of the few available

markers for genetic analysis of these viruses and facilitates rapid and accurate selection of new genetic variants (such as recombinants).

6.2. Establishment of Infection: Synthesis and Integration of Proviral DNA

Studies of the physiology of the RNA tumor virus infectious cycle culminated in the formulation of the "provirus hypothesis": RNA tumor viruses transform cells and replicate through the agency of a DNA copy of the viral genome (Temin, 1971, 1972), synthesized early in viral infection and then integrated into the DNA of host chromosomes in a manner analogous to that of DNA tumor viruses and lysogenic bacteriophage. The evidence which formed the basis of this proposal has been reviewed frequently (e.g., see Temin and Baltimore, 1972; Temin, 1971). The salient points are as follows: (1) Infection and transformation of cells by RNA tumor viruses require virus-specific DNA synthesis during the first 12 h of the infectious cycle (Bader, 1965, 1966; Temin, 1968). (2) Production of virus requires continuing DNA-dependent RNA synthesis (Bader, 1965; Temin, 1963) and structural integrity of the virus-specific DNA (Balduzzi and Morgan, 1970; Boettiger and Temin, 1970). (3) The genome of RNA tumor viruses is perpetuated as a stable genetic property of infected cells even in the absence of detectable viral replication (Coffin, 1972; Svoboda and Dourmashkin, 1969; Rowe, 1971).

The provirus hypothesis requires an enzymatic mechanism capable of copying RNA template into DNA, a requirement fulfilled by the discovery of an RNA-directed DNA polymerase in virions of RNA tumor viruses (Baltimore, 1970; Temin and Mizutani, 1970; Temin and Baltimore, 1972). Molecular studies, described below, provide definitive evidence for both the existence of provirus and the central role of provirus in viral replication and virus-induced transformation.

The major molecular predictions of the provirus hypothesis have been verified by studies in which virus-specific DNA and RNA were identified and measured by their hybridization with labeled 70S RNA or virus-specific DNA synthesized *in vitro* by virion-associated polymerases. Such studies have shown that during the first 9–12 h following infection the viral genome is transcribed into several copies of viral DNA which are then covalently inserted (or "integrated") into chromosomal DNA of the host cell (Varmus *et al.*, 1973c; Markham and Baluda, 1973). Experiments with conditional mutants suggest that the access of viral polymerase to template genome is topographically constrained; virus strains with temperature-sensitive polymerase cannot be complemented at restrictive temperatures by coinfection with wild-type virus; i.e., the polymerase gene(s) is *cis*-active (Linial and Mason, 1973). By contrast, infection with avian leukosis virus can rescue (complement) Rous sarcoma virus inactivated by chemical attack on the viral polymerase (Hung, 1973). The inconsistencies in the results from these two experimental systems are presently inexplicable.

The synthesis of viral DNA is prerequisite to both viral replication and virus-induced cellular transformation. This statement is best illustrated by experiments with the conditional mutants of Rous sarcoma virus which possess temperature-sensitive RNA-directed DNA polymerase (Linial and Mason, 1973; Baltimore et al., 1974). Infection of permissive cells by these mutants at the restrictive temperature (41°C) prevents synthesis of viral DNA at normal levels (unpublished observations of the authors, W. S. Mason, and P. K. Vogt), and there is a corresponding reduction in both viral replication and cellular transformation (Linial and Mason, 1973; Wyke and Linial, 1973). Integration of provirus is also considered to be an essential event. For example, ethidium bromide blocks integration of RSV provirus and concurrently prevents cell transformation and viral replication (see below and Table 3).

Newly synthesized viral DNA has been detected in the cytoplasm of acutely infected cells (Bishop et al., 1974b; Hatanaka et al., 1971) and in cells infected after enucleation with cytochalasin B (Varmus et al., 1974b). On the other hand, the genome of infecting virus (i.e., the template for synthesis of provirus) can be recovered from the host nucleus very shortly after infection (Dales and Hanafusa, 1972). These observations could be reconciled by supposing (1) that viral DNA is synthesized in cytoplasmic subviral particles which preserve the template during transport to the nucleus, (2) that a fraction of cytoplasmic viral DNA is an RNA–DNA hybrid which might even be integrated in this form (Leis et al., 1973, 1974), or (3) that the viral RNA observed in the nucleus is not participating in the replicative cycle. The properties of viral DNA prior to integration have not been extensively characterized. It is at least in part duplex DNA composed of chains approximately 7500 nucleotides in length and therefore presumably transcribed from single subunits of the viral genome (unpublished data of R. R. Guntaka and the authors). Recent evidence indicates that duplex viral DNA assumes a closed circular form, and that this form is required for integration (Guntaka et al., 1975).

Provirus can be integrated in the absence of mitosis (unpublished data of H. E. Varmus), whereas cellular DNA synthesis may or may not be required for

TABLE 3

Effect of Ethidium Bromide on Infection by Rous Sarcoma Virus[a]

EtBr (μg/ml)	Viral DNA synthesis (%)	Integration (%)	Transformation	Virus production (48 h)
0	100	100	+++	100
0.15	100	30	+	30
0.5	95	15	±	10–30
1.0	85	15	±	10

[a] Duck cells were infected with the B77 strain of Rous sarcoma virus (Varmus et al., 1973c). Forty-eight hours later, the synthesis and integration of virus-specific DNA ("provirus"), the production of virus, and the transformation of infected cells were detected as described elsewhere (Hanafusa, 1969; Varmus et al., 1973c). Duck cells grow at a normal rate for at least two generations in the presence of the amounts of ethidium bromide used in these experiments (unpublished data of R. R. Guntaka and the authors).

integration (this latter issue has not been directly tested). The enzymatic mechanisms responsible for integration are not known, and there is presently no indication that viral gene products are involved. If cells are infected in the presence of ethidium bromide (a dye which intercalates into DNA molecules), viral DNA is synthesized in normal amounts and transported to the nucleus (unpublished observations of R. R. Guntaka and the authors), but the extent of integration is reduced by a factor of 5–10 (Table 3) (Guntaka *et al.*, 1975). The presence of ethidium bromide greatly reduces the amount of viral DNA in a closed circular form (Guntaka *et al.*, 1975); this may account for the failure of viral DNA to integrate.

The effect of ethidium bromide on cellular transformation (Table 3) may or may not be specific; we have yet to study critically the general toxicity of ethidium bromide for cultured avian fibroblasts. However, the dye will appreciably reduce transformation and virus production (and provirus integration) at concentrations which do not immediately suppress mitochondrial function and cell growth (e.g., 0.15 μg/ml in Table 3). Moreover, infected cells containing integrated provirus produce normal amounts of virus in the presence of ethidium bromide (1 μg/ml, Guntaka *et al.*, 1975). We cannot presently reconcile our observations (Table 3) with previous reports that ethidium bromide does not affect the replication of RNA tumor viruses in newly infected cells (Richert and Hare, 1972; A. V. Bader, 1973), although there are appreciable differences of experimental design among the several studies.

Virtually nothing is known about the sites on host DNA at which provirus integrates. Do these sites occur randomly along the host chromosome, or are they limited in number and specific? Are the proviruses of different viruses integrated at different sites? Is the site of integration a determinant of the extent to which viral genes are expressed? Are proviruses which are integrated in multiple copies arranged in tandem, or are they integrated separately? These issues are now accessible to experimental test, but no persuasive data are available.

6.3. Provirus in Nonpermissive Cells

Acute infection of nonpermissive cells by Rous sarcoma virus leads to the synthesis and integration of provirus as described for permissive cells (Varmus *et al.*, 1973c; also, unpublished data of H. E. Varmus). A few of the infected nonpermissive cells will convert to a neoplastic state. The remainder will display no phenotypic manifestation of infection, although a relatively large number of these cells may contain integrated provirus (Kotler, 1971; Varmus *et al.*, 1973c). The mechanism which blocks expression of viral information in these cells is not known. The situation may be analogous to abortive transformation by SV40 (Smith *et al.*, 1972) or to reversion of RSV-transformed hamster cells (Macpherson, 1971); in these cases, the viral genome is retained by the host cell (Smith *et al.*, 1972; Varmus *et al.*, 1973d; Deng *et al.*, 1974), but there is little or no phenotypic evidence of viral gene expression.

Nonpermissive cells transformed by RNA tumor viruses carry viral genes as proviral DNA (Varmus et al., 1973b; Baluda, 1972). In at least some instances, the entire viral genome is probably harbored in this manner; virus can be rescued by fusing the transformed cells with permissive cells (Coffin, 1972; Svoboda and Dourmashkin, 1969), the bulk (more than 70%) of the viral genome can be detected in the DNA of at least one line of RSV-transformed rat cells by molecular hybridization (Varmus et al., 1974), and DNA extracted from transformed nonpermissive cells can elicit the production of virus when applied to permissive cells ("transfection") (Karpas and Milstein, 1973; Hill and Hillova, 1972a, b).

The mechanisms of transfection and rescue by fusion are not known. In both instances, a permissive host is utilized to express viral genes contained in the DNA of a nonpermissive host. Rescue by fusion may depend on the prior transcription of viral genes in the nonpermissive cell; the relative yield of avian sarcoma virus recovered by fusion from infected hamster cells (nonpermissive hosts for avian viruses) is a direct function of the amount of virus-specific RNA in the nonpermissive cell (Deng et al., 1974). Since Rous sarcoma virus can be rescued by fusing infected nonpermissive cells with duck cells (which contain no Rous virus genes, see Varmus et al., 1973c), the genome of the nonpermissive cell must provide the entire set of structural genes necessary to produce virus (Svoboda, 1972). There is no doubt that transfecting DNA also contributes viral genes to virus production in permissive cells; the recovered virus possesses genetic markers (e.g., host range and conditional mutations) characteristic of the virus strain resident in the nonpermissive cell (Hill and Hillova, 1972b). However, transfection by DNA from Rous virus–transformed mammalian cells has yet to succeed with duck cells as the permissive host, the only competent host being chicken cells (which do contain genes of Rous virus; see Varmus et al., 1973c).

Transformation of nonpermissive cells by RNA tumor viruses is inefficient, but the efficiency can be augmented by prior passage of the viral genome through cells of the same species (Altaner and Temin, 1970). The mechanism is not understood, but a biochemical correlate has been observed. Synthesis of provirus in acutely infected nonpermissive cells can be detected only if the infecting virus has been subjected to prior selection on the same host (Varmus et al., 1973a, c). The "tropism" of virus for a specific species of nonpermissive cells is an unstable genetic property which is soon lost when the virus strain is propagated serially in permissive cells (Altaner and Temin, 1970). The mechanism of tropism is not known. However, the fact that avian viruses of certain subgroups are more "mammaltropic" than those of other subgroups suggests that the viral envelope plays a critical role. This inference has been substantiated by recent experiments with pseudotype virions containing the RNA genome of vesicular stomatitis virus enclosed by the envelope of various subgroups of avian sarcoma–leukosis viruses. The infectivity of the vesicular stomatitis virus pseudotypes, measured in mammalian cells, varies as a function of the subgroup of the pseudotype (R. Weiss, personal communication).

6.4. Synthesis of Viral RNA

Proviral DNA is the presumptive template for the synthesis of viral RNA (Temin, 1971). No other template (e.g., complementary RNA) has been found in infected cells (Leong *et al.*, 1972*b*; Coffin and Temin, 1972; Bishop *et al.*, 1973), and inhibition of DNA-directed RNA synthesis interrupts both the production of virus (Temin, 1971) and the synthesis of viral RNA (Temin, 1971). Newly synthesized viral RNA appears first in the host nucleus, later in the cytoplasm (Parsons *et al.*, 1973); transcription is probably effected by nucleoplasmic RNA polymerase(II) (Rymo *et al.*, 1974; Jacquet *et al.*, 1974). No viral RNA is made until the infected cell has progressed through the cell cycle (Humphries and Temin, 1972). It is generally assumed that integrated viral genes are subject to the forms of expression and regulation which operate on "cellular" genes in the chromosome. According to this view, the initial product of transcription from provirus should appear in large, heterogeneous nuclear RNA and be covalently linked to RNA transcribed from portions of the cellular genome (Weinberg, 1973). These assumptions have yet to be validated experimentally.

6.5. Viral Messenger RNA and the Synthesis of Viral Proteins

The messenger RNAs for viral protein synthesis are probably identical to the high molecular weight subunits of the viral genome (Fan and Baltimore, 1973), although smaller virus-specific RNAs have also been found in cytoplasm and polyribosomes isolated from infected cells (Leong *et al* 1972*b*, Schincariol and Joklik, 1973; Tsuchida *et al.*, 1972). Like other, authentic messenger RNAs, the subunits of 70S RNA have poly(A) at their 3'-termini (M. L. Stephenson *et al.*, 1973; also, personal communications from R. Erikson and R. Perry). This structural feature has been implicated in the transport of messenger RNAs from nucleus to cytoplasm (Adesnik *et al.*, 1972). The only experimental tests of these implications in the case of C-type viruses were carried out with cordycepin, an analogue of adenosine which apparently impedes the synthesis of poly(A) (Adesnik *et al.*, 1972). The analogue can inhibit production of virus (Wu *et al.*, 1972) and virus-induced cellular transformation (Lovinger *et al.*, 1973), but the mechanism of this inhibition has not been elucidated.

Since viral messenger is identical to viral genome and large enough to contain multiple genes, viral polypeptides are most likely translated in the form of polycistronic proteins which are subsequently cleaved to functional units by proteolytic enzymes (Baltimore, 1971*a*). This prediction is based on previous results obtained with picornaviruses; the polycistronic genomes of these viruses are translated directly into a single protein which contains all of the viral gene products (Baltimore, 1971*b*). There is provisional experimental evidence that the messenger RNAs of RNA tumor viruses are translated in a similar manner in permissive cells (Vogt and Eisenman, 1973). However, several investigators have reported the successful translation of 70S RNA into individual viral polypeptides *in vitro* (Siegert *et al.*, 1972; Gielkens *et al.*, 1972; Twardzik *et al.*, 1973). The translation was accomplished with bacterial extracts which are not known to specifically cleave polycistronic proteins of eukaryotes. This observation cannot presently be reconciled with the data reported for infected cells.

6.6. Assembly and Maturation of Virions

The ribonucleoprotein of virion cores is assembled in the cytoplasm and buds through the plasma membrane, thereby acquiring its envelope. The details of these processes are not known, but the virion which emerges is not fully matured. Structural transitions occur in extracellular virus which affect both the polypeptides of the virion (Cheung *et al.*, 1972) and the viral genome (Cheung *et al.*, 1972; Canaani *et al.*, 1973; East *et al.*, 1973). The existence of these transitions was presaged by morphological observations made several years before the recent biochemical studies (Bernhard, 1958; Sarker *et al.*, 1971*b*). Extracellular maturation has been observed with only a few representative viruses, and the reported details vary for different viruses (Cheung *et al.*, 1972; Canaani *et al.*, 1973; East *et al.*, 1973). It would be premature to conclude that all B- and C-type viruses undergo extracellular maturation, and neither the precise nature nor the significance of the structural changes has been completely elucidated in any single instance.

Maturation of Rous sarcoma virus is accompanied by the loss of 13 specific polypeptides (out of a total of 26) from the virion (Cheung *et al.*, 1972). This process apparently requires a factor or factors derived from the host cell (Cheung *et al.*, 1972). The most extensive changes in the viral genome have also been observed with a strain of Rous sarcoma virus which contains individual subunits and low molecular weight RNAs at the time of release from the cell (Canaani *et al.*, 1973). Subsequent aggregation of the various RNAs gives rise to the 70S complex considered to be the mature viral genome (Canaani *et al.*, 1973). Nothing is known about either the forces which drive this aggregation or the structural elements responsible for it, but, once formed, the complex is stabilized by hydrogen bonds between complementary sequences of nucleotides (Duesberg, 1968; Erikson, 1969). The high molecular weight subunits are probably not joined at their immediate termini; this would require regions of poly(U) to base-pair with the 3'-terminal poly(A), and sensitive tests have failed to find any poly(U) in 70S RNA (Marshall and Gillespie, 1972).

6.7. Virus Infection and Cellular Transformation in Synchronized Cells

The synthesis and integration of provirus proceed in the absence of cell division (unpublished data of H. E. Varmus). Viral RNA synthesis does not occur in cells maintained in the G_1 stage of the cell cycle (Humphries and Temin, 1972). These observations provide molecular explanations for the previous findings that the viral genome can be stably established in permissive cells arrested in G_1 ("stationary cells") but virus is produced only after the cell cycle has been reinstituted

(Temin, 1970). The failure of infected stationary cells to synthesize viral RNA contrasts with the claim that infected cells become phenotypically transformed and produce virus despite the use of periwinkle alkaloids to block cell division (Bader, 1972*b*; J. P. Bader, 1973). If viral gene products are required for transformation (few doubt that they are), the transformation of cells in the absence of mitosis could be attributed to translation of proteins from parental (input) viral genomes. The successful translation of 70S RNA *in vitro* (Siegert *et al.*, 1972; Gielkens *et al.*, 1972) makes this explanation credible. It is also possible that an event in the cell cycle prior to metaphase is required for transformation and viral replication; the postulated event would not occur in stationary cells but would progress normally in cells blocked at metaphase by alkaloids, thereby accounting for the different results obtained with the two experimental procedures.

6.8. Viral Replication in Synchronized Cells

Several major events in viral growth are apparently related to specific phases of the cell cycle. Synchronization of infected permissive cells synchronizes the release of virus (Temin, 1967; Hobom-Schnegg *et al.*, 1970; Leong *et al.*, 1972*a*; Panem and Kirsten, 1973) and the synthesis of viral RNA and proteins (Leong *et al.*, 1972*a*). The synchronous release of virus does not require coincident viral RNA synthesis (D. Baltimore, personal communication); the released virus must be assembled from a preexistent pool of viral genomes. There is other evidence for the existence of this pool. Infected permissive cells continue to produce virus (albeit at a gradually declining rate) for as long as 12 h after the synthesis of viral RNA has been interrupted by chemical inhibitors (unpublished data of the authors).

7. Viral Genes and Oncogenesis

7.1. Endogenous Proviruses

Ostensibly uninfected cells of many species contain the genetic capacity to synthesize C-type viruses (Lieber *et al.*, 1973). Mice also harbor the genes of B-type viruses (Nandi and McGrath, 1973; Varmus *et al.*, 1972*a*). Studies of cloned cells in culture demonstrated that endogenous viral genes are present in every member of a population of cells, although only a small proportion of the cells may actually express the genes and produce virus (Rowe *et al.*, 1971). The presence of virus-specific DNA in the genomes of uninfected cells of several species has also been demonstrated by nucleic acid hybridization (Gelb *et al.*, 1971; Varmus *et al.*, 1972*b*; Baluda, 1972; Ruprecht *et al.*, 1973; Rosenthal *et al.*, 1971; Neiman, 1972). The expression of endogenous viral genes can be either partial or complete and is subject to genetically determined regulation, the nature of which varies among different species. The most widespread example of partial expression is the presence of viral group-specific antigens in otherwise normal cells (Payne and Chubb, 1968; Taylor *et al.*, 1971). In chickens and mice, this property segregates like an autosomal trait of the cellular genotype (Payne and Chubb, 1968; Taylor *et al.*, 1971, 1973; Meier *et al.*, 1973) and correlates with the presence of RNA transcribed from endogenous provirus (Hayward and Hanafusa, 1973). Other manifestations of the expression of endogenous viral genes include the presence of virus-specific RNA in ostensibly uninfected cells lacking group-specific antigen (Hayward and Hanafusa, 1973; Benveniste *et al.*, 1973) and the ability of some normal cells to complement the replication of defective exogenous viruses (Weiss and Payne, 1971; Hanafusa *et al.*, 1972*a*). These manifestations will be discussed in subsequent chapters. Spontaneous production of endogenous virus has been observed in cells from numerous species (Lieber *et al.*, 1973), but the best-studied examples are chickens (Vogt and Friis, 1971), mice (Todaro, 1972), and cats (Livingston and Todaro, 1973).

Production of endogenous virus can often be induced by treatment of cultured cells with a variety of physical and chemical agents (Weiss *et al.*, 1971; Aaronson *et al.*, 1971; Lowy *et al.*, 1971). An example is the induction of virus production in uninfected mouse cells by the application of halogenated pyrimidines (Lowy *et al.*, 1971; Aaronson *et al.*, 1971). The capacity of cells to respond to induction is determined by one or more genetic loci in the strains of mice from which the cells are derived (Rowe *et al.*, 1972; Stephenson and Aaronson, 1973), and there is a direct correlation between the relative inducibility of any strain of mouse and the incidence of spontaneous leukemia accompanied by the production of leukemia virus. These observations have provoked speculation about the possible relationship between endogenous viruses and neoplasia, but the evidence for such a relationship is only circumstantial.

The inducing agent (halogenated pyrimidine) acts during the early S phase of the cell cycle (D. Baltimore, personal communication) and must be incorporated into host DNA to be effective (Teich *et al.*, 1973), but its mechanism of action is unknown. Induction requires the initiation (or augmentation) of transcription from the provirus of endogenous virus, and transcription is the focus of most biochemical studies on induction at present. Other inducing agents have been described, including chemical carcinogens (Weiss *et al.*, 1971; Freeman *et al.*, 1971), ionizing radiations (Weiss *et al.*, 1971), corticosteroids (Paran *et al.*, 1973), and inhibitors of protein synthesis (Aaronson and Dunn, 1973). They have not been as widely used as halogenated pyrimidines, and nothing is known of their mechanisms of action.

Neither the origin of endogenous viruses nor their ubiquity has been explained. These viruses could have evolved from a common ancestral virus whose genome was initially inserted into a primordial host chromosome (Todaro and Huebner, 1972); they could have developed independently in each species by a variety of possible mechanisms (Temin, 1972). The available (and very limited) experimental evidence favors the latter alternative. The former is unlikely since the genomes of endogenous viruses from different species are usually highly diverged; i.e., they share few if any related nucleotide sequences (see below). (Partial homology between viruses endogenous to the cat and the baboon offers an interesting exception to this general rule, Benveniste *et al.*, 1974). In addition, in several instances no homology has been observed between an endogenous virus and the DNA of species closely related to the species of origin (e.g., there is no homology between mouse mammary tumor virus RNA and the DNA of several rodents other than mice). However, speculation about the origin of these viruses is tenuous in the absence of more extensive data.

Endogenous viruses represent a genetic backdrop to exogenous infection by RNA tumor viruses. Infection can induce the expression of endogenous viral genes (Hanafusa *et al.*, 1970), and some investigators contend that it is the expression of endogenous genetic information which is ultimately responsible for conversion of cells to a neoplastic state (Huebner and Todaro, 1969; Todaro and Huebner, 1972). We will not dispute the issue here because definitive experimental data are not available. Two other types of genetic interactions between infecting and endogenous viruses have been identified. First, the products of an endogenous virus of chicken cells can provide a glycoprotein for the envelope of helper-dependent avian sarcoma viruses (Scheele and Hanafusa, 1971; Kawai and Hanafusa, 1973). Second, the genomes of infecting and endogenous viruses can recombine (Weiss *et al.*, 1973). In chicken cells, this recombination may provide the gene for RNA-directed DNA polymerase for the endogenous virus (which may, in some lines of chickens, be deficient in the enzyme; see discussion in Weissbach *et al.*, 1972) and can endow the infecting virus with the subgroup (i.e., the antigenic type and host range) of the endogenous virus (Weiss *et al.*, 1973). Recombination with endogenous virus occurs only in cells which are transcribing endogenous provirus into RNA prior to infection (Weiss *et al.*, 1973). Consequently, Weiss and his colleagues have proposed that the first step in the formation of recombinants is genetic mixing among pools of viral RNA (Weiss *et al.*, 1973); this proposal would explain the finding of heterozygote viruses as apparent intermediates in the formation of stable recombinants (Weiss *et al.*, 1973).

For taxonomic purposes, we can now define two classes of hosts for infection by B- and C-type viruses. The *homologous* host is permissive for viral replication, harbors one or more endogenous viruses closely related to the virus in question, and is considered to be the species from which that virus originated. As discussed further below, the *endogenous* virus may replicate poorly in its cell of origin and is often identified only after it infects and replicates in a heterologous host. At present, the homologous host species is best defined by the use of molecular hybridization to demonstrate homology between viral genome and host DNA (Ruprecht *et al.*, 1973; Quintrell *et al.*, 1974). The *heterologous* host may be either permissive or nonpermissive, but whatever endogenous viruses it harbors are not related to the virus in question, and there will be either limited or no homology between host DNA and the genome of the infecting virus (Ruprecht *et al.*, 1973; Varmus *et al.*, 1973*b*; Quintrell *et al.*, 1974).

Totally distinct groups of viruses may exist within single species. For example, the normal cat harbors two unrelated classes of viruses—the RD-114/CCC viruses

(Livingston and Todaro, 1973) and the feline leukemia–sarcoma viruses (Rup-recht et al., 1973; Quintrell et al., 1974). Likewise, the C-type murine leukemia virus and the B-type mouse mammary tumor virus are unrelated (Varmus et al., 1973e). In both instances, the two classes of virus from the same species have distinct group-specific antigens: the viral genomes are unrelated when studied by molecular hybridization and are independently represented in the DNA of the normal host.

Are endogenous viruses hazardous to the investigator working with ostensibly normal cells which are releasing an unsuspected (or undetected) virus? Can endogenous viruses be implicated in oncogenesis? There are no certain answers to these questions. With important exceptions (for example, Nandi and McGrath, 1973; Stephenson et al., 1974), endogenous viruses have not yet proved oncogenic in their *homologous* hosts and grow poorly (if at all) in homologous host cells. However, one or more *heterologous* hosts will support the growth of each endogenous virus discovered to date. The oncogenicity of endogenous viruses in heterologous hosts has yet to be adequately tested.

7.2. Implication of Viral Genes in Transforming Infections

Transformation by viral infection is accompanied by the introduction of new genetic information into the cell by the infecting virus. This statement is based on several independent lines of evidence: (1) Studies with molecular hybridization have shown that infection introduces new sequences of nucleotides (i.e., new genes) into the DNA of the host cell. Only a portion of the viral genome is new to a *homologous* host; the remainder of the viral genome is indistinguishable (by presently available techniques) from viral genes resident in the uninfected cells (Nieman, 1972; Scolnick et al., 1974; Varmus et al., 1974c). By contrast, *heterologous* hosts, either permissive or nonpermissive, generally contain no detectable genes homologous to those of the infecting virus. Consequently, the entire viral genome is newly inserted into host DNA as a consequence of infection (see above). (2) The genotype of the infecting virus can determine specific phenotypic properties of the transformed cell, e.g., the particular morphology assumed by the cell (Temin, 1961; Yoshii and Vogt, 1970). (3) Deletion of limited portions of the genomes of transforming viruses deletes the capacity of the virus to transform cultured fibroblasts and induce sarcomas in animals (Vogt, 1971a; Duesberg et al., 1973b). The deletion is specific because the virus can retain other aspects of oncogenicity (e.g., the potential to induce leukosis in the case of avian viruses, Biggs et al., 1973). (4) The transformed phenotype of either permissive (Martin, 1970; Kawai and Hanafusa, 1971; Bader, 1972b; Scolnick et al., 1972b) or nonpermissive (Graf and Friis, 1973) cells is conditional (i.e., temperature sensitive) when induced by viral strains which are conditional mutants in genes for transformation.

Mutants of avian sarcoma viruses which are temperature sensitive for transformation have been arranged into four complementation groups (Wyke, 1973), but more recent studies indicate that the observed complementation was due to recombination (Wyke, personal communication). The nature and function of the proteins coded by transforming genes are not known. The proteins are not homologous among different strains of avian sarcoma viruses because there is no complementation among mutants of different strains (Wyke, 1973); this surprising finding contrasts with the extensive genetic relatedness among the strains as defined by molecular hybridization and is presently unexplained.

7.3. Regulated Expression of Viral Genes

Viral genes for transformation can be present in the genome of a cell without necessary effect on the cell's phenotype. We cite these examples: (1) Many mammalian cells acutely infected by Rous sarcoma virus acquire integrated provirus in the absence of neoplastic transformation (Varmus et al., 1973a, c). (2) Cells transformed by either avian (Macpherson, 1971; J. R. Stephenson et al., 1973) or murine (Stephenson et al., 1972, 1973; Nomura et al., 1973) sarcoma viruses can segregate phenotypically reverted cells. The revertants retain provirus; viral DNA can be detected by molecular hybridization (Deng et al., 1974), the revertants can yield virus when fused with permissive cells (Boettiger, 1974) or superinfected with helper virus (Stephenson et al., 1972; Nomura et al., 1973), and the transformed state sometimes returns when clones of the revertants are propagated serially (Nomura et al., 1973). (3) The genome for an oncogenic strain of MMTV is present as provirus in the chromosomal DNA of at least one strain of mice (GR) and is transmitted through the gametes of these mice (Bentvelzen et al., 1970; Nandi and McGrath, 1973). However, virus and tumor appear only in the breasts of lactating females (Nandi and McGrath, 1973).

Implicit in these examples is the existence of regulatory mechanisms in cells which can repress the expression of oncogenic viral genes. Conventional explanations of these mechanisms usually invoke the regulation of transcription of messenger RNA from provirus, but experimental efforts to to substantiate this view have not succeeded to date. In particular, results with mutants of sarcoma viruses temperature sensitive for transformation indicate that modulation of viral gene expression at restrictive and permissive temperatures does not occur at the level of transcription (Kawai and Hanafusa, 1971; Bader, 1972b; Scolnick et al., 1972b; Somers et al., 1973). Only protein synthesis (or no macromolecule synthesis at all; see Bader, 1972b) is required for the transformation of infected cells shifted from restrictive to permissive temperatures.

7.4. Properties of Cells Transformed by RNA Tumor Viruses

Transformation is defined operationally; it is useful in the identification of virus-induced charges in cultured cells, but it is not a universal correlate of oncogenicity. Many of the properties used to define transformation can be transiently induced in normal cells by experimental manipulations, such as replacement of growth medium or treatment with proteolytic enzymes. Tumor viruses are defined by their capacity to induce neoplasms in animals. By the same token, transformed cells are neoplastic only if they can grow into tumors in an appropriate host. Nevertheless, the phenotypic changes which serve to identify transformation of cultured cells are indispensable aids in the investigation of tumor viruses. Several properties of cells transformed by RNA tumor viruses are now widely recognized. However, as the ensuing discussion will show, little is known about the molecular basis of the transformed phenotype. Although there exists a requirement for continued expression of viral genes to maintain the transformed state (Martin, 1970; Kawai and Hanafusa, 1971; Bader, 1972b; Scolnick et al., 1972b; Graf and Friis, 1973), there is still virtually nothing known about the products of these genes.

7.4.1. Morphological Alterations

The fibroblast transformed by an RNA sarcoma virus acquires a new shape and appearance; the most widely cited of these changes are a rounding of the previously spindle-shaped cell and a change in the refraction of light. The shape of the transformed cell can be determined by the genotype of the infecting virus. For example, there are variants of Rous sarcoma virus which induce a fusiform shape; other variants induce a round shape (Temin, 1961; Yoshii and Vogt, 1970). These observations were among the earliest to implicate viral genes directly in the genesis of transformation. However, shape alone is inadequate to define a transformed cell. The fusiform cells could not be recognized as transformants without further criteria.

7.4.2. Orientation of Growth

The arrangement of cells on a solid surface is altered by transformation. The ordered growth of fibroblasts in parallel arrays is converted to a random and overlapping array. Efforts have been made to measure this parameter objectively (e.g., by enumerating the overlap of nuclei, Levinson et al., 1971), but these procedures have not supplanted subjective evaluation by microscopic examination.

7.4.3. Density of Cells at Saturation on a Solid Surface

Under defined conditions of growth, transformed cells can grow to a greater number on a given surface area than can normal cells. This is a controversial and tenuous criterion, useful only if conditions of growth are carefully controlled. The mechanisms which limit cellular multiplication are not known, but the once popular concept of inhibition due to contacts among cells has fallen into disrepute. Present opinion holds that "there is no experimental support for the concept that 'contact inhibition' . . . is responsible for cessation of growth in dense cultures" (Dulbecco and Elkington, 1973).

7.4.4. Growth Without Solid Support

Transformed cells can grow in suspension without anchorage on solid support, normal cells cannot. The mechanism responsible for this distinction is not known, but growth in suspension (most commonly in soft agar) constitutes an exceptionally valuable approach to the recognition, enumeration, and other experimental manipulations of transformed cells.

7.4.5. Reduction in the Requirement for Growth Factors in Serum

Transformed cells require less serum than do normal cells to accomplish a variety of functions, including DNA synthesis, movement, survival, mitosis, and growth to maximum densities. This fact has facilitated some of the more successful efforts to establish quantitative comparisons between normal and transformed cells (Clarke et al., 1970; Dulbecco, 1970).

7.4.6. Agglutination by Plant Lectins

Transformed cells are more readily agglutinated by plant lectins than are normal cells (Burger, 1969; Sharon and Lis, 1972). (It was originally reported that chick fibroblasts transformed by avian sarcoma viruses were not preferentially agglutinated by lectins, Moore and Temin, 1971, but this view has been superseded by subsequent studies: Burger and Martin, 1972; Kapeller and Doljanski, 1972.) Many of the lectins are glycoproteins, but some (such as concanavalin A) contain no carbohydrate (Sharon and Lis, 1972). The binding sites for individual agglutinins on cells are specific, and each site has a hapten which can compete with the lectin for binding; the haptens for wheat germ agglutinin and concanavalin A are N-acetylglucosamine and mannose, respectively (Sharon and Lis, 1972). Agglutination by lectins is not an exclusive property of neoplastic cells; it can be induced by trypsinization of normal cells (Burger, 1969) and by infection with nononcogenic (cytopathic) viruses (Poste and Reeve, 1972). Binding of agglutinin to transformed cells restores their growth pattern to that of normal cells (Burger and Noonan, 1970), but efforts to implicate the binding sites in the mechanisms which control cell growth have been inconclusive.

The increased agglutination of transformed cells was originally ascribed to the presence of more binding sites for lectins, but this explanation is now in doubt (Cline and Livingston, 1971; Ozanne and Sambrook, 1971; Arndt-Jovin and Berg, 1971; for a dissenting opinion, see Noonan and Burger, 1973). The prevailing explanation is that the binding sites on the surface of cells are redistributed as a consequence of transformation in a manner which facilitates agglutination (Nicolson, 1971).

7.4.7. Glycoproteins on the Surface of Transformed Cells

The surface membranes of both transformed (Buck et al., 1970, 1971a; Warren et al., 1972) and rapidly growing normal (Buck et al., 1971b) cells contain large glycopeptides in greater amounts than do normal cells. Furthermore, the glycopeptides in the envelopes of C-type viruses are slightly larger when the viruses are produced by transformed rather than by nontransformed cells (Lai and Duesberg, 1972). There is no evidence that viral genes are directly responsible for the additional residues of carbohydrate which account for the increased size of the glycoproteins in question.

7.4.8. Reduction of Intracellular 3',5'-Cyclic Adenosine Monophosphate (cAMP) Concentrations

Cells transformed by RNA (or DNA) tumor viruses have lowered levels of cAMP (Otten et al., 1971, 1972; Carchman et al., 1974), and several manifestations of transformation can be reversed by administration of dibutryl cAMP (the lipid-soluble analogue) or by inhibition of phosphodiesterases (which normally degrade cAMP to 5'-AMP) (Johnson et al., 1971; Pastan and Johnson, 1974). Reduced activity of membrane-associated adenyl cyclase has been measured in several instances, suggesting that the reduction in cAMP concentration is at least partially due to decreased synthesis, but increased phosphodiesterase activity or extrusion of cAMP from the cell could also be responsible (Pastan and Johnson, 1974). Studies with temperature-sensitive mutants of avian and murine viruses demonstrate that alterations in cAMP levels occur promptly after expression of viral genes (Otten et al., 1972; Carchman et al., 1974); however, it is not known whether the effects on adenyl cyclase activity are mediated directly by a viral gene product or are secondary to generalized changes in the cell membrane.

7.4.9. Stimulation of Hexose Uptake

The rate of uptake of hexose (e.g., 2-deoxyglucose) by cells is increased following transformation by RNA tumor viruses (Hatanaka and Hanafusa, 1970; Martin et al., 1971; Venuta and Rubin, 1973). This phenomenon can be used to monitor phenotypic changes after viral infection, but it is probably not a primary consequence of viral gene expression (Bader, 1972b). The mechanism which effects the increased uptake of hexose is in dispute (Venuta and Rubin, 1973; Romano and Colby, 1973), but active transport is not involved (Venuta and Rubin, 1973).

7.4.10. Increased Synthesis of Hyaluronic Acid

Cells transformed by RNA tumor viruses synthesize more hyaluronic acid than do normal cells (Temin, 1965; Bader, 1972b). The synthesis of hyaluronic acid is a manifestation rather than a cause of transformation (Bader, 1972b). Hyaluronic acid can impede the agglutination of transformed cells by plant lectins (Burger and Martin, 1972), a fact which may account for the reported failures to preferentially agglutinate cells transformed by RNA tumor viruses (Moore and Temin, 1971).

7.4.11. Induction of DNA Synthesis in Host Cells

Infection of either permissive or nonpermissive cells by tumor viruses induces the synthesis of host DNA (Green, 1970). Neither the mechanism nor the significance of the induction is known. This effect has been extensively studied with DNA tumor viruses, and an analogous event may follow infection with RNA tumor viruses (Kara, 1968; Macieiro-Coelho *et al.*, 1969). However, it is generally acknowledged that, unlike DNA tumor viruses, RNA tumor viruses cannot induce a round of DNA synthesis in host cells that have ceased to divide (Temin, 1967; Weiss, 1971).

7.4.12. Fibrinolysis by Transformed Cells

A wide variety of transformed cells contain and release a protease which can activate serum plasminogen into fibrinolysin (plasmin) (Reich, 1973). The activator is not detectable in cultures of normal cells. Fibrinolysis is essential for the genesis of at least several features of transformed cells, including changes in morphology and growth in suspension, but it is not required for cell growth (Ossowski *et al.*, 1973).

7.4.13. Surface Antigens of Cells Tranformed by RNA Tumor Viruses

RNA tumor viruses induce transplantation antigens in the plasma membrane of either permissive or nonpermissive infected cells. These antigens mediate the rejection of virus-induced tumor cells by immune hosts and are known as tumor-specific transplantation antigens (TSTA), tumor-specific surface antigens (TSSA), or virus-induced surface antigens (VISA). They are analogous to the transplantation antigens induced by DNA tumor viruses, i.e., specific to groups of viruses (e.g., all avian RNA tumor viruses apparently induce the same TSSA) (Gelderblom *et al.*, 1972; Kurth and Bauer, 1972*a*) and cross-reactive among different species of transformed cells (Kurth and Bauer, 1972*b*). It is generally assumed that part or all of the TSSA induced by RNA tumor viruses is encoded in the viral genome, but there is no definitive experimental evidence for this view.

Cells transformed by RNA tumor viruses (and other neoplastic cells as well) reexpress a variety of embryonic surface antigens (Ting *et al.*, 1972; Kurth and Bauer, 1973). According to available evidence, these antigens are encoded in the cellular genome and are all distinct from TSSA (Ting *et al.*, 1972). The significance of embryonic antigens on the surface of virus-induced and other tumor cells is not known.

8. Transduction by RNA Tumor Viruses

Lysogenic bacteriophage can transduce cellular genes from one host to another. The phenomenon arises from the fact that the phage genome integrates into the chromosome of the host cell. By analogy, RNA tumor viruses could be expected to transduce cellular genes, but only one specialized example has been found: the genome of a murine leukemia virus has acquired nucleotide sequences from the genome of an endogenous rat virus during the course of propagation in rat cells (Scolnick *et al.*, 1973). We have been unsuccessful in efforts to demonstrate transduction of host (either permissive or nonpermissive) nucleotide sequences by avian sarcoma viruses (unpublished data of H. E. Varmus).

9. Molecular Techniques in the Detection and Identification of Human RNA Tumor Viruses

We have reviewed the current information about the molecular mechanisms by which RNA tumor viruses replicate and induce cellular transformation and now ask how this information might be applied to the study of human neoplasia. Implicit in this exercise is the assumption that RNA tumor viruses from animals provide relevant analogues for the analysis of human materials. This assumption can be defended only by circumstantial arguments at present, but it has neverthe- less motivated intensive research efforts which have produced some startling and provocative results (for example, see Spiegelman *et al.*, 1974). Our purpose here is to explore the rationale of reported and prospective studies of human tumors. We will cast our discussion according to three possibilities.

1. Human tumors are induced by infection with RNA tumor viruses which replicate in the target tissue; i.e., man is a permissive host for RNA tumor viruses derived from his own kind (homologous host) or from other species (heterologous host). Virus particles should be recognizable by any of several criteria: morphol- ogy (electron microscopy) and the presence of 70S RNA and RNA-directed DNA polymerase. Molecular hybridization should detect virus-specific RNA and DNA in the neoplastic tissue. If the virus is derived from *Homo sapiens*, viral DNA (and possibly viral RNA) should also be detectable in normal tissues. If man is a heterologous host for the virus, there are several possible means for the identification of the species from which the virus derives: serological tests for known interspecies and group-specific antigens and molecular hybridization with either the genomes of identified RNA tumor viruses or the DNA from tissues of various species. All of these procedures are predicated on the initial identification and isolation of virus particles so that appropriate reagents can be prepared.

Recent studies of human leukemia have followed the preceding lines (Baxt and Spiegelman, 1973). Some leukemic cells contain RNA-directed DNA polymerase activity in particles with a density appropriate to RNA tumor viruses; DNA synthesized by this enzyme(s) anneals partially to normal human DNA but more completely to DNA from leukemic cells. The results are consistent with the view that leukemic human cells are infected with and are producing an RNA tumor virus native to man. This formulation implies that the viral agent of human leukemia is transmitted horizontally, a conclusion which conflicts with most epidemiological analyses of the disease (Fraumeni and Miller, 1966; Huebner and

Todaro, 1969). However, data from molecular studies are circumstantial and do not prove that a virus is present or that the putative virus is an etiological agent of human leukemia.

2. Human tumors are induced by infection with RNA tumor viruses which do not replicate in human tissue: man is a nonpermissive heterologous host for RNA tumor viruses derived from other species. According to this scheme, virus particles will not be available from tumor tissue for characterization and preparation. However, virus-specific DNA and RNA, and possibly viral antigens, should be present in tumors. Viral nucleic acids and antigens can be detected only if appropriate (i.e., homologous) reagents are available. This necessitates a survey with materials from available animal viruses in the hope that one can identify either the etiological agent or a related virus. Molecular studies of human neoplasia have demonstrated cross-reactions between the genomes of murine RNA tumor viruses and the RNA from certain human neoplasias (Hehlmann *et al.*, 1972; Kufe *et al.*, 1973; Gallo *et al.*, 1973). These results are surprising in view of the high order of species specificity among most genomes for RNA tumor viruses (Quintrell *et al.*, 1974; Bishop *et al.*, 1974a). A similar rationale has motivated serological studies of human carcinoma of the breast with reagents for mouse mammary tumor virus (Muller and Grossmann, 1972).

3. Human tumors are induced by the partial expression of endogenous viral genomes which do not replicate in the tumor tissue. This is the most difficult of the three assumptions to deal with, both conceptually and experimentally. The molecular biologist is limited to surveys, hoping for a fortuitious cross-reaction between the putative human virus and available laboratory strains of RNA tumor viruses. Present strategy is predicated on the possibility that endogenous human viruses will replicate in the cells of other species if induced in their presence. If this approach were to succeed, it would provide the molecular biologist with specific reagents for an analysis of human tumors.

The application of molecular hybridization to the search for human tumor viruses began with the expectation that the genomes of RNA tumor viruses from various species might share nucleotide sequences in amounts determined by phylogenetic proximity. In general, this has proven to be a false hope; RNA tumor viruses from different species do not have physically detectable genetic homology (Bishop *et al.*, 1974a). Some remarkable exceptions to this rule have been reported; for example, the nucleic acid of a putative virus particle in human leukemia cells has appreciable homology with the genomes of both murine leukemia–sarcoma viruses (Hehlmann *et al.*, 1972) and a virus isolated from woolly monkeys (Gallo *et al.*, 1973), and there is a corresponding relationship between viruses from primates (gibbon and woolly monkey) and murine leukemia–sarcoma virus (Gallo *et al.*, 1973; Scolnick *et al.*, 1974). The significance of these observations is enigmatic, because tests by molecular hybridization indicate that neither the woolly monkey virus nor the gibbon virus actually originated in primates (Scolnick *et al.*, 1974). Instead, these viruses were fortuitously found replicating in heterologous hosts. The species from which the woolly and gibbon viruses were originally derived is not presently known.

In summary, the application of molecular biology to the search for RNA tumor viruses in *Homo sapiens* is limited by both the specificity of most available reagents and the conceptual problems engendered by present animal models. The investigator must contend with the fact that the demonstration of viral genes in human cells does not necessarily implicate those genes in oncogenesis. The apparent ubiquity of endogenous, often cryptic C-type viruses in ostensibly normal cells, coupled with uncertainties regarding the role of these viruses in either experimental or natural oncogenesis, requires that molecular studies be conducted in conjunction with biological and genetic analyses of both known and yet to be discovered cancer viruses.

10. Conclusion: Issues in the Molecular Biology of RNA Tumor Viruses

10.1. The Viral Genome and Oncogenesis

The genetic complexity of the viral genome remains in dispute. A definitive answer is much in need because it bears on the mechanisms of heterozygote formation and genetic recombination, the number of genes available for viral functions, and the mechanisms for the synthesis and integration of provirus. Beyond these lie even more subtle problems, *viz.*, the enumeration and characterization of the viral genes responsible for transformation. What are the molecular correlates of the fact that transforming genes of different strains of RNA tumor viruses cannot complement one another (Wyke, 1973)? Are transforming genes present in normal cells and activated by a transforming infection, or are these genes inevitably introduced by infection? What is the relationship between viral transforming genes and viral genes which induce leukemia? Are both sets of genes present in sarcoma genomes, as suggested in a report by Biggs *et al.* (1973), and, if so, why are the leukemogenic genes quiescent in the presence of transforming genes? (If indeed they are—the issue has not been carefully studied.) The principal molecular approach to most of these problems will be based on the isolation and characterization of nucleotide sequences corresponding to various oncogenic genes of viral origin.

10.2. Viral Gene Products Responsible for Transformation

The nature and function of the proteins encoded in viral genes for transformation are not known; the isolation and characterization of these proteins is a central objective in the use of tumor viruses as experimental models for oncogenesis. Experiments with viral mutants which synthesize temperature-sensitive products of transforming genes have implicated these genes in the genesis of most of the properties which characterize a transformed cell (Martin, 1970; Kawai and Hanafusa, 1971; Bader, 1972b; Scolnick *et al.*, 1972b; Graf and Friis, 1973), but the identity of transforming gene products and the mechanism of transformation remain enigmatic.

10.3. Synthesis and Integration of Provirus

To date, RNA-directed DNA synthesis *in vitro* has failed to reconstruct the synthesis of provirus as it occurs in the infected cell (see Table 2), and the study of nascent provirus in the infected cell has proceeded slowly. Consequently, we know little about the structure of provirus prior to integration and nothing about the mechanisms of integration. In what form is viral DNA integrated—as a linear duplex, as a duplex circle, as an RNA–DNA hybrid, etc? Are viral gene functions required for integration (there is no evidence for this to date), and what cellular functions are required? (Provisional data exclude cellular DNA synthesis and mitosis as requirements.) At what sites on host DNA does integration occur? Are these sites the same for all RNA tumor viruses or specific for individual strains of viruses? Does the site of integration influence the extent to which viral genes are subsequently expressed? If integration sites are specific (as they are for many lysogenic bacteriophages), how are they identified by the mechanisms which integrate provirus, and how is provirus brought into appropriate alignment with the sites?

10.4. The Origin of C-Type Viruses

We have noted previously the ubiquity of C-type viruses and have discussed the alternative explanations of their origin. The central issue is: Why has the course of evolution perpetuated the genes of C-type viruses in normal cells? Do these genes serve some essential but presently unidentified function? Present speculation centers on the possibility that genes of endogenous viruses have a purpose during embryological development, but the evidence for this view is vague and indirect.

10.5. Control of Expression of Viral Genes; Synthesis of Viral RNA

There is evidence that cells can contain an integrated provirus for an oncogenic virus without being neoplastic or transformed. The most persuasive data come from studies on hamster cells infected with avian sarcoma virus and reverted from a transformed to a normal phenotype (Macpherson, 1971). These revertants retain provirus for the sarcoma virus; virus can be rescued by fusion of the revertants with permissive cells (Boettiger, 1974) and sarcoma virus DNA can be detected in the revertants by molecular hybridization (Varmus *et al.*, 1973*d*; Deng *et al.*, 1974). Moreover, at least a portion of the provirus is transcribed into RNA (Deng *et al.*, 1974). Why are these hamster cells not transformed? Either crucial genes are not transcribed into RNA or control factors operate at some point subsequent to transcription. Available data cannot distinguish between these alternatives. These observations, along with analogous findings for mouse cells infected by avian sarcoma virus (Bishop *et al.*, 1974*b*) and mouse mammary tumor virus in various strains of mice (Varmus *et al.*, 1973*e*), illustrate how little is known about the mechanisms which regulate the expression of viral genes integrated into cellular DNA. If transcriptional controls are responsible, they must operate on specific portions of the integrated viral genome rather than effecting either complete repression or complete expression.

Implicit in this discussion is the conviction that integrated viral genes are subject to the forms of expression and regulation which operate on normal cellular genes. The consequences of regulation are different in permissive and nonpermissive cells; comparative studies of viral RNA synthesis and processing in the two types of hosts may help to illuminate the mechanisms of control. Definition of these controls may provide a rationale for the design of therapeutic agents for use against virus-induced tumors.

ACKNOWLEDGMENTS

Research in the authors' laboratories is supported by grants from the American Cancer Society (VC-70) and the USPHS (AI 08864, CA 12380, CA 12705, AI 06862, AI 00299), and by Contract No. N01 CP 33293 within the Virus Cancer Program of the National Cancer Institute. H. E. V. is the recipient of a Research Career Development Award (CA 70193) from the National Cancer Institute. We thank B. Bickerstaff and J. Skiles for stenographic and bibliographical assistance.

11. References

AARONSON, S. A., AND DUNN, C. Y., 1973, High-frequency C-type virus induction by inhibitors of protein synthesis, *Science* **183:**422.

AARONSON, S. A., TODARO, G. J., AND SCOLNICK, E. M., 1971, Induction of murine C-type viruses from clonal lines of virus-free BALB/3T3 cells, *Science* **174:**157.

ADESNIK, M., SALDITT, M., THOMAS, W., AND DARNELL, J. E., 1972, Evidence that all messenger RNA molecules (except histone messenger RNA) contain poly(A) sequences and that the poly(A) has a nuclear function, *J. Mol. Biol.* **71:**21.

ALTANER, C., AND TEMIN, H. M., 1970, Carcinogenesis by RNA sarcoma viruses. XII. A quantitative study of infection of rat cells *in vitro* by avian sarcoma viruses, *Virology* **40:**118.

ARNDT-JOVIN, D. J., AND BERG, P., 1971, Quantitative binding of ^{125}I-concanavalin A to normal and transformed cells, *J. Virol.* **8:**716.

BADER, A. V., 1973, Role of mitochondria in the production of RNA-containing tumor viruses, *J. Virol.* **11:**314.

BADER, J. P., 1965, The requirement for DNA synthesis in the growth of Rous sarcoma and Rous-associated viruses, *Virology* **26:**253.

BADER, J. P., 1966, Metabolic requirements for infection by Rous sarcoma virus. I. Transient requirement for DNA synthesis, *Virology* **29:**444.

BADER, J. P., 1972a, Metabolic requirements for infection by Rous sarcoma virus. IV. Virus reproduction and cellular transformation without cellular division, *Virology* **48:**494.

BADER, J. P., 1972b, Temperature-dependent transformation of cells infected with a mutant of Bryan Rous sarcoma virus, *J. Virol.* **10:**267.

BADER, J. P., 1973, Virus-induced transformation without cell division, *Science* **180:**1069.

BADER, J. P., AND STECK, T. L., 1969, Analysis of the ribonucleic acid of murine leukemia virus, *J. Virol.* **4:**454.

BALDUZZI, P., AND MORGAN, H. R., 1970, Mechanism of oncogenic transformation by Rous sarcoma virus. I. Intracellular inactivation of cell-transforming ability of Rous sarcoma virus by 5-bromodeoxyuridine and light, *J. Virol.* **5:**470.

BALTIMORE, D., 1970, RNA-dependent DNA polymerase in virions of RNA tumor viruses, *Nature (Lond.)* **226**:1209.

BALTIMORE, D., 1971a, Expression of animal virus in genomes, *Bacteriol. Rev.* **35**:235.

BALTIMORE, D., 1971b, Is poliovirus dead? in: *Perspectives in Virology*, Vol. VII (M. Pollard, ed.), pp. 1–14, Academic Press, New York.

BALTIMORE, D., AND SMOLER, D. F., 1971, Primer requirement and template specificity of the DNA polymerase of RNA tumor viruses (avian myeloblastosis virus/mouse leukemia virus/*E. coli* DNA polymerase/homopolynucleotides/oligonucleotides), *Proc. Natl. Acad. Sci.* **68**:1507.

BALTIMORE, D., AND SMOLER, D. F., 1972, Association of an endoribonuclease with the avian myeloblastosis virus deoxyribonucleic acid polymerase, *J. Biol. Chem.* **247**:7282.

BALTIMORE, D., VERMA, I. M., DROST, S., AND MASON, W. S., 1974, Temperature sensitive DNA polymerase from Rous sarcoma virus mutants, *Cancer* **34**:1395.

BALUDA, M. A., 1972, Widespread presence, in chickens, of DNA complementary to the DNA genome of avian leukosis viruses, *Proc. Natl. Acad. Sci.* **69**:576.

BAXT, W. G., AND SPIEGELMAN, S., 1973, Nuclear DNA sequences present in human leukemic cells and absent in normal leukocytes, *Proc. Natl. Acad. Sci.* **70**:627.

BEEMAN, K., DUESBERG, P., AND VOGT, P., 1974, Evidence for crossing-over between avian tumor viruses based on analysis of viral RNAs, *Proc. Natl. Acad. Sci. USA* **71**:4254.

BENTVELZEN, P., DAAMS, J. H., HAGEMAN, P., AND CALAFAT, J., 1970, Genetic transmission of viruses that incite mammary tumors in mice, *Proc. Natl. Acad. Sci.* **67**:377.

BENVENISTE, R. E., TODARO, G. J., SCOLNICK, E. M., AND PARKS, W. P., 1973, Partial transcription of murine type C viral genomes in BALB/c cell lines, *J. Virol.* **12**:711.

BENVENISTE, R. E., LIEBER, M. M., LIVINGSTON, D. M., SHEN, C. J., AND TODARO, G. J., 1974, Infectious type C virus isolated from a baboon placenta, *Nature (Lond.)* **248**:17.

BERKOWER, I., LEIS, J., AND HURWITZ, J., 1973, Isolation and characterization of an endonuclease from *Escherichia coli* specific for ribonucleic acid in ribonucleic acid deoxyribonucleic acid hybrid structures, *J. Biol. Chem.* **248**:5914.

BERNHARD, W., 1960, The detection and study of tumor viruses with the electron microscope, *Cancer Res.* **20**:712.

BIGGS, P. M., MILNE, B. S., GRAF, T., AND BAUER, H., 1973, Oncogenicity of nontransforming mutants of avian sarcoma viruses, *J. Gen. Virol.* **18**:399.

BILLETER, M. A., PARSONS, J. T., AND COFFIN, J. M., 1974, The nucleotide sequence complexity of avian tumor virus RNA, *Proc. Natl. Acad. Sci. USA* **71**:3560.

BISHOP, J. M., LEVINSON, W. E., QUINTRELL, N., SULLIVAN, D., FANSHIER, L., AND JACKSON, J., 1970a, The low molecular weight RNAs of Rous sarcoma virus. I. The 4S RNA, *Virology* **42**:182.

BISHOP, J. M., LEVINSON, W. E., SULLIVAN, D., FANSHIER, L., QUINTRELL, N., AND JACKSON, J., 1970b, The low molecular weight RNAs of Rous sarcoma virus. II. The 7S RNA, *Virology* **42**:927.

BISHOP, J. M., FARAS, A. J., GARAPIN, A. C., HANSEN, C., JACKSON, N., LEVINSON, W. E., TAYLOR, J. M., AND VARMUS, H. E., 1973, RNA-directed DNA polymerase and the replication of Rous sarcoma virus, in: *Molecular Studies in Viral Neoplasia* (25th Annual M. D. Anderson Symposium on Fundamental Cancer Research, 1972, R. W. Cumley, ed.), University of Texas Press, Austin, pp. 229–254.

BISHOP, J. M., QUINTRELL, N., MEDEIROS, E., AND VARMUS, H. E., 1974a, Of birds and mice and men: Comments on the use of animal models and molecular hybridization in the search for human tumor viruses, *Cancer* **34**:1421.

BISHOP, J. M., DENG, C. T., FARAS, A. J., GOODMAN, H. M., GUNTAKA, R. R., LEVINSON, W. E., CORDELL-STEWART, B., TAYLOR, J. M., AND VARMUS, H. E., 1974b, The provirus of Rous sarcoma virus: Synthesis, integration and transcription, in: *Tumor Virus–Host Cell Interaction* (Proceedings of a NATO Advanced Study Institute, A. Kolber, ed.), in press.

BISWAL, N., MCCAIN, B., AND BENYESH-MELNICK, M., 1971, The DNA of murine sarcoma leukemia virus, *Virology* **45**:697.

BOETTIGER, D., 1974, Reversion and induction of Rous sarcoma virus expression in virus-transformed baby hamster kidney cells, *Virology* **62**:522.

BOETTIGER, D., AND TEMIN, H. M., 1970, Light inactivation of focus formation by chicken embryo fibroblasts infected with avian sarcoma virus in the presence of 5-bromodeoxyuridine, *Nature (Lond.)* **228**:622.

BOLOGNESI, D. P., AND BAUER, H., 1970, Polypeptides of avian RNA tumor viruses. I. Isolation and physical and chemical analysis, *Virology* **42**:1097.

BOLOGNESI, D. P., BAUER, H., GELDERBLOM, H., AND HUPER, G., 1972a, Polypeptides of avian RNA tumor viruses. IV. Components of the viral envelope, *Virology* **47**:551.

BOLOGNESI, D. P., GELDERBLOM, H., BAUER, H., MOLLING, K., AND HUPER, G., 1972b, Polypeptides of avian RNA tumor viruses. V. Analysis of the virus core, *Virology* **47**:567.

BONAR, R. A., SVERAK, L., BOLOGNESI, D. P., LANGLOIS, A. J., BEARD, D., AND BEARD, J. W., 1967, Ribonucleic acid components of BAI strain A (myeloblastosis) avian tumor virus, *Cancer Res.* **27**:1138.

BUCK, C. A., GLICK, M. C., AND WARREN, L., 1970, A comparative study of glycoproteins from the surface of control and Rous sarcoma virus transformed hamster cells, *Biochemistry* **9**:4567.

BUCK, C. A., GLICK, M. C., AND WARREN, L., 1971a, Glycopeptides from the surface of control and virus-transformed cells, *Science* **172**:169.

BUCK, C. A., GLICK, M. C., AND WARREN, L., 1971b, Effect of growth on the glycoproteins from the surface of control and Rous sarcoma virus transformed cells, *Biochemistry* **10**:2176.

BURGER, M. M., 1969, A difference in the architecture of the surface membrane of normal and virally-transformed cells, *Proc. Natl. Acad. Sci.* **62**:994.

BURGER, M. M., AND MARTIN, G. S., 1972, Agglutination of cells transformed by Rous sarcoma virus by wheat germ agglutinin and concanavalin A, *Nature New. Biol.* **237**:9.

BURGER, M. M., AND NOONAN, K. D., 1970, Restoration of normal growth by covering of agglutinin sites on tumor cell surface, *Nature (Lond.)* **228**:512.

CANAANI, E., AND DUESBERG, P., 1972, Role of subunits of 60 to 70S avian tumor virus ribonucleic acid in its template activity for the viral deoxyribonucleic acid polymerase, *J. Virol.* **10**:23.

CANAANI, E., HELM, K. V. D., AND DUESBERG, P., 1973, Evidence for 30–40S RNA as precursor of the 60–70S RNA of Rous sarcoma virus, *Proc. Natl. Acad. Sci.* **72**:401.

CARCHMAN, R. A., JOHNSON, G. S., PASTAN, I., AND SCOLNICK, E. M., 1974, Studies on the levels of cyclic AMP in cells transformed by wild-type and temperature-sensitive Kirsten sarcoma virus, *Cell* **1**:59.

CHEUNG, K.-S., SMITH, R. E., STONE, M. P., AND JOKLIK, W. K., 1972, Comparison of immature (rapid harvest) and mature Rous sarcoma virus particles, *Virology* **50**:851.

CLARKE, G. D., STOKER, M. G. P., LUDLOW, A., AND THORNTON, M., 1970, Requirement of serum for DNA synthesis in BHK 21 cells: Effects of density, suspension and virus transformation, *Nature (Lond.)* **227**:798.

CLINE, M. J., AND LIVINGSTON, D. C., 1971, Concanavalin A—Role in agglutinating transformed cells, *Nature New Biol.* **232**:155.

COFFIN, J. M., 1972, Rescue of Rous sarcoma virus from Rous sarcoma virus transformed mammalian cells, *J. Virol.* **10**:153.

COFFIN, J. M., AND TEMIN, H. M., 1972, Hybridization of Rous sarcoma virus deoxyribonucleic acid polymerase product and ribonucleic acid from chicken and rat cells infected with Rous sarcoma virus, *J. Virol.* **9**:766.

CRITTENDEN, L. B., 1968, Observations on the nature of genetic cellular resistance to avian tumor viruses, *J. Natl. Cancer Inst.* **41**:145.

DAHLBERG, J. E., SAWYER, R. C., TAYLOR, J. M., FARAS, A. J., LEVINSON, W. E., GOODMAN, H. M., AND BISHOP, J. M., 1974, Transcription of DNA from the 70S RNA of Rous sarcoma virus: Identification of a specific 4S RNA which serves as primer, *J. Virol.* **13**:1126.

DALES, S., AND HANAFUSA, H., 1972, Penetration and intracellular release of the genomes of avian RNA tumor viruses, *Virology* **50**:440.

DAVIS, N. L., AND RUECKERT, R. R., 1972, Properties of a ribonucleoprotein particle isolated from Nonidet P-40–treated Rous sarcoma virus, *J. Virol.* **10**:1010.

DENG, C. T., BOETTIGER, D., MACPHERSON, I., AND VARMUS, H. E., 1974, The persistence and expression of virus-specific DNA in revertants of Rous sarcoma virus-transformed BHK-21 cells, *Virology* **62**:512.

DE THÉ, G., BECKER, C., AND BEARD, J. W., 1964, Virus of avian myeloblastosis (BAI strain A). XXV. Ultracytochemical study of virus and myeloblast phosphatase activity, *J. Natl. Cancer Inst.* **32**:201.

DUESBERG, P. H., 1968, Physical properties of RSV RNA, *Proc. Natl. Acad. Sci.* **60**:1511.

DUESBERG, P. H., 1970, On the structure of RNA tumor viruses, *Curr. Top. Microbiol. Immunol.* **51**:79.

DUESBERG, P. H., AND VOGT, P. K., 1970, Differences between the ribonucleic acids of transforming and nontransforming avian tumor viruses, *Proc. Natl. Acad. Sci.* **67**:1673.

DUESBERG, P. H., AND VOGT, P. K., 1973a, Gel electrophoresis of avian leukosis and sarcoma viral RNA in formamide: Comparison of other viral and cellular RNA species, *J. Virol.* **12**:594.

DUESBERG, P. H., AND VOGT, P. K., 1973b, RNA species obtained from clonal lines of avian sarcoma and avian leukosis virus, *Virology* **54**:207.

DUESBERG, P. H., MARTIN, G. S., AND VOGT, P. K., 1970, Glycoprotein components of avian and murine RNA tumor viruses, *Virology* **41**:631.

DUESBERG, P., HELM, K. V. D., AND CANAANI, E., 1971, Comparative properties of RNA and DNA templates for the DNA polymerase of Rous sarcoma virus, *Proc. Natl. Acad. Sci.* **68**:2505.

DUESBERG, P. H., VOGT, P. K., AND MARTIN, G. S., 1973a, The 60–70S RNA of avian sarcoma and leukosis viruses: Distribution of class a and b subunits, in: Unifying Concepts of Leukemia (R. M. Dutcher, ed.), *Bibl. Haematol.* **99**:462–473.

DUESBERG, P. H., VOGT, P. K., MAISEL, J., LAI, M. M.-C., AND CANAANI, E., 1973b, Tracking defective tumor virus RNA, in: *Virus Research* (Proceedings of the Second ICN-UCLA Symposium on Molecular Biology, C. F. Fox and W. S. Robinson, eds.), pp. 327–338, Academic Press, New York and London.

DULBECCO, R., 1970, Topoinhibition and serum requirement of transformed and untransformed cells, *Nature (Lond.)* **227**:802.

DULBECCO, R., AND ELKINGTON, J., 1973, Conditions limiting multiplication of fibroblastic and epithelial cells in dense cultures, *Nature (Lond.)* **246**:197.

EAST, J. L., ALLEN, P. T., KNESEK, J. E., CHAN, J. C., BOWEN, J. M., AND DMOCHOWSKI L., 1973, Structural rearrangement and subunit composition of RNA from released Soehner–Dmochowski murine sarcoma virions, *J. Virol.* **11**:709.

ELDER, K. T., AND SMITH, A. E., 1973, Methionine transfer ribonucleic acids of avian myeloblastosis virus, *Proc. Natl. Acad. Sci.* **70**:2823.

ELDER, K. T., AND SMITH, A. E., Methionine transfer RNAs associated with avian oncornavirus 70S RNA, *Nature (Lond.)* **247**:435.

ELLERMAN, V., AND BANG, O., 1909, Experimentelle Leukämie bei Huhnern, *Z. Hyg. Infekt.* **62**:231.

EMANOIL-RAVICOVITCH, R., LARSEN, C. J., BAZIFIER, M., ROBIN, J., PÉRIÈS, J., AND BOIRON, M., 1973, Low molecular weight RNAs of murine sarcoma virus: Comparative studies of free and 70S RNA-associated components, *J. Virol.* **12**:1625.

ERIKSON, E., AND ERIKSON, R. L., 1970, Isolation of amino acid acceptor RNA from purified avian myeloblastosis virus, *J. Mol. Biol.* **52**:387.

ERIKSON, E., AND ERIKSON, R. L., 1971, Association of 4S ribonucleic acid with oncornavirus ribonucleic acids, *J. Virol.* **8**:254.

ERIKSON, E., ERIKSON, R. L., HENRY, B., AND PACE, N. R., 1973, Comparison of oligonucleotides produced by RNase T1 digestion of 7S RNA from avian and murine oncornaviruses and from uninfected cells, *Virology* **53**:40.

ERIKSON, R. L., 1969, Studies on the RNA from avian myeloblastosis virus, *Virology* **37**:124.

FAN, H., AND BALTIMORE, D., 1973, RNA metabolism of murine leukemia virus: Detection of virus-specific RNA sequences in infected and uninfected cells and identification of virus-specific messenger RNA, *J. Mol. Biol.* **80**:93.

FAN, H., AND PASKIND, M., 1974, Measurement of the sequence complexity of cloned Moloney murine leukemia virus 60–70S RNA: Evidence for a haploid genome, *J. Virol.* **14**:421.

FARAS, A. J., TAYLOR, J. M., MCDONNELL, J. P., LEVINSON, W. E., AND BISHOP, J. M., 1972, Purification and characterization of the deoxyribonucleic acid polymerase associated with Rous sarcoma virus, *Biochemistry* **11**:2334.

FARAS, A. J., GARAPIN, A. C., LEVINSON, W. E., BISHOP, J. M., AND GOODMAN, H. M., 1973a, Characterization of low molecular weight RNAs associated with the 70S RNA of Rous sarcoma virus, *J. Virol.* **12**:334.

FARAS, A. J., TAYLOR, J. M., LEVINSON, W. E., GOODMAN, H. M., AND BISHOP, J. M., 1973b, RNA-directed DNA polymerase of Rous sarcoma virus: Initiation of synthesis with 70S viral RNA as template, *J. Mol. Biol.* **79**:163.

FARAS, A. J., DAHLBERG, J. E., SAWYER, R. C., HARADA, F., TAYLOR, J. M., LEVINSON, W. E., AND BISHOP, J. M., 1974, Transcription of DNA from the 70S RNA of Rous sarcoma virus: Structure of a 4S RNA primer, *J. Virol.* **13**:1134.

FLEISSNER, E., 1971, Chromatographic separation and antigenic analysis of proteins of the oncornviruses. I. Avian leukemia–sarcoma viruses, *J. Virol.* **8**:778.

FRAUMENI, J. F., AND MILLER, R. W., 1966, Epidemiology of human leukemia: Recent observations, *J. Natl. Cancer Inst.* **38**:593.

40

J. M. BISHOP
AND
H. E. VARMUS

FREARSON, P. M., AND CRAWFORD, L. V., 1972, Polyoma virus basic proteins, *J. Gen. Virol.* **14**:141.

FREEMAN, A. E., KELLÓFF, G. J., GILDEN, R. V., LANE, W. T., SWAIN, A. P., AND HUEBNER, R. J., 1971, Activation and isolation of hamster-specific C-type RNA viruses from tumors induced by cell cultures transformed by chemical carcinogens, *Proc. Natl. Acad. Sci.* **68**:2386.

GALLAGHER, R. E., AND GALLO, R. C., 1973, Chromatographic analyses of isoaccepting tRNAs from avian myeloblastosis virus, *J. Virol.* **12**:449.

GALLO, R. C., MILLER, N. R., SAXINGER, W. C., AND GILLESPIE, D., 1973, Primate RNA tumor virus-like DNA synthesized endogenously by RNA-dependent DNA polymerase in virus-like particles from fresh human acute leukemic blood cells, *Proc. Natl. Acad. Sci.* **70**:3219.

GARAPIN, A. C., VARMUS, H. E., FARAS, A. J., LEVINSON, W. E., AND BISHOP, J. M., 1973, RNA-directed DNA synthesis by virions of Rous sarcoma virus: Further characterization of the templates and the extent of their transcription, *Virology* **52**:264.

GEERING, G., AOKI, T., AND OLD, L., 1970, Shared viral antigen of mammalian leukemia viruses, *Nature (Lond.)* **226**:265.

GELB, L. D., AARONSON, S. A., AND MARTIN, M. A., 1971, Heterogeneity of murine leukemia virus *in vitro* DNA; detection of viral DNA in mammalian cells, *Science* **172**:1353.

GELDERBLOM, H., BAUER, H., AND GRAF, T., 1972, Cell-surface antigens induced by avian RNA tumor viruses: Detection by immunoferritin technique, *Virology* **47**:416.

GIELKENS, A. L. G., SALDEM, M. H. L., BLOEMENDAL, H., AND KONIGS, R. N. H., 1972, Translation of oncogenic viral RNA and eukaryotic messenger RNA in the *E. coli* cell-free system, *FEBS Letters* **28**:348.

GILDEN, R. V., OROSZLAN, S., AND HUEBNER, R. J., 1971, Coexistence of intraspecies specific antigenic determinants on the major structural polypeptide of mammalian C-type viruses, *Nature New. Biol.* **231**:107.

GRAF, T., 1972, A plaque assay for avian RNA tumor viruses, *Virology* **50**:567.

GRAF, T., AND FRIIS, R. R., 1973, Differential expression of transformation in rat and chicken cells infected with an avian sarcoma virus ts mutant, *Virology* **56**:369.

GRANBOULAN, N., HUPPERT, J., AND LACOUR, F., 1966, Examen au microscope electronique du RNA du virus de la myeloblastose aviaine, *J. Mol. Biol.* **16**:571.

GRANDGENETT, D. P., GERARD, G. F., AND GREEN, M., 1972, Ribonuclease H: A ubiquitous activity in virions of ribonucleic acid tumor viruses, *J. Virol.* **10**:1136.

GRANDGENETT, D. P., GERARD, G. F., AND GREEN, M., 1973, A single subunit from avian myeloblastosis virus with both RNA-directed DNA polymerase and ribonuclease H activity (RNA virus/polyacrylamide gel electrophoresis), *Proc. Natl. Acad. Sci.* **70**:230.

GREEN, M., 1970, Oncogenic viruses, *Ann. Rev. Biochem.* **39**:701.

GUNTAKA, R. V., MAHY, B. W., BISHOP, J. M., AND VARMUS, H. E., 1975, Ethidium bromide inhibits the appearance of closed circular viral DNA and integration of virus-specific DNA in duck cells infected by avian sarcoma virus, *Nature*, in press.

HANAFUSA, H., 1965, Analysis of the defectiveness of Rous sarcoma virus. III. Determining influence of a new helper virus on the host range and susceptibility to interference of RSV, *Virology* **25**:248.

HANAFUSA, H., 1969, Rapid transformation of cells by Rous sarcoma virus, *Proc. Natl. Acad. Sci.* **63**:318.

HANAFUSA, H., AND HANAFUSA, T., 1971, Noninfectious RSV deficient in DNA polymerase, *Virology* **43**:313.

HANAFUSA, T., HANAFUSA, H., AND MIYAMOTO, T., 1970, Recovery of a new virus from apparently normal chick cells by infection with avian tumor viruses, *Proc. Natl. Acad. Sci.* **67**:1797.

HANAFUSA, T., HANAFUSA, H., MIYAMOTO, T., AND FLEISSNER, E., 1972a, Existence and expression of tumor virus genes in chick embryo cells, *Virology* **47**:475.

HANAFUSA, H., BALTIMORE, D., SMOLER, D., WATSON, K. F., YANIV, A., AND SPIEGELMAN, S., 1972b, Absence of polymerase protein in virions of alpha-type Rous sarcoma virus, *Science* **177**:1188.

HARTLEY, J. W., AND ROWE, W. P., 1966, Production of altered cell foci in tissue culture by defective Moloney sarcoma virus particles, *Proc. Natl. Acad. Sci.* **55**:780.

HATANAKA, M., AND HANAFUSA, H., 1970, Analysis of a functional change in membrane in the process of cell transformation by Rous sarcoma virus; alteration in the characteristics of sugar transport, *Virology* **41**:647.

HATANAKA, M., KAKEFUDA, T., GILDEN, R. V., AND CALLAN, E. A. O., 1971, Cytoplasmic DNA synthesis induced by RNA tumor viruses (mouse embryo fibroblasts/murine sarcoma virus/Rauscher murine leukemia virus/autoradiography), *Proc. Natl. Acad. Sci.* **68**:1844.

HAUSEN, P., AND STEIN, H., 1970, Ribonuclease H: An enzyme degrading the RNA moiety of RNA–DNA hybrids, *Europ. J. Biochem.* **14**:278.

HAYWARD, W. S., AND HANAFUSA, H., 1973, Detection of avian tumor virus RNA in uninfected chicken embryo cells, *J. Virol.* **11**:157.

HEHLMANN, R., KUFE, D., AND SPIEGELMAN, S., 1972, RNA in human leukemic cells related to the RNA of a mouse leukemia virus (leukocytes/RNA–DNA hybridization/Rauscher virus/polysomal RNA), *Proc. Natl. Acad. Sci.* **69**:435.

HILL, M., AND HILLOVA, J., 1972*a*, Virus recovery in chicken cells tested with Rous sarcoma cell DNA, *Nature New Biol.* **237**:35.

HILL, M., AND HILLOVA, J., 1972*b*, Recovery of the temperature-sensitive mutant of Rous sarcoma virus from chicken cells exposed to DNA extracted from hamster cells transformed by the mutant, *Virology* **49**:309.

HOBOM-SCHNEGG, B., ROBINSON, H. L., AND ROBINSON, W. S., 1970, Replication of Rous sarcoma virus in sychronized cells, *J. Gen. Virol.* **7**:85.

HUANG, A. S., BESMER, P., CHU, L., AND BALTIMORE, D., 1973, Growth of pseudotypes of vesicular stomatitis virus with N-tropic murine leukemia virus coats in cells resistant to N-tropic viruses, *J. Virol.* **12**:659.

HUEBNER, R. J., AND GILDEN, R. V., 1971, Inherited RNA viral genomes (virogenes and oncogenes) in the etiology of cancer, in: *RNA Viruses and Host Genomes in Oncogenesis* (P. Emmelot and P. Bentvelzen, eds.), pp. 197–219, North-Holland, Amsterdam, American Elsevier, New York.

HUEBNER, R. J., AND TODARO, G. J., 1969, Oncogenes of RNA tumor viruses as determinants of cancer, *Proc. Natl. Acad. Sci.* **64**:1087.

HUMPHRIES, E. H., AND TEMIN, H. M., 1972, Cell cycle-dependent activation of Rous sarcoma virus-infected stationary chicken cells: Avian leukosis virus group-specific antigens and ribonucleic acid, *J. Virol.* **10**:82.

HUNG, P. P., 1973, Rescue of chemically inactivated Rous sarcoma virus transforming activity by avian leukosis virus, *Virology*, **53**:463.

HURWITZ, J., AND LEIS, J. P., 1972, RNA-dependent DNA polymerase activity of RNA tumor viruses. I. Directing influence of DNA in the reaction, *J. Virol.* **9**:130.

ISHIZAKI, R., LUFTIG, R. B., AND BOLOGNESI, D. P., 1973, Outer membrane of avian myeloblastosis virus, *J. Virol.* **12**:1579.

JACQUET, M., GRONER, Y., MONROY, G., AND HURWITZ, J., 1974, The *in vitro* synthesis of avian myeloblastosis viral RNA sequences (RNA synthesis/avian myeloblastosis virus/chromatin), *Proc. Natl. Acad. Sci. USA* **71**:3145.

JOHNSON, G. S., FRIEDMAN, R. M., AND PASTAN, I., 1971, Restoration of several morphological characteristics of normal fibroblasts in sarcoma cells treated with adenosine-3′:5′-cyclic monophosphate and its derivatives, *Proc. Natl. Acad. Sci.* **68**:425.

KACIAN, D. L., WATSON, K. F., BURNY, A., AND SPIEGELMAN, S., 1971, Purification of the DNA polymerase of avian myeblastosis virus, *Biochim. Biophys. Acta* **246**:365.

KANG, C.-Y., AND TEMIN, H. M., 1973, Lack of sequence homology among RNAs of avian leukosis–sarcoma viruses, reticuloendotheliosis viruses, and chicken endogenous RNA–directed DNA polymerase activity, *J. Virol.* **12**:1314.

KAPELLER, M., AND DOLJANSKI, F., 1972, Agglutination of normal and Rous sarcoma virus-transformed chick embryo cells by concanavalin A and wheat germ agglutinin, *Nature New Biol.* **235**:184.

KARA, J., 1968, Induction of cellular DNA synthesis in chick embryo fibroblasts infected with Rous sarcoma virus in culture, *Biochem. Biophys. Res. Commun.* **32**:817.

KARPAS, A., AND MILSTEIN, C., 1973, Recovery of the genome of murine sarcoma virus (MSV) after infection of cells with nuclear DNA from MSV transformed non-virus producing cells, *Europ. J. Cancer* **9**:295.

KAWAI, S., AND HANAFUSA, H., 1971, The effects of reciprocal changes in temperature on the transformed state of cells infected with a Rous sarcoma virus mutant, *Virology* **46**:470.

KAWAI, S., AND HANAFUSA, H., 1972*a*, Plaque assay for some strains of avian leukosis virus, *Virology* **48**:126.

KAWAI, S., AND HANAFUSA, H., 1972*b*, Genetic recombination with avian tumor virus, *Virology* **49**:37.

KAWAI, S., AND HANAFUSA, H., 1973, Isolation of defective mutant of avian sarcoma virus, *Proc. Natl. Acad. Sci.* **70**:3493.

J. M. BISHOP
AND
H. E. VARMUS

KELLER, W., AND CROUCH, R., 1972, Degradation of DNA · RNA hybrids by ribonuclease H and DNA polymerases of cellular and viral origin, *Proc. Natl. Acad. Sci.* **69**:3360.

KOTLER, M., 1971, Interactions of avian sarcoma virus with rat embryo cells in cell culture, *J. Gen. Virol.* **12**:197.

KRONTIRIS, T. G., SOEIRO, R., AND FIELDS, B. N., 1973, Host restriction of Friend leukemia virus: Role of the viral outer coat, *Proc. Natl. Acad. Sci.* **70**:2549.

KUFE, D., HEHLMANN, R., AND SPIEGELMAN, S., 1973, RNA related to that of a murine leukemia virus in Burkitt's tumors and nasopharyngeal carcinomas, *Proc. Natl. Acad. Sci.* **70**:5.

KURTH, R., AND BAUER, H., 1972a, Cell-surface antigens induced by avian RNA tumor viruses: Detection by a cytotoxicity microassay, *Virology* **47**:426.

KURTH, R., AND BAUER, H., 1972b, Common tumor specific antigens on cells of different species transformed by avian RNA tumor viruses, *Virology* **49**:145.

KURTH, R., AND BAUER, H., 1973, Avian oncronavirus-induced tumor antigens of embryonic and unknown origin, *Virology* **56**:496.

LAI, M. M. C., AND DUESBERG, P. H., 1972, Differences between the envelope glycoproteins and glycopeptides of avian tumor viruses released from transformed and nontransformed cells, *Virology* **50**:359.

LAI, M. M.-C., DUESBERG, P. H., HORST, J., AND VOGT, P. K., 1973, Avian tumor virus RNA: A comparison of three sarcoma viruses and their transformation-defective derivatives by oligonucleotide fingerprinting and DNA–RNA hybridization, *Proc. Natl. Acad. Sci.* **70**:2266.

LEIS, J. P., AND HURWITZ, J., 1972, RNA-dependent DNA polymerase activity of RNA tumor viruses. II. Directing influence of RNA in the reaction, *J. Virol.* **9**:130.

LEIS, J. P., BERKOWER, I., AND HURWITZ, J., 1973, Mechanism of action of ribonuclease H isolated from avian myeloblastosis virus and *Escherichia coli* (RNA-dependent DNA polymerase/processive exonuclease/*E. coli* endonuclease), *Proc. Natl. Acad. Sci.* **70**:466.

LEIS, J. P., HURWITZ, J., SCHINCARIOL, A. L., AND JOKLIK, S. K., 1974, RNA dependent DNA polymerase activity of RNA tumor viruses; activities associated with AMV reverse transcriptase and their possible role in viral replication, in: *Symposium on Biology of Tumor Viruses* (34th Annual Biology Colloquium), Oregon State University, in press.

LEONG, J. A., LEVINSON, W., AND BISHOP, J. M., 1972a, Synchronization of Rous sarcoma virus production in chick embryo cells, *Virology* **47**:133.

LEONG, J. A., GARAPIN, A. C., JACKSON, N., FANSHIER, L., LEVINSON, W., AND BISHOP, J. M., 1972b, Virus specific ribonucleic acid in cells producing Rous sarcoma virus: Detection and characterization, *J. Virol.* **9**:891.

LEVINSON, W., BISHOP, J. M., QUINTRELL, N., AND JACKSON, J., 1970, Presence of DNA in Rous sarcoma virus, *Nature (Lond.)* **227**:1023.

LEVINSON, W., HEILBRON, D., AND JACKSON, J., 1971, Behavior of chick embryo cells in tissue culture when infected with Rous sarcoma virus. I. Loss of contact inhibition, *J. Natl. Cancer Inst.* **46**:323.

LEVINSON, W. E., VARMUS, H. E., GARAPIN, A. C., AND BISHOP, J. M., 1972, DNA of Rous sarcoma virus: Its nature and significance, *Science* **175**:76.

LIEBER, M. M., BENVENISTE, R. E., LIVINGSTON, D. M., AND TODARO, G. J., 1973, Mammalian cells in culture frequently release type C viruses, *Science* **182**:56.

LINIAL, M., AND MASON, W. S., 1973, Characterization of two conditional early mutants of Rous sarcoma virus, *Virology* **53**:258.

LIVINGSTON, D. M., AND TODARO, G. J., 1973, Endogenous type C virus from a cat cell clone with properties distinct from previously described feline type C virus, *Virology* **53**:142.

LOEB, L. A., TARTOF, K. D., AND TRAVAGLINI, E. C., 1973, Copying natural RNAs with *E. coli* DNA polymerase I, *Nature New Biol.* **242**:66.

LOVE, D. N., AND WEISS, R. A., 1974, Pseudotypes of vesicular stomatitis virus determined by exogenous and endogenous avian RNA tumor viruses, *Virology* **57**:271.

LOVINGER, G. G., KLEIN, R. A., GILDEN, R. V., AND HATANAKA, M., 1973, The effect of cordycepin on cell transformation by RNA tumor viruses, *Virology* **55**:524.

LOWY, D. R., ROWE, W. P., TEICH, N., AND HARTLEY, J. W., 1971, Murine-leukemia virus: High-frequency activation *in vitro* by 5-iododeoxyuridine and 5-bromodeoxyuridine, *Science* **174**:155.

MACIEIRO-COELHO, A., HIU, I. J., AND GARCIA-GIRALT, E., 1969, Stimulation of DNA synthesis in resting stage human fibroblasts after infection with Rous sarcoma virus, *Nature (Lond.)* **222**:1172.

MACPHERSON, I. A., 1971, Reversion in cells transformed by tumour viruses, *Proc. Roy. Soc. (Biol.)* **177**:41.

MAISEL, J., KLEMENT, V., LAI, M. M.-C., OSTERTAG, W., AND DUESBERG, P., 1973, *Proc. Natl. Acad. Sci.* **70**:3536.

MARKHAM, P. D., AND BALUDA, M. A., 1973, Integrated state of oncornavirus DNA in normal chicken cells and in cells transformed by avian myeloblastosis virus, *J. Virol.* **12**:721.

MARSHALL, S., AND GILLESPIE, D., 1972, Poly U tracts absent from viral RNA, *Nature New Biol.* **240**:43.

MARTIN, G. S., 1970, Rous sarcoma virus: A function required for the maintenance of the transformed state, *Nature (Lond.)* **227**:1021.

MARTIN, G. S., AND DUESBERG, P. H., 1972, The *a* subunit in the RNA of transforming avian tumor viruses. I. Occurrence in different virus strains. II. Spontaneous loss resulting in nontransforming variants, *Virology* **47**:494.

MARTIN, G. S., VENUTA, S., WEBER, M., AND RUBIN, H., 1971, Temperature-dependent alterations in sugar transport in cells infected by a temperature-sensitive mutant of Rous sarcoma virus, *Proc. Natl. Acad. Sci.* **68**:2739.

MAY, J. T., SOMERS, K. D., AND KIT, S., 1972, Defective mouse sarcoma virus deficient in DNA polymerase activity, *J. Gen. Virol.* **16**:223.

McCAFFREY, R., SMOLER, D. F., AND BALTIMORE, D., 1973, Terminal deoxynucleotidyl trasferase in a case of childhood acute lymphoblastic leukemia, *Proc. Natl. Acad. Sci.* **70**:521.

MEIER, H., TAYLOR, B. A., CHERRY, M., AND HUEBNER, R. J., 1973, Host-gene control of type C RNA tumor virus expression and tumorigenesis in inbred mice (reciprocal backcross progenies/complement-fixing antigens/dominant genes/genetic markers), *Proc. Natl. Acad. Sci.* **70**:1450.

MIZUTANI, S., AND TEMIN, H. M., 1971, Enzymes and nucleotides in virions of Rous sarcoma virus, *J. Virol.* **8**:409.

MODAK, M. J., MARCUS, S. L., AND CAVALIERI, L. F., 1973, DNA complementary to rabbit globin mRNA made by *E. coli* polymerase I, *Biochem. Biophys. Res. Commun.* **55**:1.

MOLLING, K., BOLOGNESI, D. P., BAUER, H., BUSEN, W., PLASSMANN, H. W., AND HAUSEN, P., 1971, Association of viral reverse transcriptase with an enzyme degrading the RNA moiety of RNA–DNA hybrids, *Nature New Biol.* **234**:240.

MOORE, E. G., AND TEMIN, H. M., 1971, Lack of correlation between conversion by RNA tumour viruses and increased agglutinability of cells by concanavalin A and wheat germ agglutinin, *Nature (Lond.)* **231**:117.

MULLER, M., AND GROSSMANN, H., 1972, An antigen in human breast cancer sera related to the murine mammary tumour virus, *Nature New Biol.* **237**:116.

NANDI, S., AND McGRATH, C. M., 1973, Mammary neoplasia in mice, *Advan. Cancer Res.* **17**:353.

NEIMAN, P. E., 1972, Rous sarcoma virus nucleotide sequences in cellular DNA: Measurement by RNA–DNA hybridization, *Science* **178**:750.

NERMUT, M. V., HERMANN, F., AND SCHAFER, W., 1972, Poperties of mouse leukemia viruses. III. Electron microscopic appearance as revealed after conventional preparation techniques as well as freeze-drying and freeze-etching, *Virology* **49**:345.

NICHOLS, J. L., AND WADDELL, M., 1973, Comparison of free and 80S RNA-associated RNAs of mouse L cell virions, *Nature New Biol.* **243**:236.

NICOLSON, G. L., 1971, Difference in topology of normal and tumour cell membranes shown by different surface distributions of ferritin-conjugated concanavalin A, *Nature New Biol.* **233**:244.

NOMURA, S., FISCHINGER, P. J., MATTERN, C. F. T., GERWIN, B., AND DUNN, K. J., 1973, Revertants of mouse cells transformed by murine sarcoma virus. II. Flat variants induced by fluorodeoxyuridine and colcemid, *Virology* **56**:152.

NOONAN, K. D., AND BURGER, M. M., 1973, Binding of ^{3}H concanavalin A to normal and transformed cells, *J. Biol. Chem.* **248**:4286.

NOWINSKI, R. C., OLD, L. J., SARKAR, N. H., AND MOORE, D. H., 1970, Common properties of the oncogenic RNA viruses (oncornaviruses), *Virology* **42**:1152.

NOWINSKI, R. C., FLEISSNER, E., SARKAR, N. H., AND AOKI, T., 1972*a*, Chromatographic separation and antigenic analysis of proteins of the oncornaviruses. II. Mammalian leukemia–sarcoma viruses, *J. Virol.* **9**:359.

NOWINSKI, R. C., WATSON, K. F., YANIV, A., AND SPIEGELMAN, S., 1972*b*, Serological analysis of the deoxyribonucleic acid polymerase of avian oncornaviruses. II. Comparison of avian deoxyribonucleic acid polymerases, *J. Virol.* **10**:959.

OBARA, T., BOLOGNESI, D. P., AND BAUER, H., 1971, Ribosomal RNA in avian leukosis virus particles, *Int. J. Cancer* **7:**535.

OROSZLAN, S., HATANAKA, M., GILDEN, R. V., AND HUEBNER, R. J., 1971, Specific inhibition of mammalian ribonucleic acid C-type virus deoxyribonucleic acid polymerases by rat antisera, *J. Virol.* **8:**816.

OSSOWSKI, L., QUIGLEY, J. P., KELLERMAN, G. M., AND REICH, E., 1973, Fibrinolysis associated with oncogenic transformation: Requirement of plasminogen for correlated changes in cellular morphology, colony formation in agar, and cell migration, *J. Exp. Med.* **138:**1056.

OTTEN, J., JOHNSON, G. S., AND PASTAN, I., 1971, Cyclic AMP levels in fibroblasts: Relationship to growth rate and contact inhibition of growth, *Biochem. Biophys. Res. Commun.* **44:**1192.

OTTEN, J., BADER, J. P., JOHNSON, G. J., AND PASTAN, I., 1972, A mutation in a Rous sarcoma virus gene that controls adenosine (ZH,5'-monophosphate levels and transformation, *J. Biol. Chem.* **247:**1632.

OZANNE, B., AND SAMBROOK, J., 1971, Binding of labelled Con A and wheat germ agglutinin to normal and transformed cells, *Nature New Biol.* **232:**156.

PANEM, S., AND KIRSTEN, W. H., 1973, release of mouse leukemia–sarcoma virus from synchronized cells, *J. Natl. Cancer Inst.* **50:**563.

PARAN, M., GALLO, R. C., RICHARDSON, L. S., AND WU, A. M., 1973, Adrenal corticosteroids enhance production of C-type virus induced by 5-iodo-2'-deoxyuridine from cultured mouse fibroblasts, *Proc. Natl. Acad. Sci.* **70:**2391.

PARKS, W. P., AND SCOLNICK, E. M., 1972, Radioimmunoassay of mammalian type C viral proteins: Interspecies antigenic reactivities of the major internal polypeptide, *Proc. Natl. Acad. Sci.* **69:**1766.

PARKS, W. P., SCOLNICK, E. M., ROSS, J., TDARO, G. J., AND AARONSON, S. A., 1972, Immunological relationships of reverse transcriptase from ribonucleic acid tumor viruses, *J. Virol.* **9:**110.

PARSONS, J. T., COFFIN, J. M., HAROZ, R. K., BROMLEY, P. A., AND WEISSMAN, C., 1973, Quantitative determination and location of newly synthesized virus-specific ribonucleic acid in chicken cells infected with Rous sarcoma virus, *J. Virol.* **11:**761.

PASTAN, I., AND JOHNSON, G. S., 1974, Cyclic AMP and the transformation of fibroblasts, *Advan. Cancer Res.*, in press.

PAYNE, L. N., AND CHUBB, R., 1968, Studies on the nature and genetic control of an antigen in normal chick embryos which reacts in the COFAL test, *J. Gen. Virol.* **3:**379.

PEEBLES, P. T., HAAPALA, D. K., AND GAZDAR, A. F., 1972, Deficiency of viral ribonucleic acid-dependent deoxyribonucleic acid polymerase in noninfectious virus-like particles released from murine sarcoma virus-transformed hamster cells, *J. Virol.* **9:**488.

PHILLIPS, L. A., HOLLIS, V. W., BASSIN, R. H., AND FISCHINGER, P. J., 1973, Characterization of RNA from noninfectious virions produced by sarcoma positive-leukemia negative transformed 3T3 cells, *Proc. Natl. Acad. Sci.* **70:**3002.

PIRAINO, F., 1967, The mechanism of genetic resistance of chick embryo cells to infection by Rous sarcoma virus–Bryan strain, *Virology* **32:**700.

POSTE, G., AND REEVE, P., 1972, Agglutination of normal cells by plant lectins following infection with nononcogenic viruses, *Nature New Biol.* **237:**113.

PROUDFOOT, N. J., AND BROWNLEE, G. G., 1974, Nucleotide sequence adjacent to polyadenylic acid in globin messenger RNA, *FEBS Letters* **38:**179.

QUINTRELL, N., VARMUS, H. E., BISHOP, J. M., NICOLSON, M. O., AND MCALLISTER, R. M., 1974, Homologies among the nucleotide sequences of the genomes of C-type viruses, *Virology* **58:**568.

RANDERATH, K., ROSENTHAL, L. J., AND ZAMECNIK, P. C., 1971, Base composition differences between avian myeloblastosis virus transfer RNA, and transfer RNA isolated from host cells, *Proc. Natl. Acad. Sci.* **68:**3233.

REICH, E., 1973, Tumor-associated fibrinolysis, *Fed. Proc.* **32:**2174.

RICHERT, N. J., AND HARE, J. D., 1972, Distinctive effects of inhibitors of mitochondrial function on Rous sarcoma virus replication and malignant transformation, *Biochem. Biophys. Res. Commun.* **46:**5.

RIFKIN, D. B. AND COMPANS, R. W., 1971, Identification of the spike proteins of Rous sarcoma virus, *Virology* **46:**485.

ROBINSON, W. S., HUNG, P., ROBINSON, H. L., AND RALPH, D. D., 1970, Proteins of avian tumor viruses with different coat antigens, *J. Virol.* **6:**695.

ROMANO, A. H., AND COLBY, C., 1973, SV40 virus transformation of mouse 3T3 cells does not specifically enhance sugar transport, *Science* **179:**1238.

ROSENTHAL, L. J., AND ZAMECNIK, P. C., 1973a, Minor base composition of "70-associated" 4S RNA from avian myeloblastosis virus (tumor virus/isotope derivative method/titanium fluorography), *Proc. Natl. Acad. Sci.* **70:**727.

ROSENTHAL, L. J., AND ZAMECNIK, P. C., 1973b, Amino-acid acceptor activity of the "70S-associated" 4S RNA from avian myeloblastosis virus (oncogenic RNA virus/RNA bound to 70S RNA), *Proc. Natl. Acad. Sci.* **70:**1184.

ROSENTHAL, P. N., ROBINSON, H. L., ROBINSON, W. S., HANAFUSA, T., AND HANAFUSA, H., 1971, DNA in uninfected and virus-infected cells complementary to avian tumor virus RNA, *Proc. Natl. Acad. Sci.* **68:**2336.

ROUS, P., 1911, A sarcoma of the fowl transmissible by an agent separable from the tumor cells, *J. Exp. Med.* **13:**397.

ROWE, W. P., 1971, The kinetics of rescue of the murine sarcoma virus genome from a nonproducer line of transformed mouse cells, *Virology* **46:**369.

ROWE, W. P., HARTLEY, J. W., LANDER, M. R., PUGH, W. E., AND TEICH, N., 1971, Noninfectious AKR mouse embryo cell lines in which each cell has the capacity to be activated to produce infectious murine leukemia virus, *Virology* **46:**866.

ROWE, W. P., HARTLEY, J. W., AND BREMNER, T., 1972, Genetic mapping of a murine leukemia virus–inducing locus of AKR mice, *Science* **178:**860.

RUPRECHT, R. M., GOODMAN, N. C., AND SPIEGELMAN, S., 1973, Determination of natural host taxonomy of RNA tumor viruses by molecular hybridization: Application to RD-114, a candidate human virus, *Proc. Natl. Acad. Sci.* **70:**1437.

RYMO, L., PARSONS, J. T., COFFIN, J. M., AND WEISSMANN, C., 1974, *In vitro* synthesis of Rous sarcoma virus-specific RNA is catalyzed by a DNA-dependent RNA polymerase (actinomycin D/α-amanitin/assay of virus-specific RNA), *Proc. Natl. Acad. Sci. USA* **71:**2782.

SARIN, P. S., AND GALLO, R. C., 1973, RNA directed DNA polymerase, in: *International Review of Science Series in Biochemistry*, Vol. 6 (K. Burton, ed.), Chap. 8, Butterworth, Oxford.

SARKAR, N. H., MOORE, D. H., AND NOWINSKI, R. C., 1971a, Symmetry of the nucleocapsid of the oncornaviruses, in: *RNA Viruses and Host Genome in Oncogenesis*, (P. Emmelot and P. Bentvelzen, eds.), pp. 71–79, North-Holland, Amsterdam, American Elsevier, New York.

SARKAR, N. H., NOWINSKI, R. C., AND MOORE, D. H., 1971b, Helical nucleocapsid structure of the oncogenic ribonucleic acid viruses (oncornaviruses), *J. Virol.* **8:**564.

SAWYER, R. C., AND DAHLBERG, J. E., 1973, Small RNAs of Rous sarcoma virus: Characterization by two-dimensional polyacrylamide gel electrophoresis and fingerprint analysis, *J. Virol.* **12:**1226.

SAWYER, R. C., HARADA, F., AND DAHLBERG, J. E., 1974, An RNA primer for Rous sarcoma virus DNA synthesis: Isolation from uninfected host cells. *J. Virol* **13:**1302.

SCHAFER, W., PISTER, L., HUNSMANN, G., AND MOENNIG, V., 1973, Comparative serological studies on type C viruses of various mammals, *Nature New Biol.* **245:**75.

SCHEELE, C. M., AND HANAFUSA, H., 1971, Proteins of helper-dependent RSV, *Virology* **45:**401.

SCHINCARIOL, A. L., AND JOKLIK, W. E., 1973, Early synthesis of virus-specific RNA and DNA in cells rapidly transformed with Rous sarcoma virus, *Virology* **56:**532.

SCOLNICK, E. M., PARKS, W. P., AND TODARO, G. J., 1972a, Reverse transcriptases of primate viruses as immunological markers, *Science* **177:**1119.

SCOLNICK, E. M., STEPHENSEN, J. R., AND AARONSON, S. A., 1972b, Isolation of temperature sensitive mutants of murine sarcoma virus, *J. Virol.* **10:**653.

SCOLNICK, E. M., PARKS, W. P., TODARO, G. J., AND AARONSON, S. A., 1972c, Immunological characterization of primate C-type virus reverse transcriptases, *Nature New Biol.* **235:**35.

SCOLNICK, E. M., RANDS, E., WILLIAMS, D., AND PARKS, W. P., 1973, Studies on the nucleic acid sequences of Kirsten sarcoma virus: A model for formation of a mammalian RNA-containing sarcoma virus, *J. Virol.* **12:**458.

SCOLNICK, E. M., PARKS, W., KAWAKAMI, T., KOHNE, D., OKALE, H., GILDEN, R., AND HATANAKA, M., 1974, Primates and murine type-C viral nucleic acid association kinetics: Analysis of model systems and natural tissues, *J. Virol.* **13:**363.

SHARON, N., AND LIS, H., 1972, Lectins: Cell-agglutinating and sugar-specific proteins, *Science* **177:**949.

SIEGERT, W., KONINGS, R. N. J., BAUER, H., AND HOFSCHNEIDER, P. H., 1972, Translation of avian myeloblastosis virus RNA in a cell-free lysate of *Escherichia coli*, *Proc. Natl. Acad. Sci.* **69:**888.

SILBER, R., MALATHI, V. G., SCHULMAN, L. H., HURWITZ, J., AND DUESBERG, P., 1973, Studies of the

Rous sarcoma virus RNA: Characterization of the 5'-terminus, *Biochem. Biophys. Res. Commun.* **50**:467.

SMITH, G. H., AND WIVEL, N. A., 1973, Intracytoplasmic A particles: Mouse mammary tumor virus nucleoprotein cores? *J. Virol.* **11**:575.

SMITH. H. S., GELB, L. D., AND MARTIN, M. A., 1972, Detection and quantitation of simian virus 40 genetic material in abortively transformed BALB/3T3 clones, *Proc. Natl. Acad. Sci.* **69**:152.

SMOLER, D., MOLINEUX, I., AND BALTIMORE, D., 1971, Direction of polymerization by the avian myeloblastosis virus deoxyribonucleic acid polymerase, *J. Biol. Chem.* **246**:7697.

SOMERS, K. D., MAY, J. T., AND KIT, S., 1973, Control of gene expression in rat cells transformed by a cold-sensitive murine sarcoma virus (MSV) mutant, *Intervirology* **1**:176.

SPIEGELMAN, S., AXEL, R., BAXT, W., GULATI, S. C., HEHLMAN, R., KUFE, D., AND SCHLOM, J., 1974, The relevance of RNA tumor viruses to human cancer, in: *The Sixth Miles International Symposium on Molecular Biology*, in press.

STEPHENSON, J. R., AND AARONSON, S. A., 1971, Murine sarcoma and leukemic viruses: Genetic differences determined by RNA–DNA hybridization, *Virology* **46**:480.

STEPHENSON, J. R., AND AARONSON, S. A., 1973, Segregation of loci for C-type virus induction in strains of mice with high and low incidence of leukemia, *Science* **180**:865.

STEPHENSON, J. R., SCOLNICK, E. M., AND AARONSON, S. A., 1972, Genetic stability of the sarcoma viruses in murine and avian sarcoma virus transformed nonproducer cells, *Int. J. Cancer* **9**:577.

STEPHENSON, J. R., REYNOLDS, R. K., AND AARONSON, S. A., 1973, Characterization of morphologic revertants of murine and avian sarcoma virus-transformed cells, *J. Virol.* **11**:218.

STEPHENSON, J. R., GREENBERGER, J. S., AND AARONSON, S. A., 1974, Oncogenicity of an endogenous C-type virus chemically activated from mouse cells in culture, *J. Virol.* **13**:237.

STEPHENSON, M. L., SCOTT, J. F., AND ZAMECNIK, P. C., 1973, Evidence that polyadenylic acid segment of "35S" RNA of avian myeloblastosis virus is located at the 3' OH terminus, *Biochem. Biophys. Res. Commun.* **55**:8.

STRAND, M., AND AUGUST, J. T., 1974, Structural proteins of mammalian oncogenic RNA viruses: Multiple antigenic determinants of the major internal protein and envelope glycoprotein, *J. Virol.* **13**:171.

SVOBODA, J., 1972, The biology of avian tumor viruses and the role of host cell in the modification of avian tumor virus expression, in: *RNA Viruses and Host Genome in Oncogenesis* (P. Emmelot and P. Bentvelzen, eds.), pp. 81–92, North-Holland, Amsterdam, American Elsevier, New York.

SVOBODA, J., AND DOURMASHKIN, R., 1969, Rescue of RSV from virogenic mammalian cells associated with chicken cells and treated with Sendai virus, *J. Gen. Virol.* **4**:523.

TANAKA, H., TAMURA, A., AND TSUJIMURA, D., 1972, Properties of the intracytoplasmic A particles purified from mouse tumors, *Virology* **49**:61.

TAYLOR, B. A., NEIHER, H., AND MYERS, D. D., 1971, Host-gene control of C-type RNA tumor virus: Inheritance of the group-specific antigen of murine leukemia virus, *Proc. Natl. Acad. Sci.* **63**:3190.

TAYLOR, B. A., MEIER, H., AND HUEBNER, R. J., 1973, Genetic control of the group-specific antigen of murine leukemia virus, *Nature New Biol.* **241**:184.

TAYLOR, J. M., VARMUS, H. E., FARAS, A. J., LEVINSON, W. E., AND BISHOP, J. M., 1974, Evidence for non-repetitive subunits in the genome of Rous sarcoma virus, *J. Mol. Biol.*, **84**:217.

TEICH, N., LOWY, D. R., HARTLEY, J. W., AND ROWE, W. P., 1973, Studies of the mechanism of induction of infectious murine leukemia virus from AKR mouse embryo cell lines by 5-iododeoxyuridine and 5-bromodeoxyuridine, *Virology Virology* **51**:163.

TEMIN, H. M., 1961, Mixed infections with two types of Rous sarcoma virus, *Virology* **13**:158.

TEMIN, H. M., 1963, The effects of actinomycin D on growth of Rous sarcoma virus *in vitro*, *Virology* **20**:577.

TEMIN, H. M., 1965, The mechanism of carcinogenesis by avian sarcoma viruses. I. Cell multiplication and differentiation, *J. Natl. Cancer Inst.* **35**:679.

TEMIN, H. M., 1967, Studies on carcinogenesis by avian sarcoma viruses, V. Requirement for new DNA synthesis and for cell division, *J. Cell. Physiol.* **69**:53.

TEMIN, H. M., 1968, Carcinogenesis by avian sarcoma viruses, *Cancer Res.* **28**:1835.

TEMIN, H. M., 1970, Formation and activation of the provirus of RNA sarcoma viruses, in: *The Biology of Large RNA Viruses* (R. D. Barry and B. W. J. Mahy, eds.), pp. 233–249, Academic Press, New York and London.

TEMIN, H. M., 1971, Mechanism of cell transformation by RNA tumor viruses, *Ann. Rev. Microbiol.* **25**:609.

TEMIN, H. M., 1972, The RNA tumor viruses—Background and foreground, *Proc. Natl. Acad. Sci.* **69:**1016.

TEMIN, H. M., AND BALTIMORE, D., 1972, RNA-directed DNA synthesis and RNA tumor viruses, *Advan. Virus Res.* **17:**129.

TEMIN, H. M., AND MIZUTANI, S., 1970, RNA-dependent DNA polymerase in virions of Rous sarcoma virus, *Nature (Lond.)* **226:**1211.

TING, C.-C., LAVRIN, D. H., SHIU, G., AND HARBERMAN, R. B., 1972, Expression of fetal antigens in tumor cells, *Proc. Natl. Acad. Sci.* **69:**1664.

TODARO, G. J., 1972, "Spontaneous" release from clonal lines of "spontaneously" transformed BALB/3T3 cells, *Nature New Biol.* **240:**157.

TODARO, G. J., AND GALLO, R. C., 1973, Immunological relatedness between a DNA polymerase from human acute leukemia cells and primate and mouse leukemia virus reverse transcriptase, *Nature (Lond.)* **244:**206.

TODARO, G. J., AND HUEBNER, R. J., 1972, The viral oncogene hypothesis: New evidence, *Proc. Natl. Acad. Sci.* **69:**1009.

TRAVNICEK, M., AND RIMAN, J., 1970, Chromatographic differences between lysyl-tRNA's from avian tumor virus BAI strain A and virus transformed cells, *Biochim. Biophys. Acta* **199:**283.

TRONICK, S. R., SCOLNICK, E. M., AND PARKS, W. P., 1972, Reversible inactivation of the deoxyribonucleic acid polymerase of Rauscher leukemia virus, *J. Virol.* **10:**885.

TSUCHIDA, M., RIBIN, M. S., AND GREEN, M., 1972, Viral RNA subunits in cells transformed by RNA tumor viruses, *Science* **176:**1418.

TWARDZIK, D., SIMONDS, J., OSKARSSON, M., AND PORTUGAL, F., 1973, Translation of AKR-murine leukemia viral RNA in an *E. coli* cell-free system, *Biochem. Biophys. Res. Commun.* **52:**1108.

VARMUS, H. E., LEVINSON, W. E., AND BISHOP, J. M., 1971, Extent of transcription by the RNA-dependent DNA polymerase of Rous sarcoma virus (RSV), *Nature New Biol.* **233:**19.

VARMUS, H. E., BISHOP, J. M., NOWINSKI, R., AND SARKAR, N., 1972a, Mammary tumor virus specific nucleotide sequences in DNA of high and low incidence mouse strains, *Nature New Biol.* **238:**189.

VARMUS, H. E., WEISS, R. A., FRIIS, R. R., LEVINSON, W., AND BISHOP, J. M., 1972b, Detection of avian tumour virus–specific nucleotide sequences in avian cell DNAs, *Proc. Natl. Acad. Sci.* **69:**20.

VARMUS, H. E., BISHOP, J. M., AND VOGT, P. K., 1973a, Synthesis and integration of Rous sarcoma virus-specific DNA in permissive and non-permissive hosts, in: *Virus Research* (Proceedings of the Second ICN-UCLA Symposium on Molecular Biology, C. F. Fox and W. S. Robinson, eds.), pp. 373–383, Academic Press, New York and London.

VARMUS, H. E., BISHOP, J. M., AND VOGT, P. K., 1973b, Appearance of virus-specific DNA in mammalian cells following transformation by Rous sarcoma virus, *J. Mol. Biol.* **74:**613.

VARMUS, H. E., VOGT, P. K., AND BISHOP, J. M., 1973c, Integration of deoxyribonucleic acid specific for Rous sarcoma virus after infection of permissive and nonpermissive hosts, *Proc. Natl. Acad. Sci.* **70:**3067.

VARMUS, H. E., HANSEN, C. B., MEDEIROS, E., DENG, C. T., AND BISHOP, J. M., 1973d, Detection and characterization of RNA tumor virus-specific nucleotide sequences in cell DNA, in: *Possible Episomes in Eukaryotes* (Fourth Lepetit Colloquium, L. G. Silvestri, ed.), pp. 50–60, North-Holland, Amsterdam, American Elsevier, New York.

VARMUS, H. E., QUINTRELL, N., MEDEIROS, E., BISHOP, J. M., AND NOWINSKI, R. C., 1973e, Transcription of mouse mammary tumor virus genes in tissues from high and low tumor incidence mouse strains, *J. Mol. Biol.* **79:**663.

VARMUS, H. E., STAVNEZER, J., MEDEIROS, E., AND BISHOP, J. M., 1974a, Detection and characterization of RNA tumor virus-specific DNA in cells, in: *Comparative Leukemia Research, 1973* (Y. Ito, ed.), University of Tokyo Press, in press.

VARMUS, H. E., GUNTAKA, R. V., FAN, W. J. W., HEASLEY, S., AND BISHOP, J. M., 1974b, Synthesis of viral DNA in the cytoplasm of duck embryo fibroblasts and in enucleated cells after infection by avian sarcoma virus, *Proc. Natl. Acad. Sci. USA* **71:**3874.

VARMUS, H. E., HEASLEY, S., AND BISHOP, J. M., 1974c, Use of DNA–DNA annealing to detect new virus-specific DNA sequences in chicken embryo fibroblasts after infection by avian sarcoma virus, *J. Virol.* **14:**895.

VENUTA, S., AND RUBIN, H., 1973, Sugar transport in normal and Rous sarcoma virus-transformed chick-embryo fibroblasts (3-O-methylglucose/glycose competition/efflux/facilitated diffusion/K_m, V/max), *Proc. Natl. Acad. Sci* **70:**653.

VERMA, I. M., MEUTH, N. L., BROMFELD, E., MANLY, K. F., AND BALTIMORE, D., 1971, Covalently linked RNA·DNA molecule as initial product of RNA tumour virus DNA polymerase, *Nature New Biol.* **233**:131.

VERMA, I. M., MEUTH, N. L., FAN, H., AND BALTIMORE, D., 1974, Hamster leukemia virus DNA polymerase: Unique structure and lack of demonstrable endogenous activity, *J. Virol.*, **13**:1075.

VOGT, P. K., 1971*a*, Spontaneous segregation of nontransforming viruses from cloned sarcoma viruses, *Virology* **46**:939.

VOGT, P. K., 1971*b*, Genetically stable reassortment of markers during mixed infection with avian tumor viruses, *Virology* **46**:947.

VOGT, P. K., 1973, The genome of avian RNA tumor viruses: A discussion of four models, in: *Possible Episomes in Eukaryotes* (Proceedings of the Fourth Lepetit Colloquium, L. Silvestri, ed.), pp. 35–41, North-Holland, Amsterdam.

VOGT, P. K., AND DUESBERG, P. H., 1973, On the mechanism of recombination between avian RNA tumor viruses, in: *Virus Research* (Proceedings of the Second ICN-UCLA Symposium on Molecular Biology, C. F. Fox and W. S. Robinson, eds.), pp. 505–512, Academic Press, New York and London.

VOGT, P. K., AND FRIIS, R. R., 1971, An avian leukosis virus related to RSV(0): Properties and evidence for helper activity, *Virology* **43**:223.

VOGT, V. M., AND EISENMAN, R., 1973, Identification of a large polypeptide precursor of avian oncornavirus proteins, *Proc. Natl. Acad. Sci.* **70**:1734.

WALKER, T. A., PACE, N. R., ERIKSON, R. L., ERIKSON, E., AND BEHR, F., 1974, The 7S RNA common to oncornaviruses and normal cells is associated with polyribosomes, *Proc. Natl. Acad. Sci. USA* **71**:3390.

WANG, L.-H., AND DUESBERG, P. H., 1973, DNA polymerase of murine sarcoma–leukemia virus: Lack of detectable RNase H and low activity with viral RNA and natural DNA templates, *J. Virol.* **12**:1512.

WANG, S., KOETHARI, R. M., AND TAYLOR, M., 1973, Transfer RNA activities of Rous sarcoma and Rous associated viruses, *Nature New Biol.* **242**:133.

WARREN, L., CRITCHLEY, D., AND MACPHERSON, I., 1972, Surface glycoproteins and glycolipids of chicken embryo cells transformed by temperature-sensitive mutant of Rous sarcoma virus, *Nature (Lond.)* **235**:275.

WEINBERG, R., 1973, Nuclear RNA metabolism, *Ann. Rev. Biochem.* **42**:329.

WEISS, R. A., 1971, Cell transformation induced by Rous sarcoma virus: Analysis of density dependence, *Virology* **46**:209.

WEISS, R. A., AND PAYNE, L. N., 1971, The heritable nature of the factor in chicken cells which acts as a helper virus for Rous sarcoma virus, *Virology* **45**:508.

WEISS, R. A., FRIIS, R. R., KATZ, E., AND VOGT, P. K., 1971, Induction of avian tumor viruses in normal cells by physical and chemical carcinogens, *Virology* **46**:920.

WEISS, R. A., MASON, W. S., AND VOGT, P. K., 1973, Genetic recombinants and heterozygotes derived from endogenous and exogenous avian RNA tumor viruses, *Virology* **52**:535.

WEISSBACH, A., BOLDEN, A., MULLER, R., HANAFUSA, H., AND HANAFUSA, T., 1972, Deoxyribonucleic acid polymerase activities in normal and leukovirus-infected chicken embryo cells, *J, Virol.* **10**:321.

WITTER, R., FRANK, H., MOENNING, V., HUNSMANN, G., LANGE, J., AND SCHAFER, W., 1973, Properties of mouse leukemia viruses. IV. Hemagglutination assay and characterization of hemagglutinating surface components, *Virology* **54**:330.

WIVEL, N. A., AND SMITH, G. H., 1971, Distribution of intracisternal A particles in a variety of normal and neoplastic mouse tissues, *Int. J. Cancer* **7**:167.

WIVEL, N. A., LENDERS, K. K., AND KUFF, E. L., 1973, Structural organization of murine intracisternal A particles, *J. Virol.* **11**:329.

WOLLMANN, R. L., AND KIRSTEN, W. H., 1968, Cellular origin of a mouse leukemia viral RNA, *J. Virol.* **2**:1241.

WU, A. M., TING, R. C., PARAN, M., AND GALLO, R. C., 1972, Cordycepin inhibits induction of murine leukovirus production by 5-iodo-2′-deoxyuridine, *Proc. Natl. Acad. Sci.* **69**:3820.

WYKE, J. A., 1973, Complementation of transforming functions by temperature-sensitive mutants of avian sarcoma virus, *Virology* **54**:28.

WYKE, J. A., AND LINIAL, M., 1973, Temperature-sensitive avian sarcoma viruses: A physiological comparison of twenty mutants, *Virology* **53**:152.

YOSHII, S., AND VOGT, P. K., 1970, A mutant of Rous sarcoma virus (type 0) causing fusiform cell transformation, *Proc. Soc. Exp. Biol. Med.* **135**:297.

2

Avian RNA Tumor Viruses

Hidesaburo Hanafusa

1. The Viruses

1.1. Pathogenic Classification

Avian RNA tumor viruses are a group with certain characteristics that can be defined by both pathogenic and molecular criteria. Other designations which have been used for RNA tumor virus include leukovirus, oncornavirus (oncogenic RNA), Rous virus, retravirus (reverse transcriptase positive virus), rnadna virus (RNA → DNA virus), and type C Virus. Historically, the viruses have been isolated from birds with certain diseases and so have been named after these diseases. The following viruses are considered to belong to the avian RNA tumor virus group.

1.1.1. Avian Sarcoma Virus

The prototype of the avian sarcoma viruses, Rous sarcoma virus (RSV), was isolated from chickens by P. Rous (1911), and the virus has been distributed since then throughout the world. In many cases, the history of the virus passage is not clear, but all sarcoma viruses considered to have derived from the one Rous isolated are called RSV. Perhaps because of evolution of the virus during passage, which might have been caused by mutation or some genetic interaction with other avian RNA tumor virus or host cell components during passage in different lines of chickens, the Rous sarcoma viruses maintained in several laboratories have different characteristics. These different "strains" are summarized in Table 1. In addition to RSV, some other sarcoma-including viruses have been isolated from

Hidesaburo Hanafusa ● The Rockefeller University, New York, N.Y.

tumors in chickens. They include the Fujinami sarcoma (Fujinami and Inamoto, 1914), B-77 sarcoma (Thurzo *et al.*, 1963), and Mill Hill sarcoma strains 13, 1, 14 (Begg, 1929; Foulds, 1934).

The sarcoma virus can produce neoplastic lesions within 48–72 h at the site of injection (usually wing webs are used because of the ease of identification). The cells in the lesions can be cultured in dishes, and they grow as spindle-shaped or round "transformed" cells. The tumors generally increase rapidly in size, and metastasis can often be seen in the lungs, liver, or spleen. Virus is present in these tumor cells. The age of the chickens greatly influences the pathogenesis. If embryos are inoculated with the virus, they will die before hatching. If adult chickens are inoculated with relatively small doses of RSV, tumors may appear but will often regress. The regression is due to the immunological mechanism.

Chickens inoculated with low doses of RSV often develop leukosis after tumor regression (Burmester *et al.*, 1960), and it has become clear that a single RSV

TABLE 1
Subgroups of Avian RNA Tumor Viruses[a,b]

	Virus subgroup					
	A	B	C	D	E	F
Sarcoma virus	SR-RSV-A	SR-RSV-B		SR-RSV-D		
	PR-RSV-A	PR-RSV-B	PR-RSV-C			
	MH-RSV		B-77	CZ-RSV		
			(BH-RSV)[c]	(HA-RSV)		
			(BS-RSV)	(FU-SV)		
Leukosis virus	RAV-1	RAV-2	RAV-7	RAV-50	RAV-0	RAV-61
	RAV-3		RAV-49		RAV-60	
	RAV-4				(chf)[d]	
	RAV-5					
	FAV-1					
		AMV-2				
	RIF-1	RIF-2				
	RPL-12	AEV				
	MAV-1	MAV-2				
	MC29-A	MC29-B				

[a] Results of Vogt and Ishizaki (1965, 1966), Ishizaki and Vogt (1966), Duff and Vogt (1969), T. Hanafusa *et al.* (1970b), Moscovici and Vogt (1968), Ishizaki and Shimizu (1970), Ishizaki *et al.* (1971), and T. Hanafusa and H. Hanafusa (1973) are compiled.

[b] RSV, Rous sarcoma virus; SR, Schmidt–Ruppin strain; PR, Prague strain; CZ, Carr–Zilber strain; MH, Mill Hill strain; B-77, avian sarcoma virus strain B-77; BH, Bryan high titer strain; BS, Bryan standard strain; HA, Harris strain; FU-SV, Fujinami sarcoma virus; RAV, Rous-associated virus; FAV, Fujinami-associated virus; AMV, avian myeloblastosis virus; RIF, resistance-including factor (lymphoid leukosis virus); RPL-12, avian leukosis virus strain RPL-12; MAV, myeloblastosis-associated virus; AEV, avian erythroblastosis virus; MC29, avian myelocytoma virus strain MC29.

[c] BH-RSV, BS-RSV, HA-RSV, and FU-SV are defective in the glycoprotein determining subgroup specificity. These viruses can be produced as pseudotypes of any one of the subgroups depending on the associated leukosis virus—for example, BH-RSV(RAV-1) and HA-RSV(RAV-2).

[d] Chf (chicken helper factor) is not a virus but a product of endogenous viral genes in chicken cells. The chf can provide the envelope glycoprotein for defective RSV.

virion can carry genetic information for both sarcomagenic and leukemogenic
activities (Biggs *et al.*, 1973). However, another possible reason for this phenomenon may be found in the composition of the virus preparations. The RSV used in early experiments often contained leukosis virus in large quantities. The contamination of RSV preparations with leukosis virus could be due to (1) contamination of chickens with leukosis virus, (2) defectiveness of some RSV strains which replicate only in association with leukosis virus, or (3) spontaneous mutation from sarcoma virus to leukosis virus.

Under certain conditions, some defective RSV can produce tumors from which infectious virus cannot be recovered. Such phenomena have been reproduced at the cellular level in tissue culture, and will be discussed in Section 6.

1.1.2. Avian Leukosis Viruses

Many strains of leukosis viruses have been isolated in the field, but a number of strains have also been isolated from stocks of sarcoma viruses. The pattern of neoplastic disease in chickens develops in many forms, very often associated with various forms of leukemia, sarcoma, or renal carcinoma at the same time (e.g., see Beard, 1963). The term "leukosis complex" is derived from this pathogenesis. In some cases, one type of neoplastic change is followed by the development of another form of neoplastic disorder. Involvement of more than one strain of virus in such multiple forms of manifestation has been considered and may resolve the complexity, at least to a certain extent.

Two major groups can be considered. First are viruses such as myeloblastosis virus (Beard, 1956) and erythroblastosis virus (Engelbreth-Holm and Rothe-Meyer, 1935), which cause acute leukemic changes in animals. Myelocytoma virus (Ivanov *et al.*, 1964) may also belong to this class. Infection of young chicks with these viruses results in an increase of either myeloblasts or erythroblasts in blood vessels as early as 1 wk after injection. In erythroblastosis virus-infected chickens, normal bone marrow is replaced by erythroblastic cells within 4 days. In the terminal stage of myeloblastosis, as many as 2 million myeloblasts can be found in 1 mm^3 of blood. The amount of virus released into blood is also high, and can reach a titer as high as 10^{11} particles per milliliter of plasma. This high yield in plasma is the principal reason that avian myeloblastosis virus is often used for the study of viral structural components. Infected chickens die within 10–20 days after inoculation with large doses of these viruses.

As in the case of RSV, the age of the chickens is an important factor in the "takes" of virus. In general, the younger the chickens, the higher the percentage of takes obtained.

The acute leukemic disease described above is seen relatively rarely in the field. A more frequent types of disease is known as lymphoid leukosis or visceral lymphomatosis (Burmester *et al.*, 1946).* The disease is characterized by the

---

* The most frequent type of leukosis is known as Marek's disease, a type of neurolymphomatosis. The agent responsible for this type of leukosis has been identified as a DNA containing herpes virus.

proliferation of lymphoid cells and their infiltration into the liver, lungs, or other visceral organs. Unlike infection with the acute leukemic viruses, infection with lymphoid leukosis virus does not produce early changes. The first changes, which occur about 5–8 wk after inoculation, are recognizable as a proliferation of lymphoid cells in the bursa. The lymphomatosis develops after 2–4 months. However, virus proliferation precedes the pathological changes. The disease is described as leukosis rather than leukemia because no prominent changes take place in the blood picture of infected chickens. However, in some chickens infected with lymphoid leukosis virus there may be an increase in erythroblasts in bone marrow. The principal symptoms in the developed stage are enlargement of the liver and spleen. Although horizontal infection, the spread of virus through normal contact, is known to occur, vertical transmission (primarily by congenital infection) from the mother to the embryo seems to be more important for the development of this disease (Rubin *et al.*, 1961). In the latter case, the chickens become immunologically tolerant to the virus. Thus both virus growth and the development of leukosis are far more frequent than in those infected later in life. Commercial losses of poultry from this type of virus are high, because of the long latent period and the coincidence of the development of disease with maturation of animals.

The other forms of leukosis are hemangiomatosis, osteopetrosis, and ocular lymphomatosis.

The myeloblastosis virus widely used today is BAI strain A. The virus preparation seems to contain several different types of particles (Moscovici and Zanetti, 1970). One of these, which is responsible for induction of myeloblastosis, is avian myeloblastosis virus (AMV). There are indications that AMV may be defective in replication, requiring lymphoid leukosis virus as a helper. The latter virus has been termed "myeloblastosis-associated virus" (MAV). A similar situation appears to be applicable to erythroblastosis (Ishizaki and Shimizu, 1970) and myelocytoma (Ishizaki *et al.*, 1971) viruses. Both require lymphoid leukosis virus as helper for the replication.

Characterization and purification of avian sarcoma virus led to the isolation of various strains of "leukosis" virus. Well-known examples are several strains of Rous-associated viruses (RAV) which have been isolated from various stocks of RSV (Vogt and Ishizaki, 1965). These viruses were first classified as leukosis virus on the basis of biological characteristics of the virus infection and interactions with other viruses. Later, these viruses were confirmed to be of the lymphoid leukosis type by *in vivo* infection. Another term, "RIF," has also been used for some lymphoid leukosis viruses isolated from field strains of chickens (Rubin, 1960*a*). RIF is an acronym for "resistance-inducing factor," which is now known to be one of the general characteristics of all leukosis viruses. Therefore, RAV and RIF can be considered as different isolates of lymphoid leukosis viruses. Avian leukosis viruses obtained from chick embryos are sometimes called "RAV," since this term is most frequently used to represent avian leukosis virus. RAV may be considered as "virus which can associate with RSV." The leukosis viruses are also shown in Table 1.

Both avian sarcoma and leukosis viruses can be further classified into subgroups   53
based on the characteristics of the viral envelope. The subgroup classification will   AVIAN RNA
be described in Section 2.   TUMOR VIRUSES

Both avian sarcoma and leukosis viruses can be further classified into subgroups based on the characteristics of the viral envelope. The subgroup classification will be described in Section 2.

The pathogenicity of the viruses to tissue-cultured cells will be described in Section 6.

1.2. Molecular Definition

Molecular biological aspects of infection and the structure of virions are discussed in the chapter by Bishop and Varmus. Therefore, in this section we will only briefly describe the biochemical and biological properties which characterize this group of viruses.

1.2.1. Size and Morphology of Virions

The virions contain an electron-dense inner core surrounded by less dense material with a total diameter of 80–100 nm. The particles are enveloped with a bilayer of lipid membranes. Knobby protrusions, called "spikes," can be observed by electron microscopy on the surface of the envelope in negatively stained preparations. The spikes contain a glycoprotein which determines subgroup-specific properties (Rifkin and Compans, 1971; Bolognesi *et al.*, 1972*a*). Removal of spikes results in loss of infectivity. The lipid envelope can be destroyed by lipid solvents or detergents. Mild treatment of virions with detergents can yield the inner core structure. The buoyant density (ρ) of the core is about 1.25 in sucrose gradients, which is higher than the 1.16 density of the lipid-containing intact virions.

1.2.2. RNA Components

Successful isolation of intact viral RNA is, surprisingly, a recent development in the biochemistry of RNA tumor viruses (Robinson *et al.*, 1965). With the present techniques using phenol and sodium dodecylsulfate, two components of single-stranded RNA can be obtained from all species of RNA tumor viruses. The heavier 60–70S RNA, equivalent to a molecular weight of 10–12 million daltons, is the major component and is considered to be the principal genetic material of the virus. The amounts of lighter 4–10S RNA vary with the source, the strain of virus, and the method of extraction. In addition, 28 or 18S RNA (presumably host ribosomal RNA) can sometimes be found associated with the virus. The 4–10S RNA contains RNA species which resemble transfer RNA in structure and, indeed, can be aminoacylated (Erikson and Erikson, 1970). A small fraction of these transfer RNAs are associated with 70S RNA and seem to be essential as primer molecules for transcription (reverse) of viral RNA to DNA (Canaani and Duesberg, 1972).

Like most messenger RNA of animal cells or animal viruses, the 60–70S RNA contains adenine-rich sequences, poly(A) (Lai and Duesberg, 1972). The poly(A) tracts are fairly large (100–300 nucleotides long, or about 4S). Thus viral RNA can be separated from other species of RNA using techniques which enrich specifically for poly(A)-containing polynucleotides. The high molecular weight RNA appears to be composed of smaller RNA species (35S) (Duesberg, 1968) and reportedly may be formed from the smaller subunits after the release of virions from the cells (Cheung *et al.*, 1972). The 60–70S RNA can be dissociated into 35S RNA subunits by treatments which dissociate hydrogen bonds, such as heating and treatment with dimethylsulfoxide. The 35S RNA has not been experimentally reassociated to the larger size. Strangely, the dissociated 35S RNA forms a single sharp peak in gel electrophoresis (Duesberg and Vogt, 1973). Therefore, if 35S RNA represents the segments of RNA which are somehow linked to form 60–70S RNA, the high molecular weight species would consist of three or four segments of approximately equal size. It is not known whether these subunits are genetically identical.

1.2.3. Protein Components

Analysis of viral proteins shows that all avian leukosis–sarcoma viruses have eight major components, of which two are glycosylated (Hung *et al.*, 1971; Fleissner, 1971). Avian viruses appear to contain one major protein which is absent in murine viruses. At least four proteins of all avian leukosis–sarcoma viruses have been shown to be group-specific (gs) antigens which are detectable by complement fixation with serum of hamsters infected with Rous sarcoma virus. Localization of some protein components in virions has been determined (Bolognesi *et al.*, 1972*b*).

A new nomenclature for viral proteins has been proposed (August *et al.*, 1973) in which a protein is named according to its molecular weight. For example, a protein previously called "gs1" or "gsa" is termed "p27," as its molecular weight is estimated as 27,000. A glycoprotein with molecular weight about 85,000 is called "gp85."

1.2.4. Enzymes Associated with Virions

For a long time, avian myeloblastosis virus has been known to contain adenosine triphosphatase (ATPase), and virus concentrations were often estimated by assay of ATPase. However, this is not true of other strains, or even of avian myeloblastosis virus grown in cells which contain little ATPase on the cell membranes (de Thé *et al.*, 1964). Therefore, this enzyme is not an integral component of the virus.

The most universal and characteristic enzyme associated with RNA tumor viruses is RNA-dependent DNA polymerase (Temin and Mizutani, 1970; Baltimore, 1970). This enzyme can be found in all virus strains except for noninfectious polymerase-negative mutants (see Section 6.1.2). The avian virus enzyme seems to differ from that of mammalian RNA tumor viruses, both antigenically and in ion requirement, but the polymerases associated with various strains of avian viruses are not distinguishable from each other. Thus this enzyme provides another taxonomic tool. The virion DNA polymerase molecule contains ribonuclease H (RNase H) activity (Mölling *et al.*, 1971). The two enzyme activities have not been physically separable. RNase H digests only RNA that is in a hybrid form

with complementary DNA. Other enzymes have been demonstrated in some strains of avian viruses, but the generality of their presence has not been established.

1.2.5. Homology of RNA Sequence

The discovery of RNA-dependent DNA polymerase has made it possible to synthesize DNA complementary to virus RNA. Radiolabeled virus-specific DNA can then be used as a probe to detect viral RNA sequences by molecular hybridization (Varmus *et al.*, 1971). This reaction is highly specific, and the degree of homology among various avian RNA tumor viruses can be determined. For example, avian virus–specific DNA does not hybridize with mouse or other mammalian virus RNA, nor with avian reticuloendotheliosis virus RNA. The extent of homology among RNAs of avian RNA tumor viruses is currently being studied.

1.2.6. Helper Activity

Any one of the avian leukosis–sarcoma viruses can serve as helper for defective sarcoma viruses. No such interaction has been demonstrated between avian and mammalian RNA tumor viruses. However, it has been shown that vesicular stomatitis virus grown in avian tumor virus–infected cells contains avian leukemia virus–specific proteins in the viral envelope (Zavada, 1972).

1.3. Relation to Reticuloendotheliosis Virus

Reticuloendotheliosis virus (RE virus) was isolated in 1958 from adult turkeys with leukosis-like lesions (Theilen *et al.*, 1966). The virus is quite virulent for many species of domestic birds, causing characteristic reticuloendotheliosis with a short latent period (Theilen *et al.*, 1966; Taylor and Olson, 1972). The RE virus may be classified in a second group of RNA tumor viruses (Purchase *et al.*, 1973) which includes duck infectious anemia virus (Ludford *et al.*, 1972), duck spleen necrosis virus (Trager, 1959), and chick syncytial virus (Cook, 1969). These viruses are serologically related to each other (Purchase *et al.*, 1973).

The RE virus is similar to leukosis–sarcoma viruses in the presence of RNA-dependent DNA polymerase in virions (Peterson *et al.*, 1972) and in the size of viral RNA (60–70S) (Halpern *et al.*, 1973). However, the DNA polymerase of RE virus is immunologically unrelated to the enzyme of leukosis–sarcoma viruses (Mizutani and Temin, 1973), and RE virus RNA has no homologous sequences with RNA of leukosis–sarcoma viruses (Kang and Temin, 1973). Particles of RE virus are morphologically similar but not identical to those of type C virus (Zeigel *et al.*, 1966). No identity was found in viral proteins between the two classes of viruses (Halpern *et al.*, 1973), and they are unrelated with respect to both gs antigen and neutralization antigen (Theilen *et al.*, 1966; Purchase *et al.*, 1973).

No biological interaction has been found between the two classes of viruses. The interactions examined include interference and phenotypic mixing with avian sarcoma viruses, helper function for the defective RSV, and recovery of RAV-60 from infected chicken cells (Halpern *et al.*, 1973).

Although the virus induces a neoplastic response in host animals, the virus grown in tissue culture appears to be nontumorigenic (Halpern *et al.*, 1973). Further investigation is required on the nature of this attenuation *in vitro*. Since there is no direct relationship with known leukosis and sarcoma viruses, the RE virus will not be described further in this chapter.

2. Classification of Viruses Based on the Envelope Structure

In addition to the classification based on pathogenic properties, viruses can be separated into several classes based on properties which appear to be determined exclusively by the structure of the viral envelope. This classification is basically defined by the host range of the virus, but other related properties are also used as criteria (Vogt, 1967c). A historical description of this classification has been presented previously (H. Hanafusa, 1969a). This classification system is outlined in Table 1. The viruses are currently grouped into subgroups A–F. The subgroup of *sarcoma viruses* can be determined directly by measuring focus formation on different cell types. The subgroup of *leukosis viruses* is generally determined by making a defective RSV pseudotype of a given virus, e.g., RSV(ALV), and examining its properties (see Section 6.1.2). The host range, neutralization, or interference of RSV(ALV) can be determined by measuring formation of foci of transformed cells, and these properties of RSV(ALV) are specified by the envelope of ALV.

2.1. Host Range

Interestingly, the discovery of the diversity of envelope specificities of avian RNA tumor viruses was made simultaneously with the finding of the presence of chicken cells genetically different in their susceptibility to different avian tumor viruses (H. Hanafusa, 1965; Vogt, 1965b). Susceptibility of cells seems to be determined by a single autosomal gene for each subgroup, and the gene for susceptibility is always dominant over resistance (Rubin, 1965; Payne and Biggs, 1964; Crittenden *et al.*, 1967). Thus far, no difference has been shown between susceptible and resistant chicken embryos other than the interaction with viruses. Cells derived from one embryo are homogeneous in susceptibility. Chicken embryos resistant to subgroup A are designated "C/A," those resistant to both subgroups A and E are termed "C/AE." Chicken cells susceptible to all known viruses are known as "C/O" (Vogt and Ishizaki, 1965). The host range specificity is very strict, if not absolute. In the range of multiplicities usually available, viruses cannot infect genetically resistant cells. (This is different from the degree of interference induced by virus; see below.) The block of virus infection is known to be at the level of virus penetration (adsorption takes place normally) (Piraino, 1967). In addition to chicken cells, other avian cells used in this classification are quail, duck, and pheasant. Infectivity for mammalian cells may be related to subgroup C and D specificities, but this has not been established (Duff and Vogt, 1969).

2.2. Sensitivity to Viral Interference

Interference between leukosis virus and RSV, discovered by Rubin (1960a), has been used as a powerful tool for detection or isolation of leukosis virus. Later studies showed that leukosis virus interferes with RSV that belongs to the same subgroup or a closely related one (Vogt and Ishizaki, 1966). The relationship between different leukosis viruses can also be determined by examining the interaction between one virus and RSV pseudotypes of another virus.

The technical details will not be discussed here, but this test can be performed only by first infecting cells with the leukosis virus. If the sequence is reversed, leukosis virus cannot cause interference. The "interfered" virus appears to be blocked at the penetration step as in the case of genetically resistant cells (Steck and Rubin, 1965). The prevailing view on the mechanism of viral interference is that the receptor site of the cells is occupied by the envelope antigen or viral particles of the initially infecting virus. Thus penetration by a second virus of the same subgroup, which would react with the same receptor site, is prevented. Cells infected by subgroup A leukosis virus become resistant to subgroup A sarcoma viruses or RSV pseudotypes, but are fully susceptible to viruses of subgroups B, C, D, E, and F. The degree of resistance is usually in the range of 10^{-4} to 10^{-5} in the fully infected cells (T. Hanafusa and H. Hanafusa, 1967). This implies that there is a finite probability that the second virus will infect. In the case of the genetically resistant cells described earlier, complete resistance may be due to the lack of a proper receptor structure.

The interference test is reliable. Viruses which belong to the same subgroup, based on host specificity, thus far have unfailingly caused interference with other viruses of the same subgroup. Therefore, this method is most useful in classification (e.g., see T. Hanafusa et al., 1970b).

2.3. Antigenicity

As will be described in Section 3.1.2, there is generally a relationship between specificity of virus neutralization and subgroup (Ishizaki and Vogt, 1966). However, viruses of the same subgroup can be antigenically unrelated. Therefore, this property should be used as a supplement to the others in classification.

The summary of subgroup classification A–F is shown in Table 2. In interference and antigenicity, viruses of subgroups B, D, and E show some degree of relatedness (T. Hanafusa et al., 1970b). Viruses of subgroups A–E have been found in naturally infected chickens, or in stocks of chicken sarcoma or leukosis viruses. "Normal" uninfected chicken cells have genes for gs antigen and envelope antigen for subgroup E. (The endogenous viral genes responsible for subgroup E will be discussed in Section 8.) Virus with subgroup E specificity has been recovered from these cells either spontaneously (Vogt and Friis, 1971) or following infection with viruses of other subgroups (T. Hanafusa *et al.*, 1970*b*). A virus of subgroup F has recently been isolated from pheasant embryo cells in a manner similar to that for the subgroup E virus (T. Hanafusa and H. Hanafusa, 1973).

TABLE 2
Avian RNA Tumor Virus Subgroup Specificity[a,b]

Cells	Virus subgroup					
	A	B	C	D	E	F
Host range						
Chicken C/O	S	S	S	S	S	S
C/A	R	S	S	S	S	S
C/AE	R	S	S	S	R	S
C/BE	S	R	S	S	R	NT
C/ABE	R	R	S	S	R	NT
C/E	S	S	S	S	R	S
Japanese quail	S	R	R, S[c]	S	S	S
Ringneck pheasant	S	R	R, S	S	S	S
Duck	R	R	R, S	S	R	S
Interference						
Chicken C/O preinfected with:						
Virus A	R	S	S	S	S	S
Virus B	S	R	S	Partially R	Partially R	S
Virus C	S	S	R	S	S	S
Virus D	S	Partially R	S	R	NT	S
Virus E	S	Partially R	S	Partially R	R	S
Virus F	S	S	S	S	R	R

[a] Results of Vogt and Ishizaki (1965, 1966), Duff and Vogt (1969), T. Hanafusa *et al.* (1970*b*), T. Hanafusa and H. Hanafusa (1973), and T. Hanafusa (personal communication) are compiled.
[b] S, Susceptible or not interfered; R, resistant or interfered; NT, not tested.
[c] Members of subgroup C have different host range for quail, pheasant, and duck cells.

3. Immunological Properties

3.1. Virus Antigens

3.1.1. Group-Specific (gs) Antigen

Attempts to detect virus by complement fixation using sera from chickens immunized with virus have been unsuccessful because of the high anticomplementary activity of the chicken sera. This difficulty was overcome when sera of hamsters or guinea pigs carrying tumors originally induced by the Schmidt–Ruppin (SR) strain of RSV were found suitable for this purpose (Hūebner *et al.*, 1964). The sera gave a positive reaction not only with SR-RSV but also with all other avian leukosis–sarcoma viruses. However, the sera are specific to avian viruses. Thus the antigen of viruses reactive with this type of serum was called "group-specific" (gs) antigen (Sarma *et al.*, 1964). Later it was shown that at least four viral structural proteins react with this serum, and are thus classified as gs antigens (Fleissner, 1971). These antigens can also be found in soluble forms in infected cells.

Because of its applicability to all strains of avian leukosis–sarcoma viruses, the complement fixation test is used for detection of this group of viruses, especially in chicken embryos. It should be pointed out, however, that the standard method of COFAL (complement fixation for avian leukosis virus) uses tissue culture fluids as the source of virus. As will be discussed in Section 8, cells of some COFAL-negative chicken embryos are now known to contain small amounts of gs antigen (Dougherty and DiStefano, 1966; Payne and Chubb, 1968), although these cells do not release virus and the culture fluid is thus COFAL negative. Today, such normal, COFAL-negative chicken embryos are called "gs antigen–positive" embryos.

Thus far, all intact virus particles of avian RNA tumor viruses, regardless of strain or infectiousness, appear to contain gs antigens. Also, all virus-infected cells contain gs antigen, whereas in the murine system some murine sarcoma virus–infected cells which do not produce virus also do not produce gs antigen.

The study of the structure of gs antigens (proteins p27, p19, p15, p12) has been initiated. Although the antigens of various viruses are functionally indistinguishable, minor differences in their structure have been observed (E. Fleissner, personal communication).

3.1.2. Envelope Antigen

The gs antigens are located inside the virus particle and have no relation to neutralization of virus by antibody. Two carbohydrate-containing proteins present on the surface of the envelope are considered to react as neutralizing antigens. Which of the carbohydrate or protein components determines the antigenicity is not known. Unlike gs antigens, which are common to all avian viruses, the neutralization of virus is specific to only certain groups of viruses. The relatedness in antigenicity generally correlates with the subgroup classification of viruses by their host range specificity (see Sections 2.1 and 2.3). For example, viruses which belong to the same subgroup are more likely to be antigenically related than those that belong to different subgroups. However, viruses in the same subgroup can be antigenically unrelated, and viruses in different subgroups may have cross-reactivity.

It is also important to remember that the envelope structure of the virus is subject to modification through interaction with other viruses (see Section 7.2). Therefore, the biological purity of virus or possible involvement of other viruses in a given system must be considered in evaluating immunological properties of the virus or immunological responses of the host.

3.2. Immunological Reaction in Hosts

Studies on the distribution or development of antibody in chicken flocks were important when leukosis in chickens was a major concern of the poultry industry. However, the early workers were unaware of the complexity of the antigenic makeup of various strains of virus and of the relationship between the defective Bryan strain of RSV and other leukosis viruses. Therefore, the data obtained have to be interpreted in light of present additional knowledge.

If chicks are derived from flocks in which lymphoid leukosis viruses are not eliminated, newly hatched chicks may carry neutralizing antibody to certain types of lymphoid leukosis virus. This is maternal antibody and may persist for about 2 wk (Bang and Haley, 1958). The development of an immunological defense system in chicks follows this period immediately. Injection of large doses of lymphoid leukosis virus into embryos or newly hatched chicks causes immunological tolerance, and virus replication continues throughout life (Rubin et al., 1962). Naturally, this situation can occur by the transmission of virus from mother to embryos, a mode of infection called "congenital transmission."

When immunologically competent chickens are exposed to lymphoid leukosis virus naturally or experimentally, they develop neutralizing antibody and often survive without getting leukosis. Therefore, the antiserum to lymphoid leukosis viruses is generally prepared by intravenous inoculation of virus into chicks which are about 6 wk old (H. Hanafusa et al., 1963). Apparently virus can persist in some organs of inoculated birds, and one inoculation is generally enough to maintain the production of high titers of antiserum for years.

The pattern of immunological response of chickens to sarcoma virus infection is essentially the same as that to leukosis virus infection. Young animals are more susceptible to tumor formation, while adult animals produce high titers of antibodies against the virus. Tumors induced in adult animals by sarcoma virus often regress when antibodies are formed. However, the antibody involved in the regression of tumors is different from that against viral envelope antigen (Rubin, 1962). The antigen responsible for this regression is called "transplantation antigen" (Jonsson and Sjögren, 1965) or "tumor-specific surface antigen" (Kurth and Bauer, 1972). The nature of this antigen has not been extensively studied.

To prepare antiserum against sarcoma viruses, 6-wk-old chickens are inoculated with low doses of viruses. Some tumors produced may grow too rapidly and kill the chickens before antibody is formed. Antibody-producing chickens may be found among the survivors in which tumors have regressed or are relatively small. Because the preparation of antibody against leukosis virus is easier than this procedure, use of a leukosis virus of the same envelope antigen, which can be obtained by mutation of sarcoma virus (see Section 7.1), may be worth consideration whenever possible.

4. Assay

Various properties of the virus are utilized for the assay of infectivity or for the measurement of the number of physical virus particles.

4.1. Focus Formation

Infection of chick embryo fibroblasts with sarcoma virus results in morphological changes in the cells: generally, flat fibroblasts become more refractile, with smooth cell surfaces, and cells assume a fat-spindle or round form (Manaker and Groupé, 1956; Temin and Rubin, 1958). The morphologically altered cells can continue to divide under certain conditions, such as under agar overlay, where uninfected cells cannot continue to grow. Thus sarcoma virus–infected cells form a colony of "transformed" cells which can be distinguished from the background of normal cells. These colonies are called "foci." The number of foci formed is proportional to the input virus concentration, indicating that a single infectious virus is sufficient to induce such cell transformation. Techniques for focus formation have been described by Vogt (1969). An accurate estimation of the ratio of the number of physical particles to the number of infectious units has not been obtained, but it appears to be in the range of 5–100, obviously depending on the preparation.

It is important to remember that focus formation is based on the transforming capacity of virus, but not on the multiplication. (The latter is essential for the plaque assay of ordinary animal viruses.) Once a single cell is infected and transformed, a focus can be formed solely by cell division of the initially infected cell. Defective RSV, such as Bryan strain virus, can cause cell transformation, but the transformed cells do not produce infectious virus.

Focus formation can be regarded as an extension of the *in vivo* assay for neoplastic changes: sarcoma formation in chickens and pock formation in chorioallantoic membranes of fertile eggs. Under optimal conditions, all of these techniques give similar results for infective titer.

Obviously the genetic susceptibility of the host cells to a given virus is one of the essential considerations in the assay. Chickens or cells used for the assay should be free of leukosis virus to avoid possible interference. Numerous physiological factors have been observed in the conditions for successful cell transformation (Rubin, 1960c; Vigier, 1970a). In addition to sarcoma virus, myelocytoma virus (MC29) has been shown to transform chick embryo fibroblasts in cultures and the focus assay is applicable to this virus (Langlois and Beard, 1967).

4.2. Plaque Formation

Unlike the sarcoma viruses, leukosis viruses generally produce little visible change in the infected cells. Therefore, direct assay of infectivity of leukosis virus has been limited to a method utilizing fluorescent antibody staining of an area of infected cells (Vogt and Rubin, 1963). While the interaction between chicken cells and leukosis virus is essentially noncytocidal, some strains of virus can induce cytopathic changes in cells under suboptimal conditions (H. Hanafusa and T. Hanafusa, 1966b). This has been applied to plaque formation by certain viruses which belong to subgroups B and D (Graf, 1972; Kawai and Hanafusa, 1972a). The infected areas are not lysed clearly, but become more translucent. These "plaques" can be recognized more distinctly by staining. The reason for the limitation of this phenomenon to particular viruses is not clear. Use of cells preinfected with a temperature-sensitive mutant of RSV and maintained at a nonpermissive temperature seems to give more consistent formation of plaques.

The virus titers determined by the plaque method are in good agreement with those obtained by other methods described below.

4.3. Interference Assay

As described in Section 2.2, infection of cells with leukosis viruses results in interference with secondary infection by viruses of the same subgroup. If sarcoma virus is used as the secondary virus, interference can be seen as a reduction in the number of foci in leukosis virus–infected cultures compared to the number of foci in control cultures not exposed to leukosis virus (Rubin, 1960a).

The interference can be used to determine virus titer by end-point dilution. This is done by infecting chick embryo cell cultures with serial dilutions of leukosis virus and separately subculturing each of the infected cultures at certain intervals. After several subcultures, plates originally infected with more than one infectious unit of leukosis virus eventually become fully infected due to the spread of virus. Such cultures become strongly resistant to infection by sarcoma virus of the same subgroup.

Analysis of the development of interference with time has shown that this method can also be used to directly compare the titer of leukosis virus in early passages of the subcultures, since the degree of interference is directly related to the input of leukosis virus (Rubin and Vogt, 1962). The interference test is sometimes called the "RIF test," because some leukosis viruses were designated as "resistance-inducing factor" from their capacity to induce interference.

4.4. Other Methods

4.4.1. Helper Activity

All strains of leukosis virus thus far studied act as helper for the production of an infectious form of defective RSV. The amount of infectious RSV produced from a given number of defective RSV–transformed cells is proportional to the amount of leukosis virus added to transformed cell cultures (H. Hanafusa and T. Hanafusa, 1966a). The transforming virus produced can then be assayed by focus formation. However, if the leukosis virus is allowed to multiply more than one growth cycle, a linear relationship may not be obtained.

4.4.2. Immunological Methods

The detection of gs antigen by complement fixation or by radioimmunoassay can be used in two ways. One method is to determine the terminal dilution of virus by detection of antigen-positive cultures after subculture, as described for the interference test. Second, direct measurement of the amount of antigen in virions can be used to estimate the concentration of total physical virus particles, which might contain noninfectious virus. Radioimmunoassay determines the amount of antigen in the sample by its ability to compete with the antigen–antibody precipitation of a known amount of radioactively labeled antigen. By this technique, one can detect 10^{-9} g of viral protein (Stephenson *et al.*, 1973; Suni *et al.*, 1973; Chen and Hanafusa, 1973).

Another application of the immunological method is the staining of infected cultures by fluorescent-conjugated antibody against virus-neutralizing antigen. Infected cells producing virus are stained and become fluorescent so that the virus-infected areas in the cultures can be enumerated, as with the plaque count (Vogt and Rubin, 1963).

4.4.3. Polymerase Assay

The amount of physically intact virions can also be determined by measurement of the activity of RNA-dependent DNA polymerase in virions. To increase sensitivity, an exogenous template–primer complex such as $poly(rA) \cdot oligo(dT)$ or $poly(rC) \cdot oligo(dG)$ is used, and polymerization of radioactive dTTP or dGTP is measured (Baltimore and Smoler, 1971). Under optimal conditions, this method also allows the detection of about 10^{-9} g of viral protein.

4.4.4. Detection of Viral RNA

The use of complementary DNA synthesized by RNA-dependent DNA polymerase with viral RNA as a template provides a sensitive method for the detection of viral RNA by molecular hybridization (Leong *et al.*, 1972; Hayward and Hanafusa, 1973). However, this is most useful for determination of homology, rather than quantitation of virus. Detection of viral RNA using the poly(A) sequence as a marker has also been used.

5. Growth Cycle of Virus

Since virus replication can be analyzed in detail in tissue culture systems, and the principles shown by *in vitro* studies can be largely applied to virus growth in host animals, the life cycle of virus in tissue culture cells will be discussed here.

5.1. Kinetics of Virus Reproduction

The growth cycle of RNA tumor viruses is not totally different from that of other animal viruses. In the initial step, the virus interacts with the host cell surface and enters the cell. The virus becomes disintegrated and viral genetic information appears to be transferred to DNA in the form of a provirus which is integrated into host cell DNA. Synthesis of viral RNA and proteins begins following transcription of the DNA. Viral RNA serves as messenger RNA and viral components synthesized appear to be assembled in the vicinity of the cell surface from which complete virions are released by a budding process.

The rate of synthesis of avian RNA tumor viruses is fairly rapid. The first progeny viruses can be detected as early as 12 h after infection and the virus titer reaches its maximum level within 36 h (Temin and Rubin, 1959; H. Hanafusa and T. Hanafusa, 1966a). Morphological alteration of sarcoma virus–infected cells becomes evident in 14 h and is often complete within 24–30 h in cultures infected with high multiplicities of virus (H. Hanafusa, 1969b).

Unlike cytocidal animal virus infection, cells infected with RNA tumor viruses are generally not killed. Thus once virus production reaches its maximum level, the virus titer in the culture fluid remains relatively constant. This is the result of an equilibrium between the release of virus and its heat inactivation in the fluid (Rubin, 1955). The virus titer varies with different virus strains, but usually is in the range of 10^6 to 10^8 infectious units in 1 ml of culture fluid. Virus yield is generally higher at 41°C than at 37°C.

5.2. Adsorption

The first step in virus–cell interaction is the attachment or adsorption of virus to the cell surface. This process seems to be nonspecific. Infectious forms as well as many types of noninfectious virus can be adsorbed to the cell surface, regardless of the genetic susceptibility or resistance of the cells, or even preinfection with other viruses (Piraino, 1967; Steck and Rubin, 1965). There are two classes of viruses: one group, represented by RAV-1, can be adsorbed with a relatively high efficiency (30–70% of input), while the majority of viruses, represented by RAV-2, attach very poorly under the same conditions (0.3–2%) (T. Hanafusa and H. Hanafusa, 1967). The attachment of the latter group of viruses can be enhanced to the same level as that of RAV-1 by treatment of cells with DEAE-dextran or other polycations (Vogt, 1967b; Toyoshima and Vogt, 1969a). These compounds have no effect on RAV-1 attachment. RAV-2 type virus attachment is also enhanced if the cells are preinfected with RAV-1 (T. Hanafusa and H. Hanafusa, 1967). This enhanced attachment can take place even on cells which are genetically resistant to the test virus. The virus infection is blocked at the following penetration step.

The nature of attachment is not known. The enhancement by polycations seems to suggest that an electrostatic interaction is involved in this phenomenon. This enhancement is observed with all viruses that belong to subgroups B–F. Many virus strains of subgroup A are unaffected or slightly inhibited by polycation. However, some viruses of subgroup A are susceptible to the polycation treatment, indicating that a generalization of the relationship between subgroup specificity and the efficiency of attachment cannot be made.

Virus attachment can take place at low temperatures, while penetration and further steps require incubation at a physiological temperature.

5.3. Penetration

Following attachment, there seems to be a step at the cell surface which is highly specific to certain cell–virus combinations. Studies on early events, both in genetically resistant cultures and in virus-induced resistant cells (interference), indicate that the resistance to infection is due to a block in the penetration of virus (Piraino, 1967; Steck and Rubin, 1965). Virus particles added to these resistant cells remain outside the cells and can be effectively inactivated by treatment with antibody, whereas virus particles added to susceptible cells become inaccessible to antibody. Since both the host range and the sensitivity to interference appear to be determined by the structure of the viral glycoprotein, the process of penetration must involve an interaction between the viral glycoprotein and a cell structure which has been postulated as a receptor.

The nature of this interaction and the subsequent fate of the entering virus are not satisfactorily understood. Electron microscopic work with avian virus–infected cells suggests that the virus is incorporated into cells through phagocytosis without demonstrable changes in the particles. The viral RNA can be demonstrated in nuclei as early as 20 min after the onset of virus penetration (Dales and Hanafusa, 1972). Similar work with murine viruses, however, showed that the membrane of the virus particles is removed on entrance into cells (Miyamoto and Gilden, 1971), and viral DNA synthesis is initiated in the cytoplasm of cells (Hatanaka et al., 1971). Further analysis is required.

5.4. Synthesis of Viral DNA

Synthesis of viral DNA uniquely characterizes the infectious cycle of RNA tumor viruses. In early studies by Temin, Bader, and Vigier, several lines of evidence pointed to the involvement of DNA synthesis in the growth cycle. First, the replication of RSV was shown to be blocked by treatment of the cells with actinomycin D (Temin, 1963; Bader, 1964; Vigier and Goldé, 1964). This antibiotic is known to affect DNA-dependent RNA synthesis but not RNA → RNA replication, so that replication of many RNA viruses is not blocked by this compound. Second, inhibition of DNA synthesis by various metabolic inhibitors blocks the replication of virus (Temin, 1964a; Bader, 1965). This DNA-requiring process seems to occur in the early stage of virus infection: inhibitors must be present during the first 6 h after infection. However, these experiments were not definitive for the role of a DNA intermediate in virus replication, since cellular DNA synthesis may also be essential for some steps in the growth cycle of virus. In fact, later experiments showed that both viral DNA synthesis and cell division (which can be blocked by inhibitors of DNA synthesis) are required for virus replication.

On the basis of the above information, Temin (1964*b*) presented the provirus concept. According to this concept, genetic information in viral RNA is transcribed into DNA by the synthesis of DNA complementary to viral RNA. This viral DNA is integrated into cellular DNA and is stably preserved. Viral RNA is made by transcription of the integrated DNA.

Demonstration of viral sequences in cellular DNA of infected cells is the most direct way to test this hypothesis. However, one of the difficulties encountered in this type of analysis arises from the fact that normal uninfected chicken cells contain such sequences (Harel *et al.*, 1966). (This is due to the presence of "endogenous" viral genes in chickens; see Section 8.) This problem has been overcome, however, mainly by refinement of techniques and also in some studies by the use of mammalian cells or duck cells as hosts for sarcoma virus infection (Neiman, 1972; Varmus *et al.*, 1973*a,b*). These experiments demonstrated that DNA sequences complementary to RSV RNA clearly increase or newly appear following infection.

The discovery of association of RNA-dependent DNA polymerase with the virions of RNA tumor viruses provided additional indirect but strong support for the provirus concept. However, the *in vitro* product of the polymerase reaction has a limited size (see Temin and Baltimore, 1972). How this small DNA is assembled into a high molecular weight molecule is not clear. Although no direct proof has been given for the role of the polymerase in *in vivo* virus replication, the isolation of mutants deficient in polymerase (both unconditional and conditional mutants) (H. Hanafusa and T. Hanafusa, 1971; Robinson and Robinson, 1971; Linial and Mason, 1973) and the inhibition of virus synthesis by drugs which affect polymerase (Hung, 1973) are consistent with the idea that this enzyme is essential during the early phase of the virus growth cycle.

More support for the provirus theory was provided by experiments demonstrating transforming activity in DNA extracted from virus-infected cells (Hill and Hillova, 1972). In early experiments, cell transformation took place only after cells exposed to the DNA were cultivated for several subcultures. However, in more recent studies, a higher frequency of transformation was obtained. Analyses of the nature of the DNA and the process of cell transformation are in progress.

The most recent studies suggest that viral DNA synthesized in infected cells becomes covalently linked to cellular DNA. A method to distinguish "free" DNA from "integrated" DNA has also been developed, and integration of viral DNA in infected cells has been demonstrated (Varmus *et al.*, 1973*b*; Markham and Baluda, 1973). Thus the hypothesis of formation of provirus DNA in infected cells seems to have gained sufficient support from experimental evidence.

5.5. Relationship Between Virus Infection and the Cell Cycle

The importance of cell division for the growth of virus or for cell transformation by sarcoma virus has been known for a long time. For example, it has been reported that focus formation by RSV is sharply reduced when old cultures or densely seeded cultures are exposed to virus (Temin and Rubin, 1958; Rubin,

1960*b*). Also, the capacity of cells to produce RSV is known to be highly sensitive to
ultraviolet light or X-rays compared to their capacity to support replication of
other RNA viruses (Rubin and Temin, 1959).

Analysis of the dependence of virus replication on the cell cycle has been
complicated by the apparent requirement for both viral and cellular DNA
synthesis. Both are blocked by the treatment of infected cells with inhibitors.
However, skillful experiments have successfully dissociated these two DNA
syntheses by use of cultures maintained in serum-deficient medium (Boettiger
and Temin, 1970; Baluduzzi and Morgan, 1970). Cells in such cultures are in the
G_l phase of the cell cycle and do not make cell DNA. Infection of these cells with
virus apparently results in the production of only viral DNA. However, neither
cell transformation nor virus reproduction can be seen until serum is added and
cell division takes place. Therefore, these experiments demonstrate that cellular
DNA synthesis or mitosis is necessary for some step following virus DNA
synthesis.

The integration of viral DNA into cellular DNA may take place in this following
step, but its relation to the cell cycle is not entirely clear. There is disagreement
even about the requirement for cell division. In experiments using mitotic
inhibitors, data have been presented which suggest that mitosis is not necessary
for cell transformation or for virus replication (Bader, 1972*a*). These results were
obtained with cultures infected by a high multiplicity of RSV. Under such
conditions, some fraction of the newly synthesized viral DNA might be transcribed into RNA without being integrated into chromosomal DNA, or the RNA of
parental virus might serve a messenger function directly.

5.6. Formation of Viral RNA and Protein

Since there is no proper inhibitor which selectively inhibits cellular RNA synthesis
in RNA tumor virus–infected cells, studies of viral RNA synthesis were hampered
until recently, when the RNA-dependent DNA polymerase system was developed. The polymerase can produce DNA complementary to the viral RNA
template. This DNA is used as a probe to detect viral RNA sequences in the cell by
molecular hybridization. Using this method, viral RNA can be quantitated with
great accuracy in the presence of bulk cellular RNA. It has been shown that cells
fully infected and producing virus contain 1000–4000 copies of viral RNA, which
constitutes about 0.5% of the total RNA in infected cells (Leong *et al.*, 1972;
Hayward and Hanafusa, 1973).

Since actinomycin D can inhibit virus synthesis at a late stage, RNA appears to be
transcribed from DNA. No virus-induced enzyme responsible for transcription
has been isolated. This process may be catalyzed by a cellular enzyme. From
studies using pulse labeling with radioactive RNA precursors and determination
of the amounts of RNA by hybridization with the viral DNA probe, viral RNA
seems to be formed in the nucleus and released into the cytoplasm (Parson *et al.*,

1973). No complementary strand of RNA can be found in infected cells, indicating that RNA is not synthesized through a double-stranded RNA intermediate (Coffin and Temin, 1972). This result also suggests that the viral RNA strand acts as a messenger for protein synthesis. Studies with murine leukemia virus–infected cells showed that 35S RNA is associated with polyribosomes and perhaps functions as messenger RNA (Fan and Baltimore, 1973). Other size classes of virus-specific RNA (18–20S) have been found, but high molecular weight 60–70S RNA seems to be absent inside the cell (Fan and Baltimore, 1973). This agrees with the finding that the formation of 70S RNA from 35S RNA occurs after virus particles are released from the cell (Cheung *et al.*, 1972).

Viral antigenic proteins are found in the polyribosome fraction, further supporting the idea that the polysomes are the site of translation (Vecchio *et al.*, 1973). *In vitro* translation with bacterial or animal cell protein-synthesizing systems has been attempted using viral RNA (Siegert *et al.*, 1972). The possibility that polyprotein synthesis and post-translational cleavage might occur has also been suggested (Vogt and Eisenman, 1973).

5.7. Assembly and Formation of Virions

It has been characteristic of RNA tumor viruses that virus particles or even precursors are generally undetectable inside the cell. All viral components appear to be transported to the plasma membrane, where the final assembly takes place, and virions are released from the cell membrane by a budding mechanism. The lipid composition of the virus is determined by the host cell in which the virus is formed (Quigley *et al.*, 1971). Thus some components of viral membranes probably come from cells. However, there is no direct proof that host cell protein is incorporated into the virions, indicating that the portion of the plasma membrane used for formation of viral membranes is preformed by the use of viral proteins.

In electron micrographs, the electron-dense structure of virions appears to change with time after budding from cells. Studies on virions collected shortly after formation (3–5 min) revealed that viral RNA in such virions is 35S instead of 60–70S, as found in standard virus preparations. The incubation of 3- to 5-min virus at 37°C results in conversion of 35S RNA to 60–70S RNA (Cheung *et al.*, 1972; Canaani *et al.*, 1973). Therefore, 35S RNA seems to be a precursor which is converted to the 60–70S form after completion and release of particles from cells.

The mature virus is normally released into the culture medium. However, the interaction between the cell surface and the virion seen in the attachment process appears to operate also at the stage of virus release. Viruses which attach poorly to the cell surface are released into the medium with relative ease, whereas viruses which attach efficiently have a tendency to remain on the cell surface. For example, the ratio of physical particles released into the medium to particles remaining on the cell surface is 1–2 for RAV-2 and 0.01–0.1 for RAV-1 (H. Hanafusa, unpublished results).

6. Virus–Cell Interactions

6.1. Absence of Virus Replication

A typical example of virus replication in chicken cells infected with avian RNA tumor virus has been described in the preceding section. However, this scheme is modified for some virus–cell systems, depending on the characteristics of both virus and cell.

6.1.1. Nonpermissive Cells

The nonpermissiveness of some avian cells was described in Sections 2.1 and 5.3. The virus fails to penetrate genetically resistant chicken cells. The pattern of susceptibility observed in chicken cells, however, cannot be applied directly to other avian cell systems. For example, RAV-7 of subgroup C is noninfectious for quail and duck cells while B-77 of the same subgroup C is infectious for both (Duff and Vogt, 1969). Also, infectivity for quail and duck cells is often less efficient than for chicken cells. Production of B-77 virus is about 100 times lower in quail cells than in chicken cells (Friis, 1972). The reason for this quantitative restriction is not clear.

A more profound restriction of avian RNA tumor virus infection and multiplication is found in mammalian cells. Some strains of RSV can produce tumors in a variety of mammals including mice, rats, hamsters, and guinea pigs (see Svoboda and Hlozánek, 1970). Efficiency of tumor production is extremely low. Except for rare cases, these tumor cells produce no virus particles. However, all tumor cells appear to retain the entire viral genetic information, since cell fusion of the tumor cells with normal chicken cells results in the formation of complete infectious virus (Svoboda, 1964; Machala *et al.*, 1970). The tumor cells contain some virus-specific proteins (gs antigens), but no envelope antigen seems to be formed. (Serum of hamsters bearing RSV tumors contains antibodies against gs antigens and is used for complement fixation tests.) Virus-specific RNA-dependent DNA polymerase is also absent in RSV-transformed mammalian cells (Coffin and Temin, 1972; Livingstone *et al.*, 1972). These results suggest that either transcription or translation of some cistrons of viral genes is inhibited in mammalian cells. This inhibition could be due to the lack of some initiation factor which might be added by fusion with chicken cells.

6.1.2. Infection by Defective Virus

Some strains of sarcoma virus (Bryan and Harris strains of RSV, Fujinami sarcoma virus) are defective and dependent on helper virus for the formation of infectious virus (H. Hanafusa *et al.*, 1963, 1964; Reamer and Okazaki, 1971). On the other hand, the Schmidt–Ruppin, Carr–Zilber, and Prague strains of RSV and the B-77 strain of avian sarcoma virus are known to be helper independent. A possible relationship between these two classes of viruses will be discussed in a later section. It may be noteworthy that most sarcoma viruses found in mammalian species are defective forms, and the type of interaction between these defective sarcoma viruses and helper leukemia viruses is similar to that found with the avian system.

The major defectiveness of these strains is in the synthesis of glycoprotein gp85 (Scheele and Hanafusa, 1971). Therefore, they will be called "gp85-defective viruses" to distinguish them from defective viruses of other types. Infection with gp85-defective sarcoma virus is rather complicated, because of the involvement of another virus in the formation of the infectious form. The properties of this system can be summarized as follows (see H. Hanafusa *et al.*, 1970*b*):

a. The infectious form of gp85-defective sarcoma virus can adsorb, penetrate, and transform cells. However, if chicken cells are free of the expression of endogenous viral genes (see Section 8), the transformed cells formed by the gp85-defective virus produce virions termed "RSV(−)," which are noninfectious for any cell under normal circumstances.

b. The noninfectious particles lack glycoprotein. Their noninfectiousness appears to result from a failure to penetrate the cell.

c. When the transformed cells are doubly infected with another virus, either sarcoma or leukosis virus, or when the endogenous viral genomes are expressed in the transformed cells, the gp85-defective virus is released as an infectious form. The infectious form contains gp85-defective RSV genomes with the envelope glycoprotein made by helper virus or helper factor in the cells.

d. The subgroup specificity of these RSV [they are designated RSV(ALV) or RSV(chf),* indicating RSV genome coated by the envelope of ALV or endogenous helper factor] is determined by the envelope proteins provided by the helper. The RSV(ALV) is called the "RSV pseudotypes" of the given ALV.

e. The formation of this infectious form is an extreme case of phenotypic mixing; the RSV genome remains defective for the synthesis of glycoprotein. Thus infection of the next cell with a single virion of RSV(ALV) or RSV(chf) will result in the sequence of events described in (a).

f. The noninfectious form RSV(−) described in (a) can be incorporated into host cells by the aid of inactivated Sendai virus, a cell fusion agent. Once incorporated into cells, the noninfectious virions are able to transform the cells (Robinson, 1967; T. Hanafusa *et al.*, 1970*a*). The cycle of virus growth is identical to that described in (a–e),

Thus the replication of the gp85-defective sarcoma virus is essentially a two-virus system. As a consequence of helper dependency, the gp85-defective sarcoma virus is usually maintained together with helper leukosis virus; usually the concentration of helper virus is higher than that of sarcoma virus. Therefore, infection of cultures with high titers of a defective RSV stock results in double infection by RSV and leukosis virus, and many cells will produce the infectious form of RSV. If one needs to establish RSV infection without leukosis virus

---

* RSV(chf) was called RSV(0) or RSVβ(0) in some papers; RSV(−) was called RSVβ'(0).

intervention, an extremely low titer of RSV must be used, and virus spread in the infected cultures should be suppressed. [Infection with RSV(−) as described in (f) can be used for this purpose.] The kinetics of production of infectious forms of gp85-defective RSV is obviously dependent on many factors: initial dose of each of the two virus components, rate of growth of helper virus, physiological conditions for virus spread, and time period after infection (H. Hanafusa and T. Hanafusa, 1966a).

Another defective virus is the "α type" of Bryan RSV (H. Hanafusa and T. Hanafusa, 1968). The virus, RSV α, which seems to be a mutant of the gp85-defective RSV described above, is deficient in the synthesis of both gp85 and the RNA-dependent DNA polymerase (H. Hanafusa and T. Hanafusa, 1971; Robinson and Robinson, 1971). However, the deficiency in this enzyme seems to be rather easily complemented by coinfection with other leukosis viruses, which can provide both the polymerase and the envelope glycoprotein. The complemented RSV α, RSV α (ALV), is capable of transforming cells. These transformed cells produce particles which lack glycoprotein and polymerase, unless the cells are coinfected with leukosis virus. The polymerase deficiency cannot be complemented by endogenous virus genes or by the cellular DNA polymerase.

The types of defective virus described above cannot be easily obtained from lytic virus or nontransforming virus. Because cell transformation can be observed independently of virus replication, transforming viruses deficient in replication can be identified. Among leukosis viruses, some leukemic strains known as myeloblastosis, myelocytoma, and erythroblastosis viruses can cause cell transformation in infected cells. Viruses defective in replication have recently been isolated from these transforming leukemia viruses (Ishizaki *et al.*, 1971; see also Section 1.1.2). Finally, nondefective helper-independent avian sarcoma virus seems to segregate mutants defective in glycoprotein at a relatively high frequency (see Section 7).

6.2. Cell Transformation

RNA tumor viruses produce tumors in infected animals. The alteration which accompanies this malignancy at the cellular level is called "cell transformation." As seen with avian myeloblastosis virus, which normally does not cause alterations characteristic of cell transformation in fibroblast cells but does produce transformation of cells derived from the hematopoietic system (Baluda, 1962; Moscovici, 1967), cell transformation by a virus may depend on both cell and virus. However, the mechanism of cell transformation in the sarcoma virus–fibroblast system may not be entirely parallel to that in the leukemic virus–hematopoietic cell system. Because sarcoma viruses produce solid tumors in animals and produce foci of transformed cells in chick embryo fibroblast cultures, this system is considered to be a clear example of cell transformation, and has been the subject of most studies on the process of transformation.

As often emphasized, cell transformation by sarcoma virus takes place rapidly, and is quantitatively related to infection. Under proper conditions, cells in the entire culture can be transformed in 24 h (H. Hanafusa, 1969b). Therefore, it is hoped that changes taking place in these cells can be studied by biochemical methods with proper control, uninfected cultures.

6.2.1. Characteristics of Transformed Cells

The following changes have been observed in cells transformed by sarcoma virus. These characteristics can be used as criteria for cell transformation.

a. Malignancy. Malignancy is generally tested by tumor production after inoculation of a certain number of cells into animals. Transformed avian cells produced by avian sarcoma virus always release virus particles. In some cases, the particles are noninfectious. But these noninfectious viruses contain RSV genes capable of transforming cells, as shown by cell transformation in the presence of inactivated Sendai virus. In fact, infection by "noninfectious" particles seems to take place in vivo at a very low frequency (H. Hanafusa et al., 1973). Therefore, the malignancy of these transformed cells cannot be rigorously evaluated by transplantation.

b. Morphological Changes. Morphological changes are most frequently used as criteria for cell transformation. Alteration can be seen in the shape of individual cells and in the orientation of cells in monolayer. Transformed cells in culture are more refractive than normal cells, and assume round or spindle forms with smoother cell surfaces than normal cells. Transformed cells lose the parallel orientation of normal fibroblasts, and have an increased tendency to pile up on each other or to make criss-cross patterns. These morphological changes are characteristic of each sarcoma virus strain, and are not affected by the virus subgroup.

c. Increased Multiplication. Cells in sarcomas apparently grow without restriction compared to uninfected normal tissues. However, the conditions for cell growth in tissue culture are not directly comparable with those in in vivo tissues. Under usual conditions for cell cultures, uninfected normal cells grow exponentially until they reach a certain cell density which is determined by the amounts of growth-promoting substances generally present in serum in the medium (see Temin et al., 1972). The growth rates of normal and transformed avian cells are generally the same. However, the extent of multiplication of these two types of cells may differ (Temin, 1965; Colby and Rubin, 1969; H. Hanafusa, 1969a; Balk et al., 1973). Apparently transformation alters the efficiency with which cells can utilize the growth-promoting substances, so the level at which the promoting substances become limiting is different for normal and transformed cells. Thus certain conditions permit the preferential multiplication of transformed cells. One example is the overlay by agar-containing medium used for focus formation by sarcoma virus. Here, one or more growth-promoting substances appear to be bound by sulfated polysaccharides in the agar so that the levels of these substances are too low for multiplication of uninfected cells but sufficient for growth of transformed cells. (For this reason, purified agar is not suitable for focus formation.)

Perhaps one of the variations of this phenomenon is colony formation in agar medium. It has been commonly found that only transformed cells can form colonies consisting of more than 1000 cells. This method is often used to isolate transformants (Macpherson and Montagnier, 1964; Rubin, 1966).

d. Changes in the Cell Surface. Changes in cell morphology by transformation suggest that some alteration takes place on the cell surface. Indeed, differences have been demonstrated between normal and transformed cells in a number of different properties.

Changes in structural components have been described for the glycopeptides (Warren *et al.*, 1972) and glycoproteins (Bussell and Robinson, 1973; Wickus and Robbins, 1973) on plasma membranes. The presence of different glycolipids (Hakomori *et al.*, 1971; Warren *et al.*, 1972) is also known. Increased hyaluronic acid is one of the common results of sarcoma virus infection (Kabat, 1939), caused by an increased level of hyaluronic acid synthetase in transformed cells (Ishimoto *et al.*, 1966).

Architectural changes in the membranes of transformed cells have been suggested by the increased rate of uptake of certain types of mono- or disaccharides (Hatanaka and Hanafusa, 1970; Martin *et al.*, 1971; Kawai and Hanafusa, 1971), and by increased agglutinability by lectin (Kapeller and Doljanski, 1972; Biquard and Vigier, 1972; Burger and Martin, 1972). The level of a specific activator (a protease) which converts plasminogen present in serum to plasmin was shown to increase significantly (Unkeless *et al.*, 1973*a,b*). The plasmin appears to associate with the cell surface of transformed cells. The cell shape may also be affected by the modification of the microtubule and microfiber structure in the cells. The involvement of cyclic AMP in this phenomenon has been suggested (Otten *et al.*, 1972).

An important, unresolved question is whether any one of the surface changes plays a causative role in cell transformation, or whether these are rather one of the results of secondary changes accompanying cell transformation.

e. Other Changes. Increased glycolysis in tumor cells has been noted (Burk *et al.*, 1941). Careful examination of glycolysis in normal and RSV-transformed cells showed that no significant difference could be found in these two cultures when they were growing exponentially (Steck *et al.*, 1968; Temin, 1968). However, under conditions where transformed cells can grow preferentially, as described before, increased lactic acid formation can be seen in transformed cells.

Finally, chromosomal alteration can be seen in cells of RSV-induced tumors, but this seems to be an indirect effect of infection, since no immediate karyological changes can be observed in tissue culture cells newly transformed by RSV (Pontén, 1963).

6.2.2. Viral Genes for Cell Transformation

Avian sarcoma virus can induce cell transformation in chick embryo fibroblasts. The induction of transformation and the maintenance of the transformed state in the cells require the products of sarcoma virus genes. This notion was first clearly demonstrated by the use of temperature-sensitive mutants of RSV (Martin, 1970). Cells infected with these mutants are transformed at permissive (low) temperatures but are not transformed at nonpermissive (high) temperatures (Toyoshima and Vogt, 1969b; Bader, 1972b). Generally the changes are reversible, and many of these mutants produce progeny virus at similar rates at either temperature (Kawai and Hanafusa, 1971; Biquard and Vigier, 1970). With some mutants, the presence of inhibitors of protein synthesis in the cultures blocks the development of cell transformation which would otherwise occur after the cultures have been shifted from high to low temperatures, suggesting that the synthesis of a viral protein(s) is essential for cell transformation. Coinfection of cells with certain combinations of different temperature-sensitive mutants of RSV causes transformation at nonpermissive temperatures (Kawai et al., 1972). The results suggest that the two mutants produce different temperature-sensitive proteins, both of which are required for cell transformation (Wyke, 1973).

Infection with leukosis viruses does not cause cell transformation in chick embryo fibroblasts. However, these viruses, particularly some acute leukemia viruses, can produce transformation in stem cells of the reticuloendothelial system. Obviously the difference between these leukosis viruses and the sarcoma viruses is attributable to a difference in the viral products in infected cells. It is not clear, however, whether the formation of the "transforming protein" by leukosis viruses is suppressed in fibroblast cells, or whether the leukosis viruses produce different products which are active in differentiated hematopoietic cells but not active in fibroblasts.

If leukosis viruses lack a significant portion of the genome responsible for synthesis of the "transforming protein," then the RNAs of leukosis viruses and sarcoma viruses could be different in size. A comparison of the size of viral RNAs has been made by gel electrophoresis, using 35S RNA obtained by dissociating viral 70S RNA. Although 35S RNAs of various strains of leukosis and sarcoma viruses are similar in size (2.5–3.0×10^6 daltons) (Duesberg and Vogt, 1970; Scheele and Hanafusa, 1972), there is some indication that sarcoma viruses have additional genes. As will be described later, virus which cannot transform fibroblasts can be obtained from clonal stocks of sarcoma virus. These transformation-defective (td) derivatives retain all other properties of the virus, and some of them have been shown to be leukemogenic in chickens. Careful examination by gel electrophoresis seems to indicate that the RNA of the sarcoma virus is somewhat larger than that of the td derivative of the sarcoma virus (Martin and Duesberg, 1972; Duesberg and Vogt, 1973).

Several different forms of variants have already been mentioned in previous sections. The diversity of viruses is one of the unique features of RNA tumor viruses. The various types will be catalogued in this section.

7.1. Variation

7.1.1. Nonconditional Mutants

The class of nonconditional mutants includes various defective viruses. The Bryan type RSV, which is defective in glycoprotein synthesis, has been described in Section 6.1.2. The majority of the virus population of the Schmidt–Ruppin strain of RSV is helper independent, but a small fraction seem to be deletion mutants, including one type which lacks the ability to make envelope glycoprotein (Kawai and Hanafusa, 1973). The results suggest that the defective Bryan strain might have been obtained by the same mechanism. The gp85-defective viruses cannot be converted to the nondefective, helper-independent form by recombination with other avian RNA tumor viruses.

A virus deficient in DNA polymerase can be isolated from the Bryan strain. This type of polymerase mutant has also been isolated from the newly isolated gp70-defective variant of the Schmidt–Ruppin strain of RSV. These polymerase-negative mutants have been obtained as spontaneous mutants at a frequency of 5–10%. The polymerase-negative virus does not contain protein antigenically related to the polymerase.

Both the gp85- and polymerase-defective viruses are considered as replication-defective viruses (rd virus). Another class of mutants is transformation defective (td), derived from helper-independent sarcoma virus. These viruses are sometimes called "nontransforming" (NT) derivatives of sarcoma viruses. The td virus can be obtained spontaneously (Vogt, 1971a; Kawai and Hanafusa, 1972b), or after treatment with mutagens (Goldé, 1970; Toyoshima *et al.*, 1970; Graf *et al.*, 1971). The spontaneous segregation of td virus takes place at a high frequency (about 10%). At least one of the td viruses (td-B-77) is known to be leukemogenic (Biggs *et al.*, 1973).

It is conceivable that the abovementioned defective mutants are produced as a result of gene deletion. One possible origin of the deletion would be an early termination in the transcription of DNA into RNA. Such RNA deletions would presumably occur in the terminal sequences of the RNA subunits.

The morphology of transformed cell foci is specific to the strain of sarcoma virus, but mutations affecting the focus morphology are also known. These mutants are called "RSV-morph[r]" for round foci and "RSV-morph[f]" for fusiform foci (Temin, 1960). They are convertible in either direction at a rather high frequency.

7.1.2. Conditional Mutants

Mutants which cannot replicate or cannot transform cells under certain growth conditions are called "conditional mutants." At the moment, only temperature-sensitive (ts) mutants belong to this category. The temperature-sensitive functions thus far identified are related to either replication of virus or cell transformation or both. (This last-mentioned type is most likely a double mutant.) Generally they are obtained by treatment of virus or infected cells with mutagens.

Many ts mutants in transformation have been isolated (Section 6.2.2). The ts mutants in virus replication can have defects in many different functions of the virus growth cycle. Some have a defective polymerase at high temperatures (Linial and Mason, 1973), and some possibly have defects in assembly or in structural proteins (Friis *et al.*, 1971; Wyke and Linial, 1973), so that particles produced are extremely unstable at nonpermissive temperatures. Undoubtedly, these mutants will be extremely useful for investigating the virus growth cycle.

7.2. Interaction Between Viruses

Infection of cells with leukosis virus can cause either interference with or enhancement of secondary infection by sarcoma virus (see Sections 2.1, and 5.2, respectively). As discussed before, these interactions occur at the attachment or penetration steps.

After two viruses enter the same cell, two types of interaction can take place: phenotypic mixing and recombination. Phenotypic mixing consists of the exchange of viral components between two viruses without modification of the viral genomes. On the other hand, the genomes of two viruses can interact in such a way that a portion of the genomes is exchanged to make a recombinant.

7.2.1. Phenotypic Mixing

The phenotypes but not genotypes of virus are altered as a result of phenotypic mixing. Classical phenotypic mixing, that is, the formation of virus having the phenotypes of both viruses (such as antigenicity in a mosaic form), is also known with avian RNA tumor viruses (Vogt, 1967a). Phenotypic mixing is extended to its extreme in such examples as the formation of RSV pseudotypes of gp85-defective strains (Section 6.1.2).

Phenotypic mixing of the envelope glycoprotein seems to take place with any combination of two types of either sarcoma or leukosis virus. The presence of two viruses is rarely encountered with other animal viruses, but this is not unusual with avian RNA tumor viruses because of the frequent existence of virus in the natural host, or the presence of endogenous viral genes in chicken cells.

The infectious form of the DNA polymerase–negative mutant can be considered an example of phenotypic mixing in which both envelope antigen and DNA polymerase are supplied by the coinfecting virus. In some cases, the complementation between two replication-defective mutants is a result of phenotypic mixing.

Recombination between avian RNA tumor viruses has been suggested as an explanation for genetic changes in viruses. Recombination between RSV and leukosis virus, resulting in production of RSV with the subgroup specificity of the leukosis virus, has been demonstrated (Vogt, 1971*b*; Kawai and Hanafusa, 1972*b*). The frequency of recombination is generally about 10%. This type of recombination can also be found between nondefective RSV and the endogenous viral genes present in chicken cells (Weiss *et al.*, 1973). The products are RSV with subgroup E specificity.

With some combinations, however, no recombination is obtained. Since defective strains of RSV are incapable of forming glycoprotein, it might be expected that a stable helper-independent RSV could be produced by recombination with leukosis virus at this marker. This has never been observed. It is conceivable that the gp85-defective RSV has a deletion in the genomes and the deletion itself results in the loss of the ability to recombine with other segments of RNA (Kawai and Hanafusa, 1973).

Another genetic change in which recombination may be involved is conversion of the polymerase mutant RSVα to polymerase-positive RSV. RSVα is a mutant defective in both glycoprotein and polymerase.

Cells transformed by RSVα never spontaneously produce a detectable quantity of polymerase-positive gp85-defective RSV. If these cultures are infected with leukosis virus, however, a complemented infectious form of RSV(ALV) is produced. Analysis of the genotype of RSV(ALV) showed that about 10% of the virus population was stably polymerase positive, i.e., polymerase-positive gp85-defective RSV (H. Hanafusa and T. Hanafusa, 1968; H. Hanafusa, 1970). It is interesting to see that RSVα recombines with leukosis virus in the polymerase genes but not in the glycoprotein genes. Some mechanism apparently operates to inhibit the recombination of gp85-defective RSV (including α) in the glycoprotein gene.

Recombination between the endogenous viral genomes and avian RNA tumor viruses seems also to be involved in the formation of RAV-60 (subgroup E) from chicken cells following infection with other sarcoma or leukosis viruses (T. Hanafusa *et al.*, 1970*b*) (see Section 8). In this case, the endogenous viral genes recombine with leukosis virus of gp85-defective RSV to produce leukosis-type virus with subgroup E glycoprotein which is specific to the endogenous viral genes. It is interesting that the reciprocal recombinant is not formed (i.e., gp85 + RSV). There is no direct proof that the interaction between leukosis virus or gp85-defective RSV and the endogenous genes to give rise to RAV-60 involves the same mechanism as in the interaction between helper-independent RSV and endogenous genes to produce recombinant subgroup E RSV. The significantly lower frequency of formation of RAV-60 suggests that the two types of interaction may not be entirely the same in detail.

A relatively high frequency of recombination is known with influenza virus and reovirus (Hirst, 1962; Fields and Voklik, 1969), both of which have segmented viral genomes (i.e., virions contain several pieces of RNA packaged nonrandomly). The high recombination rate is explained by the exchange or reassortment of the pieces when two strains of virus grow together in the same cell. Biochemically, avian tumor virus RNA is known to be dissociated into smaller pieces by disruption of hydrogen bonds and only the subunit RNA appears to be present in the cells. Thus the assumption that several subunits with different genetic information are present seems to be reasonable. However, the organization of genome RNA is not understood, and the validity of the subunit hypothesis has not been established. Alternatively, a crossing-over event may take place at the level of the provirus, during either integration or replication of provirus DNA.

8. Endogenous Viral Genes in Chicken Cells

Chickens selected as virus-free flocks are now available. However, these virus-free chickens, and possibly all chickens, appear to contain RNA tumor virus genetic information and the viral genes are expressed in some chickens.

The first indication of the presence of viral genes came from the observation that normal uninfected chickens sometimes contain gs antigen detectable by complement fixation (Dougherty and DiStefano, 1966). A detailed genetic study showed that there exist at least two classes of chickens, one which contains gs antigen and another which does not. By genetic crossing of the two classes of chickens, it was shown that the possession of gs antigen is a heritable characteristic of chickens, with the presence of gs antigen being dominant (Payne and Chubb, 1968).

Independently, two classes of chickens were found in studies of reproduction of gp85-defective RSV (Weiss, 1969; T. Hanafusa et al., 1970a). On transformation by gp85-defective RSV, one class of embryo cells produces virus which can transform Japanese quail cells, while the other class produces virus which is noninfectious for any host. Analysis of the system revealed that the first class of embryo cells contain the gp85 glycoprotein (presumably the subgroup E determinant), which is produced by the host-associated viral genes (H. Hanafusa et al., 1973). The second class of embryo does not produce this glycoprotein. Thus the host cell–associated viral factor was tentatively called "chicken cell–associated helper factor" (chf) (H. Hanafusa et al., 1970a). In the chapter, "chf" is used to denote an endogenous viral entity in chicken cells.

A good correlation between the presence or absence of gs antigen and helper factor in the same embryo soon became apparent. The embryos containing both gs antigen and helper factor will be called "chf(+)" cells and those negative for both will be called "chf(−)" cells.

8.1. Genetic Materials

The presence in normal cells of DNA which hybridizes with viral RNA has been known for some time. Refinements in hybridization techniques have made this

conclusion more convincing. The estimated number of copies of virus-specific
DNA per cell ranged from average 3.2 to about 15 depending on the method used
(Varmus *et al.*, 1972; Baluda, 1972). The most interesting point is that both chf(+)
and chf(−) embryos contain equal amounts of viral DNA (Rosenthal *et al.*, 1971).

The amount of viral RNA in these cells was examined by hybridization with radioactively labeled complementary DNA (made by polymerase with the endogenous viral RNA as template). The level of viral RNA in the chf(+) cells is clearly different from that in chf(−) cells (Hayward and Hanafusa, 1973). The former contain about 40 copies of RNA per cell, while the latter have less than 0.2 copy, suggesting that the difference between the two types of embryos is determined at the transcription level. However, post-transcriptional control may also be involved.

8.2. Expression

The "gs antigen" is measured by the complement fixation test and probably represents several viral proteins. It is clear that the major gs protein (p27) is present in chf(+) cells, but how many other viral proteins are synthesized in these cells is not known. It is also not known whether chf(−) cells lack all of the viral proteins, or whether some of them are formed in small quantities. Recent experiments using radioimmunoassay seem to indicate that minute amounts of viral proteins are present in chf(−) cells (Chen and Hanafusa, 1973).

Helper activity is measured by formation of infectious subgroup E RSV after infection with gp85-defective RSV (T. Hanafusa *et al.*, 1972). In addition to the general classification of embryos based on the presence or absence of helper factor, there are widely varying levels of helper activity detectable in different chf(+) embryos.

Although many viral proteins are synthesized, no viral RNA-dependent DNA polymerase has been detected in either chf(+) or chf(−) cells (Weissbach *et al.*, 1972; Kang and Temin, 1972).

8.3. Recovery of Subgroup E Virus

When chf(+) cells are infected with leukosis virus or RSV, a *leukosis virus* with subgroup E specificity is recovered in addition to the phenotypically mixed virus (T. Hanafusa *et al.*, 1970b). The virus, called "RAV-60," generally represents about 10^{-3} of the total virus yield. The formation of RAV-60 is considered to be a consequence of recombination between the endogenous viral gene and exogenous virus.

RAV-60 can also be recovered from chf(−) cells (T. Hanafusa *et al.*, 1972). The yield is extremely low, but this virus has been obtained from all chf(−) cells tested. This finding seems to lend support to the hypothesis that all chicken cells contain chf provirus DNA. The low level of expression of viral genes may be due to the escape from the control.

The recombination with endogenous virus causes a serious problem in maintaining the quality of avian RNA tumor virus preparations. A stock of virus grown in chf(+) cells would contain RAV-60, and if this stock were further propagated in cells susceptible to subgroup E the RAV-60 might become a major component in it. Rigorously speaking, contamination by RAV-60 could occur even in virus grown in chf(−) cells.

8.4. Spontaneous Production of Subgroup E Virus

Some strains of chickens produce a subgroup E virus, RAV-0, spontaneously (Vogt and Friis, 1971). RAV-0 is similar to RAV-60 in its capacity to infect C/0 or quail cells and to act as a helper for gp85-defective RSV. The major differences between the two viruses are in the amounts of viral genetic information and in the rates of replication: RAV-0 genomes contain less genetic information than normal leukosis viruses, and grow at an extremely slow rate in susceptible cells (T. Hanafusa, W. S. Hayward, and H. Hanafusa, unpublished results).

RAV-0-producing chicken cells must express certain viral genes which are not expressed in chf(+) virus–negative cells. For example, RAV-0 contains RNA-dependent DNA polymerase, which is not expressed in chf(+) cells. Since cultures spontaneously producing RAV-0 are generally genetically susceptible to subgroup E virus, the titer of RAV-0 might be expected to be uniformly high in such cultures. However, there seems to be a fairly large variation in the yield of RAV-0 among different embryos. Factors controlling this variation are not known, but the involvement of yet another regulatory gene controlling the formation of RAV-0 has been suggested (Crittenden and Smith, 1973).

8.5. Induction of Virus

It is conceivable that RAV-0 is produced from chicken cells as a result of induction of endogenous virus by an exogenous physical or chemical agent. This idea seems to be supported by the demonstration of the production of viruses similar to RAV-0 following treatment of virus-negative cells with X-rays or chemical carcinogens (Weiss et al., 1971). However, the frequency of virus production is low, and the use in these studies of pheasant cells to amplify the virus yield makes further analysis difficult. It has been noted that treatment with 5-bromo- or iododeoxyuridine, which are potent inducers of murine leukemia type virus in mice cells (Lowy et al., 1971), does not lead to production of virus in the chicken system. It has been shown in the murine system that some strains of mice are noninducible. Chicken cells thus far tested may belong to this class of host cells.

8.6. Genetic Control of Expression

As mentioned before, in most chicken embryos the presence of gs antigen and helper activity is correlated. Since the presence of gs antigen is inherited as a

dominant character over the absence, it was originally thought that the structural
gene for endogenous virus was present only in gs(+) cells, and was integrated into
cellular chromosomes. However, the presence of viral DNA in all chickens, the
recovery of RAV-60 from chf(−) cells, and the finding of low levels of viral
products in chf(−) cells by sensitive assay methods suggest that the chf provirus
structural gene is present in all chicken cells. This suggests that the expression of
the endogenous provirus is controlled by a regulatory gene which may be
different in chf(+) and chf(−) cells (Weiss and Payne, 1971; T. Hanafusa *et al.*,
1972).

In addition to the above generalized controlling system, there may be another
more specific mechanism regulating the expression of chf provirus. In some
chickens, high helper activity can be found without gs antigen (Hayward and
Hanafusa, 1973). The pattern of inheritance of this regulation has not been
determined.

8.7. Significance of the Endogenous Virus in Carcinogenesis

Embryos of chf(+) type have been obtained from leukosis-free flocks of chickens.
Therefore, it seems likely that the endogenous viral genes do not express the
functions which lead to leukosis in the host. However, no experimental data have
been reported concerning the effect of RAV-0 on various avian hosts. It may be
premature to judge the significance of the endogenous genes in carcinogenesis
now, since it is possible that the types of regulation could be different in different
strains of chickens. There may be some strains of chickens in which the complete
set of viral information is induced, including leukemogenic activity, as seen in the
AKR strain of mice induced by bromodeoxyuridine. Further, it is possible that
there are other endogenous viruses having other subgroup specificities. The
possible presence of endogenous virus in pheasants has been indicated by the
isolation of RAV-61 from RSV(−)-infected pheasant cells. The mechanism
involved in the production of RAV-61 may be comparable to that of RAV-60, i.e.,
recombination of exogenous and endogenous viral genes (T. Hanafusa and H.
Hanafusa, 1973).

Perhaps the most interesting problem related to the endogenous viral genes is
the mechanism of regulation of viral gene expression. Since viral RNA and viral
protein can be analyzed with great accuracy using new techniques, this system
provides a good opportunity to study the regulatory mechanisms operating on the
viral genes integrated into cellular chromosomes.

FURTHER READING

The literature citations in this chapter have been kept to a minimum by limiting
them to representative papers. The author is responsible for the possible failure to
refer to more pertinent or important papers. There are several good reviews on

avian RNA tumor viruses, and readers may find more complete citations in these reviews. Comprehensive reviews on the basic biology of viruses have been presented by Vogt (1965a), Vigier (1970b), Temin (1971, 1973), Darcel (1973), and Tooze (1973). Descriptions of RNA tumor viruses in a book by Fenner *et al.* (1974) may also be useful. Early history and virus transmission have been described by Gross (1970), Beard (1963), and Burmester (1971). Virus ultrastructure has been reviewed by Haguenau and Beard (1962). Interaction with mammalian cells is discussed by Svoboda and Hlozánek (1970) and Simkovic (1972). H. Hanafusa (1969a) describes phenotypic mixing and variants of RSV. An excellent review on DNA polymerase is also available (Temin and Baltimore, 1972). Macpherson (1970) has reviewed the characteristics of transformed cells. Finally, Volume 17 of *National Cancer Institute Monographs* (1964) contains a collection of papers on avian RNA tumor viruses.

9. References

AUGUST, J. T., BOLOGNESI, D. P., FLEISSNER, E., GILDEN, R. V., AND NOWINSKI, R. C., 1973, A proposed nomenclature for virion proteins of oncogenic RNA viruses, *Virology* **60**:595–601.

BADER, J. P., 1964, The role of deoxyribonucleic acid in the synthesis of Rous sarcoma virus, *Virology* **22**:462–468.

BADER, J. P., 1965, The DNA requirement of Rous sarcoma and Rous-associated viruses, *Virology* **26**:253–261.

BADER, J. P., 1972a, Metabolic requirements for infection by Rous sarcoma virus. IV. Virus reproduction and cellular transformation without cellular division, *Virology* **48**:494–501.

BADER, J. P., 1972b, Temperature-dependent transformation of cells infected with a mutant of Bryan Rous sarcoma virus, *J. Virol.* **10**:267–276.

BALDUZZI, P., AND MORGAN, H. R., 1970, Mechanism of oncogenic transformation by Rous sarcoma virus. I. Intracellular inactivation of cell-transforming ability of Rous sarcoma virus by 5-bromodeoxyuridine and light, *J. Virol.* **5**:470–477.

BALK, S. D., WHITFIELD, J. F., YOUDALE, T., AND BRAUN, A. C., 1973, Role of calcium, serum, plasma, and folic acid in the control of proliferation of normal and Rous sarcoma virus–infected chicken fibroblasts, *Proc. Natl. Acad. Sci.* **70**:675–679.

BALTIMORE, D., 1970, RNA-dependent DNA polymerase in virions of RNA tumor viruses, *Nature (Lond.)* **226**:1209–1211.

BALTIMORE, D., AND SMOLER, D., 1971, Primer requirement and template specificity of the DNA polymerase of RNA tumor viruses, *Proc. Natl. Acad. Sci.* **68**:1507–1511.

BALUDA, M. A., 1962, Properties of cells infected with avian myeloblastosis virus, *Cold Spring Harbor Symp. Quant. Biol.* **27**:415–425.

BALUDA, M. A., 1972, Widespread presence, in chickens, of DNA complementary to the RNA genome of avian leukosis viruses, *Proc. Natl. Acad. Sci.* **69**:576–580.

BANG, F. B., AND HALEY, R., 1958, The appearance and disappearance of antibodies to Rous virus in normal chickens, *J. Natl. Cancer Inst.* **20**:329–338.

BEARD, J. W., 1956. Virus of avian myeloblastic leukosis, *Poultry Sci.* **35**:203–223.

BEARD, J. W., 1963, Avian virus growths and their etiologic agents, *Advan. Cancer Res.* **7**:1–127.

BEGG, A. M., 1929, A filtrable fibrosarcoma of the fowl, *Brit. J. Exp. Pathol.* **10**:322.

BIGGS, P. M., MILNE, B. S., GRAF, T., AND BAUER, H., 1973, Oncogenicity of non-transforming mutants of avian sarcoma viruses, *J. Gen. Virol.* **18**:399–403.

BIQUARD, J. M., AND VIGIER, P., 1970, Isolement et etude d'un mutant conditionnel du virus de Rous a capacite transformante thermosensible, *Compt. Rend. Acad. Sci. Paris* **D271**:2430–2433.

BIQUARD, J. M., AND VIGIER, P., 1972, Agglutination par la concanavaline A des fibroblastes d'embryon de poule transforme par le virus de Rous (SR-RSV) et un mutant thermosensible de ce virus, *Compt. Rend. Acad. Sci. Paris* **D274**:144–147.

BOETTIGER, D., AND TEMIN, H. M., 1970, Light inactivation of focus formation by chicken embryo fibroblasts infected with avian sarcoma virus in the presence of 5-bromodeoxyuridine, *Nature (Lond.)* **228:**622–624.

BOLOGNESI, D. P., BAUER, H., GELDERBLOM, H., AND HÜPER, G., 1972a, Polypeptides of avian RNA tumor viruses. IV. Components of the viral envelope *Virology* **47:**551–566.

BOLOGNESI, D. P., GELDERBLOM, H., BAUER, H., MÖLLING, K., AND HÜPER, G., 1972b, Polypeptides of avian RNA tumor viruses. V. Analysis of the virus core, *Virology* **47:**567–578.

BURGER, M. M., AND MARTIN, G. S., 1972, Agglutination of cells transformed by Rous sarcoma virus by wheat germ agglutinin and concanavalin A, *Nature New Biol.* **237:**9–12.

BURK, D., SPRINCE, H., SPANGELER, J. M., KABAT, E. A., FURTH, J., AND CLAUDE, A., 1941, The metabolism of chicken tumors, *J. Natl. Cancer Inst.* **2:**201–240.

BURMESTER, B. R., 1971, Viruses of the leukosis/sarcoma group, in: *Poultry Diseases and World Economy* (R. F. Gordon and B. M. Freeman, eds.), pp. 135–152, British Poultry Science, Edinburgh.

BURMESTER, B. R., PRICKETT, C. O., AND BELDING, T. C., 1946, A filtrable agent producing lymphoid tumours and osteopetrosis in chickens, *Cancer Res.* **6:**189–196.

BURMESTER, B. R., FONTES, A. K., WATERS, N. F., BRYAN, W. R., AND GROUPÉ, V., 1960, The response of several inbred lines of white leghorns to inoculation with the viruses of strain RPL12 visceral lymphomatosis-erythroblastosis and of Rous sarcoma, *Poultry Sci.* **39:**199–215.

BUSSELL, R. H., AND ROBINSON, W. S., 1973, Membrane proteins of uninfected and Rous sarcoma virus–transformed avian cells, *J. Virol.* **12:**320–327.

CANAANI, E., AND DUESBERG, P., 1972, Role of subunits of 60–70S avian tumor virus ribonucleic acid in its template activity for the viral deoxyribonucleic acid polymerase, *J. Virol.* **10:**23–31.

CANAANI, E., HELM, K. V. D., AND DUESBERG, P., 1973, Evidence for 30–40S RNA as precursor of the 60–70S RNA of Rous sarcoma virus, *Proc. Natl. Acad. Sci.* **70:**401–405.

CHEN, J. H., AND HANAFUSA, H., 1973, Detection of a protein of avian leukoviruses in uninfected chick cells by radioimmunoassay, *J. Virol.* **13:**340–346.

CHEUNG, K. S., SMITH, R. E., STONE, M. P., AND JOKLIK, W. K., 1972, Comparison of immature (rapid harvest) and mature Rous sarcoma virus particles, *Virology* **50:**851–864.

COFFIN, J. M., AND TEMIN, H. M., 1972, Hybridization of Rous sarcoma virus DNA polymerase product and RNA from chicken and rat cells infected with Rous sarcoma virus, *J. Virol* **9:**766–775.

COLBY, C., AND RUBIN, H., 1969, Growth and nucleic acid synthesis in normal cells and cells infected with Rous sarcoma virus, *J. Natl. Cancer Inst.* **43:**437–444.

COOK, M. K., 1969, Cultivation of a filtrable agent associated with Marek's disease, *J. Natl. Cancer Inst.* **43:**203–212.

CRITTENDEN, L. B., AND SMITH, E. J., 1973, Genetic control of spontaneous RAV-0 production, in: *Possible Episomes in Eukaryotes* (L. Silvestri, ed.), North-Holland, Amsterdam.

CRITTENDEN, L. B., STONE, H. A., REAMER, R. H., AND OKAZAKI, W., 1967, Two loci controlling genetic cellular resistance to avian leukosis–sarcoma viruses, *J. Virol.* **1:**898–904.

DALES, S., AND HANAFUSA, H., 1972, Penetration and intracellular release of the genomes of avian RNA tumor viruses, *Virology* **50:**440–458.

DARCEL, C. LE Q., 1973, *Tumor Viruses of the Fowl*, Monograph No. 8, Canadian Department of Agriculture, Ottawa.

DE THÉ, G., BECKER, C., AND BEARD, J. W., 1964, Virus of avian myeloblastosis (BAI strain A). XXV. Ultracytochemical study of virus and myeloblast phosphatase activity, *J. Natl. Cancer Inst.* **32:**201–237.

DOUGHERTY, R. M., AND DISTEFANO, H. S., 1966, Lack of relationship between infection with avian leukosis virus and the presence of COFAL antigen in chick embryos, *Virology* **29:**586–595.

DUESBERG, P. H., 1968, Physical properties of Rous sarcoma virus RNA, *Proc. Natl. Acad. Sci.* **60:**1511–1518.

DUESBERG, P. H., AND VOGT, P. K., 1970, Differences between the ribonucleic acids of transforming and non-transforming avian tumor viruses, *Proc. Natl. Acad. Sci.* **67:**1673–1680.

DUESBERG, P. H., AND VOGT, P. K., 1973, RNA species obtained from clonal lines of avian sarcoma and from avian leukosis virus, *Virology* **54:**207–219.

DUFF, R. G., AND VOGT, P. K., 1969, Characteristics of two new avian tumor virus subgroups, *Virology* **39:**18–30.

ENGELBRETH-HOLM, J., AND ROTHE-MEYER, A., 1935, On the connection between erythroblastosis (haemocytoblastosis), myelosis and sarcoma in chicken. *Acta Pathol. Microbiol. Scand.* **12:**352–365.

ERIKSON, E., AND ERIKSON, R. L., 1970, Isolation of amino acid acceptor RNA from purified avian myeloblastosis virus, *J. Mol. Biol.* **52**:387–390.

FAN, H., AND BALTIMORE, D., 1973, RNA metabolism of murine leukemia virus, *J. Mol. Biol.* **80**:93–117.

FENNER, F., MCAUSLAN, B. R., MIMS, C. A., SAMBROOK, J., AND WHITE, D. O., 1974, *The Biology of Animal Viruses*, 2nd ed., Academic Press, New York.

FIELDS, B. N., AND JOKLIK, W. K., 1969, Isolation and preliminary genetic and biochemical characterization of temperature-sensitive mutants of reovirus, *Virology* **37**:335–342.

FLEISSNER, E., 1971, Chromatographic separation and antigenic analysis of proteins of oncornaviruses. I. Avian leukosis–sarcoma viruses, *J. Virol.* **8**:778–785.

FOULDS, L., 1934, The growth and spread of six filterable tumours of the fowl, transmitted by grafts, *Imperial Cancer Research Fund, 11th Scientific Report*, pp. 15–25.

FRIIS, R. R., 1972, Abortive infection of Japanese quail cells with avian sarcoma viruses, *Virology* **50**:701–712.

FRIIS, R. R., TOYOSHIMA, K., AND VOGT, P. K., 1971, Conditional lethal mutants of avian sarcoma viruses. I. Physiology of ts 75 and ts 149, *Virology* **43**:375–389.

FUJINAMI, A., AND INAMOTO, K., 1914, Ueber Geschwülste bei japanischen Haushühnern insbesondere über einen transplantablen Tumor, *Z. Krebsforsch.* **14**:94.

GOLDIÉ, A., 1970, Radio-induced mutants of the Schmidt–Ruppin strain of Rous sarcoma virus, *Virology* **40**:1022–1029.

GRAF, T., 1972, A plaque assay for avian RNA tumor viruses, *Virology* **50**:567–578.

GRAF, T., BAUER, H., GELDERBLOM, H., AND BOLOGNESI, D. P., 1971, Studies on the reproductive and cell-converting abilities of avian sarcoma viruses, *Virology* **43**:427–441.

GROSS, L., 1970, *Oncogenic Viruses*, 2nd ed., Pergamon Press, New York.

HAGUENAU, F., AND BEARD, J. W., 1962, The avian sarcoma–leukosis complex: Its biology and ultrastructure, in: *Tumors Induced by Viruses: Ultrastructural Studies* (A. J. Dalton and F. Haguenau, eds.), pp. 1–59, Academic Press, New York.

HAKOMORI, S., SAITO, T., AND VOGT, P. K., 1971, Transformation by Rous sarcoma virus: Effects on cellular glycolipids, *Virology* **44**:609–621.

HALPERN, M. S., WADE, E., RUCKER, E., BAXTER-GABBARD, K. L., LEVINE, A. S., AND FRIIS, R. R., 1973, A study of the relationship of reticuloendotheliosis virus to the avian leukosis–sarcoma complex of viruses, *Virology* **53**:287–299.

HANAFUSA, H., 1965, Analysis of the defectiveness of Rous sarcoma virus. III. Determining influence of a new helper virus on the host range and susceptibility to interference of RSV, *Virology* **25**:248–255.

HANAFUSA, H., 1969a, Replication of oncogenic viruses in virus-induced tumor cells—Their persistence and interaction with other viruses, *Advan. Cancer Res.* **12**:137–165.

HANAFUSA, H., 1969b, Rapid transformation of cells by Rous sarcoma virus, *Proc. Natl. Acad. Sci.* **63**:318–325.

HANAFUSA, H., 1970, Virus production by Rous sarcoma cells, *Curr. Top. Microbiol. Immunol.* **51**:114–123.

HANAFUSA, H., AND HANAFUSA, T., 1966a, Analysis of defectiveness of Rous sarcoma virus. IV. Kinetics of RSV production, *Virology* **28**:369–378.

HANAFUSA, H., AND HANAFUSA, T., 1966b, Determining factor in the capacity of Rous sarcoma virus to induce tumors in mammals, *Proc. Natl. Acad. Sci.* **55**:532–538.

HANAFUSA, H., AND HANAFUSA, T., 1968, Further studies on RSV production from transformed cells, *Virology* **34**:630–636.

HANAFUSA, H., AND HANAFUSA, T., 1971, Noninfectious RSV deficient in DNA polymerase, *Virology* **43**:313–316.

HANAFUSA, H., HANAFUSA, T., AND RUBIN, H., 1963, The defectiveness of Rous sarcoma virus, *Proc. Natl. Acad. Sci.* **49**:572–580.

HANAFUSA, H., HANAFUSA, T., AND RUBIN, H., 1964, Analysis of the defectiveness of Rous sarcoma virus. II Specification of RSV antigenicity by helper virus, *Proc. Natl. Acad. Sci.* **51**:41–48.

HANAFUSA, H., MIYAMOTO, T., AND HANAFUSA, T., 1970a, A cell-associated factor essential for formation of an infectious form of Rous sarcoma virus, *Proc. Natl. Acad. Sci.* **66**:314–321.

HANAFUSA, H., HANAFUSA, T., AND MIYAMOTO, T., 1970b, Avian leukosis–sarcoma viruses: Complementation and rescue, in: *The Biology of Oncogenic Viruses* (Second Lepetit Colloquium, L. G. Silvestri, ed.), pp. 170–175, North-Holland, Amsterdam.

HANAFUSA, H., AOKI, T., KAWAI, S., MIYAMOTO, T., AND WILSNACK, R. E., 1973, Presence of antigen common to avian tumor viral envelope antigen in normal chick embryo cells, *Virology* **56**:22–32.

HANAFUSA, T., AND HANAFUSA, H., 1967, Interaction among avian tumor viruses giving enhanced infectivity, *Proc. Natl. Acad. Sci.* **58**:818–825.

HANAFUSA, T., AND HANAFUSA, H., 1973, Isolation of leukosis-type virus from pheasant embryo cells: Possible presence of viral genes in cells, *Virology* **51**:247–251.

HANAFUSA, T., MIYAMOTO, T., AND HANAFUSA, H., 1970a, A type of chick embryo cell that fails to support formation of infectious RSV, *Virology* **40**:55–64.

HANAFUSA, T., HANAFUSA, H., AND MIYAMOTO, T., 1970b, Recovery of a new virus from apparently normal chick cells by infection with avian tumor viruses, *Proc. Natl. Acad. Sci.* **67**:1797–1803.

HANAFUSA, T., HANAFUSA, H., MIYAMOTO, T., AND FLEISSNER, E., 1972, Existence and expression of tumor virus genes in chick embryo cells, *Virology* **47**:475–482.

HAREL, J., HAREL, L., GOLDÉ, A., AND VIGIER, P., 1966, Homologie entre génome du virus du sarcome de Rous (RSV) et génome cellulaire, *Compt. Rend. Acad. Sci. Paris* **263**:745.

HATANAKA, M., AND HANAFUSA, H., 1970, Analysis of a functional change in membrane in the process of cell transformation by Rous sarcoma virus; alteration in the characteristics of sugar transport, *Virology* **41**:647–652.

HATANAKA, M., KAKEFUDA, T., GILDEN, R. V., AND CALLAN, E. A. O., 1971, Cytoplasmic DNA synthesis induced by RNA tumor viruses, *Proc. Natl. Acad. Sci.* **68**:1844–1847.

HAYWARD, W. S., AND HANAFUSA, H., 1973, Detection of avian tumor virus RNA in uninfected chick embryo cells, *J. Virol* **11**:157–167.

HILL, M., AND HILLOVA, H., 1972, Virus recovery in chicken cells tested with Rous sarcoma cell DNA, *Nature New Biol.* **237**:35–39.

HIRST, G. K., 1962, Genetic recombination with Newcastle disease virus, poliovirus, and influenza, *Cold Harbor Symp. Quant. Biol.* **27**:303–309.

HUEBNER, R. J., ARMSTRONG, D., OKUYAN, M., SARMA, P. S., AND TURNER, H. C., 1964, Specific complement-fixing viral antigens in hamster and guinea pig tumors induced by the Schmidt–Ruppin strain of avian sarcoma, *Proc. Natl. Acad. Sci.* **51**:742–750.

HUNG, P. P., 1973, Rescue of chemically inactivated Rous sarcoma virus transforming activity by avian leukosis virus, *Virology* **53**: 463–467.

HUNG, P. P., ROBINSON, H. L., AND ROBINSON, W. S., 1971, Isolation and characterization of proteins from Rous sarcoma virus, *Virology* **43**:251–266.

ISHIMOTO, N., TEMIN, H. M., AND STROMINGER, J. L., 1966, Studies on carcinogenesis by avian sarcoma viruses. II. Virus-induced increase in hyaluronic acid synthetase in chicken fibroblasts, *J. Biol. Chem.* **241**:2052–2057.

ISHIZAKI, R., AND SHIMIZU, T., 1970, Heterogeneity of strain R avian erythroblastosis virus, *Cancer Res.* **30**:2827–2831.

ISHIZAKI, R., AND VOGT, P. K., 1966, Immunological relationships among envelope antigens of avian tumor viruses, *Virology* **30**:375–387.

ISHIZAKI, R., LANGLOIS, A. J., CHABOT, J., AND BEARD, J. W., 1971, Component of strain MC29 avian leukosis virus with the property of defectiveness, *J. Virol.* **8**:821–827.

IVANOV, X., MLADENOV, Z., NEDYALKOV, S., TODOROV, T. G. AND YAKIMOV, M., 1964, Experimental investigations into avian leucoses. V. Transmission, haematology and morphology of avian myelocytomatosis, *Bull. Inst. Pathol. Comp. Anim.* **10**:5–38.

JONSSON, N., AND SJÖGREN, H. O., 1965, Further studies on specific transplantation antigens in Rous sarcoma of mice, *J. Exp. Med.* **122**:403–421.

KABAT, E. A., 1939, A polysaccharide in tumors due to a virus of leucosis and sarcoma of flows, *J. Biol. Chem.* **130**:143–147.

KANG, C. Y., AND TEMIN, H. M., 1972, Endogenous RNA–directed DNA polymerase activity in uninfected chicken embryos, *Proc. Natl. Acad. Sci.* **69**:1550–1554.

KANG, C. Y., AND TEMIN, H. M., 1973, Lack of sequence homology among RNAs of avian leukosis–sarcoma viruses, reticuloendotheliosis viruses, and chicken endogenous RNA–directed DNA polymerase activity, *J. Virol.* **12**:1314–1324.

KAPELLER, M., AND DOLJANSKI, F., 1972, Agglutination of normal and Rous sarcoma virus–transformed chick embryo cells by concanavalin A and wheat germ agglutinin, *Nature New Biol.* **235**:184–185.

KAWAI, S., AND HANAFUSA, H., 1971, The effects of reciprocal changes in temperature on the transformed state of cells infected with a Rous sarcoma virus mutant, *Virology* **46**:470–479.

KAWAI, S., AND HANAFUSA, H., 1972a, Plaque assay for some strains of avian leukosis virus, *Virology* **48**:126–135.

KAWAI, S., AND HANAFUSA, H., 1972b, Genetic recombination with avian tumor virus, *Virology* **49**:37–44.

KAWAI, S., AND HANAFUSA, H., 1973, Isolation of defective mutant of avian sarcoma virus, *Proc. Natl. Acad. Sci.* **70**:3493–3497.

KAWAI, S., METROKA, C. E., AND HANAFUSA, H., 1972, Complementation of functions required for cell transformation by double infection with RSV mutants, *Virology* **49**:302–304.

KURTH. R., AND BAUER, H., 1972, Common tumor-specific surface antigens on cells of different species transformed by avian RNA tumor viruses, *Virology* **49**:145–159.

LAI, M. M. C., AND DUESBERG, P. H., 1972, Adenylic acid–rich sequence in RNAs of Rous sarcoma virus and Rauscher mouse leukaemia virus, *Nature (Lond.)* **235**:383–386.

LANGLOIS, A. J., AND BEARD, J. W., 1967, Converted-cell focus formation in culture by strain MC29 avian leukosis virus, *Proc. Soc. Exp. Biol. Med.* **126**:718–722.

LEONG, J., GARAPIN, A., JACKSON, N., FANSHIER, L., LEVINSON, W., AND BISHOP, J. M., 1972, Virus-specific ribonucleic acid in cells producing Rous sarcoma virus: Detection and characterization, *J. Virol.* **9**:891–902.

LINIAL, M., AND MASON, W. S., 1973, Characterization of two conditional early mutants of Rous sarcoma virus, *Virology* **53**:258–273.

LIVINGSTON, D. M., PARKS, W. P., SCOLNICK, E. M., AND ROSS, J., 1972, Affinity chromatography of avian type C viral reverse transcriptase: Studies with Rous sarcoma virus transformed rat cells, *Virology* **50**:388–395.

LOWY, D. R., ROWE, W. P., TEICH, N., AND HARTLEY, J. W., 1971, Murine leukemia virus: High frequency activation *in vitro* by 5-iododeoxyuridine and 5-bromodeoxyuridine, *Science* **174**:155–156.

LUDFORD, C. G., PURCHASE, H. G., AND COX, H. W., 1972, Duck infectious anemia virus associated with *Plasmodium lophurae*, *Exp. Parasitol.* **31**:29–38.

MACHALA, O., DONNER, L., AND SVOBODA, J., 1970, A full expression of the genome of Rous sarcoma virus in heterokaryons formed after fusion of virogenic mammalian cells and chicken fibroblasts, *J. Gen. Virol.* **8**:219–229.

MACPHERSON, I., 1970, The characteristics of animal cells transformed *in vitro*, *Advan. Cancer Res.* **13**:169–215.

MACPHERSON, I., AND MONTAGNIER, L., 1964, Agar suspension culture for the selective assay of cells transformed by polyoma virus, *Virology* **23**:291–294.

MANAKER, R. A., AND GROUPÉ, V., 1956, Discrete foci of altered chick embryo cells associated with Rous sarcoma virus in tissue culture, *Virology* **2**:838–840.

MARKHAM, P. D., AND BALUDA, M. A., 1973, The integrated state of oncornavirus DNA in normal chicken cells and in cells transformed by avian myeloblastosis virus, *J. Virol.* **12**:721–732.

MARTIN, G. S., 1970, Rous sarcoma virus: A function required for the maintenance of the transformed state, *Nature (Lond.)* **227**:1021–1023.

MARTIN, G. S., AND DUESBERG, P. H., 1972, The a subunit in the RNA of transforming avian tumor viruses. I. Occurrence in different virus strains. II. Spontaneous loss resulting in non-transforming variants, *Virology* **47**:494–497.

MARTIN, G. S., VENUTA, S., WEBER, M., AND RUBIN, H., 1971, Temperature-dependent alterations in sugar transport in cells infected by a temperature-sensitive mutant of Rous sarcoma virus, *Proc. Natl. Acad. Sci.* **68**:2739–2741.

MIYAMOTO, K., AND GILDEN, R. V., 1971, Electron microscopic studies of tumor viruses. I. Entry of murine leukemia virus into mouse embryo fibroblasts, *J. Virol.* **7**:395–406.

MIZUTANI, S., AND TEMIN, H. M., 1973, Lack of serological relationship among DNA polymerases of avian leukosis–sarcoma viruses, reticuloendotheliosis viruses, and chicken cells, *J. Virol.* **12**:440–448.

MÖLLING, K., BOLOGNESI, D. P., BAUER, H., BÜSEN, W., PLASSMANN, H. W., AND HAUSEN, P., 1971, Association of viral reverse transcriptase with an enzyme degrading the RNA moiety of RNA–DNA hybrids, *Nature New Biol.* **234**:240–243.

MOSCOVICI, C., 1967, A quantitative assay for avian myeloblastosis virus, *Proc. Soc. Exp. Biol. Med.* **125**:1213–1215.

MOSCOVICI, C., AND VOGT, P., 1968, Effects of genetic cellular resistance on cell transformation and virus replication in chicken hematopoietic cell cultures infected with avian myeloblastosis virus (BAI-A), *Virology* **35**:487–497.

MOSCOVICI, C., AND ZANETTI, M., 1970, Studies of single foci of hematopoietic cells transformed by avian myeloblastosis virus, *Virology* **42**:61–67.

NEIMAN, P. E., 1972, Rous sarcoma virus nucleotide sequence in cellular DNA: Measurement by RNA–DNA hybridization, *Science* **178**:750–752.

OTTEN, J., BADER, J., JOHNSON, G. S., AND PASTAN, I., 1972, A mutation in a Rous sarcoma virus gene that controls adenosine 3′,5′-monophosphate levels and transformation, *J. Biol. Chem.* **247**:1632–1633.

PARSON, J. T., COFFIN, J. M., HAROZ, R. K., BROMLEY, P. A., AND WEISSMANN, C., 1973, Quantitative determination and location of newly synthesized virus-specific ribonucleic acid in chicken cells infected with Rous sarcoma virus, *J. Virol.* **11**:761–774.

PAYNE, L. N., AND BIGGS, P. M., 1964, Differences between highly inbred lines of chickens in the response to Rous sarcoma virus of the chorioallantoic membrane and of embryonic cells in tissue culture, *Virology* **24**:610–616.

PAYNE, L. N., AND CHUBB, R. C., 1968, Studies on the nature and genetic control of an antigen in normal chick embryos which reacts in the COFAL test, *J. Gen. Virol.* **3**:379–391.

PETERSON, D. A., BAXTER-GABBARD, K. L., AND LEVINE, A. S., 1972, Avian reticuloendotheliosis (strain T). V. DNA polymerase, *Virology* **47**:251–254.

PIRAINO, F., 1967, The mechanism of genetic resistance of chick embryo cells to infection by Rous sarcoma virus—Bryan strain (BS-RSV), *Virology* **32**:700–707.

PONTÉN, J., 1963, Chromosome analysis of three virus-associated chicken tumors: Rous sarcoma, erythroleukemia, and RPL12 lymphoid tumor, *J. Natl. Cancer Inst.* **30**:897–921.

PURCHASE, H. G., LUDFORD, C., NAZARIAN, K., AND COX, H. W., 1973, A new group of oncogenic viruses: Reticuloendotheliosis, chick syncytial, duck infectious anemia, and spleen necrosis viruses, *J. Natl. Cancer Inst.* **51**:489–499.

QUIGLEY, J. P., RIFKIN, D. B., AND REICH, E., 1971, Phospholipid composition of Rous sarcoma virus, host cell membranes and other enveloped RNA viruses, *Virology* **46**:106–116.

REAMER. R. H., AND OKAZAKI, W., 1971, Evidence for the defectiveness of the Harris strain of Rous sarcoma virus, *J. Natl. Cancer Inst.* **44**:763–767.

RIFKIN, D. B., AND COMPANS, R. W., 1971, Identification of the spike proteins of Rous sarcoma virus, *Virology* **46**:485–489.

ROBINSON, H. L., 1967, Isolation of non-infectious particles containing Rous sarcoma virus RNA from the medium of Rous sarcoma virus–transformed nonproducer cells, *Proc. Natl. Acad. Sci.* **57**:1655–1662.

ROBINSON, W. S., AND ROBINSON, H. L., 1971, DNA polymerase in defective Rous sarcoma virus, *Virology* **44**:456–462.

ROBINSON, W. S., PITKANEN, A., AND RUBIN, H., 1965, The nucleic acid of the Bryan strain of Rous sarcoma virus: Purification of the virus and isolation of the nucleic acid, *Proc. Natl. Acad. Sci.* **54**:137–144.

ROSENTHAL, P. N., ROBINSON, H. L., ROBINSON, W. S., HANAFUSA, T., AND HANAFUSA, H., 1971, DNA in uninfected and virus-infected cells complementary to avian tumor virus RNA, *Proc. Natl. Acad. Sci.* **68**:2336–2340.

ROUS, P., 1911, A sarcoma of the fowl transmissible by an agent separable from the tumor cells, *J. Exp. Med.* **13**:397–411.

RUBIN, H., 1955, Quantitative relations between causative virus and cell in the Rous no. 1. chicken sarcoma, *Virology* **1**:445–473.

RUBIN, H., 1960a, A virus in chick embryos which induces resistance *in vitro* to infection with Rous sarcoma virus, *Proc. Natl. Acad. Sci.* **46**:1105–1119.

RUBIN, H., 1960b, An analysis of the assay of Rous sarcoma cells *in vitro* by the infective center technique, *Virology* **10**:29–49.

RUBIN, H., 1960c, The suppression of morphological alterations in cells infected with Rous sarcoma virus, *Virology* **12**:14–31.

RUBIN, H., 1962, The immunological basis for non-infective Rous sarcomas, *Cold Spring Harbor Symp. Quant. Biol.* **27**:441–452.

RUBIN, H., 1965, Genetic control of cellular susceptibility to pseudotypes of Rous sarcoma virus, *Virology* **26**:270–276.

RUBIN, H., 1966, The inhibition of chick embryo cell growth by medium obtained from cultures of Rous sarcoma cells, *Exp. Cell Res.* **41**:149–161.

RUBIN, H., AND TEMIN, H. M., 1959, A radiological study of cell–virus interaction in the Rous sarcoma, *Virology* **7**:75–91.

RUBIN, H., AND VOGT, P. K., 1962, An avian leukosis virus associated with stocks of Rous sarcoma virus, *Virology* **17**:184–194.

RUBIN, H., CORNELIUS, A., AND FANSHIER, L., 1961, The pattern of congenital transmission of an avian leukosis virus, *Proc. Natl. Acad. Sci.* **47**:1058–1069.

RUBIN, H., FANSHIER, L., CORNELIUS, A., AND HUGHES, W. F., 1962, Tolerance and immunity to chickens after congenital and contact infection with an avian leukosis virus, *Virology* **17**:143–156.

SARMA, P. S., TURNER, H. C., AND HUEBNER, R. J., 1964, An avian leukosis group-specific complement fixation reaction: Application for the detection and assay of non-cytopathogenic leukosis viruses, *Virology* **23**:313–321.

SCHEELE, C. M., AND HANAFUSA, H., 1971, Proteins of helper-dependent RSV, *Virology* **45**:401–410.

SCHEELE, C. M., AND HANAFUSA, H., 1972, Electrophoretic analysis of the RNA of avian tumor viruses, *Virology* **50**:753–764.

SIEGERT, W., KONINGS, R. N. H., BAUER, H., AND HOFSCHNEIDER, P. H., 1972, Translation of avian myeloblastosis virus RNA in a cell-free lysate of *Escherichia coli*, *Proc. Natl. Acad. Sci.* **69**:888–891.

SIMKOVIC, D., 1972, Characteristics of tumors induced in mammals, especially rodents, by viruses of the avian leukosis sarcoma group, *Advan. Virus Res.* **17**:95–127.

STECK, F. T., AND RUBIN, H., 1965, The mechanism of interference between an avian leukosis virus and Rous sarcoma virus. II. Early steps of infection by RSV of cells under conditions of interference, *Virology* **29**:642–653.

STECK, T. L., KAUFMAN, S., AND BADER, J. P., 1968, Glycolysis in chick embryo cell cultures transformed by Rous sarcoma virus, *Cancer Res.* **28**:1611–1619.

STEPHENSON, J. R., AND AARONSON, S. A., 1972, A genetic locus for inducibility of C-type virus in Balb/c cells: The effect of a nonlinked regulatory gene on detection of virus after chemical activation, *Proc. Natl. Acad. Sci.* **69**:2798–2801.

STEPHENSON, J. R., WILSNACK, R. E., AND AARONSON, S. A., 1973, Radioimmunoassay for avian C-type virus group specific antigen: Detection in normal and virus transformed cells, *J. Virol.* **11**:893–899.

SUNI, J., VAHERI, A., AND RUOSLAHTI, E., 1973, Radioimmunoassay of avian RNA tumor virus group-specific antigen, *Intervirology* **1**:119–126.

SVOBODA, J., 1964, Malignant interaction of Rous virus with mammalian cells *in vivo* and *in vitro*, *Natl. Cancer Inst. Monogr.* **17**:277–292.

SVOBODA, J., AND HLOZÁNEK, I., 1970, Role of cell association in virus infection and virus rescue, *Advan. Cancer Res.* **13**:217–269.

TAYLOR, H. W., AND OLSON, L. D., 1972, Spectrum of infectivity and transmission of the T-virus, *Avian Dis.* **16**:330–335.

TEMIN, H. M., 1960, The control of cellular morphology in embryonic cells infected with Rous sarcoma virus *in vitro*, *Virology* **10**:182–197.

TEMIN, H. M., 1963, The effect of actinomycin D on growth of Rous sarcoma virus *in vitro*, *Virology* **20**:577–582.

TEMIN, H. M., 1964a, The participation of DNA in Rous sarcoma virus production, *Virology* **23**:486–494.

TEMIN, H. M., 1964b, The nature of the provirus of Rous sarcoma, *Natl. Cancer Inst. Monogr.* **17**:557–570.

TEMIN, H. M., 1965, The mechanism of carcinogenesis by avian sarcoma viruses. I. Cell multiplication and differentiation, *J. Natl. Cancer Inst.* **35**:679–693.

TEMIN, H. M., 1968, Studies on carcinogenesis by avian sarcoma viruses. VIII. Glycolysis and cell multiplication, *Int. J. Cancer* **3**:273–282.

TEMIN, H. M., 1971, Mechanism of cell transformation by RNA tumor viruses, *Ann. Rev. Microbiol.* **25**:609–648.

TEMIN, H. M., 1973, The cellular and molecular biology of RNA tumor viruses, especially avian leukosis–sarcoma viruses, and their relatives, *Advan. Cancer Res.* **19**:47–104.

TEMIN, H. M., AND BALTIMORE, D., 1972, RNA-directed DNA synthesis and RNA tumor viruses, *Advan. Virus Res.* **17**:129–186.

TEMIN, H. M., AND MIZUTANI, S., 1970, RNA-dependent DNA polymerase in virions of Rous sarcoma virus, *Nature (Lond.)* **226**:1211–1213.

TEMIN, H. M., AND RUBIN, H., 1958, Characteristics of an assay for Rous sarcoma virus and Rous sarcoma cells in tissue culture, *Virology* **6**:669–688.

TEMIN, H. M., AND RUBIN, H., 1959, A kinetic study of infection of chick embryo cells *in vitro* by Rous sarcoma virus, *Virology* **8**:209–222.

TEMIN, H. M., PIERSON, R. W., JR., AND DULAK, N. C., 1972, The role of serum in the control of multiplication of avian and mammalian cells in culture, in: *Growth, Nutrition, and Metabolism of Cells in Culture*, Vol. 1 (G. H. Rothblat and V. J. Cristofalo, eds.), pp. 49–81, Academic Press, New York.

THEILEN, G. H., ZEIGEL, R. F., AND TWIEHAUS, M. J., 1966, Biological studies with RE virus (strain T) that induces reticuloendotheliosis in turkeys, chickens, and Japanese quail, *J. Natl. Cancer Inst.* **37**:731–743.

THURZO, V., SMIDA, J., SMIDOVA-KOVAROVA, V., AND SIMKOVIC, D., 1963, Some properties of the fowl virus tumor B77, *Acta Unio Int. Contra Cancrum* **19**:304–305.

TOOZE, J. (ed.), 1973, The molecular biology of tumor viruses, Cold Spring Harbor Laboratory, Cold Spring Harbor, New York.

TOYOSHIMA, K., AND VOGT, P. K., 1969*a*, Enhancement and inhibition of avian sarcoma viruses by polycations and polyanions, *Virology* **38**:414–426.

TOYOSHIMA, K., AND VOGT, P. K., 1969*b*, Temperature sensitive mutants of an avian sarcoma virus, *Virology* **39**:930–931.

TOYOSHIMA, K., FRIIS, R. R., AND VOGT, P. K., 1970, The reproductive and cell-transforming capacities of avian sarcoma virus B77: Inactivation with UV light, *Virology* **42**:163–170.

TRAGER, W., 1959, A new virus of ducks interfering with development of malaria parasite (*Plasmodium lophurae*), *Proc. Soc. Exp. Biol. Med.* **101**:578–582.

UNKELESS, J. C., TOBIA, A., OSSOWSKI, L., QUIGLEY, J. P., RIFKIN, D. B., AND REICH, E., 1973*a*, An enzymatic function associated with transformation of fibroblasts by oncogenic viruses. I. Chick embryo fibroblast cultures transformed by avian RNA tumor viruses, *J. Exp. Med.* **137**:85–111.

UNKELESS, J. C., DANØ, K., KELLERMAN, G. M., AND REICH, E., 1973*b*, Fibrinolysis associated with oncogenic transformation: Partial purification and characterization of the cell factor—a plasminogen activator, *J. Biol. Chem.* **249**:4295–4305.

VARMUS, H. E., LEVINSON, W. E., AND BISHOP, J. M., 1971, Extent of transcription by the RNA dependent DNA polymerase of Rous sarcoma virus, *Nature New Biol.* **233**:19–21.

VARMUS, H. E., WEISS, R. A., FRIIS, R. R., LEVINSON, W., AND BISHOP, J. M., 1972, Detection of avian tumor virus–specific nucleotide sequences in avian cell DNA, *Proc. Natl. Acad. Sci.* **69**:20–24.

VARMUS, H. E., BISHOP, J. M., AND VOGT, P. K., 1973*a*, Appearance of virus-specific DNA in mammalian cells following transformation by Rous sarcoma virus, *J. Mol. Biol.* **73**:613–626.

VARMUS, H. E., VOGT, P. K., AND BISHOP, J. M., 1973*b*, Integration of Rous sarcoma virus–specific DNA following infection of permissive and non-permissive hosts, *Proc. Natl. Acad. Sci.* **70**:3067–3071.

VECCHIO, G., TSUCHIDA, N., SHANMUGAM, G., AND GREEN, M., 1973, Virus specific messenger RNA and nascent polypeptides in polyribosomes of cells replicating murine sarcoma–leukemia viruses, *Proc. Natl. Acad. Sci.* **70**:2064–2068.

VIGIER, P., 1970*a*, Effect of agar, calf embryo extract, and polyanions on production of foci of transformed cells by Rous sarcoma virus, *Virology* **40**:179–192.

VIGIER, P., 1970*b*, RNA oncogenic viruses: Structure, replication, and oncogenicity, *Prog. Med. Virol.* **12**:240–283.

VIGIER, P., AND GOLDÉ, A., 1964, Effects of actinomycin D and of mitomycin C on the development of Rous sarcoma virus, *Virology* **23**:511–519.

VIGIER, P., AND SVOBODA, J., 1965, Etude, en culture, de la production du virus de Rous par contact entre les cellules du sarcome XC du rat et les cellules d'embryon de poule, *Compt. Rend. Acad. Sci. Paris* **261**:4278–4281.

VOGT, P. K., 1965*a*, Avian tumor viruses, *Advan. Virus Res.* **11**:293–385.

VOGT, P. K., 1965*b*, A heterogeneity of Rous sarcoma virus revealed by selectively resistant chick embryo cells, *Virology* **25**:237–247.

VOGT, P. K., 1967*a*, Phenotypic mixing in the avian tumor virus group, *Virology* **32**:708–717.

VOGT, P. K., 1967*b*, DEAE-dextran enhancement of cellular transformation induced by avian sarcoma viruses, *Virology* **33**:175–177.

VOGT, P. K., 1967*c*, Virus-directed host responses in the avian leukosis and sarcoma complex, in: *Perspectives in Virology*, Vol. V (M. Pollard, ed.), pp. 199–228, Academic Press, New York.

VOGT, P. K., 1969, Focus assay of Rous sarcoma virus, in: *Fundamental Techniques in Virology* (K. Habel and N. P. Salzman, eds.), pp. 198–211, Academic Press, New York.

VOGT, P. K., 1971a, Spontaneous segregation of non-transforming viruses from cloned sarcoma viruses, *Virology* **46:**939–946.

VOGT, P. K., 1971b, Genetically stable reassortment of markers during mixed infection with avian tumor viruses, *Virology* **46:**947–952.

VOGT, P. K., AND FRIIS, R. R., 1971, An avian leukosis virus related to RSV(0): Properties and evidence for helper activity, *Virology* **43:**223–234.

VOGT, P. K., AND ISHIZAKI, R., 1965, Reciprocal patterns of genetic resistance to avian tumor viruses in two lines of chickens, *Virology* **26:**664–672.

VOGT, P. K., AND ISHIZAKI, R., 1966, Patterns of viral interference in the avian leukosis and sarcoma complex, *Virology* **30:**368–374.

VOGT, P. K., AND RUBIN, H., 1963, Studies on the assay and multiplication of avian myeloblastosis virus, *Virology* **19:**92–104.

VOGT, V. M., AND EISENMAN, R., 1973, Identification of a large polypeptide precursor of avian oncornavirus proteins, *Proc. Natl. Acad. Sci.* **70:**1734–1738.

WARREN, L., CRITCHLEY, D., AND MACPHERSON, I., 1972, Surface glycoproteins and glycolipids of chicken embryo cells transformed by a temperature-sensitive mutant of Rous sarcoma virus, *Nature (Lond.)* **235:**275–277.

WEISS, R. A., 1969, The host range of Bryan strain Rous sarcoma virus synthesized in the absence of helper virus, *J. Gen. Virol.* **5:**511–528.

WEISS, R. A., AND PAYNE, L. N., 1971, The heritable nature of the factor in chicken cells which acts as a helper virus for Rous sarcoma virus, *Virology* **45:**508–515.

WEISS, R. A., FRIIS, R. R., KATZ, E., AND VOGT, P. K., 1971, Induction of avian tumor viruses in normal cells by physical and chemical carcinogens, *Virology* **46:**920–938.

WEISS, R. A., MASON, W. S., AND VOGT, P. K., 1973, Genetic recombinants and heterozygotes derived from endogenous and exogenous avian RNA tumor viruses, *Virology* **52:**535–552.

WEISSBACH, A., BOLDEN, A., MULLER, R., HANAFUSA, H., AND HANAFUSA, T., 1972, Deoxyribonucleic acid polymerase activities in normal and leukovirus-infected chicken embryo cells, *J. Virol.* **10:**321–327.

WICKUS, G. G., AND ROBBINS, P. W., 1973, Plasma membrane proteins of normal and Rous sarcoma virus–transformed chick embryo fibroblasts, *Nature New Biol.* **245:**65–67.

WYKE, J. A., 1973, Complementation of transforming functions by temperature-sensitive mutants of avian sarcoma virus, *Virology* **54:**28–36.

WYKE, J. A., AND LINIAL, M., 1973, Temperature-sensitive avian sarcoma viruses: A physiological comparison of twenty mutants, *Virology* **53:**152–161.

ZAVADA, J., 1972, VSV pseudotype particles with the coat of avian myeloblastosis virus, *Nature New Biol.* **240:**122–124.

ZEIGEL, R. F., THEILEN, G. H., AND TWIEHAUS, M. J., 1966, Electron microscopic observations on RE virus (strain T) that induces reticuloendotheliosis in turkeys, chickens, and Japanese quail, *J. Natl. Cancer Inst.* **37:**709–729.

3

Mammalian Type C RNA Viruses

MICHAEL M. LIEBER AND GEORGE J. TODARO

1. Introduction

Type C RNA viruses are a distinct class of vertebrate viruses which share a common morphology, protein composition, and viral life cycle, have single-stranded RNA as their viral genome, and contain an RNA-directed DNA polymerase (reverse transcriptase).

Type C viruses have been shown to cause a variety of naturally occurring vertebrate neoplastic diseases including leukemias and sarcomas of chickens, lymphomas and related hematopoietic neoplasms of mice, and lymphosarcomas and fibrosarcomas of domestic cats. Additional type C viruses have been isolated from other mammalian species such as rats, guinea pigs, hamsters, cattle, domestic pigs, woolly monkeys, gibbons, and baboons, but, as yet, the relationship between these viruses and neoplastic diseases of their host species is not clear (Table 1). There have been reports of electron microscopic observation of typical type C viral particles in tissues from certain other mammalian species, including dogs, horses, and rhesus monkeys, and from human placentas and certain human neoplasms, but such viruses have not yet been isolated *in vitro* and biochemically characterized.

The genetic information for the production of vertebrate type C viruses is commonly transmitted "vertically" from parent to progeny as DNA integrated in the cellular genome, without full expression of the viral genes. Such "endogenous" type C "virogenes" or "proviruses" have now been directly demonstrated in the DNA from chickens and a variety of mammalian species, including species of

MICHAEL M. LIEBER and GEORGE J. TODARO ● Viral Leukemia and Lymphoma Branch, National Cancer Institute, National Institutes of Health, Bethesda, Maryland.

Old World monkeys. Because of their wide prevalence among vertebrate species, it seems likely that endogenous type C virogenes must generate a selective advantage in the species carrying them. However, what physiological functions such endogenous type C virogenes generally perform and the relationship of endogenous type C virogenes to neoplastic disease in their natural hosts are unclear at present. It seems certain that various type C viruses can also be naturally transmitted "horizontally," from one animal to another, by virus-containing respiratory droplets, saliva, urine, and milk, and also by congenital infection *in utero*. Such exogenous infection patterns, now established for avian and feline leukemia viruses, may also occur with the woolly monkey sarcoma virus (SSV-1) and the gibbon lymphosarcoma virus (Scolnick *et al.*, 1974; Benvenisre *et al.*, 1974*a*).

At the present time, there have been no confirmed isolations of infectious type C virus from human tissues. Nevertheless, even without the direct clinical relevance that would be provided by such human isolates, it is evident that mammalian type C viruses provide challenging possibilities for understanding the molecular basis of certain mammalian neoplastic diseases and may, eventually, be shown to be the etiological agents responsible for certain human tumors.

TABLE 1

Mammalian Type C RNA Virus Isolates

Species	Description
Mouse (*Mus musculus*)	Many well-studied laboratory strain murine leukemia and sarcoma viruses (MuLV, MSV); large variety of endogenous viruses
Rat (*Rattus norvegicus*)	Endogenous viruses released from numerous rat cell lines in culture; poorly infectious
Chinese hamster (*Cricetulus griseus*) and Syrian (or golden) hamster (*Mesocricetus auratur*)	Poorly infectious viruses released from cells in culture
Guinea pig (*Cavies* spp.)	Type C virus induced from cultured cells and associated with spontaneous and transmissible leukemia
Domestic cat (*Felis catus*)	Two distinct classes: (a) feline leukemia and sarcoma viruses (FeLV, FeSV); (b) RD-114/CCC family of endogenous feline viruses
Pig (*Sus scrofa*)	Endogenous viruses released from cell lines in culture
Cattle (*Bos taurus*)	Infectious type C viruses isolated from lymphosarcoma tissue
Woolly monkey (*Lagothrix* spp.)	Simian sarcoma virus (SSV-1)
Baboon (*Papio cynocephalus*)	Endogenous viruses which replicate well in cells from heterologous species
Gibbon (*Hylobates lar*)	Gibbon lymphosarcoma virus (GALV)

All mammalian type C viruses isolated so far have a common ultrastructural appearance and common biochemical and antigenic properties which define them as a class. These common characteristics are listed in Table 2.

2.1. Morphology

The development of ultrathin sectioning techniques permitted the first significant electron microscopic characterization of mammalian type C viruses (Dmochowski and Grey, 1957; Bernhard, 1958). Tissues from mice with spontaneous leukemia or leukemia induced by inoculation of virus filtrates were found to contain in their intercellular spaces spherical viral particles with a diameter of approximately 100 nm. Bernhard (1958) described a system of morphological classification of mammalian RNA tumor viruses which is still in use. The morphological form of virion invariably associated with preparations of murine leukemia viruses was called a "C-type" particle. All subsequent biochemically related mammalian viruses have been found to share the same morphology and mechanism of assembly. C-type or type C particles are always located extracellularly near the surface of cells or in intracytoplasmic vacuoles and consist of a spherical core of about 70 nm diameter surrounded by a viral envelope, giving an outside diameter

TABLE 2

Common Properties of Mammalian Type C RNA Viruses

Ultrastructure (type C particles): 90- to 110-nm spherical viral particles with central symmetrical electron-dense nucleoid of approximately 70 nm diameter; viral surface generally possesses short spikes or knobs

Assembly: Typical "condensation" of electron-dense nucleoid beneath surface of cytoplasmic cell membrane with subsequent "budding" of type C particle from cell surface

Viral genome: Single-stranded RNA which sediments at 60–70S (probably about 1×10^7 daltons molecular weight); denaturation yields subunits sedimenting at 30–40S (probably about $3–4 \times 10^6$ daltons molecular weight)

Reverse transcriptase: Transcribes single-stranded RNA into homologous copies of DNA; molecular weight generally 70,000

Group-specific antigens: Antigenic determinants carried on the major internal viral protein (mol wt 25,000–30,000) and on other viral proteins; there now appear to be type-specific, intraspecies, and interspecies antigenic reactivities on several different proteins of the mammalian type C viral isolates studied so far

In vitro replication: Most isolates generally produce no detectable cytopathic effect in culture; however, sarcoma viruses can transform fibroblasts

Pseudotype formation: Can form pseudotype virions with genomes of various mammalian sarcoma viruses; can rescue the sarcoma virus genome from "nonproducer" sarcoma virus–transformed cell lines

Miscellaneous:
Density ~1.16 g/ml
Inactivated by ether and detergents

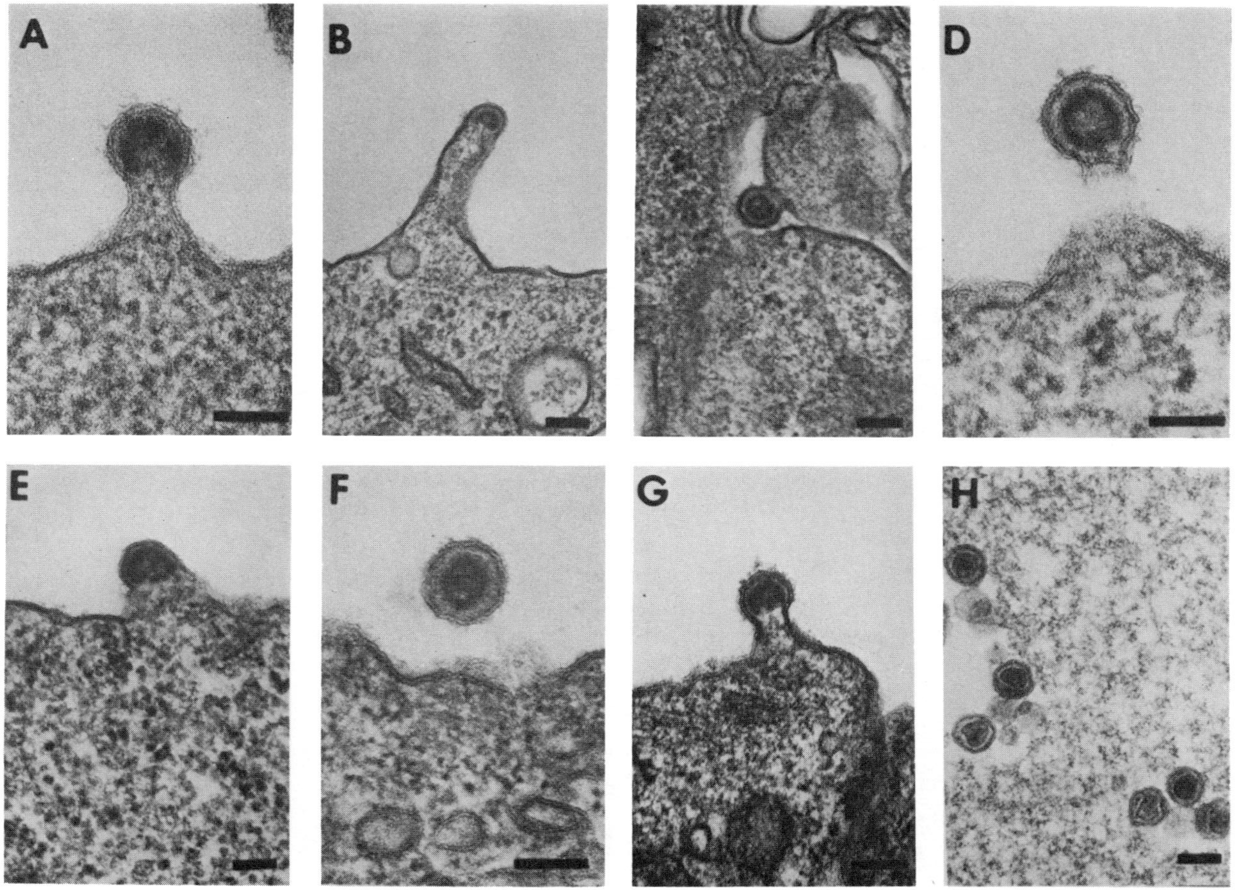

M. M. LIEBER
AND
G. J. TODARO

FIGURE 1. Electron micrographs of type C virions released by mammalian cell lines. (A) Budding particle from the Chinese hamster NCTC 4206 (CCL 14.2) cell line. (B,C) Budding particles from the Chinese hamster CHO-K1 (CCL 61) cell line 5 days after treatment with 5-iododeoxy-uridine (30 g/ml) for 48 h. (D,E) Free and budding virions from the rat RR1022 (CCL 47) cell line. (F) A free type C particle from the fetal cat FFc2K cell strain. (G,H) Free and budding particles from the pig PK(15) (CCL 33) cell line. The scale represents 100 nm.

of 90–110 nm (Bernhard, 1973, see Fig. 1). [B-type particles have been regularly

associated with mouse mammary tumor virus (MMTV) preparations and are similar-sized particles but with an eccentric core and prominent surface spikes (Sarkar *et al.*, 1973, Fig. 1); A-type particles are double-shelled spheres of about 70 nm diameter which are commonly found in the cytoplasm and endoplasmic reticulum cisternae of various murine solid tumors and leukemias. It is not clear whether A-type particles, which are very similar morphologically to the cores of type C particles, are in fact related to type C viruses.]

Type C particles are assembled in the cytoplasm and bud from the cell membrane. At the earliest stage, a protrusion of the cell surface is associated with a crescent of electron-dense material. As the bud elongates into a microvillus-like structure, the crescent curves into a circle and becomes the viral core, while the plasma membrane is gradually transformed into a spherical viral envelope. These pinched-off "immature" type C particles resemble enveloped A-type particles. Subsequently, the center of the viral core becomes electron dense, and such particles are called "mature" type C particles.

Recently, Nermut *et al.* (1972) have carefully studied the morphology of Rauscher, Gross, and Friend murine leukemia viruses (MuLV) by a combination of negative-staining, freeze-drying, and freeze-etching techniques. These techniques demonstrate that the surface of MuLV virions is covered with "knobs" of about 80 Å diameter which are weakly bound to the viral membrane; the knobs are commonly lost when other techniques of fixation and staining are used. Viral cores liberated by ether or detergent treatment showed a regular surface pattern of hexagonally arranged subunits with a diameter of about 60 Å; together with the occasional observation of pentons, this evidence suggests that the viral core has an icosahedral shape. The internal "nucleoid" or nucleocapsid component of the viral core was found to be a filamentous structure which might possess helical symmetry. Similar data about the fine structure of avian type C particles have also been published (Gelderblom *et al.*, 1972), suggesting a common morphology for vertebrate type C particles in general.

2.2. Chemical Composition

2.2.1. Viral Genome

When RNA is extracted from mammalian type C viruses and sedimented through neutral sucrose gradients, a major component is found which sediments at 60–70S. The 60–70S RNA is believed to be the viral genome and has a molecular weight, from hydrodynamic considerations, of $10–13 \times 10^6$ daltons (Duesberg and Robinson, 1966). The 60–70S viral RNA is fully susceptible to digestion with pancreatic ribonuclease and its base composition is consistent with a single-stranded structure (Duesberg and Robinson, 1966). When the 60–70S RNA is denatured by heating or by exposure to urea, formaldehyde, or dimethylsulfoxide, it sediments slower than the original viral RNA (30–40S), and migrates faster during electrophoresis in polyacrylamide gels. The conclusion drawn is that the viral genome is composed of RNA subunits, each with a molecular weight of $3–4 \times 10^6$ daltons, assembled through weak interactions (Duesberg, 1970). Such results are consistent with similar studies of avian type C viruses.

The 60–70S RNA component of mammalian type C virions cannot be detected in the cytoplasm of virus-producing cells, whereas a 30–40S component is present within such cells (Watson, 1971). Fan and Baltimore (1973), using molecular hybridization techniques and a labeled DNA transcript of Moloney MuLV, have shown that 35S RNA serves as the virus-specific messenger RNA in Moloney MuLV–infected cells. Thus the 60–70S RNA component is probably formed during virion assembly at the cell surface and release from the cell. Finally, although the 30–40S RNA subunits of newly synthesized MuLV are homogeneous in size, RNA subunits from virions aged for a period of hours at 37°C are of heterogeneous sizes, presumably representing degradative products of the 30–40S subunit (Bader and Steck, 1969; Watson, 1971). Thus the "maturation" of mammalian type C virions observed by electron microscopic studies may reflect the intravirion disruption of the viral RNA genome (Bader and Steck, 1969).

Kakefuda and Bader (1969) have directly observed the RNA viral genome of Rauscher MuLV using the protein monolayer technique and electron microscopy. Purified viral 60–70S RNA appeared as long straight filaments 6–14 μm long, but when denatured the viral RNA collapsed into tangled filaments. No suggestion of subunit structure could be detected. In contrast, Kung *et al.* (1974) studied the RNA genome of the RD-114 endogenous cat type C virus by electron microscopy under denaturing conditions and reported the presence of large subunits of about 5.0×10^6 molecular weight (3.7 μm in length) with a characteristic "rabbit ears" secondary structure near the center of the genome.

The 60–70S viral RNA of most murine leukemia–sarcoma viruses has been shown to contain poly(A)-rich sequences of over 90% adenylic acid in stretches from 150 to 250 nucleotides long. These sequences sediment at 4–5S; each 60–70S viral genome probably contains three to eight poly(A) sequences (Lai and Duesberg, 1972; Green and Cartas, 1972; Ross *et al.*, 1972). Such sequences have also been identified in messenger RNA and heterogeneous nuclear RNA fractions of mammalian cells (Lim and Canellakis, 1970; Edmonds *et al.*, 1971; Darnell *et al.*, 1971; Lee *et al.*, 1971) and in viral RNA of cells infected with the DNA viruses vaccina (Kates, 1970) and adenovirus (Phillipson *et al.*, 1971). The function these poly(A)-rich sequences serve in viral RNAs has not been determined.

2.2.2. Reverse Transcriptase

All mammalian type C viruses possess an RNA-directed DNA polymerase or "reverse transcriptase" which can synthesize homologous DNA from single-stranded RNA templates (Baltimore, 1970; Temin and Mitzutani, 1970). The conversion of the viral RNA genome into DNA permits unique interactions between type C viruses and their vertebrate cellular hosts (i.e., the integration of type C virus–specific sequences into the chromosomal DNA) so that the reverse transcription mechanism appears to be the key element in the biology of type C viruses (Temin, 1971). The molecular biology of reverse transcriptases is thoroughly reviewed in the chapter by Bishop and Varmus. For our purposes, certain properties of type C viral reverse transcriptases need emphasis.

The presence of reverse transcriptase activity is a definitive property of mammalian type C viruses, and since this activity can be measured *in vitro* using synthetic templates and primers, biochemical assays to detect the presence of type C virus in tissue cultures and other specimens have been developed (Ross *et al.*, 1971; Kelloff *et al.*, 1972). These assays are rapid and very sensitive, so that testing for viral reverse transcriptase activity is a common technique for identifying the presence of type C virus (Lieber *et al.*, 1973a). The mammalian enzymes studied so far have molecular weights of about 70,000, in contrast to a molecular weight of about 160,000 for the avian type C viral polymerase (Ross *et al.*, 1971; Kacian *et al.*, 1971). Mammalian type C reverse transcriptases are antigenically distinct from both the avian type C viral polymerases and the RNA-directed DNA polymerases of mammalian B-type viruses (mouse mammary tumor virus) and certain other mammalian RNA viruses such as foamy viruses, Mason-Pfizer viruses, and visna virus (Parks *et al.*, 1972). Thus, antisera directed against polymerases from mammalian type C viruses can be used to classify reverse transcriptases as mammalian type C viral in origin. In addition, antipolymerase sera directed toward species-specific determinants on the reverse transcriptases can be used to identify the species of origin of unknown mammalian type C viruses (Aaronson *et al.*, 1971a; Scolnick *et al.*, 1972a).

Finally, of considerable recent importance has been the refinement in technique permitting the generation of highly labeled DNA transcripts of type C viral RNAs through the use of the reverse transcriptase enzyme *in vitro*. These DNA products can be used in nucleic acid hybridization studies to determine the relatedness of given DNAs and RNAs. Such nucleic acid hybridization techniques have permitted rapid advances in understanding the taxonomy and molecular biology of mammalian type C viruses, as indicated in the subsequent sections of this chapter.

2.2.3. Proteins

Those mammalian type C viruses which have been characterized biochemically have been found to possess six major structural proteins (in addition to the reverse transcriptase) (Nowinski *et al.*, 1972; August *et al.*, 1974). Two proteins are glycoproteins and are structural elements of the viral coat and knobs (Witte *et al.*, 1973). Immunological assays for various viral structural proteins are the major means at present used for classification of given mammalian type C viral isolates. Three classes of antigenic determinants present on mammalian type C viral proteins have been defined: type specific, group specific, and interspecies. Type-specific antigens, which distinguish different viruses derived from the same species of animal, have been characterized chiefly by studies of virus neutralization (Eckner and Steeves, 1972; Gomard *et al.*, 1972). Group-specific antigens have been identified as those that are common to different viruses of the same species. Several viral components showing group-specific antigenicity have been detected by immunodiffusion analysis of degraded virions or by partial purification of the viral proteins (Geering et al., 1966; Hartley et al., 1965; Nowinski et al., 1972; Schäfer et al., 1972). Included among these is the major structural protein of the type C viruses, with a molecular weight of about 27,000–30,000 ("p27–p30"), which has been extensively purified and characterized and is an internal element of the virion. Interspecies antigens, first described by Geering et al. (1968, 1970), are defined as those that are common among type C viruses of different animal species. At this time, three components of mammalian type C viruses are known to possess such determinants: the major internal protein (p30), the viral RNA–dependent DNA polymerase, and the glycopeptide ("gp69–71") which appears to be an element of the viral envelope (Strand and August, 1974). Whether there exist interspecies determinants common to all mammalian type C viruses has not been determined.

A variety of immunological tests to detect the structural proteins of mammalian type C viruses have been developed. For example, at present, highly sensitive radioimmunoassays exist for the 30,000 molecular weight protein (p30) of all known mammalian type C viruses. Radioimmunoassays also exist for the approximately 12,000 molecular weight protein of murine viruses ("p12") (Stephenson et al., 1974b) and for the high molecular weight glycoprotein of murine type C viruses (Strand and August, 1974). Such assays will detect nanogram amounts of viral proteins.

3. Biological Properties in Vitro

Mammalian type C viruses generally can be grown in vitro in cell lines from homologous or heterologous mammalian species. For example, type C viruses can be readily isolated from murine lymphomatous tumors and grown in murine fibroblast cultures; similarly, type C viruses isolated from feline lymphosarcomas replicate to high titer in fibroblast cultures of cat cells, as well as in cells from canine, human, and other primate species. Such "leukemia" viruses, as well as the "endogenous" mammalian type C viruses (see below), generally produce no cytopathic effect when replicating in fibroblasts, so that infected and uninfected cultures appear identical by light microscopy, and special methods must be used to detect and titer such viruses (Table 3). However, it has proved difficult to find permissive host cell lines for type C viruses released from cells of certain mammalian species. The endogenous viruses released from rat, hamster, and pig cell lines, even though they are spontaneously released in high titer and have reverse transcriptase activity, have not yet been shown to be infectious for other cell lines (Lieber et al., 1973a).

The type C viruses isolated from fibrosarcomas of mice, cats, and a woolly monkey, which cause sarcomas when inoculated into animals, cause fibroblasts to transform in vitro. This property can be used for the ready detection and quantification of "sarcoma" viruses, since transformed foci of cells are generally distinct morphologically from the surrounding field of uninfected cells. Figures 2 and 3 show photographs of typical murine sarcoma virus–transformed fibroblasts. The use of contact-inhibited cell lines in these focus formation assays further permits easier recognition of the transformed foci and ease in cloning the resultant transformed cells (Jainchill *et al.*, 1969).

With standard preparations of transforming DNA viruses, such as SV40 or polyoma, there is a linear or "one-hit" relationship between the number of transformed colonies and the virus dilution. In early studies of murine sarcoma virus (MSV), however, Hartley and Rowe (1966) and others (O'Connor and Fischinger, 1968; Yoshikura *et al.*, 1968; Parkman *et al.*, 1970) described a different pattern for focus formation in mouse cells. Here, the number of detectable foci falls as the square of the virus dilution (a "two-hit" titration pattern). The addition of optimal levels of "helper" murine leukemia virus (MuLV), which itself does not produce morphological alteration, changes the titration pattern from two-hit to one-hit. This two-hit pattern for focus formation led to the conclusion that MSV is defective and requires a "helper" leukemia virus for focus formation. Subsequently, it has been shown that all mammalian type C sarcoma viruses (mouse, feline, and woolly monkey) are transforming, replication-defective viruses. These transforming viruses require coinfection with nontransforming "helper" type C virus in order to generate productive infections. Thus mammalian type C sarcoma viruses are markedly different from most Rous sarcoma virus isolates among the avian type C viruses, since, in general, Rous sarcoma virus isolates can transform cells *and* replicate.

Most preparations of MSV contain a large excess of nontransforming helper type C viruses. However, the existence of certain preparations of MSV with only a small excess of helper type C virus has permitted study of the cellular events

TABLE 3

Commonly Used Assay Techniques for Detection of Nontransforming Mammalian Type C RNA Viruses

1. Electron microscopic demonstration of typical extracellular and budding particles
2. Assay of reverse transcriptase activity in tissue culture fluid
3. Detection of group-specific antigens (species specific or interspecies) by radioimmunoassay, complement fixation, immunodiffusion, or fluorescent antibody techniques
4. Labeling of viral RNA with radioactive ribonucleotides with the subsequent demonstration of label in particles with a density of 1.16 g/ml and in 60–70S single-stranded RNA
5. Demonstration of rescue of a mammalian sarcoma virus genome from a "nonproducer" cell line by a transformed focus formation assay
6. Interference with a focus formation assay by appropriate sarcoma virus or sarcoma pseudotype (thus preinfection with a related "helper" type C virus interferes with subsequent focus formation by the homologous sarcoma virus pseudotype)
7. Pseudotype formation with vesicular stomatitis virus (VSV) genomes
8. *In vitro* tests for murine leukemia viruses:
   XC plaque test (Klement *et al.*, 1969*b*; Rowe *et al.*, 1970)
   S^+L^- plaque test (Bassin *et al.*, 1971*b*)
9. Nucleic acid hybridization techniques using labeled viral RNA or labeled DNA transcripts of the viral RNA genome

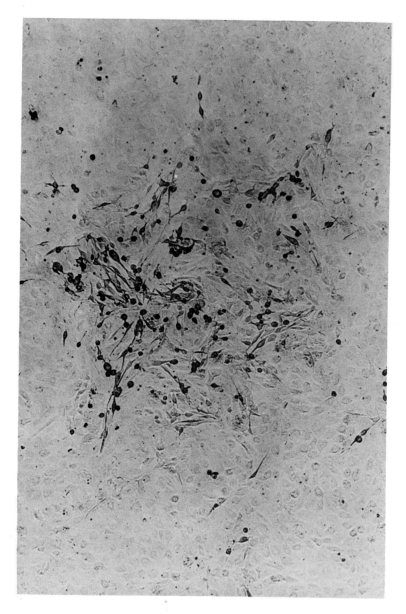

FIGURE 2. Transformed focus induced in BALB/3T3 cells by infection with Moloney murine sarcoma virus 7 days previously. × 49.

transpiring after infection of fibroblasts *in vitro* with the transforming, nonreplicating MSV genome alone. Such "nonproducer" MSV foci are transformed morphologically, but are generally much smaller in size and appear at a later time than productively infected MSV foci, which is why these foci were not detected in the studies cited above. The difference in focus size occurs because the nonproducer foci acquire more cells only by cell division, whereas producer foci enlarge also by infectious cell-to-cell transmission of the MSV genome. The

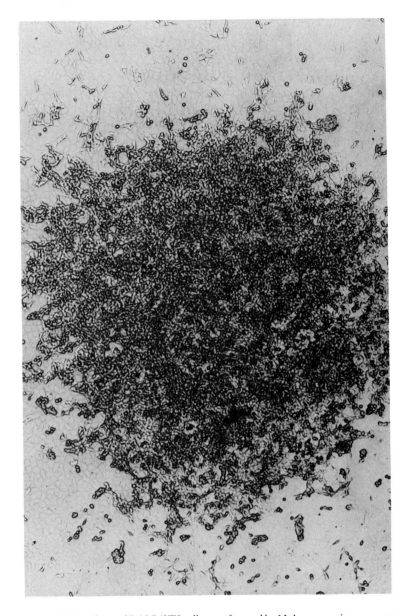

FIGURE 3. A colony of BALB/3T3 cells transformed by Moloney murine sarcoma virus, 4 wk after infection. × 49.

production of nonproducer foci follows "one-hit" kinetics, demonstrating that one mammalian sarcoma genome is sufficient to transform an infected cell (Aaronson and Rowe, 1970; Aaronson *et al.*, 1970).

If nonproducer foci of cells are isolated by growth in agar or by picking transformed foci from monolayer cultures infected with sarcoma viruses, it is possible to establish permanent cell lines of morphologically transformed cells (Todaro and Aaronson, 1969; Aaronson and Rowe, 1970). These cells will cause sarcomas if inoculated into appropriate strains of host animals. Moreover, if a sarcoma virus–transformed nonproducer cell line can be infected with a given helper type C virus, the sarcoma virus genome will be *rescued* by the infecting type C virus. The resulting sarcoma virus particles behave as though they possess the host range for infectivity and neutralization properties of the helper virus which rescued them. Thus, for example, when an MSV-transformed nonproducer cell line derived from hamster fibroblasts is cocultivated with cat embryo cells releasing feline leukemia virus (FeLV), it is possible to recover focus-forming virus in the tissue culture medium (Sarma *et al.*, 1970). This focus-forming virus will grow in cat, dog, and human cell cultures but not in mouse cells. This is the host range for the FeLV, whereas the MSV (plus helper MuLV) used to generate the hamster nonproducer cell line replicates only in murine cells. Similarly, the resulting focus-forming virus is neutralized by antisera raised against FeLV and not by antisera raised against MSV(MuLV) (Sarma *et al.*, 1970). Such results are typical of all mammalian type C viruses studied so far and are compatible with a model in which the sarcoma genome is contained in the coat of the rescuing helper type C virus. Such viruses are called "pseudotype" viruses; in the example given above, the resulting focus-forming virus would be called an "FeLV pseudotype of MSV"—MSV(FeLV), for short.

The ability to rescue to the MSV genome from nonproducer cell lines has been widely used as a sensitive test for the presence of putative type C helper virus, and has resulted in the detection of certain new mammalian type C virus isolates (e.g., Klement *et al.*, 1969*a*). Similarly, the possibility of rescuing the MSV genome in various mammalian nonproducer cell lines by inducing endogenous helper type C viruses from their generally nonexpressed state has been used to identify a variety of inducible endogenous type C viral genomes (Aaronson, 1971; Klement *et al.*, 1971). Sarcoma virus pseudotypes can also be used to detect the presence of helper type C viruses in an interference assay. The interference assay depends on the observation that a preinfected culture replicating a given type C helper virus will interfere with focus formation by sarcoma virus genomes "pseudotyped" by related helper type C virus (Sarma *et al.*, 1967). For example, feline embryo fibroblasts preinfected with FeLV will prevent focus formation by FeLV pseudotypes of feline sarcoma virus or MSV. The preinfecting helper virus is believed to generate products which block membrane receptors necessary for attachment and penetration of the homologous pseudotype sarcoma virus.

In a conceptually related system, Zavada has shown the mammalian type C helper viruses can also pseudotype the vesicular stomatitis virus (VSV) RNA genome (Zavada, 1972*a,b*). VSV infection rapidly generates lytic foci in many mammalian monolayer cell lines. If a culture of mammalian cells producing type C virus is infected briefly with VSV, a small percentage of pseudotype virions are formed with type C viral coats and VSV genomes. These minority pseudotype particles can be detected either by neutralizing the normally coated VSV particles with specific antisera or by originally using a VSV mutant with temperature-dependent coat functions. Such type C pseudotypes of VSV can be used to study the mechanism of type C viral attachment and penetration as well as to detect the covert production of type C virus in a given culture.

Although the MSV and simian sarcoma virus (SSV) nonproducer cell lines studied so far do not release infectious focus-forming virus (by definition), considerable variation exists in expression of other viral functions besides transformation. On one hand, there are MSV and SSV "pure" nonproducer cell lines which show no detectable expression of viral structural proteins or demonstrable viral particles by electron microscopic study (Aaronson *et al.*, 1972; Aaronson, 1973; Scolnick and Parks, 1973). Other nonproducer cell lines show both expression of viral structural proteins and small numbers of viral particles by electron microscopy (Bassin *et al.*, 1971a). These latter nonproducers have been called "sarcoma-positive, leukemia-negative" or "S^+L^-" nonproducer cell lines. The molecular mechanisms responsible for this variation in expression of viral functions are not understood at present.

Several reports have described a variety of experiments with flat revertants of MSV-transformed nonproducer cell lines (Fischinger *et al.*, 1972; Nomura *et al.*, 1972, 1973). These revertants occurred spontaneously or after treatment with mutagens (fluorodeoxyuridine, colcemid) and were similar in growth properties to the original nontransformed cell lines. Of considerable interest was the fact that the MSV genome could not be rescued from the flat revertants by superinfection with MuLV, or by cell fusion. However, the flat revertants remained susceptible to MuLV and MSV infection. Certain revertant cell lines spontaneously retransformed; certain of the retransformants contained rescuable MSV genomes and others did not. In many of the MSV flat revertants, loss of expression of transformation was associated with a marked increase in chromosome number, but this was not invariable. These studies indicate that both phenotypic expression and rescuability of the MSV genome can be regulated in various ways by certain, presumably cellular, genes.

Other reports have described studies of the MSV genome by biochemical techniques. Maisel *et al.*, (1973) demonstrated that certain murine sarcoma virus preparations (Kirsten, Moloney, and Harvey and defective Friend spleen focus–forming virus) contain two sizes of genomic RNA. In contrast, only the larger-sized RNA component was found when pure preparations of the MuLV helper virus were tested. This suggests that RNA genomes of replication-defective MSV transforming viruses are somewhat smaller than those of helper viruses which can replicate, and provides a molecular explanation for the defectiveness. Smaller genomes (relative to helper-independent Rous sarcoma virus) have been previously found in the avian system both for nontransforming, replicating type C virus and for transforming, replication-defective isolates (see the chapter by Varmus and Bishop). Recent molecular hybridization studies with Kirsten MSV suggest (1) that the viral genome expressed in the RNA of MSV-transformed nonproducer rat and mouse cells is approximately 50% homologous to the Kirsten MuLV helper virus (Benveniste and Scolnick, 1973), and (2) that other sequences in the RNA are homologous to rat type C viral sequences, suggesting that the Kirsten MSV genome may have formed by recombination of Kirsten MuLV with endogenous rat type C virus during passage through rats (Scolnick *et al.*, 1973). In contrast, Moloney MSV–transformed cells contained only mouse type C–specific sequences, and Moloney MSV(MuLV) had not been passaged through rats.

4. Endogenous Type C Viruses

Many well-studied avian and mammalian type C viruses are "typical" infectious viruses which can be transmitted from animal to animal and from culture to culture via cell-free filtrates. However, certain unusual features of the biology of vertebrate type C viruses led a series of investigators to propose that type C viral genetic information could also be transmitted "vertically," in an unexpressed form, from parent to progeny (animal or cell), along with the host's genetic information (Lwoff, 1960; Latarjet and Duplan, 1962; Bentvelzen *et al.*, 1968; Huebner and Todaro, 1969; Temin, 1971). During the past 5 years, much evidence has accumulated supporting the reality of this hypothesis for a variety of vertebrate species, so that the postulated existence of *unexpressed endogenous vertically transmitted type C virogenes* is a necessary conceptual tool for understanding present research with mammalian type C viruses.

Murine cell lines maintained in culture commonly begin to produce typical type C viral particles biochemically and antigenically related to the type C viruses isolated from the tumor tissues of leukemic mice (Kindig and Kirsten, 1967; Hall *et al.*, 1967; Aaronson *et al.*, 1969). To demonstrate that such viruses were endogenous viruses of the sort hypothesized above, it was necessary to prepare virus-free murine cell lines from single-cell clones and then demonstrate the induced or spontaneous release of type C viruses from such a virus-free cell line. Such experiments were patterned after the bacteriophage induction experiments of Lwoff *et al.* (1950), and were intended to demonstrate that the virus was indeed carried in an unexpressed form in each cell, with cloning serving to eliminate the possibility of low-level initial viral contamination as an explanation for the eventual appearance of virus in the cell cultures.

In 1971, Lowy *et al.* and Aaronson *et al.* (1971*b*) prepared such virus-negative single-cell clones of murine cells, and then showed that the halogenated pyrimidines 5-iododeoxyuridine and 5-bromodeoxyuridine operated as highly efficient inducing agents of typical murine type C viral particles from these "virus-negative" cell lines. These experiments conclusively demonstrated the reality of endogenous type C virogenes in mouse cells. Klement *et al.*, (1971) and Aaronson (1971) subsequently showed that halogenated pyrimidines would also induce the production of type C virus from "virus-free" rat cell clones, and Rowe *et al.* (1971) and Todaro (1972) demonstrated that mouse clones could also *spontaneously* begin to release their endogenous type C viruses. These results have now been confirmed and extended by many research groups, and endogenous type C viruses have been obtained spontaneously or induced from virus-free single-cell clones of Chinese and Syrian hamster (Lieber *et al.*, 1973*a*), guinea pig

(Nayak and Murray, 1973), and cat (Livingston and Todaro, 1973; Fischinger *et al.*, 1973) cells.

Most endogenous type C viruses are restricted from replicating in their cell of origin and in closely related cells. The most prevalent virus induced from BALB/c mouse cells after 5-bromodeoxyuridine treatment is unable to replicate in all mouse cells tested so far but does replicate to high titer in rabbit, rat, dog, and mink cells (Benveniste *et al.*, 1974*c*). The endogenous feline viruses of the RD-114/CCC class are restricted from replicating in most cat cell lines and strains tested so far, but do replicate in human, rhesus monkey, horse, and dog cells (Livingston and Todaro, 1973). Similarly, the endogenous baboon viruses obtained from a variety of normal baboon tissues do not replicate in the baboon cells tested so far, but do replicate in bat, dog, rhesus monkey, pig, and human cells (Benveniste *et al.*, 1974*b*). Of interest is the analogous existence of similar inducible host-restricted endogenous type C viruses in the chicken system (Weiss *et al.*, 1971); these viruses (subgroup E) will not replicate in most chicken cells but will replicate in cells from turkeys, ring-necked pheasants, and Japanese quail.

When the endogenous viruses are grown *in vitro* to high titer, it is possible to obtain enough virus to make *in vitro* ^{3}H-DNA transcripts of the viral RNA using the viral reverse transcriptase. When such labeled transcripts are hybridized with the DNA of their original species of origin, multiple copies of the viral genome have been found in the DNA of each cell, in every individual, for the various species tested (mouse, rat, pig, cat, baboon) (Benveniste and Todaro, 1974*b*). The virogenes are found, as predicted, in cells and tissues which are not producing virus. In contrast, gene sequences of exogenously infecting type C viruses are present in only one copy per haploid cellular genome of the infected cells. This technique allows direct confirmation of the species of origin of a given virus and suggests which viruses are endogenous in a given species.

Finally, the demonstrated existence of endogenous type C virogenes in the cells from a variety of mammalian species can complicate experiments with such cells. Many commonly used mouse, rat, hamster, pig, and certain feline cell lines spontaneously release large quantities of endogenous type C virus without the appearance of a cytopathic effect and without changes in the growth pattern of the cultures (Lieber *et al.*, 1973*a*). The release of such viruses evidently must change the cellular physiology and probably modifies the cellular antigenicity of these cultures. If such endogenous viruses replicate in human cells, the cell lines releasing such viruses may pose a biohazard to research workers and necessitate utilization of extensive containment procedures and equipment.

5. Murine Type C Viruses

Murine leukemia and sarcoma viruses have been much more extensively studied than any other mammalian type C viruses and are the prototypes upon which knowledge of the behavior of mammalian type C viruses, as a general class, has been based. Because of space limitations, we have chosen not to discuss most of the vast topic of the pathogenesis of murine leukemia and sarcoma virus experimentally induced disease in laboratory animals. This topic is admirably reviewed in Gross's monograph, *Oncogenic Viruses* (1970). Rather, we shall discuss certain areas of murine type C virus research of current "virological interest," with emphasis on studies of the naturally occurring endogenous murine viruses.

5.1. *"Infectious Viruses"*

In 1951, Ludwick Gross produced evidence which suggested that murine leukemia might be of viral origin. Extracts of leukemic tissues from Ak strain mice were passed through filter pads impervious to *Escherichia coli*. Among 25 newborn C3H strain mice injected with these leukemic extracts, seven (28%) developed generalized lymphatic luekemia within 9 months. In contrast, noninoculated C3H strain control animals had a very low incidence of spontaneous leukemia, less than 0.5% (Gross, 1951). In the following decade, using newborn animals as a bioassay system, other investigators confirmed the possibility of transmitting murine leukemia by using ultrafiltrates of diseased tissue. "Murine leukemia virus" (MuLV) was found in extracts of serially transplanted murine sarcomas and carcinomas by Graffi (1957), Friend (1957), Moloney (1960), Rauscher (1962), and many other investigators and in extracts of transplantable lymphoid tumors by Schoolman *et al.* (1957), Tennant (1962), and Kirsten *et al.* (1967). Gross *et al.* (1958) and Lieberman and Kaplan (1959) demonstrated that extracts of radiation-induced lymphoid tumors of mice also contained murine leukemia virus. The neoplasms caused by these various isolates of murine leukemia virus consisted of a wide variety of lymphoreticular and hematological diseases, including lymphatic, myeloid, monocytic, and stem cell leukemias, localized (thymic) or generalized lymphosarcomas, reticulum cell sarcoma, and an erythroblastosis syndrome characterized by marked hepatosplenomegaly (Friend, Rauscher, and Kirsten MuLVs). In general, the various MuLV isolates caused similar diseases when inoculated into newborn or suckling rats (Gross, 1970).

Harvey in 1964 observed that newborn BALB/c mice injected with plasma from rats in which murine leukemia virus was being passaged developed, instead of leukemia, sarcomas at the injection site (Harvey, 1964). Subsequently, Moloney described the development of rhabdomyosarcomas in newborn BALB/c mice following injection of Moloney strain murine leukemia virus (Moloney MuLV) (Moloney, 1966), and Kirsten and his associates described the induction of pleomorphic sarcomas following inoculation of plasma or spleen extracts from rats previously injected with Kirsten MuLV (Kirsten and Mayer, 1967). Filtered extracts of these sarcomas were generally able to cause sarcomas in rats, hamsters, and certain other rodent species.

Subsequently, it has been shown that the filtrable agents in the leukemogenic and sarcomagenic extracts described above are all type C RNA viruses and constitute a family of related viruses by antigenic and biochemical criteria. All murine leukemia and sarcoma viruses have common group-specific antigens on their viral structural proteins, and contain reverse transcriptases with common antigenic determinants. Nucleic acid hybridization studies also demonstrate that there is partial viral genome sequence homology among the various MuLVs (infectious and endogenous) and MSVs studied so far (Callahan *et al.*, 1974).

The early isolates of murine leukemia and sarcoma viruses have been developed through serial animal or tissue culture passage into laboratory strains of virus with wide host range, which replicate to high titer and rapidly cause disease when injected into newborn mice and rats. Most biochemical studies of mammalian type C viruses have been performed with these laboratory strains of MuLV and the basic biology of mammalian type C viruses has been studied predominantly with these strains.

5.2. Host Range Determinants

From the early experiments of Gross and Tennant, it was known that the susceptibility of various inbred strains of mice to infection with a given MuLV isolate varied markedly. Because of the ease of studying mice with spleen foci induced by Friend MuLV (Axelrad and Steeves, 1964), such variations in viral host range were most carefully characterized with the Friend virus. Two host range variants of Friend MuLV were widely studied. F-S virus, carried in DBA/2 mice, is about a hundred fold more efficient in inducing spleen foci in mouse strains such as DBA/2, C3H, and AKR than in BALB/c and A strain animals; however, F-S virus passaged in BALB/c mice induces spleen foci in BALB/c and A strains as efficiently as in DBA/2. Genetic experiments *in vivo* showed that these patterns of susceptibility to Friend virus disease are governed by a single genetic locus called *Fv-1* (Odaka, 1969).

In 1970, Hartley *et al.* determined that previously studied isolates of MuLV could be classified into one of three *in vitro* host range categories: cells from NIH Swiss mice are more sensitive to infection with "N-tropic" viruses than are cells from BALB/c mice, whereas BALB/c cells are more sensitive than NIH Swiss cells to infection by "B-tropic" viruses. "NB-tropic" viruses replicate equally well in NIH Swiss and BALB/c cells. (It is now known that there is an additional host range class of murine type C viruses which are restricted from replicating in all mouse cells; see below.) When cells from a large number of inbred mouse strains were tested *in vitro*, it was found that the cells from each strain were either more susceptible to N-tropic virus or more susceptible to B-tropic virus. Hybrid animals were resistant to both virus types. Similar studies with cells from appropriately backcrossed animals revealed that a single genetic locus was responsible for determining resistance to *in vitro* infection with N- and B-tropic MuLVs (Pincus *et al.*, 1971*a, b*). Of considerable interest was the finding that cells from all strains of mice which were susceptible to F-S Friend virus *in vivo* showed N-type susceptibility when tested *in vitro*, while cells from F-S virus–resistant strains showed B-type susceptibility *in vitro*. Further genetic experiments have confirmed that the *Fv-1* genetic locus which controls infection with Friend MuLV *in vivo* is the same locus which determines tissue culture sensitivity to N- or B-type MuLVs (Pincus *et al.*, 1971*a*). Subsequently, the *Fv-1* locus has been mapped on linkage group VIII (chromosome 4) (Rowe *et al.*, 1973). Recent studies with MuLV pseudotypes of vesicular stomatitis virus suggest that the regulation of infection by N- and B-type cells does not occur during attachment and penetration, since N- or B-type pseudotypes of VSV infect both types of cells equally well (Krontiris *et al.*, 1973; Huang *et al.*, 1973). Additional genetic studies have demonstrated that the *Fv-1* locus markedly regulates the horizontal spread (from cell to cell in the animal) of spontaneously activated N- and B-tropic endogenous MuLVs (Rowe, 1972; Rowe and Hartley, 1972).

Another genetic locus responsible for certain limitations of murine type C virus replication in mouse cells has also been identified. This locus (*Fv-2*) has been mapped on linkage group II of the mouse genome (Lilly, 1970). Repeated passage of Friend virus in rats leads to loss of the erythroid cell specificity of the virus. Such virus induces lymphoid leukemia similar to Gross virus disease and is known as lymphatic leukemia virus (LLV). The component responsible for spleen focus–forming activity (SFFV) is lost during passage in rats. SFFV is defective and will not induce erythroleukemia in the absence of infection with LLV. Mice which are homozygous or heterozygous for the *Fv-2* allele are highly sensitive to SFFV; mice homozygous for the recessive allele *Fv-2* are highly resistant to SFFV. In contrast, replication of the LLV component of Friend virus disease is regulated by the *Fv-1* locus described above. The mechanism by which the *Fv-2* locus acts and its relevance to natural murine leukemogenesis have not been elucidated (Lilly, 1972).

Within the past 2 years, another major host range class of MuLVs has been described: these are MuLVs unable to replicate in any mouse cells so far tested, but able to replicate well in cells from heterologous species such as rats, rabbits, monkeys, and humans (Todaro *et al.*, 1973*a*; Aaronson and Stephenson, 1973; Levy, 1973; Benveniste *et al.*, 1974*c*). Such mouse-restricted MuLVs have been characterized as "xenotropic" by Levy (1973). It is now clear that viruses of this type can be isolated from a large number of inbred strains, including NIH Swiss and NZB, strains which previously had failed to yield endogenous "mouse-tropic" virus. Xenotropic viruses can be readily induced from certain strains of cells *in vitro* by halogenated pyrimidine treatment (Aaronson and Stephenson, 1973; Benveniste *et al.*, 1974*c*) and also by immunological reactions involving splenocytes both *in vitro* and *in vivo* (Sherr *et al.*, 1974*b*). Weanling animals from inbred strains with a low incidence of leukemia contain readily isolated xenotropic MuLV in their spleens. In contrast, none of the standard animal-passaged leukemogenic preparations of MuLV contains xenotropic virus (Lieber *et al.*, 1974). What role, if any, this virus class plays in normal murine physiology and whether it is leukemogenic remain to be determined.

The spontaneous appearance of high titers of leukemogenic type C virus in multiple tissues of healthy young animals of the high leukemic inbred mouse strains AKR and C58 has been known for the past 20 years (Gross, 1970). Rowe and Pincus have quantitated the appearance of the AKR virus by XC plaque titers; their studies demonstrate that high levels of infectious virus appear in embryos just prior to birth and then continue to rise subsequently (Rowe and Pincus, 1972). Studies of the *Fv-1* locus provide a partial explanation of these events. The virus spontaneously activated from AKR and C58 cells *in vivo* and *in vitro* with high probability is an N-tropic virus. AKR and C58 cells are N-type cells, i.e., permissive for N-type virus, so that horizontal spread of type C virus occurs. AKR hybrid animals heterozygous at *Fv-1* show much lower titers of virus than age-matched AKR controls (Rowe, 1972). AKR and C58 strain mice thus provide one of the few known examples among vertebrates in which the most readily activated endogenous type C virus is able to replicate with ease in the animals' own cells.

In contrast, a large epidemiological study of spontaneous tumor occurrence in natural populations of wild mice (*Mus musculus*) has been made by Gardner *et al.* (1973*b*). Spontaneous tumors were rare until after $2\frac{1}{2}$ yr of age, and type C virus expression in spleens was undetectable in younger mice. In mice older than $2\frac{1}{2}$ yr, lymphomas, pulmonary adenomas, fibrosarcomas, and granulocytic neoplasms occurred spontaneously. Type C virus group-specific antigens and particles were found in the lymphomas of the older mice and in spleens of certain nontumorous older mice, but not in the spontaneous sarcomas or pulmonary adenomas. These data, in comparison with similar studies of inbred mouse strains described below, indicate that feral mice, in general, have "powerful natural repression" of their endogenous type C viral genomes. However, Gardner *et al.* also have described two local populations of wild mice trapped in Los Angeles County which have a high spontaneous incidence of lymphoma and type C virus expression. Of considerable interest has been their demonstration that the type C virus isolated from such mice can cause a lower motor neuron disease similar to amyotropic lateral sclerosis (Officer *et al.*, 1973; Gardner *et al.*, 1973*a*). Type C virus can be isolated from the embryos of such animals, and has both N-tropic and xenotropic host range properties, suggesting the presence of a mixture of viruses (Lieber *et al.*, 1974). Whether this virus is endogenous or is spread by horizontal infection *in vivo* has not yet been determined.

A variety of recent studies have described the extent of natural expression of type C virus in various inbred mouse strains with low leukemia incidence. Electron microscopic studies have described the general appearance of type C particles in the embryos of all strains of mice examined (Vernon *et al.*, 1973; Chase and Pikó, 1973). It has been proposed that full expression of endogenous type C information fulfills normal functions in embryogenesis (Gilden *et al.*, 1970), but evidence for this hypothesis is lacking at present. In postnatal animals, natural expression of xenotropic virus can be detected in weanlings from a variety of strains (Lieber *et al.*, 1974). In the low leukemia BALB/c strain, which has been studied most carefully, B-tropic virus able to replicate in the animals' own cells has been isolated only from older animals (Peters *et al.*, 1972); BALB/c cells both *in vivo* and *in vitro* show a much "tighter control" of the autoinfectious B-type virus than of the endogenous N-tropic and xenotropic viruses present in their cells (Benveniste *et al.*, 1974c). Recent experiments demonstrate that the naturally occurring BALB/c B-tropic virus will cause lymphomas when injected into newborn BALB/c mice, whereas the N-tropic virus does not (Peters *et al.*, 1973a, b). The mean latent period for induction of lymphoma was quite long (about 15 months), and no solid tumors were induced at a statistically significant level.

Further evidence concerning the relationship between expression of endogenous type C virus and oncogenesis is provided by the genetic study of Meier *et al.* (1973). Hybrid and backcrossed animals between AKR and the low leukemic strain C57L were observed for the expression of type C virus in their spleens and for tumor development. Young animals which expressed either type C viral group-specific antigen or complete viral particles in their spleens had a predictable association of later developing lymphoma and related mesenchymal tumors. The presence or absence of endogenous type C viral expression could be used to predict whether or not an animal would develop a certain group of tumors, and suggested that the extent of expression of the endogenous type C viral genomes is a major determinant of developing lymphoid tumors in these mice.

Recent studies indicate that inbred mouse strains are not "immunologically tolerant" of their endogenous type C viruses. Kidneys from AKR mice contain type C viral antigens and antibodies against viral structural proteins and the reverse transcriptase (Oldstone *et al.*, 1972; Hollis *et al.*, 1974). Other strains of mice with a known high incidence of spontaneous type C virus expression also have a high incidence of immune complex glomerulonephritis believed to be caused by glomerular deposition of viral antigens and antibody. Ihle *et al.* (1973) have shown that natural antibody to type C virus occurs in the sera of AKR, BALB/c, and (C57BL × C3H)F₁ hybrid mice, and Aaronson and Stephenson (1974) have shown that most mouse strains possess neutralizing antibodies against the xenotropic endogenous type C virus. What role such humoral immunity serves in regulating the expression and spread of the endogenous type C viruses and in the occurrence of natural neoplasms remains to be determined.

In summary, recent studies in various types of mice strongly suggest a *natural* etiological association between murine endogenous type C viruses and lymphoreticular neoplasms. (Thymic lymphosarcomas and reticulum cell sarcoma are the histological types of disease commonly associated with type C viruses in mice.) Genetic studies have begun to delineate the genetic loci which regulate spontaneous activation and spread of the endogenous viruses and thus determine the probabilities of tumorigenesis. Moreover, immunological studies indicate that mice are not immunologically tolerant of their endogenous type C viruses. However, the exact molecular pathophysiology of type C virus infections in generating lymphoreticular neoplasms has not clearly been described, since the endogenous viruses will not transform the fibroblastic cell lines available for study *in vitro*. The development of suitable culture systems for murine thymic and

lymphoid cells should permit much progress in understanding the exact cellular
mechanism of murine type C viral leukemogenesis (e.g. Sklar *et al.*, 1974).

5.4. In Vitro Studies of Endogenous Murine Type C Viruses

The halogenated pyrimidines 5-iododeoxyuridine and 5-bromodeoxyuridine
have been widely used to induce endogenous type C viruses from mouse
cells previously virus free. With cells from certain strains and with certain
transformed cell lines, treatment with these agents induces rapid production of
virus in an exponential fashion (see Fig. 4) (Lieber *et al.*, 1973*b*). Experiments with
metabolic inhibitors suggest that 5-iododeoxyuridine and 5-bromodeoxyuridine
must be incorporated in the cellular DNA for induction to occur (Teich *et al.*,
1973). Since even highly inducible murine cell lines do not contain complete
viral-specific sequences of RNA prior to induction, transcriptional controls
probably are involved in the initiation of new endogenous virus release (Benveniste *et al.*, 1973). Aaronson and Dunn (1974*b*) have shown that inhibitors of

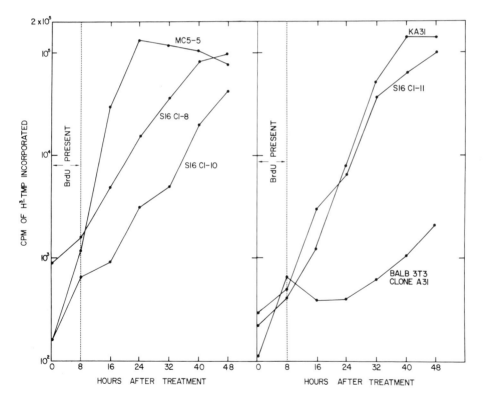

FIGURE 4. Induction of endogenous type C virus from murine BALB/3T3 and transformed cell
lines derived from BALB/3T3 by brief treatment with 5-bromodeoxyuridine (BrdU). S16Cl-8,
S16Cl-10, and S16Cl-11 are spontaneous transformants, MC5-5 is a methylcholanthrene-derived
transformant, and KA31 is a Kirsten MSV nonproducer transformant. The extracellular production of virus is measured by an *in vitro* supernatant reverse transcriptase assay and demonstrates
that induced virus release is exponential in character. For details, see Lieber *et al.* (1973*b*).

protein synthesis (cycloheximide, puromycin) will also induce production of endogenous type C virus from mouse cells.

Cell lines derived from BALB/c embryo cells have been most carefully studied regarding induction of endogenous virus. After 5-bromodeoxyuridine treatment, such cells release two host range classes of endogenous type C virus, N-tropic virus and xenotropic virus; the latter virus is induced in large excess (Aaronson and Stephenson, 1973; Benveniste *et al.*, 1974*c*). Experiments with cell lines derived from BALB/c and NIH Swiss hybrid and backcrossed animals have demonstrated that two separate loci regulate inducible expression of these two host range classes of virus in BALB/c animals (Aaronson and Stephenson, 1973). Since BALB/c cells themselves are B-type for virus susceptibility, the N-tropic and xenotropic endogenous viruses released cannot autoinfect the culture releasing them, and expression of endogenous virus disappears gradually when the inducing agent is removed. In contrast, when cells derived from AKR or C58 embryos are induced, the resulting endogenous viruses are autoinfectious, and a permanent virus-producing culture results (Rowe *et al.*, 1971; Stephenson and Aaronson, 1972). Genetic experiments suggest that C58 animals have more than two loci regulating the inducibility of endogenous type C virus (Stephenson and Aaronson, 1973). Recently, it has been shown that the type C virus from C58 × NIH Swiss hybrid cells induced *in vitro* is leukemogenic when injected into newborn NIH Swiss mice (Stephenson *et al.*, 1974*a*).

Endogenous type C viruses can also begin to be spontaneously released in high titer from previously virus-free clones of cells in culture. With BALB/c-derived cells, spontaneous release of N-tropic and/or xenotropic viruses occurs (Todaro, 1972; Aaronson and Dunn, 1974*a*), and the probability of virus release seems to be higher for transformed cell lines than for "contact-inhibited" cell lines (Lieber and Todaro, 1973).

Murine cells *in vivo* can also spontaneously begin to release endogenous type C viruses. Mice of the high leukemia incidence strains AKR and C58 spontaneously release endogenous virus early in life, and since their cells are susceptible to infection with their homologous type C virus, rapid spread of virus occurs, so that high titers of endogenous virus can be cultured from young animals of these strains. It is presumed that such spontaneous activation and spread of endogenous type C virus are in part responsible for the high incidence of leukemia in these strains, since genetic experiments which introduce a resistance allele at the *Fv-1* locus markedly reduce and delay the subsequent titer of endogenous virus in the animals' tissues (Rowe, 1972; Rowe and Hartley, 1972). Rowe and his colleagues have identified two unlinked autosomal loci which regulate the spontaneous activation of N-tropic AKR endogenous type C virus *in vivo*, and one of these loci, called *V1*, has been mapped on linkage group I (Rowe, 1972).

Besides spontaneous and chemical induction of type C viruses *in vitro*, it also seems likely that specific immunological activation of virus can occur. Mixed lymphocyte reactions *in vitro* have been found to activate type C viruses (Hirsch *et al.*, 1972; Sherr *et al.*, 1974*b*). Since such viruses are not activated by the mitogen, phytohemagglutinin, alone, it appears that specific immunological mechanisms may be required. The *in vivo* correlate of the mixed lymphocyte culture is the graft vs. host (GVH) reaction, and such *in vivo* experiments have also been shown to activate endogenous type C viruses (Hirsch *et al.*, 1972). Animals undergoing chronic GVH reactions tend to have a much higher incidence of lymphoid neoplasms, and extracts of such tumors are leukemogenic when transmitted as cell-free filtrates (Armstrong *et al.*, 1973).

6. Feline Type C Viruses

6.1. Infectious Virus

Lymphosarcoma is the most frequent neoplasm of domestic cats. Jarrett and associates demonstrated that presumed cell-free filtrates of a feline lymphosarcoma could transmit the disease (Jarrett *et al.*, 1964*b*) and also that typical type C viral particles could be identified in the induced case (Jarrett *et al.*, 1964*a*; Laird *et al.*, 1968*b*). Subsequently, type C particles were commonly observed in tissues from cats with spontaneous lymphosarcoma (Rickard *et al.*, 1967, 1969; Laird *et al.*, 1968*a*) and other feline diseases such as myeloproliferative diseases, infectious peritonitis, and certain anemias.

Present evidence strongly suggests that feline leukemia virus (FeLV) is spread horizontally by contact or contagion among domestic cats, just as the avian type C viruses may be spread horizontally among chickens (Rubin *et al.*. 1961). Thus apparent contact infections with FeLV have occurred in laboratory cat colonies (Rickard, 1969; Jarrett, 1971), and there are also numerous reported cases of household clusters of feline lymphosarcoma among unrelated cats. Using an immunofluorescence test for FeLV structural protein antigens in peripheral blood leukocytes, Hardy *et al.* (1973) have shown that FeLV infection is very common among cats in a household with another cat having lymphosarcoma or another FeLV-related disease (33%), whereas FeLV infection is rare (0.14%) among cats not housed with other diseased animals. Subsequently, 24% of FeLV-infected cats developed lymphosarcoma; a smaller number also developed the anemia associated with FeLV infection. Additional evidence for the horizontal spread of FeLV is the fact that cats raised in an isolated colony have not developed lymphosarcoma spontaneously (Rickard *et al.*, 1973); also, "germ-free" cats do not have detectable levels of antibody against FeLV antigens, whereas normal cat populations generally do (Olsen and Yohn, 1972).

Spontaneous feline fibrosarcomas also contain typical type C viral particles, and cell-free extracts of such tumors can transmit sarcomatous tumors to other cats (Snyder and Theilen, 1969; Gardner *et al.*, 1971). Although fibrosarcomas are not common feline tumors, they comprise a substantial fraction of mesenchymal soft tissue malignancies; they tend to occur in older cats, grow slowly, and metastasize infrequently. Feline sarcoma virus (FeSV) can experimentally generate sarcomas in many other species as well, including dogs, rabbits, sheep fetuses, white-lipped marmosets, macaque monkeys, and squirrel monkeys.

FeLV can be readily isolated *in vitro* from feline lymphosarcoma tissues. It replicates readily in most cat cell strains and cell lines; secondary and tertiary cultures of feline embryo fibroblasts (FEF) have generally been used for such isolations. Canine cells and human cells also will support replication of certain FeLV isolates. No cytopathic change identifies infection of fibroblast cultures with FeLV. In contrast, infection of feline, canine, and human cell strains and cell lines with extracts of feline fibrosarcomas (feline sarcoma virus, FeSV) generally results in the generation of foci of transformed fibroblasts. Cultures of Snyder–Theilen (ST) or Gardner–Arnstein (GA) FeSV have been found to invariably contain a marked excess of associated nontransforming type C virus similar to FeLV, analogous to the murine MSV(MuLV) system. Similarly, it has been possible to isolate "nonproducer" clones of cells transformed by ST FeSV (Chan *et al.*, 1974; Henderson *et al.*, 1974), and then rescue the FeSV genome with a variety of nontransforming mammalian type C viruses.

All *in vitro* isolates of type C virus from feline lymphosarcomas and the FeSV-associated type C virus have been found to share common antigenic determinants which permit the classification of FeLVs. Such viruses share immunologically similar reverse transcriptases and p30 proteins. Of considerable interest has been the cross-reaction observed between FeLV p30 antigens and antisera prepared against MuLV p30 antigens (Geering *et al.*, 1968) and vice versa. This reaction has defined an interspecies determinant on the p30 proteins, which has allowed the detection and classification of certain other mammalian type C viruses.

FeLV pseudotypes of MSV have been prepared by several techniques. Fischinger and O'Conner (1967, 1970) prepared aggregates of MSV and FeLV by ultracentrifugation. Infection with such aggregates permitted MSV to enter and multiply in normally unsusceptible feline embryo fibroblast cells. The product of such infection was the MSV genome in an FeLV coat. It could be neutralized with antisera to FeLV and showed the broad host range of FeLV for replication (and transformation) of cat, dog, and human, but not mouse, cells; cat embryo cultures preinfected with FeLV showed interference with focus formation by MSV(FeLV). Sarma *et al.* prepared similar MSV(FeLV) virions either by *in vitro* cocultivation of MSV-transformed hamster tumor cells with cat embryo cultures infected with FeLV or by inoculation of such tumor cells into FeLV-infected newborn cats (Sarma *et al.*, 1970).

The existence of FeLV pseudotypes of MSV and of FeSV(FeLV) which could also generate foci *in vitro* was used for the subgroup classification of FeLV isolates into three classes based on neutralization and viral interference tests (Sarma and Log, 1971, 1973). All FeLVs appear to have distinct viral envelope antigens responsible for type-specific neutralizing antibodies. The viral interference patterns are also controlled by these same viral envelope antigens. Thus the virus–host cell relationship for FeLVs appears to be similar to that found among the avian type C viruses, in which all viruses with the same envelope antigen use a specific viral receptor for attachment and penetration (Vogt and Ishizaki, 1965).

6.2. *Endogenous Feline Viruses*

In 1971, McAllister and associates (McAllister *et al.*, 1971) reported the hetero-transplantation of human tumor cells into cats. Cultured human embryonal rhabdomyosarcoma cells of the RD cell line were injected into fetal cats; three of five surviving kittens and one stillborn animal developed disseminated rhabdomyosarcomas with the human karyotype of the original RD cell line. Although the original RD cell line did not have detectable type C virus, electron microscopic studies of two of the cat tumors and of a cell line established from one of the tumors revealed typical type C virions. Subsequent characterization of the "RD-114" virus (McAllister *et al.*, 1972) further demonstrated the presence of reverse transcriptase activity, 70S viral RNA, and an interspecies antigenic determinant on the p30 protein characteristic of mammalian type C viruses. However, it was not possible to demonstrate feline leukemia virus–specific p30 antigens in RD-114 virus, nor to demonstrate neutralization of RD-114 by antisera directed against FeLV, nor interference with focus formation of FeSV(FeLV) pseudotypes in cultures preinfected with RD-114. The p30 and envelope antigens of RD-114 were distinctly different from known feline type C viruses. The RD-114 reverse transcriptase was also antigenically different from the FeLV polymerase (Scolnick *et al.*, 1972*b*). Since there had been no previous examples of a single species having two distinct classes of type C viruses, and since RD-114 and feline leukemia virus were antigenically unrelated, it was at the time reasonable to suspect that RD-114 virus might be of human origin.

Subsequent studies, however, have shown RD-114 to be a second distinct class of cat type C viruses. Livingston and Todaro (1973) characterized a type C virus released spontaneously from the CCC line of fetal feline kidney fibroblasts; this virus possessed p30 protein and reverse transcriptase immunologically cross-reactive with the analogous proteins from RD-114. Moreover, a virus with similar antigenic properties could be activated from a cloned line of non-virus-producing CCC cells by treatment with 5-iododeoxyuridine. Virus-negative CCC cells and other fetal cat cells were resistant to exogenous infection with either the spontaneously released or the induced CCC virus. Thus the CCC virus and, by implication, the RD-114 virus are representatives of a distinct class of endogenous feline type C viruses (Livingston and Todaro, 1973). Fischinger and associates also studied the CCC spontaneously released and inducible type C viruses. They demonstrated that the host range, helper functions, interference properties, and specific neutralization of CCC and RD-114 and their respective MSV pseudotypes were closely similar if not identical (Fischinger *et al.*, 1973). Sarma *et al.* (1973) confirmed the isolation of an RD-114-like virus from the CCC cell line. Nucleic acid hybridization studies also demonstrated that RD-114 was an endogenous feline virus and not an endogenous human virus (Gillespie *et al.*, 1973; Okabe *et al.*, 1973; Baluda and Roy-Burman, 1973; Neiman, 1973; Ruprecht *et al.*, 1973).

At the present time, domestic cats are known to possess at least two distinct classes of type C RNA viruses. Feline leukemia viruses (FeLVs) appear to be highly infectious, horizontally spread viruses which are widely prevalent among domestic cats. They are associated with feline lymphosarcoma and certain other common feline diseases, and pseudotype FeSV genomes when such sarcoma viruses are isolated from fibrosarcomas. Whether FeLVs are endogenous feline viruses has not yet been fully resolved either by virological or by nucleic acid hybridization studies. No one has yet reported the isolation of FeLV from virus-negative clones of normal cat cells either spontaneously or after various chemical induction treatments. In contrast, most normal cat cell strains and cell lines have been shown to have endogenous type C viruses of the RD-114/CCC class (Todaro *et al.*, 1973*b*). Such viruses do not appear to be frequently expressed in cats *in vivo* or to be related to feline neoplasms tested so far. Thus Sarma *et al.* (1973) reported failure to identify RD-114 p30 antigens in 100 naturally occurring feline tumors and lack of detection of RD-114 neutralizing antibodies in the serum of 24 normal cats and of 20 cats with neoplastic diseases. However, such viruses can readily be isolated *in vitro* by cocultivating a wide variety of feline cell lines with the appropriate permissive cell lines from heterologous species (Todaro *et al.*, 1973*b*).

If FeLV and FeSV are endogenous viruses of domestic cats, full expression of these virogenes is very tightly controlled in the cat cells so far studied. Teleologically, such tight control of viruses potentially infectious for the cat's own cells makes good sense, whereas looser control of expression of a virus such as RD-114 which is restricted from replicating in most feline cells seems reasonable. The general picture is similar to the situation in murine BALB/c cells in which the autoinfectious B-type virus present in the cellular genome is under tight control and is not frequently activated spontaneously or after treatment with inducing agents.

7. Primate Type C Viruses

7.1. Infectious Viruses

In 1971, Theilen and associates reported the presence of type C viral particles in a naturally occurring fibrosarcoma of a 3-yr-old woolly monkey. Cell-free filtrates of this tumor produced fibrosarcomas in marmosets and transformed marmoset, cat, and human cells *in vitro* (Wolfe *et al.*, 1971). This virus was called "simian sarcoma virus No. 1" (SSV-1). Subsequently, as with the other known natural mammalian sarcoma virus isolates, SSV-1 was shown to be accompanied by an excess of a nontransforming "sarcoma-associated" type C virus (SSAV-1) (Wolfe *et al.*, 1972). In 1972, Kawakami *et al.* reported the isolation of a type C virus from

suspension cultures of lymphosarcoma cells taken from a diseased gibbon. This
gibbon lymphosarcoma virus, or GALV, does not produce foci in tissue culture
but will replicate in certain mammalian cell lines such as rat, human, and pig.

These two primate type C virus isolates are closely related to one another by
immunological and nucleic acid hybridization criteria. RNA·DNA hybridization
reveals approximately 50% nucleic acid homology (Benveniste and Todaro,
1973), and the antigenic determinants on the 30,000 dalton molecular weight
protein (p30) are essentially identical for both viruses (Parks *et al.*, 1973; Gilden *et
al.*, 1974). The viruses also share antigenic determinants on their reverse
transcriptases (Scolnick *et al.*, 1972*a,b*). SSV-1 focus-forming virus has been used
to prepare cloned transformed nonproducer cell lines of rat cell origin (Scolnick
and Parks, 1973; Aaronson, 1973). These cell lines show the range of variability in
the expression of type C viral functions associated with MSV-transformed mouse
and rat nonproducer clones. Certain clones show no viral particles, no p30
antigens, and no supernatant reverse transcriptase activity, whereas other clones
appear more like S^+L^- MSV-transformed mouse cells in showing SSV-1 p30
antigen expression and small numbers of viral particles by electron microscopy.
Both classes of nonproducers do not yield infectious virus, but focus-forming
virus can be rescued from SSV-1-transformed nonproducers using various
mammalian helper viruses. As expected, the rescued virus has the host range and
neutralization properties of the helper virus used to infect the SSV-1 nonproducer cell lines.

Of considerable interest are recent nucleic acid hybridization studies which fail
to show sequences homologous to SSV-1 and GALV in the DNA of uninfected
woolly monkeys and gibbons (Scolnick *et al.*, 1974; Benveniste *et al.*, 1974*a*). These
studies strongly suggest that these "primate" viruses may have originated from
endogenous viruses of another species and are now horizontally transmitted type
C viruses among certain primates. At the present time, the natural "homologous"
host or source of SSV-1 and GALV is not known, but DNA·RNA as well as
DNA·DNA hybridization studies suggested that the viruses are most closely
related to mouse type C viruses (Benveniste and Todaro, 1973).

7.2. Endogenous Primate Viruses

Electron micrographs of placentas from various primates, including rhesus
monkeys (Schidlovsky and Ahmed, 1973), baboons (Kalter *et al.*, 1973*a*), and
humans (Kalter *et al.*, 1973*b*), have demonstrated the appearance of particles
morphologically resembling type C viruses. When placental tissue from a baboon
was cocultivated with cell lines from a variety of mammalian species, a type C virus
was isolated after several months from cultures of dog, bat, human, and rhesus
monkey cells (Benveniste *et al.*, 1974*b*). Immunological studies demonstrated that
the baboon type C virus was distinctly different from previously described type C
viruses (Sherr *et al.*, 1974*b*; Sherr and Todaro, 1974*a*), and nucleic acid hybridization studies showed that viral-specific sequences were present in the DNA of

normal baboon liver tissue (Benveniste *et al.*, 1974*a,b*). These data strongly suggested that the baboon isolate was an endogenous primate virus. Subsequently, additional isolates of baboon type virus have been obtained by cocultivating various other normal baboon tissues (lung, kidney, testes) with permissive host cell lines (Todaro *et al.*, 1974*b*). Nucleic acid hybridization studies have demonstrated baboon type C viral specific sequences in other Old World monkey and ape species including humans, with the degree of relatedness roughly correlating with the presumed evolutionary diversity of the species (Benveniste and Todaro, 1974*a*). Antigens related to those of baboon virus p30 protein have also been identified in tissues from other Old World monkey species (Sherr *et al.*, 1974*a*) and in human tumors (Sherr and Todaro, 1974*b*).

Of marked interest is the immunological and nucleic acid relatedness shown between the endogenous baboon viruses and the endogenous feline viruses of the RD-114/CCC group (approximately 20% homology by DNA · RNA hybridization) (Sherr *et al.*, 1974*c*; Benveniste *et al.*, 1974*a,b*; Sherr and Todaro, 1974*a*). It does not seem possible to explain such relatedness on the basis of evolutionary divergence. Recent nucleic acid hybridization experiments demonstrate that the RD-114/CCC viruses represent the residue of infection of cats by a virus from Old World monkeys which has now become endogenous in domestic cats (Benveniste and Todaro, 1974*c*).

8. Other Mammalian Type C Isolates

8.1. Pigs

Typical type C particles have been detected in several permanent cell lines derived from porcine tissue, including the widely used pig kidney cell line PK(15) (Breese, 1970; Armstrong *et al.*, 1971). The PK(15) virus is a typical type C virus but is immunologically different from other species of type C virus studied so far (Todaro *et al.*, 1974*a*). Nucleic acid hybridization studies with PK(15) viral probes further demonstrate that the pig viruses are unrelated to other known mammalian type C viruses and also that viral-specific sequences can be detected in the DNA of normal pig liver cells (but not in the RNA), strongly suggesting that pig type C viruses are endogenous viruses (Todaro *et al.*, 1974*a*). The release of type C virus particles from a permanent cell line derived from the tissues of a leukemic pig after treatment with 5-bromodeoxyuridine and dimethylsulfoxide has been described (Strandström *et al.*, 1974; Moenning *et al.*, 1974).

8.2. Guinea Pigs

For several years, typical type C particles have been observed in the leukocytes of leukemic guinea pigs (Opler, 1967; Nadel *et al.*, 1967), but such particles could not be demonstrated in cultured guinea pig cells. More recently, however, Hsiung (1972), Nayak and Murray (1973), and Rhim *et al.*, (1973) have demonstrated that type C viral particles can be induced in high titer from cultured guinea pig cells by halogenated pyrimidine treatment. Such viruses have not been shown to be infectious as yet, and are presumably endogenous viruses also. There have been no direct demonstrations that the guinea pig type C virus is leukemogenic *in vivo*, although guinea pig leukemia is transmissible by cell-free filtrates (Gross, 1970, p. 611).

8.3. Rats

There have been approximately a dozen separate reports of the appearance of type C viral particles in cultures of rat cells serially propagated *in vitro*, often associated with morphological transformation of the culture (e.g., see Gazzolo *et al.*, 1971; Bergs *et al.*, 1970, 1972). Indeed, several of the most commonly used standard rat cell lines are spontaneously producing high titers of rat type C virus (Lieber *et al.*, 1973*a*). Endogenous rat type C viruses can also be induced from rat cell lines by 5-iododeoxyuridine and 5-bromodeoxyuridine treatment (Klement *et al.*, 1971; Aaronson, 1971). Both the spontaneously released and the induced viruses have not been infectious for a variety of mammalian cell lines tested (Lieber *et al.*, 1973*a*), but, like the pig virus (and the hamster viruses, see below), the rat type C virus can rescue the MSV genome from transformed nonproducer rat cell lines and convey it into other rat cells from certain strains (Klement *et al.*, 1971, 1972; Aaronson, 1971). Thus certain replication-defective mammalian type C viruses can still rescue and transduce the MSV genome, so that they presumably can attach to and penetrate certain mammalian cells. Molecular hybridization techniques indicate that rat type C viruses and murine type C viruses are completely unrelated, although both species are members of the same taxonomic family of Muridea (Benveniste and Todaro, 1973).

8.4. Hamsters

Typical type C viral particles have been observed in Syrian hamster cells *in vivo* and *in vitro* (Graffi *et al.*, 1968; Kelloff *et al.*, 1970*a*; Freeman *et al.*, 1971). There is some evidence that the hamster type C virus is leukemogenic in hamsters and can also rescue the MSV genome from nonproducer transformed hamster cells and carry the genome into nontransformed hamster cells (Kelloff *et al.*, 1970*b*). The hamster type C virus carries unique p30 antigens (Kelloff *et al.*, 1970*a*), and a recent report by Verma *et al.*, (1974) demonstrates that the hamster type C reverse transcriptase appears unique in that it will not carry out an "endogenous reaction" in which the 60–70S viral RNA acts as template; the reverse transcriptase enzyme appears to be made up of two polypeptides, one with a molecular weight of 68,000 and one with a molecular weight of 53,000. As noted previously, other mammalian type C viral polymerases have been found to consist of a single polypeptide chain of approximately 70,000 molecular weight. Halogenated pyrimidine treatment also will induce type C virus from "virus-free" Chinese and Syrian hamster cell lines (Lieber *et al.*, 1973*a*).

8.5. Cattle

A variety of epidemiological and clinical evidence has for many years suggested that bovine lymphosarcoma might be an infectious disease (Gross, 1970, p. 623; Dutcher *et al.*, 1964, 1967). Type C virus was first consistently associated with bovine lymphosarcoma when Miller *et al.* (1969) described typical type C virions in short-term lymphocyte suspension cultures treated with phytohemagglutinin. Subsequently, monolayer cell cultures derived from lymphosarcomatous bovine tissues have also been shown to release typical type C particles (Van Der Maaten *et al.*, 1974). Inocula prepared from these cultures have induced lymphoid tumors in sheep (Kawakami *et al.*, 1970; Olson *et al.*, 1972) and have been shown to replicate in newborn calves (Van Der Maaten, 1974). Initial serological studies of the bovine type C virus have also been performed (Ferrer *et al.*, 1972).

9. Search for Human Type C Viruses

As yet, there have been no confirmed isolations of infectious type C virus from normal or transformed human tissues. Multiple efforts to obtain such viruses are under way using the virological techniques which have worked successfully for the known mammalian type C viruses. However, several groups have recently reported the identification in human tumor tissue of nucleic acid sequences or reverse transcriptase activities which appear biochemically related to RNAs or the reverse transcriptases from known well-characterized mammalian type C viruses. Spiegelman's laboratory has demonstrated that RNA sequences homologous to certain sequences of Rauscher MuLV can be detected in a wide variety of human neoplasms, including leukemias (Hehlmann *et al.*, 1972*a*), lymphomas (Hehlmann *et al.*, 1972*b*; Kufe *et al.*, 1973), sarcomas (Kufe *et al.*, 1972), and brain tumors (Cuatico *et al.*, 1973). Gallo and his associates have isolated an enzyme from peripheral blood leukemic leukocytes with biochemical properties similar to those of the reverse transcriptase of mammalian type C viruses (Sarngadharan *et al.*, 1972), and Todaro and Gallo (1973) have shown that this polymerase activity is inhibited by antisera directed against the woolly monkey and gibbon type C viral polymerases. DNA synthesized endogenously by this human polymerase and its associated RNA has also been shown by Gallo *et al.* (1973), using nucleic acid hybridization techniques, to be related to RNA isolated from certain mammalian type C viruses (woolly monkey and murine type C viruses).

While such results are of great interest, it seems clear that rapid progress in unraveling the possible association between type C viruses and human neoplastic disease must await the isolation of infectious type C virus from human tissues or at least the identification of a human cell culture which releases human type C virus

in high titer.

ACKNOWLEDGMENTS

We thank Dr. Charles Sherr for his helpful discussion and review of the manuscript and Mrs. Patt Nichol for her skillful assistance assembling the text and references.

10. References

AARONSON, S. A., 1971, Chemical induction of focus-forming virus from nonproducer cells transformed by murine sarcoma virus, *Proc. Natl. Acad. Sci.* **68**:3069.

AARONSON, S. A., 1973, Biologic characterization of mammalian cells transformed by a primate sarcoma virus, *Virology* **52**:562.

AARONSON, S. A., AND DUNN, C. Y., 1974a, Endogenous C-type viruses of BALB/c cells: Frequencies of spontaneous and chemical induction, *J. Virol.* **13**:181.

AARONSON, S. A., AND DUNN, C. Y., 1974b, High-frequency C-type virus induction by inhibitors of protein synthesis, *Science* **183**:422.

AARONSON, S. A., AND ROWE, W. P., 1970, Nonproducer clones of murine sarcoma virus transformed BALB/3T3 cells, *Virology* **42**:9.

AARONSON, S. A., AND STEPHENSON, J. R., 1973, Independent segregation of loci for activation of biologically distinguishable RNA C-type viruses in mouse cells, *Proc. Natl. Acad. Sci.* **70**:2055.

AARONSON, S. A., AND STEPHENSON, J. R., 1974, Widespread natural occurrence of high titered neutralizing antibodies to a specific class of endogenous mouse type C virus, *Proc. Natl. Acad. Sci.* **71**:1783.

AARONSON, S., HARTLEY, J., AND TODARO, G. J., 1969, Mouse leukemia virus: "Spontaneous" release by mouse embryo cells after long term *in vitro* cultivation, *Proc. Natl. Acad. Sci.* **64**:87.

AARONSON, S., JAINCHILL, J., AND TODARO, G. J., 1970, Murine sarcoma virus transformation of BALB/3T3 cells: Lack of dependence on murine leukemia virus, *Proc. Natl. Acad. Sci.* **66**:1236.

AARONSON, S. A., PARKS, W. P., SCOLNICK, E. M., AND TODARO, G. J., 1971a, Antibody to the RNA-dependent DNA polymerase of mammalian C-type RNA tumor viruses, *Proc. Natl. Acad. Sci.* **68**:920.

AARONSON, S. A., TODARO, G. J., AND SCOLNICK, E. M., 1971b, Induction of mouse C-type viruses from clonal lines of virus-free BALB/3T3 cells, *Science* **174**:157.

AARONSON, S. A., BASSIN, R. H., AND WEAVER, C., 1972, Comparison of murine sarcoma viruses in nonproducer and S^+L^- transformed cells, *J. Virol.* **9**:701.

ARMSTRONG, J. A., PORTERFIELD, J. S., AND DE MADRID, A. T., 1971, C-type virus particles in pig kidney cell lines, *J. Gen. Virol.* **10**:195.

ARMSTRONG, M. Y. K., RUDDLE, N. H., LIPMAN, M. B., AND RICHARDS, F. F., 1973, Tumor induction by immunologically activated murine leukemia virus, *J. Exp. Med.* **137**:1163.

AUGUST, J. T., BOLOGNESI, D. P., FLEISSNER, E., GILDEN, R. V., AND NOWINSKI, R. C., 1974, A proposed nomenclature for the virion proteins of oncogenic RNA viruses, *Virology* **60**:595.

AXELRAD, A. A., AND STEEVES, R. A., 1964, Assay for Friend leukemia virus: Rapid quantitative method based on enumeration of macroscopic spleen foci in mice, *Virology* **24**:513.

BADER, J. P., AND STECK, T. L., 1969, Analysis of the ribonucleic acid of murine leukemia virus, *J. Virol.* **4**:454.

BALTIMORE, D., 1970, RNA-dependent DNA polymerase in virions of RNA tumor viruses, *Nature (Lond.)* **226**:1209.

BALUDA, M. A., AND ROY-BURMAN, P., 1973, Partial characterization of RD114 virus by DNA–RNA hybridization studies, *Nature New Biol.* **244**:59.

BASSIN, R. H., PHILLIPS, L. A., KRAMER, M. J., HAAPALA, K. D., PEEBLES, P. T., NOMURA, S., AND FISCHINGER, P. J., 1971a, Transformation of mouse 3T3 cells by murine sarcoma virus: Release of virus-like particles in the absence of replicating murine leukemia helper virus, *Proc. Natl. Acad. Sci.* **68:**1520.

BASSIN, R., TUTTLE, N., AND FISCHINGER, P. J., 1971b, Rapid cell culture assay technique for murine leukaemia viruses, *Nature (Lond.)* **229:**564.

BENTVELZEN, P., TIMMERMANS, A., DAAMS, J. H., AND VAN DER GUGTEN, A., 1968, Genetic transmission of mammary tumor inciting viruses in mice: Possible implications for murine leukemia, *Bibl. Haematol.* **31:**101.

BENVENISTE, R. E., AND SCOLNICK, E. M., 1973, RNA in mammalian sarcoma virus transformed nonproducer cells homologous to murine leukemia virus RNA, *Virology* **51:**370.

BENVENISTE, R. E., AND TODARO, G. J., 1973, Homology between type C viruses of various species as determined by molecular hybridization, *Proc. Natl. Acad. Sci.* **70:**3316.

BENVENISTE, R. E., AND TODARO, G. J., 1974a, Evolution of type C viral genes. I. Nucleic acid from baboon type C virus as a measure of divergence among primate species, *Proc. Natl. Acad. Sci.* **71:**4513.

BENVENISTE, R. E., AND TODARO, G. J., 1974b, Multiple divergent copies of endogenous type C virogenes in mammalian cells, *Nature (Lond.)* **252:**170.

BENVENISTE, R. E., AND TODARO, G. J., 1974c, Evolution of C-type viral genes: Inheritance of exogenously acquired viral genes, *Nature (Lond.)* **252:**456.

BENVENISTE, R. E., TODARO, G. J., SCOLNICK, E. M., AND PARKS, W. P., 1973, Partial transcription of murine type C viral genomes in BALB/c cell lines, *J. Virol.* **12:**711.

BENVENISTE, R. E., HEINEMANN, R., WILSON, G. L., CALLAHAN, R., AND TODARO, G. J., 1974a, Detection of baboon type C viral sequences in various primate tissues by molecular hybridization, *J. Virol.* **14:**56.

BENVENISTE, R. E., LIEBER, M. M., LIVINGSTON, D. M., SHERR, C. J., TODARO, G. J., AND KALTER, S. S., 1974b, Infectious type C virus isolated from a baboon placenta, *Nature (Lond.)* **248:**17.

BENVENISTE, R. E., LIEBER, M. M., AND TODARO, G. J., 1974c, A distinct class of inducible murine type C viruses which replicate in the rabbit SIRC cell line, *Proc. Natl. Acad. Sci.* **71:**602.

BERGS, V. V., BERGS, M., AND CHOPRA, H. C., 1970, A virus (RMTDV) derived from chemically induced rat mammary tumors. I. Isolation and general characteristics, *J. Natl. Cancer Inst.* **44:**913.

BERGS, V. V., PEARSON, G., CHOPRA, H. C., AND TURNER, W., 1972, Spontaneous appearance of cytopathology and rat C-type virus (SF-1) in a rat embryo cell line, *Int. J. Cancer* **10:**165.

BERNHARD, W., 1958, Electron microscopy of human cells and tumor viruses: A review, *Cancer Res.* **18:**491.

BERNHARD, W., 1973, Oncornaviruses. 2. Type A and C virus particles in murine and other mammalian leukemias and sarcomas, in: *Ultrastructure of Animal Viruses and Bacteriophages,* Vol. 5 (A. J. Dalton and F. Hagnenau, eds.), p. 283, Academic Press Inc., New York.

BREESE, S. S., JR., 1970, Virus-like particles occurring in cultures of stable pig kidney cell lines, *Arch. Ges. Virusforsch.* **30:**401.

CALLAHAN, R., BENVENISTE, R. E., LIEBER, M. M., AND TODARO, G. J., 1974, Nucleic acid homology of murine type C viral genes. *J. Virol.* **14:**1394.

CHAN, E. W., SCHIOP-STANSLY, P. E., AND O'CONNOR, T. E., 1974, Rescue of cell-transforming virus from a non-virus-producing bovine cell culture transformed by feline sarcoma virus, *J. Natl. Cancer Inst.* **52:**469.

CHASE, D. G., AND PIKÓ, L., 1973, Expression of A- and C-type particles in early mouse embryos, *J. Natl. Cancer Inst.* **51:**1971.

CUATICO, W., CHO, R., AND SPIEGELMAN, S., 1973, Particles with RNA of high molecular weight and RNA-directed DNA polymerase in human brain tumors, *Proc. Natl. Acad. Sci.* **70:**2789.

DARNELL, J. E., WALL, R., AND TUSHINSKI, R. J., 1971, An adenylic acid–rich sequence in messenger RNA of HeLa cells and its possible relationship to reiterated sites in DNA, *Proc. Natl. Acad. Sci.* **68:**1321.

DMOCHOWSKI, L., AND GREY, C. E., 1957, Electron microscopy of tumours of known and suspected viral etiology, *Texas Rep. Biol. Med.* **15:**256.

DUESBERG, P. H., 1970, On the structure of RNA tumor viruses, *Curr. Top. Microbiol. Immunol.* **51:**79.

DUESBERG, P. H., AND ROBINSON, W. S., 1966, Nucleic acid and proteins isolated from the Rauscher mouse leukemia virus (MLV), *Proc. Natl. Acad. Sci.* **55:**219.

DUTCHER, R. M., LARKIN, E. P., AND MARSHAK, R. R., 1964, Virus-like particles in cow's milk from a herd with a high incidence of lymphosarcoma, *J. Natl. Cancer Inst.* **33:**1055.

DUTCHER, R. M., LARKIN, E. P., TUMILOWICS, J. J., NAZERIAN, K., EUSEBIO, C. P., STOCK, N. D., GUEST, G. B., AND MARSHAK, R. R., 1967, Evidence in support of a virus etiology for bovine leukemia, *Cancer* 20:851.

ECKNER, R. J., AND STEEVES, R. A., 1972, A classification of the murine leukemia viruses: Neutralization of pseudotypes of Friend spleen focus-forming virus by type-specific murine antisera, *J. Exp. Med.* 136:832.

EDMONDS, M. P., VAUGHAN, M. H., JR., AND NAKAZATO, H., 1971, Polyadenylic acid sequences in the heterogeneous nuclear RNA and rapidly-labeled polyribosomal RNA of HeLa cells: Possible evidence for a precursor relationship, *Proc. Natl. Acad. Sci.* 68:1336.

FAN, H., AND BALTIMORE, D., 1973, RNA metabolism of murine leukemia virus; detection of virus-specific RNA sequences in infected and uninfected cells and identification of virus-specific messenger RNA, *J. Mol. Biol.* 80:93.

FERRER, J. F., AVILA, L., AND STOCK, N. D., 1972, Antigenic comparison of bovine type C virus with murine and feline leukemia viruses, *Cancer Res.* 32:1871.

FISCHINGER, P. J., AND O'CONNOR, T. E., 1969, Viral infection across species barriers: Alteration of murine sarcoma virus for growth in cat cells, *Science* 165:714.

FISCHINGER, P. J., AND O'CONNOR, T. E., 1970, Productive infection and morphologic alteration of human cells by a modified sarcoma virus, *J. Natl. Cancer Inst.* 44:429.

FISCHINGER, P. J., NOMURA, S., PEEBLES, P. T., HAAPALA, D. K., AND BASSIN, R. H., 1972, Reversion of murine sarcoma virus transformed mouse cells: Variants without a rescuable sarcoma virus, *Science* 176:1033.

FISCHINGER, P. J., PEBBLES, P. T., NOMURA, S., AND HAAPALA, D. K., 1973, Isolation of an RD-114-like oncornavirus from a cat cell line, *J. Virol.* 11:978.

FREEMAN, A. E., KELLOFF, G. J., GILDEN, R. V., LANE, W. T., SWAIN, A. P., AND HUEBNER, R. J., 1971, Activation and isolation of hamster-specific C-type RNA viruses from tumors induced by cell cultures transformed by chemical carcinogens, *Proc. Natl. Acad. Sci.* 68:2386.

FRIEND, C., 1957, Cell-free transmission in adult Swiss mice of a disease having the character of a leukemia, *J. Exp. Med.* 105:307.

GALLO, R. C., MILLER, N. R., SAXINGER, W. C., AND GILLESPIE, D., 1973, Primate RNA tumor virus–like DNA synthesized endogenously by RNA-dependent DNA polymerase in virus-like particles from fresh human acute leukemic blood cells, *Proc. Natl. Acad. Sci.* 70:3219.

GARDNER, M. B., ARNSTEIN, P., JOHNSON, E., RONGEY, R. W., CHARMAN, H. P., AND HUEBNER, R. J., 1971, Feline sarcoma virus tumor induction in cats and dogs, *J. Am. Vet. Med. Assoc.* 158:1046.

GARDNER, M. B., HENDERSON, B. E., OFFICER, J. E., RONGEY, R. W., PARKER, J. C., OLIVER, C., ESTES, J. D., AND HUEBNER, R. J., 1973a, A spontaneous lower motor neuron disease apparently caused by indigenous type-C RNA virus in wild mice, *J. Natl. Cancer Inst.* 51:1243.

GARDNER, M. B., HENDERSON, B. E., RONGEY, R. W., ESTES, J. D., AND HUEBNER, R. J., 1973b, Spontaneous tumors of aging wild house mice: Incidence, pathology and C-type virus expression, *J. Natl. Cancer Inst.* 50:719.

GAZZOLO, L., SIMKOVIC, D., AND MARTIN-BERTHELON, M. C., 1971, The presence of C-type RNA virus particles in a rat embryo cell line spontaneously transformed in tissue culture, *J. Gen. Virol.* 12:303.

GEERING, G., OLD, L. J., AND BOYSE, E. A., 1966, Antigens of leukemias induced by naturally occurring murine leukemia virus: Their relation to the antigens of Gross virus and other murine leukemia viruses, *J. Exp. Med.* 124:753.

GEERING, G., HARDY, W. D., JR., OLD, L. J., AND DEHARVEN, E., 1968, Shared group-specific antigen of murine and feline leukemia viruses, *Virology* 36:678.

GEERING, G., AOKI, T., AND OLD, L. J., 1970, Shared viral antigen of mammalian leukaemia viruses, *Nature (Lond.)* 226:265.

GELDERBLOM, H., BAUER, H., BOLOGNESI, D. P., AND FRANK, H., 1972, Morphogenese und Aufbau von RNS-Tumorviren: Elektronenoptische Untersuchungen an Viruspartikeln vom C-typ, *Zentralbl. Bakteriol. Parasitenk. Infektionskr. Hyg. Abt. 1 Orig.* 220:79.

GILDEN, R. V., OROSZLAN, S., MEIER, H., MYERS, D. D., AND PETERS, R. L., 1970, Group-specific antigen expression during embryogenesis of the genome of the C-type RNA tumor virus: Implications for ontogenesis and oncogenesis, *Proc. Natl. Acad. Sci.* 67:366.

GILDEN, R. V., TONI, R., HANSON, M., BOVA, D., CHARMAN, H. P., AND OROSZLAN, S., 1974, Immunochemical studies of the major internal polypeptide of woolly monkey and gibbon ape type C viruses, *J. Immunol.* 112:1250.

GILLESPIE, D., GILLESPIE, S., GALLO, R. C., EAST, J. L., AND DMOCHOWSKI, L., 1973, Genetic origin of RD114 and other RNA tumour viruses assayed by molecular hybridization, *Nature New Biol.* **244:**51.

GOMARD, E., LECLERC, J. C., AND LEVY, J. P., 1972, Murine leukemia and sarcoma viruses: Further studies on the antigens of the viral envelope, *J. Natl. Cancer Inst.* **50:**955.

GRAFFI, A., 1957, Chloroleukemia of mice, *Ann. N.Y. Acad. Sci.* **68:**540.

GRAFFI, A., SCHRAMM, T., BNEDER, E., GRAFFI, I., HORN, K. H., AND BIERWOLD, D., 1968, Cell free transmissible leukosis in Syrian hamster, probably of viral aetiology, *Brit. J. Cancer* **22:**577.

GREEN, M., AND CARTAS, M., 1972, The genome of RNA tumor viruses contains polyadenylic acid sequences, *Proc. Natl. Acad. Sci.* **69:**791.

GROSS, L., 1951, "Spontaneous" leukemia developing in C3H mice following inoculation in infancy, with A-K leukemic extracts, or AK embryos, *Proc. Soc. Exp. Biol. Med.* **76:**27.

GROSS, L., 1958, Attempt to recover filterable agent from X-ray-induced leukemia, *Acta Haematol.* **19:**353.

GROSS, L., 1970, *Oncogenic Viruses*, 2nd ed., Pergamon Press, Oxford.

HALL, W. T., ANDRESEN, W. F., SANFORD, K. K., EVANS, V., AND HARTLEY, J. W., 1967, Virus particles and murine leukemia virus complement-fixing antigen in neoplastic and non-neoplastic cell lines, *Science* **156:**85.

HARDY, W. D., JR., OLD, L. J., HESS, P. W., ESSEX, M., AND COTTER, S., 1973, Horizontal transmission of feline leukaemia virus, *Nature (Lond.)* **244:**266.

HARTLEY, J. W., AND ROWE, W. P., 1966, Production of altered cell foci in tissue culture by defective Moloney sarcoma virus particles, *Proc. Natl. Acad. Sci.* **55:**780.

HARTLEY, J. W., ROWE, W. P., CAPPS, W. I., AND HUEBNER, R. J., 1965, Complement fixation and tissue culture assays for mouse leukemia viruses, *Proc. Natl. Acad. Sci.* **53:**931.

HARTLEY, J. W., ROWE, W. P., AND HUEBNER, R. J., 1970, Host-range restrictions of murine leukemia viruses in mouse embryo cell cultures, *J. Virol.* **5:**221.

HARVEY, J. J., 1964, An unidentified virus which causes the rapid production of tumours in mice, *Nature (Lond.)* **204:**1104.

HEHLMANN, R., KUFE, D., AND SPIEGELMAN, S., 1972a, RNA in human leukemic cells related to the RNA of a mouse leukemia virus, *Proc. Natl. Acad. Sci.* **69:**435.

HEHLMANN, R., KUFE, D., AND SPIEGELMAN, S., 1972b, Viral-related RNA in Hodgkins' disease and other human lymphomas, *Proc. Natl. Acad. Sci.* **69:**1727.

HENDERSON, I. C., LIEBER, M. M., AND TODARO, G. J., 1974, Mink cell line MvlLu (CCL 64): Focus formation and the generation of "nonproducer" transformed cell lines with murine and feline sarcoma viruses, *Virology* **60:**282.

HIRSCH, M. S., PHILLIPS, S. M., SOLNIK, C., BLACK, P. H., SCHWARTZ, R. S., AND CARPENTER, C. B., 1972, Activation of leukemia viruses by graft-versus-host and mixed lymphocyte reactions *in vitro, Proc. Natl. Acad. Sci.* **69:**1069.

HOLLIS, V. W., JR., AOKI, T., BARRERA, O., OLDSTONE, M. B. A., AND DIXON, F. J., 1974, Detection of naturally occurring antibodies to RNA-dependent DNA polymerase of murine leukemia virus in kidney eluates of AKR mice, *J. Virol.* **13:**448.

HSIUNG, G. D., 1972, Activation of guinea pig C-type virus in cultured spleen cells by 5-bromo-2'-deoxyuridine, *J. Natl. Cancer Inst.* **49:**567.

HUANG, A. S., BESMER, P., CHU, L., AND BALTIMORE, D., 1973, Growth of pseudotypes of vesicular stomatitis virus with N-tropic murine leukemia virus coats in cells resistant to N-tropic viruses, *J. Virol.* **12:**659.

HUEBNER, R., AND TODARO, G. J., 1969, Oncogenes of RNA tumor viruses as determinants of cancer, *Proc. Natl. Acad. Sci.* **64:**1087.

IHLE, J. N., YURCONIC, M., JR., AND HANNA, M. G., JR., 1973, Autogenous immunity to endogenous RNA tumor virus, *J. Exp. Med.* **138:**194.

JAINCHILL, J., AARONSON, S., AND TODARO, G. J., 1969, Murine sarcoma and leukemia viruses: Assay using clonal lines of contact inhibited cells, *J. Virol.* **4:**549.

JARRETT, W. F. H., 1971, Feline leukaemia, *Int. Rev. Exp. Pathol.* **10:**243.

JARRETT, W. F. H., CRAWFORD, E. M., MARTIN, W. B., AND DAVIE, F., 1964a, Leukaemia in the cat: A virus-like particle associated with leukaemia (lymphosarcoma), *Nature (Lond.)* **202:**567.

JARRETT, W. F. H., MARTIN, W. B., CRIGHTON, G. W., DALTON, R. G., AND STEWART, M. F., 1964b, Leukaemia in the cat: Transmission experiments with leukaemia (lymphosarcoma), *Nature (Lond.)* **202:**566.

KACIAN, D. L., WATSON, K. F., BURNY, A., AND SPIEGELMAN, S., 1971, Purification of the DNA polymerase of avian myeloblastosis virus, *Biochim. Biophys. Acta* **246**:365.

KAKEFUDA, T., AND BADER, J. P., 1969, Electron microscopic observations on the ribonucleic acid of murine leukemia virus, *J. Virol.* **4**:460.

KALTER, S. S., HELMKE, R. J., PANIGEL, M., HEBERLING, R. L., FELSBURG, P. J., AND AXELROD, L. R., 1973a, Observations of apparent C-type particles in baboon (*Papio cynocephalus*) placentas, *Science* **179**:1332.

KALTER, S. S., HELMKE, R. J., HEBERLING, R. L., PANIGEL, M., FOWLER, A. K., STRICKLAND, J. E., AND HELLMAN, A., 1973b, C-type particles in normal human placentas, *J. Natl. Cancer Inst.* **50**:1081.

KATES, J., 1970, Transcription of the vaccinia virus genome and the occurrence of polyribadenylic acid sequences in messenger RNA, *Cold Spring Harbor Symp. Quant. Biol.* **35**:743.

KAWAKAMI, T. G., MOORE, A. L., THEILEN, G. H., AND MUNN, R. J., 1970, Comparisons of virus-like particles from leukotic cattle to feline leukosis virus, in *Leukemia in Animals and Man* (R. M. Dutcher, ed.), p. 471, Karger, Basel.

KAWAKAMI, T., HUFF, S. D., BUCKLEY, P. M., DUNGWORTH, D. L., SNYDER, S. P., AND GILDEN, R. V., 1972, C-type virus associated with gibbon lymphosarcoma, *Nature New Biol.* **235**:170.

KELLOFF, G., HUEBNER, R. J., CHANG, N. H., LEE, Y. K., AND GILDEN, R. V., 1970a, Envelope antigen relationships among three hamster specific sarcoma viruses and a hamster specific virus, *J. Gen. Virol.* **9**:19.

KELLOFF, G., HUEBNER, R. J., LEE, Y. K., TONI, R., AND GILDEN, R., 1970b, Hamster-tropic sarcomagenic and non-sarcomagenic viruses derived from hamster tumors induced by the Gross pseudotypes of Moloney sarcoma virus, *Proc. Natl. Acad. Sci.* **65**:310.

KELLOFF, G. J., HATANAKA, M., AND GILDEN, R. V., 1972, Assay of C-type virus infectivity by measurement of RNA-dependent DNA polymerase activity, *Virology* **48**:266.

KINDIG, D. A., AND KIRSTEN, W. H., 1967, Virus-like particles in established murine cell lines: Electron microscopic observations, *Science* **155**:1543.

KIRSTEN, W. H., AND MAYER, L. A., 1967, Morphologic responses to a murine erythroblastosis virus, *J. Natl. Cancer Inst.* **39**:311.

KIRSTEN, W. H., MAYER, R. A., WOLLMANN, R. L., AND PIERCE, M. I., 1967, Studies on a murine erythroblastosis virus, *J. Natl. Cancer Inst.* **38**:117.

KLEMENT, V., HARTLEY, J. W., ROWE, W. P., AND HUEBNER, R. J., 1969a, Recovery of a hamster-specific, focus-forming, and sarcomagenic virus from a "non-infectious" hamster tumor induced by the Kirsten mouse sarcoma virus, *J. Natl. Cancer Inst.* **43**:925.

KLEMENT, V., ROWE, W. P., HARTLEY, J. W., AND PUGH, W. E., 1969b, Mixed culture cytopathogenicity: A new test for growth of murine leukemia viruses in tissue culture, *Proc. Natl. Acad. Sci.* **63**:753.

KLEMENT, V., NICOLSON, M. O., AND HUEBNER, R. J., 1971, Rescue of the genome of focus forming virus from rat non-productive lines by 5'-bromodeoxyuridine, *Nature New Biol.* **234**:12.

KLEMENT, V., NICOLSON, M. O., GILDEN, R. V., OROSZLAN, S., SARMA, P. W., RONGEY, R. W., AND GARDNER, M. B., 1972, Rat C-type virus induced in rat sarcoma cells by 5-bromodeoxyuridine, *Nature New Biol.* **238**:234.

KRONTIRIS, T. G., SOEIRO, R., AND FIELDS, B. N., 1973, Host restriction of Friend leukemia virus: Role of the viral outer coat, *Proc. Natl. Acad. Sci.* **70**:2549.

KUFE, D., HEHLMANN, R., AND SPIEGELMAN, S., 1972, Human sarcomas contain RNA related to the RNA of a mouse leukemia virus, *Science* **175**:182.

KUFE, D., HEHLMANN, R., AND SPIEGELMAN, S., 1973, RNA related to that of a murine leukemia virus in Burkitt's tumors and nasopharyngeal carcinomas, *Proc. Natl. Acad. Sci.* **70**:5.

KUNG, H.-J., BAILEY, J. M., DAVIDSON, N., NICOLSON, M. O., AND McALLISTER, R. M., 1974, Structure and molecular length of the large subunits of RD-114 viral RNA, *J. Virol.*, **14**:170.

LAI, M. M. C., AND DUESBERG, P. H., 1972, Adenylic acid–rich sequence in RNAs of Rous sarcoma virus and Rauscher mouse leukaemia virus, *Nature (Lond.)* **235**:383.

LAIRD, H. M., JARRETT, O., CRIGHTON, G. W., AND JARRETT, W. F. H., 1968a, An electron microscopic study of virus particles in spontaneous leukemia in the cat, *J. Natl. Cancer Inst.* **41**:867.

LAIRD, H. M., JARRETT, O., CRIGHTON, G. W., JARRETT, W. F. H., AND HAY, D., 1968b, Replication of leukemogenic-type virus in cats inoculated with feline lymphosarcoma extracts, *J. Natl. Cancer Inst.* **41**:879.

LATARJET, R., AND DUPLAN, J.-F., 1962, Experiment and discussion on leukaemogenesis by cell-free extracts of radiation-induced leukaemia in mice, *Int. J. Radiat. Biol.* **5**:339.

LEE, Y., MENDECKI, J., AND BRAWERMAN, G., 1971, A polynucleotide segment rich in adenylic acid in the rapidly-labeled polyribosomal RNA component of mouse sarcoma 180 ascites cells, *Proc. Natl. Acad. Sci.* **68:**1331.

LEVY, J. A., 1973, Xenotropic viruses: Murine leukemia viruses associated with NIH Swiss, NZB, and other mouse strains, *Science* **182:**1151.

LIEBER, M. M., AND TODARO, G. J., 1973, Spontaneous and induced production of endogenous type C RNA virus from a clonal line line of spontaneously transformed BALB/3T3, *Int. J. Cancer* **11:**616.

LIEBER, M. M., BENVENISTE, R. E., LIVINGSTON, D. M., AND TODARO, G. J., 1973*a*, Mammalian cells in culture frequently release type C viruses, *Science* **182:**56.

LIEBER, M. M., LIVINGSTON, D. M., AND TODARO, G. J., 1973*b*, Superinduction of endogenous type C virus by 5-bromodeoxyuridine from transformed mouse clones, *Science* **181:**443.

LIEBER, M. M., SHERR, C. J., AND TODARO, G. J., 1974, S-tropic murine type C viruses: Frequency of isolation from continuous cell lines, leukemic virus preparations and normal spleens, *Int. J. Cancer,* **13:**587.

LIEBERMAN, M., AND KAPLAN, H. S., 1959, Leukemogenic activity of filtrates from radiation-induced lymphoid tumors of mice, *Science* **130:**387.

LILLY, F., 1970, Fv-2: Identification and location of a second gene governing the spleen focus response to Friend leukemia virus in mice, *J. Natl. Cancer Inst.* **45:**163.

LILLY, F., 1972, Mouse leukemia: A model of a multiple-gene disease, *J. Natl. Cancer Inst.* **49:**927.

LIM, L., AND CANELLAKIS, E. S., 1970, Adenine-rich polymer associated with rabbit reticulocyte messenger RNA, *Nature (Lond.)* **227:**710.

LIVINGSTON, D. M., AND TODARO, G. J., 1973, Endogenous type C virus from a cat clone with properties distinct from previously described feline type C viruses, *Virology* **53:**142.

LOWY, D. R., ROWE, W. P., TEICH, N., AND HARTLEY, J. W., 1971, Murine leukemia virus: High-frequency activation *in vitro* by 5-iododeoxyuridine and 5-bromodeoxyuridine, *Science* **174:**155.

LWOFF, A., SIMINOVITCH, L., AND KJELDGAARD, N., 1950, Induction de la production de bacteriophages chez une bacterie lysogène, *Ann. Inst. Pasteur* **79:**815.

LWOFF, A., 1960, Tumor viruses and the cancer problem: A summation of the conference, *Cancer Res.* **20:**820.

MAISEL, J., KLEMENT, V., LAI, M. M-.C., OSTERTAG, W., AND DUESBERG, P., 1973, Ribonucleic acid components of murine sarcoma and leukemia viruses, *Proc. Natl. Acad. Sci.* **70:**3536.

MCALLISTER, R. M., NELSON-REES, W. A., JOHNSON, E. Y., RONGEY, R. W., AND GARDNER, M. B., 1971, Disseminated rhabdomyosarcomas formed in kittens by cultured human rhabdomyosarcoma cells, *J. Natl. Cancer Inst.* **47:**603.

MCALLISTER, R. M., NICOLSON, M., GARDNER, M. B., RONGEY, R. W., RASHEED, S., SARMA, P. S., HUEBNER, R. J., HATANAKA, M., OROSZLAN, S., GILDEN, R. V., KABIGTING, A., AND VERNON, L., 1972, C-type virus released from cultured human rhabdomyosarcoma cells, *Nature New Biol.* **235:**3.

MEIER, H., TAYLOR, B. A., CHERRY, M., AND HUEBNER, R. J., 1973, Host-gene control of type-C RNA tumor virus expression and tumorigenesis in inbred mice, *Proc. Natl. Acad. Sci.* **70:**1450.

MILLER, J. M., MILLER, L. D., OLSON, C., AND GILLETTE, K. G., 1969, Virus-like particles in phytohemagglutinin stimulated lymphocyte cultures with reference to bovine lymphosarcoma, *J. Natl. Cancer Inst.* **43:**1297.

MOENNIG, V., FRANK, H., HUNSMANN, G., OHMS, P., SCHWARZ, H., SCHÄFER, W., AND STRANDSTRÖM, H.; 1974, C-type particles produced by a permanent cell line from a leukemic pig. II. Physical, chemical and serological characterization of the particles, *Virology* **57:**179.

MOLONEY, J. B., 1960, Biological studies on a lymphoid-leukemia virus extracted from sarcoma 37. I. Origin and introductory investigations, *J. Natl. Cancer Inst.* **24:**933.

MOLONEY, J. B., 1966, A virus-induced rhabdomyosarcoma of mice, in: *Conference on Murine Leukemia,* p. 139, National Cancer Institute Monograph No. 22, U.S. Public Health Service, Bethesda, Md.

NADEL, E., BANFIELD, W., BURSTEIN, S., AND TOUSIMIS, A. J., 1967, Virus particles associated with strain 2 guinea pig leukemia (L2C/N-B), *J. Natl. Cancer Inst.* **38:**979.

NAYAK, D. P., AND MURRAY, P. R., 1973, Induction type C viruses in cultured guinea pig cells, *J. Virol.* **12:**177.

NEIMAN, P. E., 1973, Measurement of RD114 virus nucleotide sequences in feline cellular DNA, *Nature New Biol.* **244:**62.

NERMUT, M. V., HERMANN, F., AND SCHÄFER, W., 1972, Properties of mouse leukemia viruses. III. Electron microscopic appearance as revealed after conventional preparation techniques as well as freeze-drying and freeze-etching, *Virology* **49:**345.

NOMURA, S., FISCHINGER, P. J., MATTERN, C. F. T., PEEBLES, P. T., BASSIN, R. H., AND FRIEDMAN, G. P., 1972, Revertants of mouse cells transformed by murine sarcoma virus. I. Characterization of flat and transformed sublines without a rescuable murine sarcoma virus, *Virology* **50:**51.

NOMURA, S., FISCHINGER, P. J., MATTERN, C. F. T., GERWIN, B. I., AND DUNN, K. J., 1973, Revertants of mouse cells transformed by murine sarcoma virus. II. Flat variants induced by fluorodeoxyuridine and colcemid, *Virology* **56:**152.

NOWINSKI, R. C., FLEISSNER, E., SARKAR, N. H., AND AOKI, T., 1972, Chromatographic separation and antigenic analysis of proteins of the oncornaviruses. II. Mammalian leukaemia–sarcoma viruses, *J. Virol.* **9:**359.

O'CONNOR, T. E., AND FISCHINGER, P. J., 1968, Physical properties of competence defective states of murine sarcoma (Moloney) virus, *J. Natl. Cancer Inst.* **43:**487.

ODAKA, T., 1969, Inheritance of susceptibility to Friend mouse leukaemia virus, *J. Virol.* **3:**543.

OFFICER, J. E., TECSON, N., ESTES, J. D., FONTANILLA, E., RONGEY, R. W., AND GARDNER, M. B., 1973, Isolation of a neurotropic type C virus, *Science* **181:**945.

OKABE, H., GILDEN, R. V., AND HATANAKA, M., 1973, Extensive homology of RD114 virus DNA with RNA feline cell origin, *Nature New Biol.* **244:**54.

OLDSTONE, M. B., AOKI, T., AND DIXON, F. J., 1972, The antibody response of mice to murine leukemia virus in spontaneous infection: Absence of classical immunologic tolerance, *Proc. Natl. Acad. Sci.* **69:**134.

OLSEN, R. G., AND YOHN, D. S., 1972, Demonstration of antibody in cat sera to feline oncornavirus by complement-fixation inhibition, *J. Natl. Cancer Inst.* **49:**395.

OLSON, C., MILLER, L. D., MILLER, J. M., AND HOSS, H. E., 1972, Transmission of lymphosarcoma from cattle to sheep, *J. Natl. Cancer Inst.* **49:**1463.

OPLER, S. R., 1967, Observations on a new virus associated with guinea pig leukemia: Preliminary note, *J. Natl. Cancer Inst.* **38:**797.

PARKMAN, R., LEVY, J. A., AND TING, R. C., 1970, The question of defectiveness of murine sarcoma virus, *Science* **168:**387.

PARKS, W. P., SCOLNICK, E. M., ROSS, J., TODARO, G. J., AND AARONSON, S. A., 1972, Immunologic relationships of reverse transcriptases from RNA tumor viruses, *J. Virol.* **9:**110.

PARKS, W. P., SCOLNICK, E. M., NOON, M. C., WATSON, C. J., AND KAWAKAMI, T. G., 1973, Radioimmunoassay of mammalian type-C polypeptides. IV. Characterization of woolly monkey and gibbon viral antigens, *Int. J. Cancer* **12:**129.

PETERS, R. L., HARTLEY, J. W., SPAHN, G. J., RABSTEIN, L. S., WHITMIRE, C. E., TURNER, H. C., AND HUEBNER, R. J., 1972, Prevalence of the group-specific (gs) antigen and infectious virus expressions of the murine C-type RNA viruses during the life span of BALB/cCr mice, *Int. J. Cancer* **10:**283.

PETERS, R. L., SPAHN, G. J., RABSTEIN, L. S., KELLOFF, G. J., AND HUEBNER, R. J., 1973*a*, Murine C-type RNA virus from spontaneous neoplasms: *In vitro* host range and oncogenic potential, *Science* **181:**665.

PETERS, R. L., SPAHN, G. J., RABSTEIN, L. S., KELLOFF, G. J., AND HUEBNER, R. J., 1973*b*, Oncogenic potential of murine C-type RNA virus passaged directly from naturally occurring tumors of the BALB/cCr mouse, *J. Natl. Cancer Inst.* **51:**621.

PHILLIPSON, L., WALL, R., GLICKMAN, R., AND DARNELL, J. E., 1971, Addition of polyadenylate sequences to virus-specific RNA during adenovirus replication, *Proc. Natl. Acad. Sci.* **68:**2806.

PINCUS, T., HARTLEY, J. W., AND ROWE, W. P., 1971*a*, A major genetic locus affecting resistance to infection with murine leukemia viruses. II. Apparent identity to a major locus described for resistance to Friend murine leukemia virus, *J. Exp. Med.* **133:**1234.

PINCUS, T., ROWE, W. P., AND LILLY, F., 1971*b*, A major genetic locus affecting resistance to infection with murine leukemia viruses. I. Tissue culture studies of naturally occuring viruses, *J. Exp. Med.* **133:**1219.

RAUSCHER, F. J., 1962, A virus-induced disease of mice characterized by erythrocytopoiesis and lymphoid leukemia, *J. Natl. Cancer Inst.* **29:**515.

RHIM, J. S., DUH, F. G., CHO, H. Y., WUU, K. D., AND VERNON, M. L., 1973, Activation by 5-bromo-2'-deoxyuridine of particles resembling guinea-pig leukemia virus from guinea-pig nonproducer cells, *J. Natl. Cancer Inst.* **51:**1327.

RICKARD, C. G., 1969, Feline leukemia (Lymphosarcoma Symposium), *J. Small Anim. Pract.* **10:**615.

RICKARD, C. G., BARR, L. M., NORONHA, F., DOUGHERTY, E., 3RD, AND POST, J. E., 1967, C-type virus particles in spontaneous lymphocytic leukemia in a cat, *Cornell Vet.* **57**:302.

RICKARD, C. G., POST, J. E., NORONHA, F., AND BARR, L. M., 1969, A transmissible virus-induced lymphocytic leukemia of the cat, *J. Natl. Cancer Inst.* **42**:937.

RICKARD, C. G., POST, J. E., NORONHA, F., DOUGHERTY, E., III, AND BARR, L. M., 1973, Feline tumor viruses, in: *Biohazards in Biological Research*, p. 166, Cold Spring Harbor Laboratory, Cold Spring Harbor, N.Y.

ROSS, J., SCOLNICK, E. M., TODARO, G. J., AND AARONSON, S. A., 1971, Separations of murine cellular and murine leukemia virus DNA polymerase, *Nature New Biol.* **231**:163.

ROSS, J., TRONICK, S. R., AND SCOLNICK, E. M., 1972, Polyadenylate rich RNA in the 70S RNA of murine leukemia–sarcoma virus, *Virology* **49**:230.

ROWE, W. P., 1972, Studies of genetic transmission of murine leukemia virus by AKR mice. I. Crosses with $Fv-1^n$ strains of mice, *J. Exp. Med.* **136**:1272.

ROWE, W. P., AND HARTLEY, J. W., 1972, Studies of genetic transmission of murine leukemia virus by AKR mice. II. Crosses with $Fv-1^b$ strains of mice, *J. Exp. Med.* **136**:1286.

ROWE, W. P., AND PINCUS, T., 1972, Quantitative studies of naturally occurring murine leukemia virus infection of AKR mice, *J. Exp. Med.* **135**:429.

ROWE, W. P., PUGH, W. E., AND HARTLEY, J. W., 1970, Plaque assay techniques for murine leukemia viruses, *Virology* **42**:1136.

ROWE, W. P., HARTLEY, J. W., LANDER, M. R., PUGH, W. E., AND TEICH, N., 1971, Noninfectious AKR mouse embryo cell lines in which each cell has the capacity to be activated to produce infectious murine leukemia virus, *Virology* **46**:866.

ROWE, W. P., HUMPHREY, J. B., AND LILLY, F., 1973, A major genetic locus affecting resistance to infections with murine leukemia viruses. III. Assignment of the $Fv-1$ locus to linkage group VIII of the mouse, *J. Exp. Med.* **137**:850.

RUBIN, H., CORNELIUS, A., AND FANSHIER, L., 1961, The pattern of congenital transmission of an avian leukosis virus, *Proc. Natl. Acad. Sci.* **47**:1058.

RUPRECHT, R. M., GOODMAN, N. C., AND SPIEGELMAN, S., 1973, Determination of natural host taxonomy of RNA tumor viruses by molecular hybridization: Application to RD-114, a candidate human virus, *Proc. Natl. Acad. Sci.* **70**:1437.

SARKAR, N. H., MOORE, D. H., KRAMARSKY, G., AND CHOPRA, H. C., 1973, Oncornaviruses. 3. The mammary tumor virus in: *Ultrastructure of Animal Viruses and Bacteriophages*, Vol. 5 (A. J. Dalton and F. Hagnenau, eds.), p. 307. Academic Press Inc., New York.

SARMA, P. S., AND LOG, T., 1971, Viral interference in feline leukemia–sarcoma complex, *Virology* **44**:352.

SARMA, P. S., AND LOG, T., 1973, Subgroup classification of feline leukemia and sarcoma viruses by viral interference and neutralization tests, *Virology* **54**:160.

SARMA, P. S., CHEONG, M. P., HARTLEY, J. W., AND HUEBNER, R. J., 1967, A viral interference test for mouse leukemia viruses, *Virology* **33**:180.

SARMA, P. S., LOG, T., AND HUEBNER, R. J., 1970, Trans-species rescue of defective genomes of murine sarcoma virus from hamster tumor cells with helper feline leukemia virus, *Proc. Natl. Acad. Sci.* **65**:81.

SARMA, P. S., TSENG, J., GILDEN, R., AND LEE, Y. K., 1973, Virus similar to RD-114 virus in cat cells, *Nature New Biol.* **244**:56.

SARNGADHARAN, M., SARIN, P., REITZ, M., AND GALLO, R. C., 1972, Reverse transcriptase activity of human acute leukemic cells: Purification of the enzyme, response to AMV 70S RNA, and characterization of the DNA product, *Nature New Biol.* **240**:67.

SCHÄFER, W., FISCHINGER, P. J., LANGE, J., AND PISTER, L., 1972, Properties of mouse leukemia viruses. I. Characterization of various antisera and serological identification of viral components, *Virology* **47**:197.

SCHIDLOVSKY, G., AND AHMED, M., 1973, C-type virus particles in placentas and fetal tissues of rhesus monkeys, *J. Natl. Cancer Inst.* **51**:225.

SCHOOLMAN, H. M., SPURRIER, W., SCHWARTZ, S. O., AND SZANTS, P. B., 1957, Studies in leukemia. VII. The induction of leukemia in Swiss mice by means of cell-free filtrates of leukemic mouse brain, *Blood* **12**:694.

SCOLNICK, E. M., AND PARKS, W. P., 1973, Isolation and characterization of a primate sarcoma virus: Mechanism of rescue, *Int. J. Cancer* **12**:138.

SCOLNICK, E. M., PARKS, W. P., AND TODARO, G. J., 1972a, Reverse transcriptases of primate viruses as immunological markers, *Science* **177**:1119.

SCOLNICK, E. M., PARKS, W. P., TODARO, G. J., AND AARONSON, S. A., 1972b, Primate C-type virus reverse transcriptases: Immunological properties, *Nature New Biol.* **235**:35.

SCOLNICK, E. M., RANDS, E., WILLIAMS, D., AND PARKS, W. P., 1973, Studies on the nucleic acid sequences of Kirsten sarcoma virus: A model for formation of a mammalian RNA-containing sarcoma virus, *J. Virol.* **12**:458.

SCOLNICK, E. M., PARKS, W., KAWAKAMI, T., KOHNE, D., OKABE, H., GILDEN, R., AND HATANAKA, M., 1974, Primate and murine type-C viral nucleic acid association kinetics: Analysis of model systems and natural tissues, *J. Virol.* **13**:363.

SHERR, C. J., AND TODARO, G. J., 1974, Radioimmunoassay of the major group specific protein of endogenous baboon type C viruses: Relation to the RD-114/CCC group and detection of antigen in normal baboon tissues, *Virology*, **61**:168.

SHERR, C. J., AND TODARO, G. J., 1974b, Type C viral antigens in man. I. Antigens related to endogenous primate virus in human tumors, *Proc. Natl. Acad. Sci.* **71**:4703.

SHERR, C. J., BENVENISTE, R. E., AND TODARO, G. J., 1974a, Type C viral expression in primate tissues, *Proc. Natl. Acad. Sci.* **71**:3721.

SHERR, C. J., LIEBER, M. M., AND TODARO, G. J., 1974b, Mixed splenocyte cultures and graft versus host reactions selectively induce an "S-tropic" murine type C virus, *Cell* **1**:55.

SHERR, C. J., LIEBER, M. M., BENVENISTE, R. E., AND TODARO, G. J., 1974c, Endogenous baboon type C virus (M7): Biochemical and immunologic characterization, *Virology* **58**:476.

SKLAR, M. D., WHITE, B. J., AND ROWE, W. P., 1974, Initiation of oncogenic transformation of mouse lymphocytes *in vitro* by Abelson leukemia virus, *Proc. Natl. Acad. Sci.* **71**:4077.

SNYDER, S. P., AND THEILEN, G. H., 1969, Transmissible feline lymphosarcoma, *Nature (Lond.)* **221**:1074.

STEPHENSON, J. R., AND AARONSON, S. A., 1972, Genetic factors influencing C-type RNA virus induction, *J. Exp. Med.* **136**:175.

STEPHENSON, J. R., AND AARONSON, S. A., 1973, Segregation of loci for C-type virus induction in strains of mice with high and low incidence of leukemia, *Science* **180**:865.

STEPHENSON, J. R., GREENBERGER, J. S., AND AARONSON, S. A., 1974a, Oncogenicity of an endogenous C-type virus chemically activated from mouse cells in culture, *J. Virol.* **13**:237.

STEPHENSON, J. R., TRONICK, S. R., AND AARONSON, S. A., 1974b, Analysis of type specific antigenic determinants of two structural polypeptides of mouse RNA C-type viruses, *Virology* **58**:1.

STRAND, M., AND AUGUST, J. T., 1974, Structural proteins of mammalian oncogenic RNA viruses: Multiple antigenic determinants of the major internal protein and envelope glycoprotein, *J. Virol.* **13**:171.

STRANDSTRÖM, H., VEIJALAINENE, P., MOENNIG, V., HUNSMANN, G., SCHWARZ, H., AND SCHÄFER, 1974, C-type particles produced by a permanent cell line from a leukemic pig. I. Origin and properties of the host cells and some evidence for the occurrence of C-type-like particles, *Virology* **57**:175.

TEICH, N., LOWY, D. R., HARTLEY, J. W., AND ROWE, W. P., 1973, Studies of the mechanism of induction of infectious murine leukemia virus from AKR mouse embryo cell lines by 5-iododeoxyuridine and 5-bromodeoxyuridine, *Virology* **51**:163.

TEMIN, H. M., 1971, Mechanism of cell transformation by RNA tumor viruses, *Ann Rev. Microbiol.* **25**:609.

TEMIN, H., AND MIZUTANI, S., 1970, RNA-dependent DNA polymerase in virions of Rous sarcoma virus, *Nature (Lond.)* **226**:1211.

TENNANT, J. R., 1962, Derivation of a murine lymphoid leukemia virus, *J. Natl. Cancer Inst.* **28**:1291.

THEILEN, G. H., GOULD, D., FOWLER, M., AND DUNGWORTH, D. L., 1971, C-type virus in tumor tissue of a woolly monkey (*Lagothrix* spp.) with fibrosarcoma, *J. Natl. Cancer Inst.* **47**:881.

TODARO, G. J., 1972, "Spontaneous" release of type C viruses from clonal lines of "spontaneously" transformed BALB/3T3 cells, *Nature New Biol.* **240**:157.

TODARO, G. J., AND AARONSON, S., 1969, Properties of clonal lines of murine sarcoma virus transformed BALB/3T3 cells, *Virology* **38**:174.

TODARO, G. J., AND GALLO, R. C., 1973, Immunologic relatedness between a DNA polymerase from human acute leukaemia cells and primate and mouse leukaemia virus reverse transcriptase, *Nature (Lond.)* **244**:206.

TODARO, G. J., ARNSTEIN, P., PARKS, W. P., LENNETTE, E. H., AND HUEBNER, R. J., 1973a, A type C virus in human rhabdomyosarcoma cells after inoculation into antithymocyte serum–treated NIH Swiss mice, *Proc. Natl. Acad. Sci.* **70**:859.

TODARO, G. J., BENVENISTE, R. E., LIEBER, M. M., AND LIVINGSTON, D. M., 1973b, Infectious type C viruses released by normal cat embryo cells, *Virology* **55**:505.

TODARO, G. J., BENVENISTE, R. E., LIEBER, M. M., AND SHERR, C. J., 1974a, Characterization of a type C virus released from the porcine cell line PK(15), *Virology* **58:**65.

TODARO, G. J., SHERR, C. J., BENVENISTE, R. E., LIEBER, M. M., AND MELNICK, J. L., 1974b, Type C viruses of baboons: Isolation from normal cell cultures, *Cell,* **2:**55.

VAN DER MAATEN, M. J., MILLER, J. M., AND BOOTHE, A. D., 1974, Replicating type-C virus particles in monolayer cell cultures of tissues from cattle with lymphosarcoma, *J. Natl. Cancer Inst.* **52:**491.

VERMA, I. M., MEUTH, N. L., FAN, H., AND BALTIMORE, D., 1974, Hamster leukemia virus DNA polymerase: Unique structure and lack of demonstrable endogenous activity, *J. Virol.* **13:**1075.

VERNON, M. L., LANE, W. T., AND HUEBNER, R. J., 1973, Prevalence of type-C particles in visceral tissues of embryonic and newborn mice, *J. Natl. Cancer Inst.* **51:**1171.

VOGT, P. K., AND ISHIZAKI, R., 1965, Reciprocal patterns of genetic resistance to avian tumor viruses in two lines of chickens, *Virology* **26:**664.

WATSON, J. D., 1971, The structure and assembly of murine leukemia virus: Intracellular viral RNA, *Virology* **45:**586.

WEISS, R. A., FRIIS, R. R., KATZ, E., AND VOGT, P. K., 1971, Induction of avian tumor viruses in normal cells by physical and chemical carcinogens, *Virology* **46:**920.

WITTE, N. O., WEISSMAN, I. L., AND KAPLAN, H. S., 1973, Structural characteristics of some murine RNA tumor viruses studied by lactoperoxidase iodination, *Proc. Natl. Acad. Sci.* **70:**36.

WOLFE, L. G., DEINHARDT, F., THEILEN, G. H., RUBIN, H., KAWAKAMI, T., AND BUSTAD, L. K., 1971, Induction of tumors in marmoset monkeys by simian sarcoma virus type 1 (*Lagothrix*): A preliminary report, *J. Natl. Cancer Inst.* **47:**1115.

WOLFE, L. G., SMITH, R. K., AND DEINHARDT, F., 1972, Simian sarcoma virus, type 1 (*Lagothrix*): Focus assay and demonstration of nontransforming associated virus, *J. Natl. Cancer Inst.* **48:**1905.

YOSHIKURA, H., HIROKAWA, Y., TKAWA, Y., AND SUGANO, H., 1968, Transformation of a mouse cell line by murine sarcoma virus (Moloney), *Int. J. Cancer* **3:**743.

ZAVADA, J., 1972a, Pseudotypes of vesicular stomatitis virus with the coat of murine leukaemia and of avian myeloblastosis virus, *J. Gen. Virol.* **15:**183.

ZAVADA, J., 1972b, VSV pseudotypes particles with the coat of avian myelobastosis virus, *Nature New Biol.* **240:**122.

4

Mammary Tumor Virus

DAN H. MOORE

1. Introduction

Two hundred years ago, Bernard Peyrilhe of Perpignan, France, believing that cancer might be caused by "a specific virus,"* injected subcutaneously, into a dog, fluid from a human breast carcinoma. This was 25 years before Edward Jenner inoculated an 8-year-old boy with "matter from cow-pox vesicles" which successfully protected him against a later inoculation with smallpox virus. Although the experiment of Peyrilhe was itself not successful, the idea was kept alive in the minds of a few investigators until the present century, and now viruses as etiological agents in cancer are known to be commonplace.

Throughout history, several species have been used for experimentation with cancer, but the mouse has been the animal most extensively used in experimental investigations of cancer of the mammary gland because it is quite prone to mammary tumors, has a short life, and can be easily maintained in large numbers. It is not known precisely when the mouse began to be used as an experimental animal, but man and mouse have been coinhabitants of the same domicile throughout recorded history and they may have served as food for each other in prehistoric times.

Mention of their tumors is made in the first book of Samuel, which records an incident that happened more than 3000 years ago. The Philistines had carried off

---

* Perhaps a word should be said about the shift in meaning of the term "virus" that has taken place since the time of Peyrilhe. At that time, "virus" meant any substance "developed by morbid processes within an animal body" capable of transmitting a specific disease. Bacteria, after they were discovered, fell into this category; later, smaller transmitting agents that passed through filters which held back bacteria were called "filterable viruses." Now, of course, in most cases the difference between viruses and other transmitting agents is distinct.

DAN H. MOORE ● Institute for Medical Research, Camden, New Jersey.

the Ark of the Covenant and with the booty went pestilence and plague. After 7 months, they went to their own priests and asked with what guilt offering they might return the Ark. The priests answered, "Five golden tumors and five golden mice, according to the number of the lords of the Philistines, for the same plague was upon all of you and upon your lords . . . . And they put the Ark of the Lord on the cart, and the box with the golden mice and the images of their tumors" (I Samuel 6: 4 and 11).

To the Greeks, the mouse was sacred. In the temples of Apollo-Smintheus, domesticated white mice were kept at public expense, according to Aelian. "Under the altar white mice are hidden and on the tripod of Apollo a white mouse is standing."

It is believed that the laboratory mouse used today is a descendent of the sacred Greek mouse.

2. Breast Cancer Research Before 1930

Systematic experimentation on mammary tumors in mice began early in this century. From the initial experiments and from those that were performed during the following 25 years, it was concluded that heredity was a principal factor in mammary tumorigenesis. Between 1910 and 1930, numerous homozygous mouse strains were developed, some with a low mammary tumor incidence and others with a very high incidence (see Section 10 for a description of mouse strains). During this period, it became quite clear to most investigators that mammary tumors were an inherited characteristic, although some had ideas of an infectious agent.

Since nematodes and cestodes are common parasites in mice, some investigators thought they might be involved in mammary tumor causation. Borrel (1910) even suggested that the parasites might be carriers of a tumor virus. Gaylord and Clowes (1907) suspected infected cages, and Loeb (1907/1908) placed nontumorous mice in cages which had not been cleaned since they were occupied by mice bearing tumors. No tumors developed, but they were observed for only 3 months. Further experimentation indicated that if animals were kept long enough in either clean or dirty cages some of them developed mammary tumors. While others were thinking of infectious agents, Tyzzer (1909) came out strongly in favor of the hereditary influences, and Bashford (1909) pointed out that there was not satisfactory evidence for epidemics of tumors among mice housed together, suggesting that the cause of the high tumor incidence was more likely to be the result of inbreeding of cancer stock. By 1911, both Bashford and Murray had come to the conclusion that mammary tumors were inherited. Murray's observations between 1906 and 1911 are classical (Murray, 1911). Out of his careful work came the conclusion that if the mother or grandmother of a mouse had a mammary tumor, her risk was significantly higher than that of one whose mother or grandmother did not. The breeding experiments of Slye (1914, 1920, 1926, 1928) and Lathrop and Loeb (1913, 1915) confirmed the strong influence of hereditary factors. By the time the milk influence was discovered in 1936, Slye had studied approximately 100,000 mice and had reached the conclusion that this disease was primarily hereditary.

The nature of the genetic factors influencing mammary tumor development became an important question, and waves of opinions ensued. Slye (1914, 1920, 1926, 1928), Dobrovolskaia-Zavadskaia (1930, 1933), and Bernstein (1937) stressed the recessiveness of tumor inheritance, while later workers (Little, 1928, 1936; Lynch, 1924; Bittner, 1938) suggested dominant inheritance. Tumor inheritance studies were obstructed, however, by the concept that all tumors could be grouped as a single character. Using highly inbred strains, Little (1928) and others showed that tumors seemed to be inherited as separate characters. In other sections, we will look into present concepts of viral and hormonal involvement in mammary tumor incidence.

3. Discovery of the Milk Influence

Just at the time the hereditary nature of mouse mammary cancer was being universally accepted as firmly established, new data were beginning to flow from two laboratories: (1) the Jackson Memorial Laboratory in Maine and (2) the National Cancer Institute in Amsterdam. Under the direction of Dr. C. C. Little, the Staff of the Jackson Laboratory (1933) conducted a number of reciprocal crossbreeding experiments between high and low tumor strains. They found that the inheritance of cancer of the mammary gland did not follow the laws of Mendelian genetics, but that the incidence depended primarily on the mother. Rummert Korteweg made similar observations in Amsterdam. These early crossbreeding experiments are summarized in Table 1. Korteweg (1936) postulated that the influence might be transmitted through the cytoplasm of the ovum (cytoplasmic inheritance), through the placenta (intrauterine influence), or through the milk (milk influence). Korteweg favored cytoplasmic inheritance (1936). Fekete and Little (1942) undertook the problem of intrauterine influence, but before either of the other two means had been tested, a young geneticist at the Jackson Laboratory, Dr. John Bittner (1936), had done a simple foster-nursing experiment which indicated that the mammary tumor influence was transmitted in milk. He foster-nursed nine newborn strain A females on CBA mothers. Normally eight of the nine A females should have developed tumors, but only three did. The CBA stock had a mammary tumor incidence of 10%; thus the incidence of the fostered mice lay between the incidences of the real and foster mothers. Although the number of animals employed in this experiment was dangerously small, the new information gained from it has remained unchallenged over the years. This new information was that (1) the so-called extrachromosomal factor, indicated by reciprocal crosses of high and low mammary tumor strains, was at least partially transmitted in the milk, and (2) there were other factors affecting mammary tumor incidence that were not dependent on the milk. The details of these "other factors" will be discussed later, but let it be said here that foster-nursing newborns or even near-term fetuses removed by caesarian section has never annihilated the disease from high tumor strains, even when the foster mothers are of a strain that has zero or near zero incidence (Heston and Levillain, 1950; Heston, 1958; Pullinger and Iversen, 1960).

Most of the early work on trying to rid mice of the mammary tumor agent by foster-nursing was done with strain C3H or RIII fostered on C57BL. More recently, several other strains have been used. Heston (1958) reported that from the sixth to the twenty-fifth generation his C3Hf subline with a total of 911 females had an average tumor incidence of 22% at an average tumor age of 19.9 months. A litter of these C3Hf mice (F_9 generation) was removed by caesarian section and foster-nursed again on a C57BL mother, creating a doubly fostered substrain, C3Hff. From the F_1 to the F_7 generation, the incidence (118 females) was 29% at an average tumor age of 18.9 months. Pullinger and Iversen (1960) found a much lower incidence in RIIIf sublines which were also started by fostering litters of RIII newborn on C57BL mothers. In 544 females, the incidence was 2.6% at a mean age of 16.2 months. (Table 2 gives the incidence and the mean age at which the tumors occur in several strains and substrains maintained at I.M.R.). After removal of the milk-transmitted agent, the occurrence of mammary tumors was completely random—the progeny of mothers that developed tumors were at no greater risk than the progeny of mothers that did not have tumors. The incidence in families could not be changed by selective breeding.

TABLE 1

Early Demonstrations of Maternal Influence

Source of data and crosses	Number of females[a]	Percent with tumors
Staff Jackson Laboratory (1933):		
DBA female × C57BL male	113 V	39.82
C57BL female × DBA male	379 V	6.06
A female × CBA male	44 B	90.90
CBA female × A male	16 B	18.80
C3H female × I male	36 B	91.70
I female × C3H male	10 B	0.00
Bittner and Little (1937):		
C3H female × N male	46 B	97.90
N female × C3H male	18 B	27.80
Korteweg (1936):		
DBA female × C57BL male	7	100.00
C57BL female × DBA male	67	2.99
DBA female × F_1 male (C57BL female × DBA male)	63	82.54
F_1 female (C57BL female × DBA male) × DBA male	30	10.00

From Heston (1945).
[a] V, Virgin; B, Breeder.

Although Bittner discovered the milk factor, his training as a geneticist and his strong belief that heredity was a major factor in the development of mammary tumors influenced most of his experimentation. In addition to the genetic and milk factors, he pointed out the important role of hormones. It is now believed that immune response and environmental factors must be considered as well. An immune response to tumors or to the milk agent has long been suspected, but such a response was not established until relatively recently (for reviews of this area, see Blair, 1968, 1971).

4.1. Immunological Factors

With few exceptions, until recently it was held that immunity did not constitute an important mechanism in the control of oncogenesis, although it is now considered to be a major factor. One of the earliest reports of the cross-antigenicity of mammary tumors was made by Gross in 1947. He showed that intracutaneous or subcutaneous inoculations of mammary tumor cells from one tumor immunized the mouse against challenge with mammary tumor cells from another mouse. Since this cross-immunization did not occur with chemically induced tumors, Gross concluded that the immunization must have been due to the mammary tumor agent (presumably a virus) which was common to all the mammary tumors. This conclusion has been borne out by numerous more recent studies (Weiss *et al.*, 1966; Weiss, 1967; Morton, 1969; Morton *et al.*, 1969). These studies have not only shown the presence of such tumor antigenicity but have also demonstrated that it exists in preneoplastic lesions and in the normal mammary gland (Lavrin *et al.*, 1966; Dezfulian *et al.*, 1967).

That the mammary tumor agent could be neutralized by serum from rabbits immunized with mouse mammary tumor tissue was shown as early as 1944 (Andervont and Bryan), and later confirmed by Blair (1963), but the demonstration of antibodies in the serum of either tumor-bearing or immunized mice did not occur until relatively recently (Blair *et al.*, 1966; Blair and Pitelka, 1966). By immunodiffusion techniques, Blair and coworkers showed that antibodies against MTV were present in some of the sera of mice immunized with extracts or implants of MTV-containing tissue and/or challenged with MTV-containing mammary tumor tissue. They also demonstrated, by electron microscopy, that the agar area containing the precipitin line also contained clumps of the virus particles. Nowinski *et al.* (1967) demonstrated antibodies in immunized (BALB/c × DBA/2)F_1 hybrids and I strain mice.

Earlier attempts to show humoral antibodies to MTV in mice based on neutralization, cytotoxicity, or complement fixation were unsuccessful (Dmochowski and Passey, 1952; Dmochowski, 1958; Gorer and Law, 1949; Imagawa *et al.*, 1950).

Although most of the mammary tumor antibody in mice is directed against the virus (MTV), at least some mammary tumors have been shown to possess, in addition to the MTV-associated antigenicity, a characteristic antigenicity which does not cross-react with that of other mammary tumors (Heppner and Pierce, 1969; Heppner, 1969; Vaage, 1968a, b; Morton et al., 1969). It is similar to the tumor-specific antigenicity usually associated with tumors induced by chemical carcinogens. These tumor-specific antigens do not seem to represent a reexpression of embryonic antigens (Blair, 1970) but may be organ-specific antigens that are permitted to arise from the partially protected and privileged nature of the mammary fat pad (Weiss, 1969; Moretti and Blair, 1966).

Throughout the literature on the immunology of mice to MTV and to mammary tumors, there is frequent reference to strains or substrains of mice that are free of MTV. It is now supposed that all or nearly all mice (Moore, 1963; Bentvelzen et al., 1970) carry an MTV genome and that in some strains it is expressed early or in a high percentage of the animals while in other strains it is expressed late or not at all. In the high mammary tumor strains, the newborn mice are infected via virus carried in the mother's milk and tumors appear early (Table 2), but when the milk-borne virus is removed by foster-nursing on MTV-free milk, viral antigen is found in the milk only at later lactations and the tumors occur late in life.

TABLE 2

Tumor Incidence, Tumor Age, and MTV Antigen in Mouse Strains[a]

Mouse strain[b]	Tumor incidence	Average tumor age (months)	Immuno-diffusion
A/Bi	97	7.8	1:64[c]
Af[d]	46	18.5	10/58 pos.[e]
RIII/Haag	96	8.8	1.128
RIIIf	10	18.0	neg.
BALB/cfC3H/Crgl (C[+])	97	7.2	1:16
BALB/c/Crgl (C[-])	27	19.0	neg.
C3H/He	98	6.6	1:64
C57fRIII	92	12.0	all pos.
C57BL/Haag	0	—	neg.
GR/Mul	100	7.0	1:128
GRf	100	7.0	1:128
DD/He	95	7.5	—

[a] Strains maintained at the Institute for Medical Research.
[b] Bi, Bittner, University of Minnesota; Haag, Haagensen, Columbia University; He, Heston, National Cancer Institute; Mul, Mühlbock, Amsterdam.
[c] End-point titer of MTV antigen in third lactation milk.
[d] f, Foster-nursed on C57BL except for BALB/cfC3H/Crgl.
[e] Ten of 58 Af mice showed MTV antigen at the third lactation; not titered for end point. In the high mammary tumor strains, A, RIII, C[+], C3H, GR, GRf, DBA-R, and DD, approximately 100% of the mice are positive by the immunodiffusion test at the third lactation. Compared to infectivity, the immunodiffusion test is relatively insensitive.

ovariectomized mouse is different in the various inbred strains. It is seven times higher for DBA mice than for C57BL (Mühlbock and Boot, 1959). From this and other observations, it may be concluded that the ovaries of DBA mice produce more estrogenic hormones than C57BL. Since it appears that the sensitivity of the mammary glands to estrogenic hormones is the same in the two strains, the glands of the mice of the DBA strain are under stronger hormonal stimulation. This, no doubt, influences their susceptibility to breast cancer. It is through such mechanisms that strains may acquire the reputation of being susceptible or resistant to mammary tumors.

5. Speculations on the Meaning of Susceptibility and Resistance of Mouse Strains to MTV

There is a great difference in the apparent susceptibility of different mouse strains to MTV and to the development of mammary tumors. This susceptibility has generally been thought to be due to the body genes of the mouse, but it may be due to a weak immune response so that the real reason for the low or high susceptibility is immune response, which, however, may in turn be determined genetically, at least in part. It was suggested by the work of Mühlbock (1951, 1956) that the susceptibility of some strains of mice to MTV infection depended on which strain was used as a source of virus. More recent data (Moore *et al.*, 1974) indicate that susceptibility or resistance may depend almost entirely on the kind and quantity of virus (Fig. 1). Thus C57BL mice are susceptible to RIII virus but more resistant to C3H virus, particularly if the C3H virus was carried in BALB/c mice (BALB/cfC3H). However, when C57BL mice are inoculated with large doses of RIII virus, the incidence of infection is usually lower. This might be explained by assuming that the high dose stimulates the immune reaction to reject the virus before it can effectively replicate. A strong immune response is found in the C57BL mice after MTV inoculation. With a killed vaccine, they can be solidly immunized against future challenge with live virus (Charney and Moore, 1972).

It has always been thought that when MTV is introduced into the C57BL mice through foster-nursing on strains that carry the virus, no or very few mammary tumors occur in the fostered (F_0) females or in their inbred descendents (Andervont, 1945). By foster-nursing very susceptible hybrids on fostered (F_0) C57BL, it was shown that the F_0 generation transmits MTV, but the F_1 C57BL females transmitted very little virus in their milk and succeeding generations transmitted none at all (Mühlbock, 1956; Andervont, 1964).

In contrast to these results, if RIII virus instead of C3H, as Andervont used, is introduced into C57BL mice, they (F_0) have a high incidence of infection and about 80% of those infected develop mammary tumors (Fig. 2). When C57BL newborns were foster-nursed on RIII mothers for 24 h and then returned to their own C57BL mothers, 15 of 23 (65%) showed MTV antigen in their milk at the third lactation and nine of 22 (41%) developed tumors. When RIII newborns were transferred after 24 h from their own mothers to C57BL, the MTV antigen

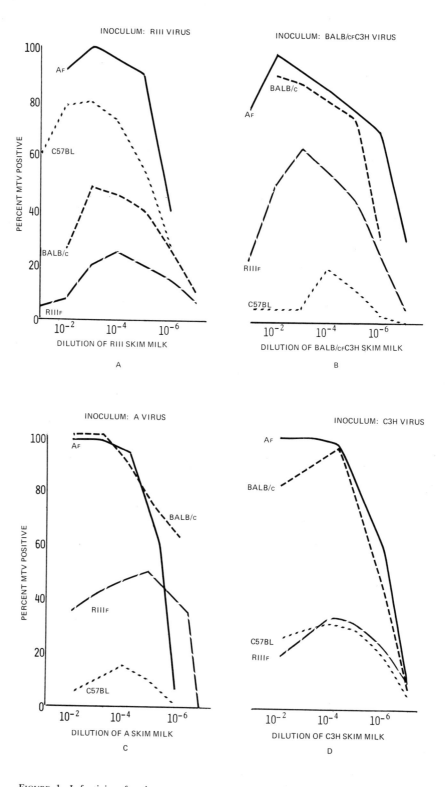

FIGURE 1. Infectivity of various mouse strains as a function of dose and source of virus.

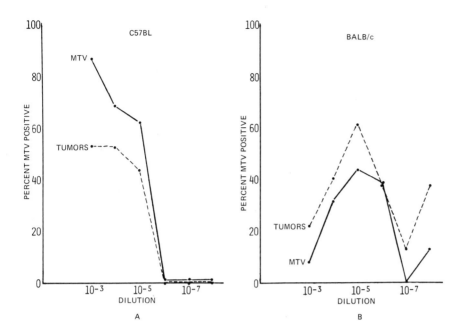

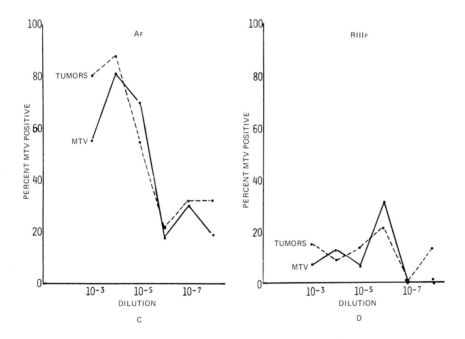

FIGURE 2. Correlation of infectivity with tumor formation in various mouse strains as a function of dose and source of virus.

incidence at the third lactation was 9/22 (41%) and the eventual tumor incidence was 7/21 (33%). The F_1 and subsequent generations of C57BL mice seem no more likely to lose the virus than does the RIII line itself. RIII mice have a tendency to lose their MTV (Andervont and Dunn, 1959, 1962, 1965). In another experiment, an infected subline of C57BL was started by inoculating a 4-wk-old female with RIII milk. Her progeny now at the F_5 generation showed the following MTV antigen incidence in third lactation milk: F_1, 6/7; F_2, 7/7; F_3, 5/6; F_4, 9/9. The tumor incidences in the F_1 and F_2 generations were 5/6 and 5/5, respectively. The tumor incidences in the F_3 and F_4 generations are not yet available, but the C57BL mice are certainly giving no indication of losing the RIII virus with progressive generations. In order to maintain a high tumor incidence in either the RIII or C57BL strain, it is necessary to save breeders from late litters (third or later) (Moore et al., 1974).

On the other hand, BALB/c mice are quite susceptible to C3H virus but are more resistant to RIII. Therefore, the resistance or susceptibility of different strains that used to be attributed to genetic differences now seems more likely to be due to immune responses to viruses with slightly different antigenic characteristics, although this explanation is only tentative.

Perhaps the strongest evidence that resistance to MTV infection is not entirely genetic is the observation that when the milk-transmitted virus is removed from the RIII line by foster-nursing on C57BL mothers and a subline of RIIIf is established with a tumor incidence of 5–10%, this subline is poorly receptive to reinfection with RIII virus. Before being foster-nursed, the mammary tumor incidence in the RIII females is 97% at an average age of $8\frac{1}{2}$ months, but after being foster-nursed the genetically identical subline so established responds very poorly to reinoculation of the same virus that was removed from it (Fig. 1a).

One, but perhaps not the only, explanation for the resistance is that the low-grade infection which the RIIIf mice receive through the gametes conveys an immunity against superinfection with the immunologically similar but biologically much more potent milk-transmitted virus. Viral antigen in the milk of RIIIf mice does not become detectable until the sixth to tenth lactation. Against this hypothesis, however, is the fact that Af mice, which also carry low infectivity gamete-transmitted virus, are quite susceptible to infection by MTV from A and other strains. However, many A mice secrete MTV antigen earlier (Table 2).

As to the question of whether susceptibility or resistance is determined by the whole animal or is restricted to just the mammary gland, Dux and Mühlbock (1966) performed an elegant experiment. If susceptible mammary glands and resistant mammary glands could be grown in genetically identical hosts, then it should be possible to determine whether or not the tumor incidence depends on the genotype of the host or on the transplanted mammary gland. Dux used the so-called highly susceptible strain C3Hf and the resistant strain 020 as donors of the mammary glands and the F_1 hybrids, C3Hf × 020, as the hosts. One group of completely mammectomized F_1 hybrids received mammary glands from 5-day-old C3Hf females; other mammectomized hybrids received mammary glands from 5-day-old 020 females. If the hybrids were given MTV (by fostering on C3H) and extra hormonal stimulation by hypophyseal transplants, tumors developed in practically 100% of all transplanted glands whether they were from susceptible C3Hf or resistant 020 donors, but there was a significant difference in the time required. In the transplanted C3Hf mammary glands the average tumor age was 233 days (8 months), and in the transplanted 020 glands the average tumor age was 323 days (11 months). When the so-called agent-free (not fostered on C3H) hybrids were used as hosts 11 out of 13 transplanted C3H mammary glands developed tumors in an average of 492 days (16 months), while in the 020 glands only two out of 18 developed tumors in an average of 511 days (17 months). These differences in tumor age could be interpreted as being due to the genetic differences in the mammary glands from the two mouse strains, but it is now believed that there are two types of mammary tumor viruses in C3H mice (Pitelka *et al.*, 1964) and at least one in the 020 mice (Bentvelzen *et al.*, 1970). In the C3H strain, one of the viruses is transmitted via the milk and causes a high incidence of mammary tumors at an early age; the other virus is transmitted via the gametes and causes a low incidence of tumors at a late age. In the 020 strain, only the latter virus is present and is usually occult or inactive. Differences in tumor development that may appear to result from genetic susceptibility may actually result from the kind of virus involved.

This possibility is further indicated by experiments of Bittner (1956). He observed the tumor incidence and average tumor age of two families of C3H mice, Z(C3H) and a subline of Z(C3H) which had been started by foster-nursing a newborn litter of the Z(C3H) on a strain A mother. Since strain A is also a high tumor strain whose tumors appear early, the subline ZfA was carrying two viruses [Z(C3H) and A]. The tumor incidence in Z(C3H) breeders was 96.8% at an average age of 272 days, but in the fostered line, ZfA, it was 92.5% (321 days); in virgin Z(C3H), it was 87.0% (386 days), but in ZfA virgins it was 71.8% (397 days). Fostering the newborn C3H mice on strain A, whose milk probably has even more virus than that of their own C3H mothers, but with somewhat different characteristics, seems to have lowered the incidence, particularly in the nonbreeders, and delayed the age at tumor onset. Bittner commented that the tumors appeared later in the ZfA with each succeeding generation. Here the mice are carrying three kinds of MTV, two milk transmitted and one gamete transmitted. This makes it very difficult to draw a conclusion as to what influences the incidence or age of tumors, but the ZfA subline, which is genetically C3H, seems to be taking on the characteristics of strain A insofar as the effect of parity is concerned.

Blair (1960) observed other evidence for control of the age at tumor onset by milk-transmitted MTV. Strain A mice from Heston had been maintained in Berkeley for 85 generations, and the mean tumor age in breeders had consistently been about 12 months. Suddenly it was discovered that breeding females in one branch of the stock were developing tumors at about 8 months of age. Reciprocal crossbreeding and also cross-foster-nursing experiments between the two branches showed that the tumor age depended entirely on a milk-transmitted agent.

An indication that mammary tumor viruses may control tumor characteristics that were once thought to be under genetic control of the host comes from the observations of Squartini (1963). Squartini foster-nursed low tumor BALB/c mice on RIII and on C3H mothers and then maintained each BALB/c family as an inbred line. The line started by foster-nursing newborn BALB/c mice on RIII mothers had tumors with RIII characteristics, while those fostered on C3H mothers had tumors with C3H characteristics. These differences are listed in Table 4.

TABLE 4

Characters of Mammary Tumors in BALB/c Female Mice Foster-Nursed by C3H and RIII Mothers

	C3H (donor)→	BALB/cf (C3H)	BALB/cf (RIII)	RIII ←(donor)
Clinical duration (days)	49	59	104	103
Growth rate (cm/wk)	0.238	0.231	0.125	0.135
Partial regressions (%)	27	34	60	59
Type of growth (regular: %)	64.3	61.5	25	30
Responsiveness to pregnancy (%)	0[a]	19	82	80.3
Histological origin (prevalent)	Nodules	Nodules	Plaques	Plaques
Morphological picture (prevalent)	Pure	Pure	Varied	Varied

From Squartini (1963).

[a] Because of the low fertility of these animals at the age of tumor appearance, this figure concerns only a few tumors.

It cannot be concluded, however, that the genotype of the host has no effect on tumor development. Host factors greatly influence the propagation of the virus and the eventual development of mammary tumors. This influence may be mediated through immune reaction, hormone levels, or other means, but these in turn are under genetic control—at least at the present time we have no reason to believe that they are not. There is, however, some indication that MTV may influence both the hormonal milieu and the hormonal sensitivity of the mammary gland of the infected mouse (Blair, 1971). It has also been observed that BALB/c mice infected with MTV undergo general immunological reactivity impairment as they age (Blair *et al.*, 1971).

6. Biological Nature of MTV

Since the tumors in C3Hf (Heston, 1958) and RIIIf (Pullinger and Iversen, 1960) mice occurred completely at random and since their occurrence could be greatly influenced by the administration of estrogens, mammotropin, or somatotropin—that is, they were hormone dependent—it was postulated that the viral genome must be integrated in the host cells and express itself only under certain conditions (Moore, 1963). It was also postulated that although they appeared identical in the electron microscope there must be two viruses, one

which occurs in C3H tumors and milk and is transmissible by ingestion or
inoculation and another which occurs in C3Hf tumors and is transmissible only via the gametes (Pitelka *et al.*, 1964). The virions found in the tumors or milk of C3Hf, RIIIf, or Af mice have not yet been shown to be infectious. Since the B particles were found in precancerous hypoplastic nodules of the C3Hf mammary glands, this nontransmissible virus was called "nodule-inducing virus" (NIV) (Pitelka *et al.*, 1964). More recently, it has been designated as MTV-L for "virus with low activity" (Bentvelzen *et al.*, 1970). Two milk-transmitted viruses have so far been recognized (Bentvelzen *et al.*, 1970); one is carried in the C3H stock and produces nodules of high tumor potential, the other is carried in RIII and DD mice, DBA, and others and produces plaques from which the tumors apparently form. It now seems likely that there may be other variations of MTV. The factors which go into making MTV transmissible with very high tumor-producing potential or apparently nontransmissible with low tumor-producing potential are as yet unknown. RIIIf mice have a particle corresponding to NIV or MTV-L of the C3H stock which when extracted from the late-appearing tumors has not been found to be infectious, but the right conditions for its infectivity may not have been used. Milk-transmitted virus from RIII mothers is also not very infectious if tested in RIIIf mice, whereas it is more infectious if inoculated into C57BL or BALB/c and highly infectious in Af mice. Most of the testing for activity of the C3Hf virus has been done in BALB/c mice. It may be that the milk-transmitted C3H virus is very infectious in BALB/c whereas the virus of C3Hf might be more infectious in some other strains. We do not yet understand the conditions necessary to show the horizontal transmissibility of these various viruses.

The MTV of GR mice is transmitted via both the milk and the gametes. Foster-nursing newborns on MTV-free mothers has no effect on the tumor incidence; it remains 100% (Mühlbock, 1965). Reciprocal crossbreeding with BALB/c mice gives F_1 hybrids which also have a 100% mammary tumor incidence at an early age, and Bentvelzen indicates that the virus is as readily transmitted by the father as by the mother. GR mice are extremely susceptible to the GR virus, but so are mice of the C57BL strain (Moore, Charney, and Holben, unpublished data). Studies by Mühlbock and Bentvelzen (1968), Bentvelzen *et al.* (1970), Bentvelzen (1968), and Zeilmaker (1969) indicate that the GR host genome is necessary for nonmilk transmission of GR MTV, because introduction of this virus into other mouse strains does not lead to male transmission by the new host. GR virus has the same infectivity in GR mice whether it is milk or gamete transmitted—that is, the virus appears to have the same properties in GR and GRf mice—but when transferred to another strain it seems to be only milk transmitted.

6.1. MTV Genome Ubiquitous

In addition to hormones, irradiation and chemicals have been demonstrated to increase the occurrence of mammary tumors in many of the low tumor strains. It was originally thought by most investigators that a virus was not involved in the onset of these tumors, but now it seems unlikely that mammary tumors occur in mice without the presence of the mouse mammary tumor virus or at least without its genome. In fact, there is a great deal of evidence (Moore, 1963; Bentvelzen, 1968; Bentvelzen *et al.*, 1970; Varmus *et al.*, 1972, 1973) that every mouse contains genetic information for a mammary tumor virus and that aging, hormones, irradiation, and chemicals partially or fully activate the virus. Even the C57BL strain, which normally never has overt mammary tumors, shows by nucleic acid hybridization the presence of at least portions of the viral genome in multiple copies in host cells (Varmus *et al.*, 1972).

Using DNA probes synthesized from MuMTV RNA by means of virion-associated RDDP,* Varmus *et al.* (1973) found, by specific hybridization experiments, various amounts of MuMTV RNA in mice of various strains and in the various tissues of mice of the same strain. For example, BALB/c and C57BL mice contained low amounts of viral RNA per cell compared to the tissues of high mammary tumor strains and lactating mammary gland cells contained more than liver or spleen cells, suggesting that hormonal responsiveness and/or cellular differentiation may have regulatory roles in the expression of viral information. There were consistent significant differences found in the amount of virus-specific RNA of lactating glands from several low mammary tumor incidence strains, indicating that unidentified hereditary factors may also influence transcription of the viral genes and may regulate tumor formation. C57BL mice, which rarely or never have tumors, showed more viral RNA per cell than BALB/c mice, which usually have an appreciable tumor incidence late in life. Mammary glands which produce detectable virus at the first lactation showed much higher levels of viral RNA than those from mice of strains that have detectable viral antigen only at late lactations. The absence of MuMTV-like virus sequences in the DNA of species closely related to the mouse such as the rat, hamster, and European field vole makes it unlikely that the MuMTV-like virus sequences are cellular and not viral genes. As we shall see in Section 8, some human tumors contain a small amount of RNA which hybridizes with a large proportion of MuMTV probes, indicating that the mammary tumor viral genome exists in some humans.

6.2. Resistance of MTV to Irradiation

The amount of the viral genome required for oncogenicity is not known. Irradiation studies of MTV employing X-rays and γ-rays have shown that an unexpectedly high dose was required to inactivate the virus so that it no longer produced tumors when inoculated into mice (Ardashnikov and Spasskaia, 1949; Moore *et al.*, 1959, 1962; Gorka *et al.*, 1972). In fact, doses under 10^6 R usually enhanced the tumor incidence in inoculated mice. This indicates that possibly only a small fraction of the viral nucleic acid is required for cellular transformation. Irradiation of DNA viruses also caused enhancement of oncogenicity, but decreased infectivity and complement-fixing antigens and DNA synthesis in tissue cultures (Defendi and Jensen, 1967; Latarjet *et al.*, 1967). Adenovirus 7–SV40

* RNA-directed DNA polymerase.

hybrid virus was able to transform African green monkey cells after the irradiation had completely destroyed its ability to replicate. Such experiments cannot be done with MTV because of its inability to infect cells *in vitro*, but the oncogenic activity of both RNA and DNA viruses is much more resistant to irradiation than would be expected from infectivity data on any virus. In fact, it was at one time argued that the mouse mammary tumor agent could not be a virus because of its very high resistance to irradiation (Ardashnikov and Spasskaia, 1949).

6.3. Methods for Assay of MTV

Three methods are available for the assay of MTV: (1) detection of tumors, (2) detection of nodules (Pullinger, 1947; Nandi, 1963), and (3) detection of viral replication by the presence of viral antigen in the milk (Nowinski *et al.*, 1967; Charney *et al.*, 1969). Noduligenesis in BALB/c mice has been compared with tumorigenesis in C57BL mice. The infectivity of RIII milk titrated by these two methods indicates no significant difference (Moore *et al.*, 1969a). Similarly, the presence of viral antigen at the third lactation in inoculated C57BL mice has been compared with the eventual development of tumors. About 85% of the infected mice eventually develop tumors, but very few tumors develop in mice that do not show viral antigen at the third lactation. C57BL mice are much more susceptible to virus from RIII mice than to virus from C3H or A mice. The time required for tumor development is 10–20 months, for nodule development 16–18 wk, and for antigen development 12–16 wk. The antigen test requires antiserum which is prepared in rabbits by intramuscularly inoculating purified MTV combined with complete Freund's adjuvant at monthly intervals. The fourth and last dose is given without adjuvant, and the rabbits are bled out 3 days later. The antigen test requires 24–48 h and is made in a micro-Ouchterlony diffusion plate.

The effect of inoculation age on infection in C57BL mice was measured and correlated with the eventual development of mammary tumors (Moore *et al.*, 1970). Over the age range of 2–10 wk, the total lapsed time from inoculation to the appearance of antigen in the milk or the development of tumors was approximately constant irrespective of age at inoculation. Inoculation at 12 wk of age gave a relatively low incidence of infection and tumor development. All age groups had a gradual increase in antigen incidence from the first to the third lactation. Force-breeding to the second or third lactation of mice inoculated at age 10–12 wk did not shorten the lapsed time for obtaining equivalent antigen incidence. Inoculation during first pregnancy gave inconsistent antigen assay results on the milk of inoculated mice at the third lactation, but pregnant animals seem to be less susceptible than younger, nonpregnant ones. Inoculating newborn mice sometimes gave, unlike leukemia virus, a poor incidence of infection. Inoculating mice at between 4 and 10 wk of age, mating them at 10–12 wk of age, and testing their milk at the third lactation gave a practical assay requiring about 15 wk. With this schedule, dose–response regression curves were obtained typical of other virus end-point dilution assays, and 50% Reed–Muench end points could be estimated (Charney *et al.*, 1969) on milks from the same mouse strain. End points, however, vary appreciably from one experiment to another.

There are two established cell lines (Sykes *et al.*, 1968; Lasfargues *et al.*, 1972) made from mouse mammary tumor cells that continuously produce MTV at a low rate, but it has not yet been possible to infect normal cells *in vitro*. New methods of enzymatic dissociation have made possible the cultivation of normal mammary cells isolated from virgin mice or mice in early stages of the pregnancy cycle. Hormonal stimulation of these cells is not essential, but helps to provide a physiological environment favorable to virus replication.

Cultures derived from normal mouse mammary glands have been inoculated with milk from MTV-infected mice, with mammary tumor extracts, and with purified virions from milk. In every case, a growth stimulation of the inoculated cells was obtained. Virus particles have been found by electron microscopy in thin sections of the inoculated cells. The virions were type C particles and were identified as leukemia virus, not MTV (Lasfargues *et al.*, 1970*a*).

Studies on the time of penetration of the B particle into the cells demonstrated much slower kinetics than for the C particle. Attempts were made, therefore, to accelerate the penetration of the viral particles by a modification of the cell membrane (Lasfargues *et al.*, 1970*b*). DEAE-dextran, reported to enhance the focus-forming titer of a murine sarcoma virus, was used. Purified RIII virions with DEAE-dextran induced nuclear alterations earlier than in nontreated control cells, but the replicating virus found by electron microscopy was still the type C particle. Apparently, an inoculum completely free of leukemia virus is required to give information on the infective capability of the B particle. This made the use of a LV-free MTV compulsory for all experimental inoculations and raised the problem of the relationship between MTV and LV.

6.5. Changes in MTV Virions on Ingestion

Virions washed from the small intestine of young high mammary tumor strain mice and from the peritoneal cavity of intraperitoneally inoculated mice of a low mammary tumor strain were found to be disrupted to varying degrees. Structural changes in the virions were observed as early as 15 min after intraperitoneal inoculation, and disruption increased with time. These findings indicate that decoating of the virions occurs in both routes of infection. The absence of one or more extracellular decoating enzymes in cell cultures might help to explain why MTV does not infect *in vitro* (Kramarsky *et al.*, 1971).

7. Chemical and Physical Properties of MTV

Procedures have been devised for separating MTV virions from mouse milk in what appears to be a fairly pure form (Lyons and Moore, 1965; Sarkar and Moore, 1968). In the process, the cream, which constitutes about 30% of mouse milk, is removed. Although the cream contains a considerable amount of virus and viral antigen, it is not easy to recover intact particles from it. The skim milk is diluted with buffer and the casein is solubilized by treating with EDTA. Pelletized, partially purified resuspended virus is laid over a continuous gradient of Ficoll, sucrose, potassium citrate or cesium chloride, and a large percentage of the virions form a recoverable band. This purification procedure depends on both sedimentation rate and buoyant density, but prolonged centrifugation does not concentrate all of the virus into a single band; both the virions and bioactivity are found elsewhere throughout the gradient tube (Moore *et al.*, 1969a). It is not yet known whether the different densities result from the intrinsic nature of the virus or whether they are due to adherence of lighter or heavier materials. Electron microscopy indicates that the virus has a great tendency to adhere to other particles and to form aggregates with itself. Coalesced large syncytial particles are found in all fractions (Sarkar *et al.*, 1969). As to buoyant density, there is a peak of bioactivity and particles at a density of 1.18 g/cm^3. Buoyant densities of the virus as determined in a variety of gradient materials are recorded in Fig. 3. Rauscher leukemia virus has a mean density of 1.16 g/cm^3 (Sarkar and Moore, 1974a). The RNA has a mononucleotide composition as follows: UMP, 28.9%; GMP, 30.2%; CMP, 21.6%; AMP, 19.3% (Lyons and Moore, 1965).

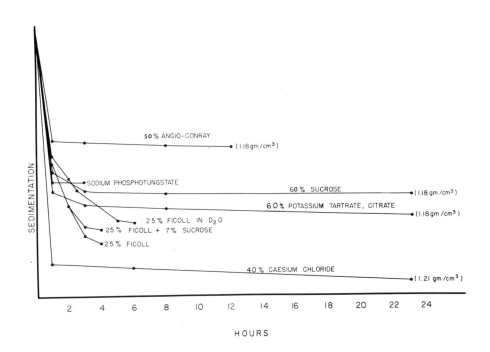

FIGURE 3. Sedimentation–time curves for MTV in various gradients. In most of the gradients, the virion band approached equilibrium at density 1.18 g/cm^3 (in CsCl, 1.22 g/cm^3). In Ficoll gradients, most of the particles were injured on prolonged centrifugation so that in no case could equilibrium be reached.

7.1. Structure of MTV Virions

DAN H. MOORE

The MTV virion is easily recognized by its membrane and the protrusions (spikes) extending from its outer surface, as shown by negative-contrast electron microscopy (Fig. 4) (Sarkar *et al.*, 1969, 1971, 1973*a*). Myxoviruses and the paramyxoviruses also have surface protrusions, but they are quite different in structure and dimensions (Horne *et al.*, 1969). Mitochondria and some cell membranes contain

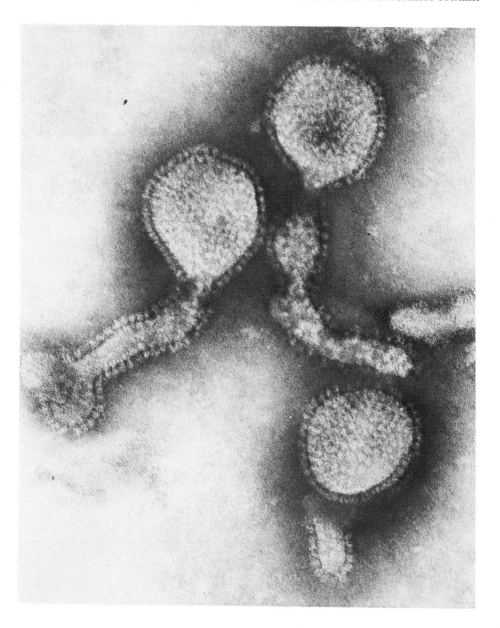

FIGURE 4. Electron micrographs of MTV virions in negative stain. × 100 000. Courtesy of Dr. William Manthey.

protrusions (Fernández-Morán *et al.*, 1964), but these are easily distinguishable from the B particle spikes. Some electron micrographs show short peripheral spikes on avian myeloblastosis virus, but there are no other structures known that correspond in detail to the mammary tumor virus. On MTV, the spikes are mostly distributed in a six-coordinated array; that is, each spike is surrounded by six others. In virions whose spikes are damaged or detached from the membrane, a network structure resembling a honeycomb is observed on the membrane. Thus it seems that the spikes are superimposed on the reticular structure of the membrane. The center-to-center spacing of the projections is about 74 Å compared to 60 Å for the influenza virion. The knob-shaped distal end of the B particle spike has an average diameter of about 45 Å, and the stalk between the knob and the membrane is only 10–20 Å in diameter. The total length of the spikes is about 95 Å, ranging from 80 to 100 Å (Sarker and Moore, 1974*b*).

The internal components of the B particle released after a variety of treatments reveal a number of interesting structures (Sarkar and Moore, 1968, 1970; Sarkar *et al.*, 1971). The intact naked nucleoids have a diameter of about 45 nm. Unraveled nucleoids show double helical structures 80–90 Å in diameter and single strands having a diameter of 30–40 Å with a pitch of about 126 Å. The double helices are considered to be the basic components of the nucleocapsid of the virions, and the single strands are the uncoiled elements of the double helices. The diameter of the single helical strand is about 33 Å. After treatment of purified virions with phenol in the presence of pronase, filamentous RNA was prepared. Rotary shadowed preparations were examined in the electron microscope. The length distribution of the RNA filaments showed peaks at 1.2, 2.4, and 3.6 μm (Sarkar and Moore, 1970). The molecular weight of the longest molecule was estimated at 3.6×10^6 daltons, although sedimentation analysis of extracted RNA indicated a molecular weight of 10×10^6 daltons (Duesberg and Blair, 1966).

7.2. Structural Components of MTV

Treatment of the MTV virion with Tween 80 and ether results in disruption of the viral membrane and release of three structural components—the nucleoid, large fragments of membranes, and short pieces of membrane that appear as rosettes (Sarkar *et al.*, 1971). These structural components have been isolated by density gradient centrifugation. The buoyant density of the nucleoid in potassium citrate or tartrate is 1.24 g/cm^3, as compared to 1.18 g/cm^3 for the untreated virus. The isolated nucleoids contain 4.4% RNA, as compared to 1.9% for the whole virion. RNase treatment of the nucleoid causes little or no structural alteration. The nucleoid membrane is resistant to protease and can be isolated from trypsinized nucleoids at a density of 1.14. The isolated nucleoids are not infective in inoculated mice. Trypsin treatment of the intact virus results in the loss of spikes from some but not all virions. Tween 80–ether treatment does not effectively remove the spikes from the viral membranes, but occasionally structures resembling free spikes are observed.

Soluble proteins have been separated from Tween 80-ether treated MTV by Sephadex G200 chromatography and used for immunization of rats (Nowinski *et al.*, 1971). These antisera have identified five viral antigens. Polyacrylamide gel electrophoresis of MTV in sodium dodecyl sulfate shows seven major polypeptide components in the virion. Figure 5 shows patterns of MTV for three different mouse strains and, for comparison, of Rauscher leukemia virus, Mason–Pfizer monkey virus, and R-35, a virus found in a rat mammary tumor. The molecular weights of the polypeptides are p1, 90,000; p2, 70,000; p3, 50,000–60,000; p4, 34,000; p5, 28,000; p6, 18,000; and p7, 12,000 daltons. A major component of the viral protein is p3, which is very broad and actually consists of several components. One is glycopeptide, molecular weight 55,000 daltons, which is easily removed from the virion with acid. It appears to be associated with the spikes which are not visible after acid treatment. Other components of p3 are also associated with the surface of the virion, but their precise location has yet to be determined. In addition, purified viral cores and A particles which are related to viral cores contain a polypeptide of molecular weight of approximately 52,000 daltons. The multiple nature of p3 was not originally recognized and it was classified as wholly

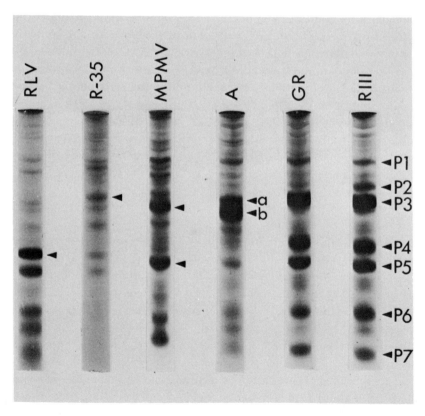

FIGURE 5. Polyacrylamide gel electrophoresis patterns of the structural proteins of Rauscher leukemia virus (RLV), a virus from a rat mamary tumor (R-35), a virus from a rhesus monkey mammary tumor (MPMV), and mammary tumor virus from three strains of mice (A, GR, and RIII). Courtesy of A. S. Dion.

core protein. The component p4 also contains a carbohydrate and is likely to be a
constituent of the viral membrane.

Antisera prepared against isolated MTV polypeptides are also used in immunofluorescence tests to determine the intracellular disposition of MTV antigens. These studies suggest that all MTV structural proteins are synthesized cytoplasmically. Screening of a variety of neoplasms by immunofluorescence and immunodiffusion tests demonstrates MTV infection in only three types of neoplastic diseases—mammary tumors, ML leukemias, and Leydig cell tumors of MTV-infected mice. Whereas mammary tumors synthesize all viral structural proteins, the synthesis of MTV proteins in the leukemias and Leydig cell tumors is limited to certain antigens. Electron microscopic examination of these tissues confirms that the synthesis results in an accumulation of viral nucleocapsids (A particles) without the production of budding virions.

7.3. Effect of pH on MTV

The electrophoretic mobility at various pH values, the isoelectric point, and the bioactivity of MuMTV at various pH values have been determined (Sarkar *et al.*, 1973*b*). Recovery of fractions after electrophoresis in a Tiselius cell shows bioactivity distributed in all fractions as are the B particles. With a high concentration of virus a peak will remain visible long enough to obtain a mobility measurement (Moore and Lyons, 1963). The pH mobility curve indicates an isoelectric point at pH 2.5. Infectivity in mice shows little loss of bioactivity between pH 5 and 11 (Fig. 6). There is a close correlation between the injury to the B particles, as seen in the electron microscope, and the decrease in bioactivity at low and high (pH 12) pH values.

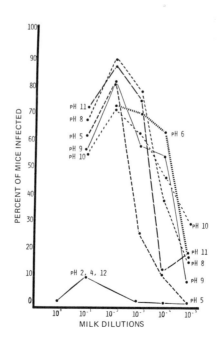

FIGURE 6. The effect of pH on the infectivity (in strain C57BL) of mouse mammary tumor virus (in milk from strain RIII).

Hemagglutination activity of MTV has not yet been demonstrated. A variety of erythrocytes have been used to test hemagglutination of MTV. The cells were tested at 4, 25, and 37°C as 25% or 5% suspensions in 0.85% NaCl or in phosphate-buffered saline. The MTV preparation employed was defatted mouse milk or virus partially purified by electrophoresis or density gradient centrifugation. The erythrocytes tested were from the following animals: calf, cat, chick, dog, duck, goat, goose, guinea pig, hamster, horse, human, monkey, mouse, ox, pigeon, rabbit, rat, sheep, swine, and turkey. MTV concentrations were calculated to be in excess of 10^8 particles/ml. No hemagglutination was observed (Came and Moore, 1966).

8. Putative Human Breast Cancer Virus

The idea of infectious agents in human cancer is not new; for centuries there have been ripples of evidence that such agents exist, but these have been swept away by major tides of dissent. Why is it so difficult to prove or disprove the existence of an infectious agent in cancer? In the first place, the development of cancer is one of the most complex events in nature. There are many complex events in biology, e.g., the clotting of blood, but in such phenomena events take place rapidly and the results of any experiment can quickly be evaluated so that a future experiment can be planned. The process of cancer, like the process of aging, takes place very slowly, and thus does not lend itself to quick experimentation.

As to the etiology of human breast cancer, there seems no longer to be a question of whether or not there is a virus in humans that is closely related to MuMTV, but we do not know whether it is involved in the etiology of breast cancer, nor do we know how it is transmitted. On the long path from conception to the eventual appearance of the tumor there are many factors that go into determining this relatively rare event. These factors are the general genetic makeup of the host, the hormonal milieu at various stages of life, the quantity and quality of the diet, environmental and psychological stress factors, and the whole relationship of the host to her environment.

The ultimate and definitive test for a human cancer virus, the infectivity test, cannot be made, and since the mouse mammary tumor virus has not yet infected any other species it is not likely that a human MTV would cross the species barrier either, although this has certainly not been ruled out. The evidence for a human MTV must therefore, at present, be obtained indirectly, and there are now many approaches for doing this. The main approach used until recently has been to search for virions in human milk or mammary tissues that correspond to those found in mouse milk. Several such searches have been recorded: Gross *et al.* (1950), Passey *et al.* (1951), Lunger *et al.* (1964), Feller and Chopra (1968), Seman *et al.* (1969), Moore *et al.* (1969*b*, 1971). During the period of these searches, techniques for preparing specimens and for examining them in the electron microscope have continually improved. Particles somewhat resembling MuMTV were reported in all of these publications, but as techniques improved the evidence became more convincing. At first, it was thought that there was a correlation between families or patients with breast cancer and the presence of the particles, but extensive examinations of milk have now indicated no such correlation (Sarkar and Moore, 1972). Particles identical to the mouse virus, as characterized by negative-staining procedures, have been found rarely. In milks from more than 1000 women studied recently, only 16 have shown unequivocal B particles by negative-staining procedures.* Possible reasons for the low content of particles in human milk are many. In the high cancer strains of inbred mice where the incidence approaches 100%, the concentration of virions in the milk is approximately 10^{12} particles/ml. Human milk rarely has more than one-millionth this concentration of virions, which is at the limit of detectability with the electron microscope. There are no high breast cancer inbred strains in human populations. Human populations seem to be more like the low mammary tumor strains of mice, and in these the virions are rarely found in milk until late in life (see Table 2). Another factor influencing the concentration of virions in human milk is their instability. The virus particles are quite stable in mouse milk, but they are unstable in most human milks because of the presence of factors which cause rapid deterioration of the mouse virus when added to human milk (Sarkar *et al.*, 1973c). This degradation of virions is not limited to MuMTV but also occurs with avian myeloblastosis virus and the mouse leukemia viruses.

There is now much other evidence for the existence of a human mammary tumor virus. New biochemical, molecular biological, and immunological means have all supplied strong evidence for the existence of a virus similar to MuMTV in human milk and tumors. The discovery of a RNA-directed DNA polymerase (RDDP) in RNA tumor viruses (Temin and Mizutani, 1970; Baltimore, 1970) has opened up a new approach for the detection of this type of virus. Soon after the reports of B particles in human milk had appeared, Spiegelman and collaborators started examining human milk specimens for the presence of RDDP (Schlom *et al.*, 1971; Axel *et al.*, 1972). In some milks, RDDP was found. A little later, Schlom and Spiegelman (1971) and Schlom *et al.* (1972) devised a procedure for the simultaneous detection of RDDP and its association with high molecular weight (60–70S or 35S) RNA, which is another characteristic of the RNA tumor viruses.

The presence in human milk of RDDP and 70S RNA was indicative of an oncornavirus but did not define its exact nature. From extensive animal studies, the most likely contaminant would be the leukemia–sarcoma type C viruses, and type C particles were often found in human milk. It thus became essential to separate the two types. It was shown (Moore *et al.*, 1973) that the buoyant density of MuMTV (type B particles) in a variety of gradients (sucrose, potassium tartrate, Angio-Conray) was 1.18 g/ml, although there was some scatter of particles above and below the main band. In CsCl, the isopycnic density of MuMTV was about

---

* Because of the unique characteristics of the MTV virion coat and the length, spacing, and shape of the surface protrusion, this particular particle can be more reliably identified by the negative-staining procedure than by thin sectioning.

1.21 g/ml. In sucrose or potassium tartrate or cesium chloride, the type C particles banded at density 1.16 g/ml (Sarkar and Moore, 1974a), making separation of B and C particles possible.

In human milk, RDDP was usually associated with particles having a buoyant density of 1.18 in sucrose and higher in CsCl, although there was not a good correlation between the RDDP values and the type of particle found by means of electron microscopy. Why was this correlation so poor? The explanation might be that the "needle in haystack" approach inherent in electron microscopy did not provide significant particle incidence data when the concentration of the particles was at the borderline of detectability. Out of the milk specimens examined from more than 1000 women, only four milks had a significant number of B particles or what appeared to be injured B particles; the RDDP in these milks was of a different order of magnitude from that in the other milks. Another explanation for the discrepancy between the presence of RDDP and B particles could be that whole virions do not remain intact very long after they are synthesized and liberated into the milk ducts. The viral cores may, however, be more stable. There is now much evidence for this kind of particle injury (Sarkar and Moore, 1972). The extent and celerity of damage caused vary from one human milk sample to another.

By using the endogenous RNA template, which has a sedimentation constant of 35S or 70S, RDDP has been found in human milks by all laboratories involved in these investigations (Vaidya, 1973). An exogenous synthetic template, poly(rC)·oligo(dG), can be used as a highly specific sensitive template for determining the presence and quantity of RDDP in RNA tumor viruses (Smith

TABLE 5

Ratios of [^{3}H]dGTP Incorporation Directed by Poly(rC)·oligo(dG) in the Presence of Mg^{2+} or Mn^{2+}

Virus	Type	Host	Mg^{2+}/Mn^{2+} [a]
R-35	C	Rat	0.07
MSV	C	Mouse	0.10
RLV	C	Mouse	0.18
FLV	C	Cat	0.19
GAL	C	Gibbon	0.44
SSV	C	Woolly monkey	0.56
RSV	C	Chicken	4.21
AMV	C	Chicken	4.8
C3H	B	Mouse	5.3
RIII	B	Mouse	12.8
GR	B	Mouse	15.5
A	B	Mouse	18.6
MPMV	C-B	Rhesus monkey	21.2
Human milk: pool of 7		Human	5.11

[a] Ratio of cpm. Values were obtained from Mg^{2+} or Mn^{2+} optimal concentrations or from an average of plateau points.

and Gallo, 1972; McCaffrey *et al.*, 1973). For activation of this enzyme a cation is required, and it has been found that the RDDP of some tumor viruses is more active in the presence of Mg^{2+} while this enzyme from other viruses is more active in the presence of Mn^{2+}. As is shown in Table 5, the mammary tumor viruses from several strains of mice have a strong preference for Mg^{2+}, whereas the leukemia–sarcoma type C particles have a preference for Mn^{2+}. The RDDP of human milk particles prefers Mg^{2+} (Dion and Vaidya, 1974).

More evidence for the existence of a HuMTV is the homology found between the nucleic acid of MuMTV and that of human materials. The relationship of the RNA of MuMTV to the RNA found in polysomes of tissue has been investigated by means of molecular hybridization experiments. Axel *et al.* (1972) reported that 70S RNA associated with RDDP in particles with a buoyant density 1.16–1.19 g/ml from human breast carcinomas was able to synthesize a DNA that at least to some extent complexed with MuMTV RNA. This occurred in 30 of 38 human mammary adenocarcinomas but not in four normal breast tissues and six fibroadenomas. In other homology experiments, ^{3}H-DNA probes were prepared from MuMTV and Rauscher leukemia virus RNAs and tested against monosomal and polysomal RNA from human breast carcinomas. The monosomal RNA did not react. The polysomal RNA hybridized only with the MuMTV ^{3}H-DNA and not with RLV ^{3}H-DNA (Spiegelman *et al.*, 1972).

In still another investigation carried out by M. R. Das *et al.* in Bombay (1972), DNA probes made by using reverse transcriptase and RNA from isolated human milk particles were reacted with polysomal RNA from human breast tumors. The RNA from one of three breast tumors, an undifferentiated carcinoma, showed considerable homology with the DNA probes. Neither mouse embryos, human placenta, nor normal human breast showed any measurable homology with the DNA probes.

Vaidya *et al.* (1974) employed single-strand specific nuclease S_1 for detecting RNA sequences in human tumors homologous with MPMV and MuMTV DNA probes (Varmus *et al.*, 1973). Out of 15 tumors tested, none showed homology with MPMV, while five tumors had RNA which hybridized from 18 to 77% of the MTV DNA at C_rt^* values of from 2.2 to 5.1×10^4 mole-s/liter. All five of these tumors were carcinomas of the breast; three were *in situ* types, one was an infiltrating carcinoma with extensive *in situ* areas, and the other was an invasive carcinoma. Estimation of the number of MuMTV-related RNA molecules per cell from $C_rt_{1/2}$ values of the test RNAs and of MuMTV 70S RNA indicated from one to ten MuMTV-related RNA molecules, a rather low number, but melting temperature studies indicated only 5% mismatching of the base sequences for the molecules of the two species. These hybridization results support and help to explain the immunological cross-reactivity observed in other studies (Charney and Moore, 1971; Black *et al*, 1974a, b; Hoshino *et al.*, 1973).

Additional evidence for the similarity of the putative human mammary tumor virus and the mouse virus is that 25% of all human sera tested (now more than

---

* C_rt is the product of RNA concentration and time of hybridization corrected to 0.12 M [Na^+]; see Britten and Smith (1970), Leong *et al.* (1972), and Varmus *et al.* (1973).

100) showed a neutralizing effect on MuMTV irrespective of whether the sera came from breast cancer patients or not (Charney and Moore, 1974). Some of the sera completely neutralized the RIII mouse virus. The serum component responsible for the neutralization is precipitated as a globulin by ammonium sulfate and is not affected by absorption with MuMTV-free C57BL milk or mammary gland extract.

In other experiments, Black *et al.* (1974*b*) have shown a specific relatedness of human breast tumor components to MuMTV by utilizing a leukocyte migration procedure for the demonstration of cellular hypersensitivity responses to human breast cancer tissue. Cellular hypersensitivity responses were found in 70% of tests against autologous *in situ* breast cancer, 29% of tests against autologous invasive breast cancer, 33% of tests against homologous *in situ* breast cancer, and 16% of tests against homologous invasive breast cancer. When leukocytes from unselected breast cancer patients were tested against RIII milk containing MuMTV, positive responses were obtained in 25 (31%) of 80 tests. Leukocytes which were responsive to *in situ* breast cancer tissue cross-reacted with MuMTV-containing RIII milk, but not with MuMTV-free RIIIf and C57BL milk in 18 (66%) of 27 tests. Conversely, when leukocytes responsive to MuMTV were tested against homologous *in situ* breast cancer, positive responses were found in 37 (60%) of 61 tests. Leukocytes which failed to respond to MuMTV rarely (10/108 or 9%) responded to homologous *in situ* breast cancer tissues. It appears that an appreciable proportion of human *in situ* breast cancers contain a component similar to a component of MuMTV.

Additional evidence that cross-reacting antigens exist in the two species is furnished by Priori *et al.* (1972), who found by immunofluorescence that 50% of the sera from breast cancer patients could react positively with mouse mammary tumor cells. Müller *et al.* (1972) have confirmed these observations on frozen sections of mouse mammary tumors.

In other experiments using peroxidase-coupled anti-human globulin, Hoshino *et al.* (1973) have shown that sera from breast cancer patients formed a virus-specific precipitate in thin sections of mouse mammary tumor examined with the electron microscope. This appeared to be a specific antigen–antibody reaction between the mouse virus and the component in the human sera.

9. Culture of Human Mammary Tumor Cells

Cultures of cells derived from human mammary carcinomas are being studied in many laboratories with the hope of finding evidence for the production of a mammary tumor virus. It is now possible to prepare cultures of pure mammary epithelial cells that survive for long periods. The epithelial cells can be freed of connective tissue and adipose cells by employing several techniques such as use of collagenase, slicing the tumor tissue under culture medium so that the spilled cells which are epithelial can be collected separately, and selecting epithelial cells

through the differential rate of attachment to the flasks. Fibroblasts settle to the   159
floor of the flask in a few hours, while the epithelial cells remain in suspension for   MAMMARY
48 h or longer. By these procedures, it is easy to collect epithelial cell populations   TUMOR VIRUS
that are viable for many months (Lasfargues, 1974). A serum substitute consisting
of peptones, dextrose, lactalbumin hydrolysate, and polyvinylpyrrolidone has
been developed (Lasfargues *et al.*, 1973). This mixture, which has the appearance
and many properties of serum, is autoclavable and therefore free of adventitious
viruses and mycoplasmas. It is also free of hormones and inhibitors, which are
uncontrollable factors in serum. By use of these and many other procedures,
hundreds of human breast tumors have been screened for the presence of a
mammary tumor virus. Although not a single budding B particle has been found,
there is evidence that the viral genome exists in these cells. Virus-like particles are
often found in high-speed centrifugation pellets of culture supernatants. Some of
these particles have an external membrane with spikes comparable to those of the
mouse mammary tumor virus. Others have a smooth surface like that of the
leukemia viruses. It appears significant that such particles have not been observed
in culture fluids of normal human cells, but the meaning of these virus-like
particles is difficult to assess. One primary culture, BT-271, has shown sufficient
amounts of reverse transcriptase and 70S RNA to support the idea that in human
materials, like in the mouse, there is production of viral components. The
detection of a reverse transcriptase and 70S RNA in milk, tumor biopsies, and
tissue cultures from breast cancer patients constitutes a strong evidence in favor of
a tumor virus in man. The finding in culture supernatants of virus-like particles
comparable in size and morphology to murine viruses is strongly suggestive that
an oncogenic agent of the same type exists.

10. Summary of Evidence for a Mouse-Related Virus in Man

1. Type B particles are occasionally found in human milk.
2. RNA-directed DNA polymerase (RDDP) is found in many human milks,
   although because of destroying factor(s) not evident in mouse or cow's milk
   its presence usually depends on freshness and/or on the amount of destroying factor.
3. The RDDP is associated with particles having the same buoyant density as
   mouse MuMTV, 1.18 vs. 1.16 g/ml for type C particles.
4. The RDDP is associated with a 35S or 70S RNA, which is a characteristic of
   RNA tumor viruses.
5. The human RDDP responds to Mg^{2+} for activity with a synthetic template,
   poly(rC)·oligo(dG$_{12-18}$), in agreement with MuMTV, whereas the RT of
   mouse leukemia virus type C particles requires Mn^{2+}.
6. Extensive hybridization studies using different procedures in several
   laboratories indicate a relationship between MuMTV RNA and human
   breast cancer RNA.

7. Of 100 human sera tested for neutralization of mouse MTV, 25 showed a neutralizing effect, and some completely neutralized the mouse virus. (Absorption of human sera with MTV-free C57BL milk or mammary tissue had no effect on its neutralizing ability.)

8. Cellular hypersensitivity responses of human leukocytes to homologous *in situ* breast cancer tissue are correlated with responsiveness to MuMTV.

9. Sera from some human breast cancer patients contain material that precipitates specifically on the membrane of budding MuMTV virions as demonstrated with peroxidase-coupled anti-human globulin.

11. Appendix: Mouse Strains

Of the many different isologous mouse strains used in breast cancer research, only seven of the most widely used ones will be mentioned here (see Chapt. 2 by Heston in Volume 1 for further details).

DBA: DBA (dilute brown nonagouti) was started by Clarence C. Little in 1909 (see Murray, 1934); it was the first isologous line established by brother × sister mating. It is a high mammary tumor strain in both breeders and virgins.

C3H: C3H was started by Leonell C. Strong in 1920 by mating a female obtained from Halsey Bagg's colony of albinos (BALB) with a male of Little's DBA strain (Strong, 1935). The mammary tumor incidence in these mice is little affected by breeding. The mammary tumor incidence is usually above 90% in all the many laboratories that have used this strain. Even after foster-nursing on agent-free strains such as C57BL, the incidence may be as much as 50%. There is both male and female gamete transmission of the MTV genome.

A: Strain A was started by Strong in 1921, by mating a mouse from Bagg's albino stock with one from Little's stock (Strong, 1936). Breeders of this strain have a high incidence of mammary tumors, but virgins have a very low incidence. Of all the high mammary tumor strains used, the tumors in A are the most dependent on breeding.

BALB/c: Strain BALB/c is a continuation of one of the branches of Bagg's original albino stock and was established by MacDowell in 1923. It is considered a low mammary tumor strain, although the incidence is appreciable (5–30%) in most laboratories. The mammary tumors usually come late in life, and unlike the tumors in other strains they do not seem to contain the usual type B particles. When inoculated as weanlings, BALB/c mice respond well to virus from C3H or A donors but poorly to the virus from RIII donors.

C57BL: Little originated the C57 black line in 1920 by mating two genetically heterogeneous mice he obtained from Lathrop (Snell, 1941). The offspring of this mating segregated into black and brown mice, and both lines have been propagated. The black line has been used extensively for mammary tumor

studies. It normally has a very low mammary tumor incidence (under 1%), and some colonies have gone for years without a single spontaneous mammary tumor. It is quite resistant to infection with virus from C3H or A mice but susceptible to RIII or GR virus. Its resistance to C3H virus has given it the reputation of being genetically resistant to mammary tumors, but it is more susceptible to RIII virus than is the BALB/c stock. With RIII virus and breeding from the third or later litters, a high mammary tumor line of C57BL mice has been maintained through the F_4 generation (Moore, 1973, unpublished).

RIII: The RIII strain originated in the Institute de Radium, Paris, in the late 1920s, when N. Dobrovolskaia-Zavadskaia (1933) mated "two cancerous adenoma of the mammary gland" sisters to a male with characteristic short tail who had a cancer case in his ancestry four generations back. RIII is a high mammary tumor strain, some colonies having an incidence of almost 100%, but it has a tendency to lose the mammary tumor virus (Andervont and Dunn, 1962). Breeding from the third or later litters and selection of only the progeny of mothers that develop tumors seem to be responsible for maintaining a high incidence.

GR: Strain GR was developed in the early 1960s by Otto Mühlbock in Amsterdam from a pair of mice from Zurich. It has always been a high mammary tumor strain. The stock now called GR was derived from a pair taken from the uterus and foster-nursed on a C57BL mother (Dux and Mühlbock, 1968). The GR strain has the characteristic of retaining the same high tumor incidence (approximately 100%) after being foster-nursed on MTV-free C57BL mice. GR mice carry a very virulent milk-transmitted and gamete-transmitted virus. Tumors appear early, and the life span of females is short. They are relatively poor milk producers. C57BL females have a high incidence of infection when inoculated with GR milk.

12. References

ANDERVONT, H. B., 1945, Fate of C3H milk influence in mice of strains C and C57 black mice, *J. Natl. Cancer Inst.* **5**:383.

ANDERVONT, H. B., 1964, Fate of the C3H mammary tumor agent in mice of strains C57BL, I and BALB/c, *J. Natl. Cancer Inst.* **32**:1189.

ANDERVONT, H. B., AND BRYAN, W. R., 1944, Properties of the mouse mammary-tumor agent, *J. Natl. Cancer Inst.* **5**:143.

ANDERVONT, H. B., AND DUNN, T. B., 1948, Mammary tumors in mice presumably free of the mammary tumor agent, *J. Natl. Cancer Inst.* **8**:227.

ANDERVONT, H. B., AND DUNN, T. B., 1959, Disappearance of the mammary tumor agent in strain RIII mice, *Acta Unio Int. Contra Cancrum* **15**:124.

ANDERVONT, H. B., AND DUNN, T. B., 1962, Studies of the mammary tumor agent of strain RIII mice, *J. Natl. Cancer Inst.* **28**:159.

ANDERVONT, H. B., AND DUNN, T. B., 1964, Occurrence of mammary tumors in castrated agent-free male mice after limited or repeated exposure to diethylstilbestrol, *J. Natl. Cancer Inst.* **33**:143.

ANDERVONT, H. B., AND DUNN, T. B., 1965, Further studies of the mammary tumor agent of strain RIII mice, *J. Natl. Cancer Inst.* **35**:39.

ARDASHNIKOV, S. N. AND SPASSKAIA, I. G., 1949, Employment of biophysical methods for determining the nature of the so-called milk factor, *J. Microbiol. Epidemiol. Immunobiol. U.S.S.R.* **9**:44.

AXEL, R., GULATI, C., AND SPIEGELMAN, S., 1972, Particles containing RNA-instructed DNA polymerase and virus-related RNA in human breast cancers, *Proc. Natl. Acad. Sci.* **69**:3133.

BALTIMORE, D., 1970, Viral RNA–dependent DNA polymerase in virions of RNA tumor viruses, *Nature (Lond.)* **226**:1209.

BASHFORD, E. F., 1909, The incidence of cancer in mice of known age, *Roy. Soc. Lond. Proc.* **81**:310.

BENTVELZEN, P., 1968, *Genetical Control of the Vertical Transmission of the Mühlbock Mammary Tumour Virus in the GR Mouse Strain*, Hollandia, Amsterdam.

BENTVELZEN, P., DAAMS, J. H., HAGEMAN, P., AND CALAFAT, J., 1970, Genetic transmission of viruses that incite mammary tumor in mice, *Proc. Natl. Acad. Sci.* **67**:377.

BERNSTEIN, F., 1937, The factors of heredity, age and acquired hypersensitiveness in relation to cancer, *Occas. publ. AAAS Suppl.* **85**:45.

BITTNER, J. J., 1936, Some possible effects of nursing on the mammary gland tumor incidence in mice (preliminary report), *Science* **84**:162.

BITTNER, J. J., 1938, The genetics of cancer in mice, *Quart. Rev. Biol.* **13**:51.

BITTNER, J. J., 1956, Mammary cancer in C3H mice of different sublines and their hybrids, *J. Natl. Cancer Inst.* **16**:1263.

BITTNER, J. J., AND LITTLE, C. C., 1937, The transmission of breast and lung cancer in mice, *J. Hered.* **28**:117.

BLACK, M. M., LEIS, H. P., JR., SHORE, B., AND ZACHRAU, R. E., 1974a, Cellular hypersensitivity to breast cancer: Assessment by a leukocyte migration procedure, *Cancer*, **33**:952.

BLACK, M. M., MOORE, D. H., SHORE, B., ZACHRAU, R. E., AND LEIS, H. P., JR., 1974b, Effect of mouse mammary tumor virus containing milk and human breast tissues on human leukocyte migration, *Cancer Res.* **34**:1954.

BLAIR, P. B., 1960, A Mutation in the Mouse Mammary Tumor Virus, *Cancer Res.* **20**:635.

BLAIR, P. B., 1963, Neutralization of mouse mammary tumour virus by rabbit antisera against C3Hf tissues, *Cancer Res.* **23**:381.

BLAIR, P. B., 1968, The mammary tumor virus (MTV), *Curr. Top. Microbiol. Immunol.* **45**:1.

BLAIR, P. B., 1970, Search for cross-reacting antigenicity between MTV-induced mammary tumors and embryonic antigens: Effect of immunization on development of spontaneous mammary tumors, *Cancer Res.* **30**:1199.

BLAIR, P. B., 1971, Immunological aspects of the relationship between host and oncogenic virus in the mouse mammary tumor system, *Israel J. Med. Sci.* **7**:161.

BLAIR, P. B., AND PITELKA, D. R., 1966, Immunology of the mouse mammary tumor virus: Correlation of the immunodiffusion precipitate line with the type-B virus particles, *J. Natl. Cancer Inst.* **37**:261.

BLAIR, P. B., LAVRIN, D. H., DEZFULIAN, M., AND WEISS, D. W., 1966, Immunology of the mouse mammary tumor virus (MTV): Identification *in vitro* of mouse antibodies against MTV, *Cancer Res.* **26**:647.

BLAIR, P. B., KRIPKE, M. L., LAPPÉ, M. A., BONHOG, R. S., AND YOUNG, L., 1971, Immunologic deficiency associated with the mammary tumor virus (MTV) infection in mice: Hemagglutinin response and allograft survival, *J. Immunol.* **106**:364.

BOOT, L. M., AND MÜHLBOCK, O., 1956, The mammary tumor incidence in the C3H mouse-strain with and without the agent (C3H; C3Hf; C3He), *Acta Univ Int. Contra Cancrum* **12**:569.

BORREL, A., 1910, Parasitisme et tumeurs, *Ann. Inst. Pasteur* **24**:778.

BRITTEN, R. J., AND SMITH, J., 1970, A bovine genome, *Carnegie Inst. Wash. Year Book* **68**:378.

CAME, P. E., AND MOORE, D. H., 1966, Unpublished observations.

CHARNEY, J., AND MOORE, D. H., 1971, Neutralization of murine mammary tumour virus by sera of women with breast cancer, *Nature (Lond.)* **229**:627.

CHARNEY, J., AND MOORE, D. H., 1972, Immunization studies with mammary tumor virus, *J. Natl. Cancer Inst.* **48**:1125.

CHARNEY, J., AND MOORE, D. H., 1974, MTV-neutralizing activity of human sera, In preparation.

CHARNEY, J., PULLINGER, B. D., AND MOORE, D. H., 1969, Development of an infectivity assay for mouse mammary-tumor virus, *J. Natl. Cancer Inst.* **43**:1289.

DAS, M. R., SADISIVAN, E., KOSHY, R., VAIDYA, A. B., AND SIRSAT, S. M., 1972, Homology between RNA from human malignant breast tissue and DNA synthesized by milk particles, *Nature New Biol.* **239**:92.

DEFENDI, V., AND JENSEN, F., 1967, Oncogenicity by DNA tumor viruses: Enhancement after ultra violet and cobalt-60 radiations, *Science* **157**:703.

DEZFULIAN, M., LAVRIN, D. H., SHEN, A., BLAIR, P. B., AND WEISS, D. W., 1967, Immunology of spontaneous mammary carcinomas in mice: Studies on the nature of the protective antigens, in: *Carcinogenesis: A Broad Critique*, pp. 365–388, Williams and Wilkins, Baltimore.

DION, A. S., VAIDYA, A. B., AND FOUT, G. S., 1974, Cation preferences for poly(rC) · oligo(dG)-directed DNA synthesis by RNA tumor viruses and human milk particulates, *Cancer Res.* **34**:3509.

DMOCHOWSKI, L., 1958, The importance of studies on the mammary tumor–inducing virus in the problem of breast cancer, in: *International Symposium on Mammary Cancer* (L. Severi, ed.), pp. 655–708, Division of Cancer Research, Perugia.

DMOCHOWSKI, L., AND PASSEY, R. D., 1952, Attempts at tumor virus isolation, *Ann. N.Y. Acad. Sci.* **54**:1035.

DOBROVOLSKAIA-ZAVADSKAIA, N., 1930, Sur une lignee de souris, riche en adenocarcinome de la mammelle, *Compt. Rend. Soc. Biol.* **104**:1193.

DOBROVOLSKAIA-ZAVADSKAIA, N., 1933, Heredity of cancer susceptibility in mice, *J. Genet.* **27**:181.

DUESBERG, P. H., AND BLAIR, P. B., 1966, Isolation of the nucleic acid of mouse mammary tumor virus (MTV), *Proc. Natl. Acad. Sci.* **55**:1490.

DUX, A., AND MÜHLBOCK, O., 1966, Tumour incidence in mammary glands transplanted from the strains C3H and 020 into their mammectomized F$_1$-hybrids, *Int. J. Cancer* **1**:5.

DUX, A., AND MÜHLBOCK, O., 1968, Susceptibility of mammary tissues of different strains of mice to tumor development, *J. Nat. Cancer Inst.* **40**:1259.

FEKETE, E., AND LITTLE, C. C., 1942, Observations on the mammary tumor incidence of mice born from transferred ova, *Cancer Res.* **2**:525.

FELLER, W. F., AND CHOPRA, H. C. 1968, A small virus-like particle observed in human breast cancer by means of electron microscopy, *J. Natl. Cancer Inst.* **40**:1359.

FERNÁNDEZ-MORÁN, H., ODA, T., BLAIR, P. B., AND GREEN, D. E., 1964, A macromolecular repeating unit of mitochondrial structure and function: Correlated electron microscopic and biochemical studies of isolated mitochondria and submitochondrial particles of beef heart muscle, *J. Cell Biol.* **22**:63.

FURTH, J. J., 1972, Epilogue: Quo vadis? *J. Natl. Cancer Inst.* **48**:1235.

GAYLORD, H. G., AND CLOWES, G. H. A., 1907, Evidence of infected cages as the source of spontaneous cancer developing among small caged animals, *Am. Med. Assoc. J.* **48**:15.

GORER, P. A., AND LAW, L. W., 1949, An attempt to demonstrate neutralizing antibodies to the mammary tumour "milk agent" in mice, *Brit. J. Cancer* **3**:90.

GORKA, C., MISTRY, P., AND MOURIQUAND, J., 1972, Effets de hautes doses d'irradiation γ sur le virus de la tumeur mammaire murine, in: *Recherches Fondamentales sur les Tumeurs Mammaires*, pp. 163–175, Institut Nat'l de le Sante et de la Recherche Medicale, Paris.

GROSS, L., 1947, Immunological relationship of mammary carcinomas developing spontaneously in female mice of a high-tumor line, *J. Immunol.* **55**:297.

GROSS, L., GESSLER, A. E., AND MCCARTY, K. S., 1950, Electron microscopic examination of human milk particularly from women having family record of breast cancer, *Proc. Soc. Exp. Biol. Med.* **75**:270.

HALL, W. T., AND MOORE, D. H., 1966, Effects of estrogenic hormones on the mammary tissue of agent-free and agent-bearing male mice, *J. Natl. Cancer Inst.* **36**:181.

HEPPNER, G. H., 1969, Studies on serum-mediated inhibition of cellular immunity to spontaneous mouse mammary tumors, *Int. J. Cancer* **4**:608.

HEPPNER, G. H., AND PIERCE, G., 1969, *In vitro* demonstration of tumor-specific antigens in spontaneous mammary tumors in mice, *Int. J. Cancer* **4**:212.

HESTON, W. E., 1945, Genetics of mammary tumors in mice, in: *A Symposium on Mammary Tumors in Mice* (F. R. Moulton, ed.), pp. 55–84, Science Press, Lancaster, Pa.

HESTON, W. E., 1958, Mammary tumors in agent-free mice, *Ann. N.Y. Acad. Sci.* **71**:931.

HESTON, W. E., AND LEVILLAIN, W. D., 1950, Factors in the development of spontaneous mammary gland tumors in agent-free strain C3Hb mice, *J. Natl. Cancer Inst.* **10**:1139.

HORNE, R. W., WATERSON, A. P., WILDY, P., AND FARNHAM, A. E., 1960, The structure and composition of the myxoviruses. I. Electron microscope studies of the structure of myxovirus particles by negative staining techniques, *Virology* **11**:79.

HOSHINO, M., DMOCHOWSKI, L., AND WILLIAMS, W. C., 1973, Electron microscope study of antigens in cell of mouse mammary tumor cell lines by peroxidase-labeled antibodies in sera of mammary tumor–bearing mice and of patients with breast cancer, *Cancer Res.* **33**:2551.

IMAGAWA, D. T., BITTNER, J. J., AND SYVERTON, J. T., 1950, Cytotoxic studies on mouse mammary cancer cells, *Cancer Res.* **10**:226.

KORTEWEG, R., 1936, On the manner in which the disposition to carcinoma of the mammary gland is inherited in mice, *Genetica* **18**:350.

KRAMARSKY, B., LASFARGUES, E. Y., AND MOORE, D. H., 1971, Ultrastructural changes in mammary tumor virus upon ingestion or intraperitoneal inoculation in mice, *Proc. Am. Assoc. Cancer Res.* **12**:52 (abst.).

LASFARGUES, E. Y., 1974, New approaches to the cultivation of human breast carcinomas, in: *Human Tumor Cells in Culture* (J. Fogh, ed.), Plenum, New York.

LASFARGUES, E. Y., PILLSBURY, N., LASFARGUES, J. C., AND MOORE, D. H., 1970a, Release of leukemia C particles from murine cell lines infected with Bittner virus–containing inocula, *Cancer Res.* **30**:167.

LASFARGUES, E. Y., KRAMARSKY, B., SARKAR, N. H., LASFARGUES, J. C., PILLSBURY, N., AND MOORE, D. H., 1970b, Stimulation of mammary tumor virus production in a mouse mammary tumor cell line, *Cancer Res.* **30**:1109.

LASFARGUES, E. Y., KRAMARSKY, B., SARKAR, N. H., LASFARGUES, J. C., AND MOORE, D. H., 1972, An established RIII mouse mammary tumor cell line: Kinetics of mammary tumor virus (MTV) production, *Proc. Soc. Exp. Biol. Med.* **139**:242.

LASFARGUES, E. Y., COUTINHO, W. G., LASFARGUES, J. C., AND MOORE, D. H., 1973, A serum substitute that can support the growth of mammary tumor cells, *In Vitro* **6**:494.

LATARJET, R., CRAMER, R., AND MONTAGNIER, L., 1967, Inactivation by UV-, X-, and γ-radiations, of the infecting and transforming capacities of polyoma virus, *Virology* **33**:104.

LATHROP, A. E. C., AND LOEB, L., 1913, The incidence of cancer in various strains of mice, *Proc. Soc. Exp. Biol. Med.* **11**:34.

LATHROP, A. E. C., AND LOEB, L., 1915, Further investigations on the origin of tumors in mice: Tumor incidence and tumor age in various strains of mice, *J. Exp. Med.* **22**:646.

LAVRIN, D. H., BLAIR, P. B., AND WEISS, D. W., 1966, Immunology of spontaneous mammary carcinomas in mice. III. Immunogenicity of C3H preneoplastic hyperplastic alveolar nodules in C3Hf hosts, *Cancer Res.* **26**:293.

LEONG, J., GARAPIN, A., JACKSON, N., FANSHIER, L., LEVINSON, W., AND BISHOP, J. M., 1972, Virus-specific ribonucleic acid in cells producing Rous sarcoma virus: Detection and characterization, *J. Virol.* **9**:891.

LITTLE, C. C., 1928, Evidence that cancer is not a simple Mendelian recessive, *J. Cancer Res.* **12**:30.

LITTLE, C. C., 1936, The present status of our knowledge of heredity and cancer, *Am. Med. Assoc. J.* **106**:2234.

LOEB, L., 1907/1908, Further observations on the endemic occurrence of carcinoma and on the inoculability of tumors, *Univ. Pa. Med. Bull.* **20**:2.

LUNGER, P. D., LUCAS, J. C., JR., AND SHIPKEY, F. H., 1964, The ultramorphology of milk fractions from normal and breast cancer patients: A preliminary report, *Cancer* **17**:549.

LYNCH, C. J., 1924, Studies on the relation between tumor susceptibility and heredity, *J. Exp. Med.* **39**:481.

LYONS, M. J., AND MOORE, D. H., 1965, Isolation of the mouse mammary tumor virus: Chemical and morphological studies, *J. Natl. Cancer Inst.* **35**:549.

McCAFFREY, R., SMOLER, D. F., AND BALTIMORE, D., 1973, Terminal deoxynucleotidyl transferase in a case of childhood acute lymphoblastic leukemia, *Proc. Natl. Acad. Sci.* **70**:521.

MEITES, J., 1972, Relation of proclactin and estrogen to mammary tumorigenesis in the rat, *J. Natl. Cancer Inst.* **48**:1217.

MOORE, D. H., 1963, Mouse mammary tumour agent and mouse mammary tumours, *Nature (Lond.)* **198**:429.

MOORE, D. H., AND LYONS, M. J., 1963, Electrophoretic separation of the mouse mammary tumor virus, *J. Natl. Cancer Inst.* **31**:1255.

MOORE, D. H., LASFARGUES, E. Y., MURRAY, M. R., HAAGENSEN, C. D., AND POLLARD, E. C., 1959, Correlation of physical and biological properties of mouse mammary tumor agent, *J. Biophys. Biochem. Cytol.* **5**:85.

MOORE, D. H., POLLARD, E. C., AND HAAGENSEN, C. D., 1962, Further correlations of physical and biological properties of mouse mammary tumor agent, *Fed. Proc.* **21**:942.

MOORE, D. H., PILLSBURY, N., AND PULLINGER, B. D., 1969a, Titrations of mammary tumor virus in fresh and treated RIII milk and milk fractions, *J. Natl. Cancer Inst.* **43**:1263.

MOORE, D. H., SARKAR, N. H., KELLY, C. E., PILLSBURY, N., AND CHARNEY, J., 1969b, Type B particles in human milk, *Texas Rep. Biol. Med.* **27**:1027.

MOORE, D. H., CHARNEY, J., AND PULLINGER, B. D., 1970, Mouse mammary tumor virus infectivity as a function of age at inoculation, breeding, and total lapsed time, *J. Natl. Cancer Inst.* **45**:561.

MOORE, D. H., CHARNEY, J., KRAMARSKY, B., LASFARGUES, E. Y., SARKAR, N. H., BRENNAN, M. J., BURROWS, J. H., SIRSAT, S. M., PAYMASTER, J. C., AND VAIDYA, A. B., 1971, Search for a human breast cancer virus, *Nature (Lond.)* **229**:611.

MOORE, D. H., SARKAR, N. H., CHARNEY, J., AND KRAMARSKY, B., 1973, Some physical and biological characteristics of the mouse mammary tumor virus, *Cancer Res.* **33**:5.

MOORE, D. H., CHARNEY, J., AND HOLBEN, J. A., 1974, Titrations of various mouse mammary tumor viruses in different mouse strains, *J. Natl. Cancer Inst.*, **52**:1757.

MORETTI, R. L., AND BLAIR, P. B., 1966, The male histocompatibility antigen in mouse mammary tissue. I. Growth of the male mammary gland in female mice, *Transplantation* **4**:596.

MORTON, D. L., 1969, Acquired immunological tolerance and carcinogenesis by the mammary tumor virus. I. Influence of neonatal infection with the mammary tumor virus on the growth of spontaneous mammary adencarcinomas, *J. Natl. Cancer Inst.* **42**:311.

MORTON, D. L., GOLDMAN, L., AND WOOD, D. A., 1969, Acquired immunological tolerance and carcinogenesis by the mammary tumor virus. II. Immune responses influencing growth of spontaneous mammary adenocarcinomas, *J. Natl. Cancer Inst.* **42**:321.

MÜHLBOCK, O., 1950, Mammary tumor-agent in the sperm of high-cancer-strain male mice, *J. Natl. Cancer Inst.* **10**:861.

MÜHLBOCK, O., 1951, Comparison of the mammary-tumor agent in tumor-extracts of various high-cancer-strain of mice, *Kon. Ned. Akad. Wetenschappen Proc. Ser. C* **54(4)**:386.

MÜHLBOCK, O., 1952, Studies on the transmission of the mouse mammary tumor agent by the male parent, *J. Natl. Cancer Inst.* **12**:819.

MÜHLBOCK, O., 1956, Biological studies on the mammary tumor agent in different strains of mice, *Acta Univ Int. Contra Cancrum* **12**:665.

MÜHLBOCK, O., 1965, Note on a new inbred mouse strain GR/A, *Europ. J. Cancer* **1**:123.

MÜHLBOCK, O., 1972, Role of hormones in the etiology of breast cancer, *J. Natl. Cancer Inst.* **48**:1213.

MÜHLBOCK, O., AND BENTVELZEN, P., 1968, The transmission of the mammary tumor viruses, in: *Perspectives in Virology*, Vol. 6 (M. Pollard, ed.), Academic Press, New York, p. 75.

MÜHLBOCK, O., AND BOOT, L. M., 1959, The mechanism of hormonal carcinogenesis, in: *Ciba Foundation Symposium on Carcinogenesis: Mechanisms of Action*, J. & A. Churchill Ltd., London, p. 83.

MÜLLER, M., ZOTTER, S., GROSSMANN, H., AND KEMMER, C., 1972, Antibodies in women with mammary carcinoma or proliferating mastopathy reacting specifically with an intracellular antigen of mammary tumor virus (MTV) producing tumors of mice, in: *Recherches Fondamentales sur les Tumeurs Mammaires*, pp. 343–349, Institut Nat'l de Inst. Sante et de la Recherche Medicale, Paris.

MURRAY, J. A., 1911, Cancerous ancestry and the incidence of cancer in mice, in: *Fourth Scientific Report of the Imperial Cancer Research Fund*, London, p. 114.

MURRAY, W. S., 1934, The breeding behavior of the dilute brown stock of mice (Little dba). *Amer. J. Cancer* **20**:573.

NANDI, S., 1963. New method for the detection of mouse mammary tumor virus. I. Influence of foster nursing on incidence of hyperplastic mammary nodules in BALB/c–Crgl mice, *J. Natl. Cancer Inst.* **31**:57.

NOWINSKI, R. C., OLD, L. J., MOORE, D. H., GEERING, G., AND BOYSE, E. A., 1967, A soluble antigen of the mammary tumor virus, *Virology* **31**:1.

NOWINSKI, R. C., SARKAR, N. H., OLD, L. J., MOORE, D. H., SCHEER, D. I., AND HILGERS, J., 1971, Characteristics of the structural components of the mouse mammary tumor virus. II. Viral proteins and antigens, *Virology* **46**:21.

PASSEY, R. D., DMOCHOWSKI, L., ASTBURY, W. T., REED, R., AND EAVES, G., 1951, Electron microscope studies of human breast cancer, *Nature (Lond.)* **167**:643.

PITELKA, D. R., BERN, H. A., NANDI, S., AND DEOME, K. B., 1964, On the significance of virus-like particles in mammary tissues of C3Hf mice, *J. Natl. Cancer Inst.* **33**:867.

PRIORI, E. S., ANDERSON, D. E., WILLIAMS, W. C., AND DMOCHOWSKI, L., 1972, Immunological studies on human breast carcinoma and mouse mammary tumors, *J. Natl. Cancer Inst.* **48**:1131.

PULLINGER, B. D., 1947, Forced activation and early detection of the milk-borne agent of mammary adenomas in mice, *Brit. J. Cancer* **1**:177.

PULLINGER, B. D., AND IVERSEN, S., 1960, Mammary tumour incidence in relation to age and number of litters in C3H and RIII mice, *Brit. J. Cancer* **14**:267.

SARKAR, N. H., AND MOORE, D. H., 1968, The internal structure of mouse mammary tumor virus as revealed after Tween–ether treatment, *J. Microsc.* **7**:539.

SARKAR, N. H., AND MOORE, D. H., 1970, Electron microscopy of the nucleic acid of mouse mammary tumor virus, *J. Virol.* **5**:230.

SARKAR, N. H., AND MOORE, D. H., 1972, On the possibility of a human breast cancer virus, *Nature (Lond.)* **236**:103.

SARKAR, N. H., AND MOORE, D. H., 1974a, Separation of B and C type virions by centrifugation in gentle density gradients, *J. Virol.*, **13**:1143.

SARKAR, N. H., AND MOORE, D. H., 1974b, Surface structure of mouse mammary tumor virus, *Virology*, **61**:38.

SARKAR, N. H., CHARNEY, J., AND MOORE, D. H., 1969, Mammary tumor virion structure in mouse milk fractions, *J. Natl. Cancer Inst.* **43**:1275.

SARKAR, N. H., NOWINSKI, R. C., AND MOORE, D. H., 1971, Characteristics of the structural components of the mouse mammary tumor virus. I. Morphological and biochemical studies, *Virology* **46**:1.

SARKAR, N. H., MOORE, D. H., KRAMARSKY, B., AND CHOPRA, H. C., 1973a, Oncornaviruses. 3. The mammary tumor virus, in: *Ultrastructure of Animal Viruses and Bacteriophages: An Atlas* (A. J. Dalton, ed.), pp. 307–321, Academic Press, New York.

SARKAR, N. H., MOORE, D. H., AND CHARNEY, J., 1973b, The effect of pH on the morphology, electrophoretic mobility, and infectivity of the mouse mammary tumor virus, *Cancer Res.* **33**:2283.

SARKAR, N. H., CHARNEY, J., DION, A. S., AND MOORE, D. H., 1973c, Effect of human milk on the mouse mammary tumor virus, *Cancer Res.* **33**:626.

SCHLOM, J., AND SPIEGELMAN, S., 1971, Simultaneous detection of the reverse transcriptase and high molecular weight RNA unique to the oncogenic RNA viruses, *Science* **174**:840.

SCHLOM, J., SPIEGELMAN, S., AND MOORE, D. H., 1971, RNA-dependent DNA polymerase activity in virus-like particles isolated from human milk, *Nature (Lond.)* **231**:97.

SCHLOM, J., SPIEGELMAN, S., AND MOORE, D. H., 1972, Reverse transcriptase and high molecular weight RNA in particles from mouse and human milk, *J. Natl. Cancer Inst.* **48**:1197.

SEMAN, G., MYERS, B., WILLIAMS, W. C., GALLAGER, H. S., AND DMOCHOWSKI, L., 1969, Studies on the relationship of viruses to the origin of human breast cancer. II. Virus-like particles in human breast tumors, *Texas Rep. Biol. Med.* **27**:839.

SLYE, M., 1914, The incidence and inheritability of spontaneous tumors in mice, 2nd report, *J. Med. Res.* **39**:281.

SLYE, M., 1920, The relation of inbreeding to tumor production: Studies in the incidence and inheritability of spontaneous tumors in mice, *J. Cancer Res.* **5**:53.

SLYE, M., 1926, The inheritance behavior of cancer as a simple Mendelian recessive, *J. Cancer Res.* **10**:15.

SLYE, M., 1928, The relation of heredity to cancer, *J. Cancer Res.* **12**:83.

SMITH, G. H., 1966, Role of the milk agent in disappearance of mammary cancer in C3H/StWi mice, *J. Natl. Cancer Inst.* **36**:685.

SMITH, R. C., AND GALLO, R. C., 1972, DNA-dependent DNA polymerases I and II from normal human-blood lymphocytes, *Proc. Natl. Acad. Sci.* **69**:2879.

SNELL, G. D., 1941, *Mouse Genetics News, No. 1.*

SPIEGELMAN, S., AXEL, R., AND SCHLOM, J., 1972, Virus-related RNA in human and mouse mammary tumors, *J. Natl. Cancer Inst.* **48**:1205.

SQUARTINI, F., ROSSI, G., AND PAOLETTI, I., 1963, Characters of Mammary tumours in BALB/c female mice foster-nursed by C3H and RIII mothers, *Nature (Lond.)* **197**:505.

Staff of Roscoe B. Jackson Memorial Laboratory, 1933, The existence of nonchromosomal influence in the incidence of mammary tumors in mice, *Science* **78**:465.

STRONG, L. C., 1935, The establishment of the C3H inbred strain of mice for the study of spontaneous carcinoma of the mammary gland, *Genet.* **20**:586.

STRONG, L. C., 1936, The establishment of the "A" strain of inbred mice, *J. Hered.* **27**:21.

SYKES, J. A., WHITESCARVER, J., AND BRIGGS, L., 1968, Observations on a cell line producing mammary tumor virus, *J. Natl. Cancer Inst.* **41**:1315.

TEMIN, H. M., AND MIZUTANI, S., 1970, RNA-dependent DNA polymerase in virions of Rous sarcoma virus, *Nature (Lond.)* **226**:1211.

TYZZER, E. E., 1909, A series of spontaneous tumors in mice with observations on the influence of heredity on the frequency of their occurrence, *J. Med. Res.* **21**:479.

VAAGE, J., 1968a, Non-cross-reacting resistance to virus induced mouse mammary tumours in virus infected C3H mice, *Nature (Lond.)* **218:**101.

VAAGE, J., 1968b, Non-virus-associated antigens in virus induced mouse mammary tumors, *Cancer Res.* **28:**2477.

VAIDYA, A. B., 1973, Molecular biology of human milk, *Science* **180:**776.

VAIDYA, A. B., DION, A. S., AND MOORE, D. H., 1974, Homology of mouse mammary tumor viral RNA with RNA from human breast cancer, *Nature (Lond.)*, **249:**565.

VARMUS, H. E., BISHOP, J. M., NOWINSKI, R. C., AND SARKAR, N. H., 1972, Mammary tumour virus specific nucleotide sequences in mouse DNA, *Nature New Biol.* **238:**189.

VARMUS, H. E., QUINTRELL, N., MEDEIROS, E., BISHOP, J. M., NOWINSKI, R. C., AND SARKAR, N. H., 1973, Transcription of mouse mammary tumor virus genes in tissues from high and low tumor incidence mouse strains, *J. Mol. Biol.* **79:**663.

WEISS, D. W., 1967, Immunology of spontaneous tumors, in: *Proceedings of the 5th Berkeley Symposium on Mathematical Statistics and Probability*, University of California Press, Berkeley.

WEISS, D. W., 1969, Immunologic parameters of host–tumor relationships: Spontaneous mammary neoplasia of the inbred mouse as a model, *Cancer Res.* **29:**2368.

WEISS, D. W., LAVRIN, D. H., DEZFULIAN, M., VAAGE, J., AND BLAIR, P. B., 1966, Studies on the immunology of spontaneous mammary carcinomas of mice, in: *Viruses Inducing Cancer—Implications for Therapy* (W. J. Burdette, ed.), pp. 138–168, University of Utah Press, Salt Lake City.

ZEILMAKER, G. H., 1969, Transmission of mammary tumor virus by female GR mice: Results of egg transplantation, *Int. J. Cancer* **4:**261.

5

Feline Leukemia–Sarcoma Complex: A Model for RNA Viral Tumorigenesis

Gordon H. Theilen

1. Animal Models of RNA Viral Oncogenesis

RNA tumor viruses have been isolated from poultry, mice, cats, monkeys, and other animals, even poikilotherms, and are known to be responsible for a variety of neoplastic and nonneoplastic diseases. These RNA type C or oncornaviruses mainly cause hematopoietic and connective tissue neoplasms that in mice, poultry, cats, and monkeys have been classified as the causative agents of disease conditions in the leukemia–sarcoma complex. In addition to known tumorigenic RNA tumor virus isolates, type C virus has been suspected as the cause of leukemia in cattle, sheep, swine, dogs, and a variety of other warm-blooded animals and some cold-blooded animals.

There are many reasons why certain animal models are better than others for the study of comparative viral oncogenesis. RNA tumor viruses have been extensively studied in mice and poultry and are carefully covered in other chapters of this volume. The advantages of using small laboratory animals are obvious: they can be inbred and are relatively inexpensive, and many strains of animals with different genetic susceptibilities are readily available. The big advantage of genetic control has allowed scientists to develop principles of RNA oncogenesis far beyond what was possible before inbred animals were available for research. However, RNA viral oncogenesis in man and most outbred animals

Gordon H. Theilen ● Department of Surgery, School of Veterinary Medicine, University of California at Davis, Davis, California.

169

is still as much a hypothesis as it was several years ago, which demonstrates that manipulated research of inbred animals has its limitations.

Cattle, sheep, swine, dogs, cats, and monkeys, on the other hand, are outbred animals which have spontaneous neoplasms that frequently resemble those of humans and these animals are used in laboratory experiments as comparative models. Important food-producing animals such as cattle, sheep, swine, and poultry may have neoplastic diseases of considerable economic importance. For example, Marek's disease of chickens annually cost poultry farmers over 150 million dollars loss in income until the recent development of a vaccine. If only from an economic standpoint, the control of Marek's disease by vaccination exemplifies why it is important to study viral oncogenesis in food-producing animals. Another reason for studying neoplasms of outbred animals is to determine whether those caused by viruses have a wide host range and therefore may be of public health importance. The larger farm animals used in cancer research under laboratory conditions are expensive, have few young per year—particularly cattle—and must be housed in special facilities, making them of limited use in manipulative cancer research. Sheep may be an exception; they are relatively inexpensive, docile animals, are easy to keep in laboratory conditions, and are one of the best subjects for study of the ontogeny of immune responses. In this regard at least, they should prove to be excellent animals in the study of how a host responds to its tumor.

Monkeys are useful outbred animals in cancer research because of their close phylogenetic relationship to human beings, particularly since an RNA tumor virus has been isolated from a woolly monkey (Theilen et al., 1971; Wolfe et al., 1971) and type C virus has been isolated in cell cultures from gibbons (Kawakami et al., 1972). The disadvantages of nonhuman primate research are the difficulty of obtaining certain species for study and the extreme expense involved in maintaining and housing monkeys for viral tumorigenic studies.

It is important to know the range of animal classes from which RNA tumor viruses can be isolated and demonstrated to be cancer producing. This justifies investigations of RNA viral oncogenesis in poikilotherms as well as in different types of warm-blooded animals, but each animal model presents technical and logistic problems in the development of each new model system.

It is with investigations of RNA viral oncogenesis in smaller multiparous animals that newer approaches to studying comparative RNA tumorigenesis should be most fruitful. The dog is a good animal model because, as with humans, tumor viruses have been difficult to isolate. Many dogs with cancer are seen by practicing veterinarians and considerable information is available concerning the epidemiology and natural history of canine neoplasms. On the other hand, a study of RNA viral tumorigenesis in feral mice might prove of value because after trapping they can be maintained in the laboratory and compared with other wild populations as described by Gardner et al. (1973).

Because of recent advances in our knowledge of the etiology of feline leukemia–sarcoma complex and biological responses in spontaneous and experimental situations, cats are an excellent example of an appropriate animal model

for study of RNA viral oncogenesis. This model system has gained additional
prominence since Hardy *et al.* (1973) and W. F. H. Jarrett *et al.* (1973*a*) reported
horizontal transmission of feline leukemia and Sarma *et al.* (1973*a*), Livingston
and Todaro (1973), and Fischinger *et al.* (1973) described an endogenous
vertically transmitted type C virus, RD114. Thus cats, unlike other mammalian
species, carry more than one group of type C viruses, i.e., viruses of feline
leukemia–sarcoma complex and viruses related to RD114.

FELINE
LEUKEMIA–
SARCOMA
COMPLEX:
A MODEL FOR
RNA VIRAL
TUMORIGENESIS

2. Feline Leukemia–Sarcoma Complex: A Comparative Model for Study of Animal and Human Viral Oncogenesis

Cancer ranks as one of the important medical problems of cats, and one-third or
more of all cat tumors are of hemolymphatic origin (Priester, 1971). There is
probably no other outbred animal in which the various tumors of the blood and
blood-forming organs so closely emulate those of man. Most outbred animals
(with the possible exception of swine and some nonhuman primates) are affected
primarily with lymphoreticular neoplasms, while the cat, in addition, is subject to a
wide variety of neoplasms arising from bone marrow, including granulocytic
leukemia, and erythroleukemia, other myeloproliferative diseases, nonresponsive anemias, and myelofibrosis (Table 1). Cats kept as pets live in close association

TABLE 1
Feline Leukemia–Sarcoma Complex

Neoplasm or condition	Cell type
Hemolymphatic	
Lymphoreticular neoplasm	Lymphocyte or reticulum cell
Myeloproliferative	
Reticuloendotheliosis	Undifferentiated mononuclear cell
Granulocytic leukemia	Granulocyte
Erythroleukemia	Erythrocyte and granulocyte
Erythremic myelosis	Erythrocyte
Polycythemia vera	Erythrocyte
Megakaryocytic myelosis	Megakaryocyte
Aplastic or hypoplastic anemia	Erythrocyte
Myelofibrosis	Fibroblast
Connective tissue	
Fibrosarcoma	Fibroblast
Other	
Multiple myeloma	Plasma cell
Mast cell sarcoma (leukemia)	Mast cell

with humans in the same environment and often eat similar or identical foods, additional factors that make them useful for comparative studies.

Since the isolation of feline type C oncornaviruses (FOV) from feline lymphosarcoma (W. F. H. Jarrett *et al.*, 1964), the transmission of feline leukemia (lymphosarcoma) (Rickard *et al.*, 1968, 1969; Kawakami *et al.*, 1967; Theilen *et al.*, 1968, 1970a) and fibrosarcoma (Snyder and Theilen, 1969; Gardner *et al.*, 1970; McDonough *et al.*, 1971), and the association of this virus with other neoplasms and myeloproliferative diseases (Hertz *et al.*, 1970), feline cancer has gained international prominence. The etiology of feline leukemia–sarcoma complex is similar to that of its counterpart in birds and mice, which again exemplifies biological repetition in various species and suggests that oncornavirus may be a causative factor in some human cancers.

It is estimated that approximately one of every four households in the United States has a cat; in other words, some 50 million American people have frequent contact with cats. The press has given extensive attention to cats as possible hosts or vectors of human disease, including cancer. This publicity has caused considerable concern within both the medical and veterinary professions; however, present evidence is strictly circumstantial—that FOV can infect human cells in culture (Sarma *et al.*, 1970)—and there is no proof that feline type C viruses are agents of human cancer. It should be stressed that so far no cat oncornaviruses or viral protein components have been identified in human sera (Sarma *et al.*, 1974), and epidemiological studies have not demonstrated an association between sick cats, those with leukemia or other malignancies, and human disease (Schneider, 1970, 1972b; Hoover *et al.*, 1972; Hanes *et al.*, 1970). Boss and Gibson (1970), on the other hand, reported an association between childhood leukemia and "sick" cats, but what made the cats sick was not clear. Inasmuch as one out of every four American households has a cat, this does not seem unusual, but since the cause of childhood leukemia is unknown this report deserves additional study.

On the other hand, evidence accumulated in recent years makes it scientifically untenable to assume that feline tumor viruses are harmless species-specific entities. For instance, sarcomagenic mutant virus (the sarcoma virus) has an oncogenic spectrum in a wide variety of animal species, including rabbits, dogs, sheep, and several species of nonhuman primates (Theilen *et al.*, 1970b, 1973; Deinhardt *et al.*, 1970). The sarcoma virus will infect and transform several different types of cells from a variety of species, including human embryonic cells in culture. The high occurrence of spontaneous feline leukemia in outbred animals as well as its histological similarity to the spectrum of hematopoietic neoplasms found in human beings strongly emphasizes, if for no other reason, the value of studying cat leukemia as a comparative model.

3. Epidemiological Aspects of Feline Leukemia–Sarcoma Complex

Priester (1971) described the distribution of tumors of cats according to body system and cell type. Approximately one-third of all cat neoplasms are located in the hematopoietic tissues, which is much higher than the figure reported for dogs, cattle, and horses. The relative frequency of lymphoreticular neoplasms in cats is estimated to be higher than that in man, also (Dorn *et al.*, 1967; Hardy, 1971*a*). The true incidence of feline myeloproliferative diseases is unknown; however, we have reported that they are a frequent form of the leukemia complex and may account for about 10% of feline hemolymphatic neoplasms (Schalm and Theilen, 1970). Dorn *et al.* (1968) found a difference in the incidence of lymphosarcoma in cats by sex: 33% of all cancers in male cats and 18% in female cats were lymphatic. Spontaneous fibrosarcomas and other sarcomas are relatively rare in cats (Moulton, 1961).

173

FELINE
LEUKEMIA–
SARCOMA
COMPLEX:
A MODEL FOR
RNA VIRAL
TUMORIGENESIS

Most reports of feline leukemia–sarcoma complex have come from the United States and Europe (O. Jarrett *et al.*, 1967); however, there is little doubt that there is a worldwide distribution. The frequency of feline leukemia based on necropsy reports has varied in different animal hospitals. Holzworth (1960*a*) at Angell Memorial Animal Hospital in Boston reported a hospital frequency of 10%. Cotchin (1957) at the Royal Veterinary College in London reported a postmortem frequency of 15%, and for the last 17 years at U.C.D. we have had a frequency of 0.36% for all cat accessions to our teaching hospital. Dorn *et al.* (1968) reported the incidence rate of feline lymphoreticular neoplasms to be 46 per 100,000 cats in Alameda and Contra Costa Counties of California, and Hardy (1971*a*) indicated a high incidence of this neoplasm in the New York City area.

At the University of California, lymphosarcoma (lymphocytic leukemia) and reticulum cell sarcoma (monocytic leukemia) comprise about 90% of all cat leukemias, while the myeloproliferative diseases make up the remaining 10% and include such conditions as granulocytic leukemia, erythroleukemia, erythremic myelosis, myelofibrosis with myeloid metaplasia, reticuloendotheliosis, and polycythemia vera. Basophilic, eosinophilic, and mast cell leukemia, multiple myeloma, and miscellaneous types are rather rare, but they all have been reported. Sarcomas are relatively infrequent.

4. Clinicopathological Aspects of Feline Leukemia–Sarcoma Complex

The clinicopathological aspects of the feline leukemia–sarcoma complex will be discussed according to five categories: lymphoreticular neoplasms, myeloproliferative diseases, multiple myeloma, mast cell sarcoma, and fibrosarcoma.

4.1. Lymphoreticular Neoplasms

4.1.1. Sex and Breed Distribution

A study by Dorn *et al.* (1967) established a statistically greater frequency of lymphosarcoma in male cats. Data compiled by us support Dorn's report (Table 2); however, Nielsen (1964) found a greater frequency in females.

The incidence of lymphosarcoma in purebred cats such as Siamese may reflect a genetic susceptibility, but it probably only reflects the popularity of the breed

TABLE 2

Sex Distribution of 44 Cats with Lymphoreticular Neoplasms Seen at U.C.D. 1967–1970

Sex	Number
Female intact	3
Female spayed	8
Male intact	21
Male castrated	12

TABLE 3

Breed Distribution of 44 Cats with Lymphoreticular Neoplasms Seen at U.C.D. 1967–1970

Number	Percent	Breed
6	13	DLH
21	50	DSH
13	29	Siamese
4	8	Other[a]

[a] Two Burmese, one Persian, one Melanese.

TABLE 4

Age Distribution of 44 Cats with Lymphoreticular Neoplasms Seen at U.C.D. 1967–1970

Number	Accumulated frequency	Age[a] (yr)
1	1	1
7	8	1–2
6	14	2–3
8	22	3–4
3	25	4–5
3	28	5–6
4	32	6–7
1	33	7–8
4	37	8–9
1	38	9–10
2	40	10–11
0	40	11–12
3	43	12–13
1	44	Unknown

[a] Mean age 4.6 yr.

because both crossbred domestic long-hair (DLH) and domestic short-hair (DSH) cats frequently have leukemia (Table 3). The question of breed susceptibility on the basis of genetic predisposition is a problem that needs to be clarified by additional histological documentation of cases classified as lymphoreticular and myelogenous (including myeloproliferative) disease.

175

FELINE
LEUKEMIA–
SARCOMA
COMPLEX:
A MODEL FOR
RNA VIRAL
TUMORIGENESIS

4.1.2. Age Distribution

Cats of any age, including kittens as young as 2–3 months old, can develop lymphoreticular neoplasms. The mean age for lymphosarcoma in our study was 4.6 yr, and 41% of the animals were represented in the age group birth to 3 yr old (Table 4). Nielsen (1964) reported a mean age of 5.7 yr, with a greater frequency in the age group older than 3 yr.

4.1.3. Clusters

Multiple cases in the same household have been reported or seen by Schneider *et al.* (1967), Brodey *et al.* (1970), Hardy *et al.* (1969), and ourselves (Theilen, 1970). This clustering of disease, often involving unrelated cats, led to the hypothesis of horizontal transmission.

4.1.4. Diagnosis

Lymphosarcoma is much more common than reticulum cell sarcoma; however, it may be difficult to separate them clinically. Thus they are collectively referred to as lymphoreticular neoplasms, although they may also be more broadly designated as feline leukemia. A classification of lymphoreticular neoplasms into different clinicopathological types on the basis of anatomical location of neoplastic involvement has been reported (W. F. H. Jarrett *et al.*, 1966); the types are (1) multicentric, (2) thymic, (3) alimentary, and (4) unclassified or miscellaneous, including variations of the three main forms (Table 5). In our experience and that of Crighton (1969), the alimentary type is seen more commonly than either the thymic or the multicentric type and the latter is the least frequent (Table 6), although the thymic form was the least frequent in W. F. H. Jarrett's series (1966).

TABLE 5
Clinicopathological Types of Lymphoreticular Neoplasms in Cats Listed by Anatomical Location

Clinicopathological type	Organs involved
Alimentary	Mesenteric nodes, intestine, liver, kidneys, spleen
Thymic	Thymic mass, mediastinal lymph nodes, occasional abdominal organs, lungs and pleura
Multicentric	Lymph nodes, external and internal liver, spleen, kidneys, other visceral organs
Miscellaneous	A variety of changes with no consistent pathological pattern

TABLE 6

*Feline Lymphoreticular Neoplasms Classified by
Anatomical Location in 44 Cats Seen at U.C.D.
1967–1970*

Number	Clinicopathological type
16	Alimentary
15	Thymic
8	Multicentric
5	Miscellaneous[a]

[a] One each of lesions in spleen and liver only, spinal cord only, head and neck nodes only, eye only, and peripheral blood and bone marrow only.

A blending of the three types may be a clinical finding; however, separation into three separate clinicopathological entities is the usual situation and is a useful aid to clinicians and experimentalists alike in selecting biopsies for diagnostic purposes and properly evaluating clinical findings. Apparently, the various clinicopathological changes are different host responses to the same type C virus infection.

Just as the physical findings vary accordingly to type, so do other clinicopathological findings. A confirmatory clinical diagnosis of overt disease is based on radiographs, on blood and bone marrow studies (Schalm, 1971), on needle aspirations and biopsies of enlarged lymph nodes, masses, or tumorous organs, and on exploratory laparotomies or thoracotomies. Exploratory surgery is indicated particularly in cases where intestinal stenosis, palpable abdominal masses, or abdominal symptoms of unknown etiology are present. A summary of clinical signs classified according to clinicopathological type and anatomical site is presented in Table 7. Diagnostic X-rays are often valuable in making a presumptive diagnosis of feline lymphoreticular neoplasia (Table 8).

a. Peripheral Blood Examinations. Normal hemograms are not unusual in all clinicopathological types, although abnormal lymphocytes were found in the

TABLE 7

Clinical Signs of Feline Lymphoreticular Neoplasia

Alimentary type
 Anorexia, weakness, emaciation, straining to defecate, blood in stool, diarrhea, polydipsia, offensive breath, icterus, pale mucous membranes
Thymic type
 Open-mouth breathing, extended neck, coughing, sneezing, dysphagia, pale mucous membranes, usually excellent physical condition
Multicentric type
 Generalized lymphadenopathy, anorexia, cachexia, diarrhea, pale mucous membranes
Miscellaneous
 Edematous nictitating membranes, spontaneous fractures, posterior paresis, etc.

peripheral blood in 62% of cats with lymphosarcoma examined at U.C.D. Frank lymphocytic leukemia was encountered in 21% of the cases, whereas monocytic leukemia was relatively rare in association with reticulum cell sarcoma (Table 9).

177

FELINE
LEUKEMIA–
SARCOMA
COMPLEX:
A MODEL FOR
RNA VIRAL
TUMORIGENESIS

b. Bone Marrow Examinations. The technique of aspirating bone marrow from the femur or crest of the ilium has been described by Switzer and Schalm (1968). Bone marrow infiltration is found in 50% of cats with lymphosarcoma, but less frequently in cats with reticulum cell sarcoma. Anemia may be progressive due to a myelophthisic response or as a result of blood loss primarily from gastrointestinal hemorrhage, or hemolytic anemia of the autoimmune type may be present.

c. Examination of Pleural and Peritoneal Aspiration Fluid. To obtain fluid from coelomic cavities, the animal is positioned so that vital organs will not be punctured. This technique is often used to confirm the diagnosis of feline leukemia or to differentiate it from other diseases that have inflammatory cells in pleural and peritoneal fluid.

d. Serological Test for Diagnosis of Feline Oncornavirus Infection. Serological tests are available for detection of type C FOV infections by use of an indirect immunofluorescence (IF) test (Hardy *et al.*, 1972). This test specifically detects the

TABLE 8
*Radiological Findings in
Feline Lymphoreticular
Neoplasia*

Mediastinal mass
Hydrothorax
Abdominal mass
Ascites
Enlarged kidneys
Splenomegaly
Hepatomegaly

TABLE 9
Hematological Findings in 26 Cats with Lymphoreticular Neoplasms Seen at U.C.D.[a]

Hematological condition	Percent of cases
Nondiagnostic	38
Neoplastic cells in peripheral blood	62
Leukopenia < 5500	21
Lymphopenia < 1500	48
Subleukemic with a normal WBC	41
Leukemic WBC 20,000	21
Highest WBC 118,000	
Lowest WBC 1000	
Severe anemia	50

[a] Compliments of O. W. Schalm.

presence of group-specific (gs) antigens in peripheral blood or bone marrow cells, and it can easily be conducted on perpheral blood and bone marrow smears obtained from cats in the clinic. However, FOV-infected "clinically normal" cats as well as cats with leukemia, myeloproliferative disorders, fibrosarcoma, nonresponsive anemias, infectious peritonitis, and other conditions may be IF positive, which makes clinical interpretation of the test difficult, especially considering that many normal but infected cats and others with a variety of conditions never develop signs of leukemia or related diseases of the feline leukemia–sarcoma complex.

    e. Gross Pathology. The alimentary type of lymphoreticular neoplasm usually includes infiltrations of kidneys, liver, spleen, intestines, and mesenteric lymph nodes. Other organs are less frequently tumorous. The mediastinal type involves infiltrated thymus gland and mediastinal lymph nodes, and only rarely are other organs involved. The multicentric type includes a generalized lymphadenopathy and frequent involvement of abdominal organs, while miscellaneous neoplasms are atypical and do not fit into any of the three major groups. An extensive report on feline lymphoid neoplasms was written by Holzworth (1960*a*). The distribution of organ involvement in 65 cats with feline lymphoreticular neoplasia examined at U.C.D. is presented in Table 10.

    Multicentric type: Generalized enlarged lymph nodes are homogeneous in texture, being juicy, soft, and a glistening whitish-yellow color. Some nodes may be hemorrhagic, with areas of necrosis. The multicentric type is frequently classified histologically as reticulum cell sarcoma.

    Mediastinal type: Lymph nodes may be large and fused to make single large masses. The thymus gland is usually enlarged, particularly in younger cats. Small to large tumors may be found in parietal pleura invading intercostal muscles; occasionally the neoplastic process may be found protruding from the thoracic inlet into the posteroventral cervical neck region.

    Alimentary type: The spleen is often greatly enlarged, with prominent and circumscribed malpighian corpuscles. The liver is less frequently enlarged, but

TABLE 10

*Distribution of Organ Involvement in 65 Cats
with Feline Lymphoreticular Neoplasia Seen at U.C.D.*

Organ	Percent
Lymph nodes	100
Spleen	75
Liver	65
Thymus	55
Kidneys	45
Intestines	37
Lungs	25
Heart, musculoskeletal tissue	Low
Pancreas	Low

hepatomegaly is not uncommon; the color be reddish brown to distinctly yellow depending on the extent of the neoplastic processes and clinical duration. Conicoid tumors protruding from the surface of the liver and kidneys are not unusual. Tumorous kidneys are often enlarged $1\frac{1}{2}$–2 times their normal size. Neoplasms of the intestine appear as nodular or diffuse swellings in the wall. Muscle layers and the submucosa (Peyer's patches) are often involved, and annular thickenings are the cause of partial or complete occlusion of the intestine. Intestinal dilatation is a common finding proximal to the area of occlusion.

179

FELINE
LEUKEMIA–
SARCOMA
COMPLEX:
A MODEL FOR
RNA VIRAL
TUMORIGENESIS

f. Microscopic Pathology. The histological appearance of tumorous lymph nodes and involved visceral organs in lymphosarcoma is the same as described for other species (Nielsen, 1969). Various degrees of lymphocytic cell maturation are found within neoplastic foci of the same animal; however, usually either the blastic, prolymphocytic, or mature lymphocytic cell type predominates in a particular animal. The presence of large histiocytic macrophages spaced among many more smaller lymphocytic-type cells may give the tissue section the appearance of bright stars in a dark sky, hence the term "starry-sky effect" to describe these cytological changes. Because of the histological similarity to Burkitt's lymphoma, Squire (1966) did a comparative study of the two diseases. Some workers have used the term "feline Burkitt's lymphoma," a misnomer whose use should be discouraged.

Reticulum cell sarcoma arises from reticular cells, particularly in lymph nodes. It must be distinguished histologically from lymphosarcoma. In this group of neoplasms, cell types include reticular cells in various degrees of differentiation toward the formation of reticular fibers. Reticulum cell sarcoma is composed of undifferentiated cells that may form reticular patterns in broad sheets. Cell boundaries are difficult to discern, and cells are generally embedded in syncytial masses of reticular fibers. Reticular fibers are demonstrated by special differential stains, such as Foot's or Gordon Sweet stain.

4.1.5. Differential Diagnosis

Feline lymphoreticular neoplasia must be distinguished from a variety of other diseases (Wilkinson, 1966). When anemia is one of the main clinical findings, feline infectious anemia is a possibility, although it is becoming increasingly clear that anemia in cats is often the direct result of FeLV infection. Diseases that should be considered in differential diagnosis of the three main types of lymphoreticular neoplasia are as follows:

Multicentric type:
1. Idiopathic lymphadenitis (usually seen in young kittens).
2. Inflammatory lymphadenopathy.
3. Myeloproliferative diseases.
4. Some of the same differential diagnosis as listed above must be considered when there is alimentary of thoracic involvement accompanying the multicentric type of feline lymphosarcoma.

Mediastinal type:

1. Pneumonia arising from either bacterial, viral, fungal, or foreign body reactions, pleuritis.
2. Toxoplasmosis.
3. Feline infectious peritonitis (FIP).
4. Feline infectious anemia (FIA), emphysema, bronchiectasis, or bronchial occlusion.
5. Chylothorax, hemothorax, pyothorax, pneumothorax, diaphragmatic hernia.
6. Metastatic neoplasms.
7. Ventral neck abscesses.

Alimentary type:

1. FIP.
2. FIA—primary tumors of liver, bilary tract, pancreas, or intestine.
3. Chronic or acute nephritis, toxoplasmosis.
4. Enteritis or obstructions from foreign bodies, intussusception, or intestinal torsion.
5. Myeloproliferative diseases with splenomegely and hepatomegely.

The infrequent miscellaneous types of lymphoreticular neoplasms must be compared to other disease entities that occur in the same organ systems.

4.2. Myeloproliferative Diseases

The myeloproliferative disorders of cats consist of a group of primary bone marrow dyplasias in which the cell lines increase in number at the expense and to the eventual exclusion of other marrow cells. The abnormal cells may be present in the peripheral blood as well as in the bone marrow. Some of the abnormalities are neoplastic, some are not, and others have the combined features of neoplastic and benign or hyperplastic conditions.

Type C virus is usually found replicating in bone marrow cells, lymph nodes, liver, spleen, and elsewhere in cats with myeloproliferative diseases. Evidence is still lacking on whether these RNA viruses are causal factors in all the various entities that make up the myeloproliferative disorders, but they have been suggested as causal for some (Herz *et al.*, 1970).

Little is known about the epidemiological aspects of these diseases, although they have been reported from a variety of centers (Holzworth, 1960*b*; Gilmore *et al.*, 1964; Zawidzka *et al.*, 1964; Schalm and Theilen, 1970). Accurate sex, breed, and age distributions have not been established; however, we have demonstrated that these distributions are similar whether cats have lymphoreticular neoplasms or myeloproliferative diseases. Our data suggest that myeloproliferative diseases are common in cats up to 4 yr of age (Table 11). This contention is supported by a mean age of 4 yr, with more than 50% of our cases occurring between a few months of age to 4 yr. The data also appear to support the contention that males have a greater risk than females (Table 12). Most likely, cats of all breeds are

181

FELINE
LEUKEMIA–
SARCOMA
COMPLEX:
A MODEL FOR
RNA VIRAL
TUMORIGENESIS

TABLE 11
Age Distribution of 28 Cats with
Myeloproliferative Diseases

Number	Accumulated frequency	Age (yr)
5	5	1–2
3	8	2–3
5	13	3–4
3	16	4–5
3	19	5–6
3	22	6–7
4	26	7–8
1	27	8–9
1	28	9–10

TABLE 12
Sex Distribution of 28 Cats with
Myeloproliferative Diseases

Sex	Number
Female intact	4
Female spayed	4
Male intact	10
Male castrated	10

TABLE 13
Breed Distribution of 28 Cats with
Myeloproliferative Diseases

Number	Percent	Breed[a]
7	25	DLH
14	50	DSH
6	20	Siamese
1	5	Persian

[a] DLH, domestic long hair; DSH, domestic short hair.

susceptible, but those of the Siamese breed were the most frequently involved in our series (Table 13).

Irrespective of the cell type involved, these disorders are characterized by gradual weight loss with initial maintenance of a relatively good appetite. The disease is progressive, with extreme emaciation and anorexia being the most common complaint.

4.2.1. Diagnosis

A clinical diagnosis is usually made on the basis of the history and clinical findings that correlate with recognition of specifically abnormal hematopoietic cells in peripheral blood or bone marrow, or in both. A clinical diagnosis cannot be made without blood and bone marrow studies (as described by Schalm and Theilen, 1970). The spleen and liver are usually palpably enlarged, while lymph nodes are rarely larger than normal.

A characteristic feature of these diseases is progressive anemia that is eventually unresponsive to therapy; however, long-term therapeutic remissions are not uncommon. Clinically, mucous membranes are pale pink to whitish in color, and tachycardia is a frequent finding depending on the severity of anemia. The presence of primitive cells in peripheral blood and bone marrow is the most frequent clinical finding. Primitive cells may be completely undifferentiated, thereby giving no hint as to the cell type involved; this condition has been referred to as reticuloendotheliosis (RE) by Gilmore *et al.* (1964) (see Fig. 1). Nielsen (1969) classified reticuloendotheliosis as a separate entity not included in the myeloproliferative diseases. We have demonstrated that RE is associated with type C virus, just as other myeloproliferative diseases are, and we suggest that RE be classified as a myeloproliferative disease. It is noteworthy, however, that a histologically similar disease of poultry called reticuloendotheliosis is etiologically distinct from avian lymphoid erythroblastosis and myeloblastosis (Theilen *et al.*, 1966). The poultry RE type C virus is also morphologically and antigenically distinct from viruses causing avian leukemias and sarcomas (Zeigel *et al.*, 1966; Purchase *et al.*, 1973). Therefore, one should be aware that reticuloendotheliosis of cats similarly may be a distinct entity, as suggested by Nielsen (1969).

Differentiation may be indicative of abnormalities in the erythrocytic maturation series, which has been called erythremic myelosis (Zawidzka *et al.*, 1964), or there may be an excessive red blood cell count (polycythemia vera). A combination of erythrocytic and granulocytic primitive cells occurring together is called erythroleukemia (Ward *et al.*, 1969) and is similar to Di Guglioma's syndrome in man; or differentiation may be strictly of the granulocytic cell type, which is called granulocytic leukemia (Holzworth, 1960*b*).

A review of myeloproliferative diseases (by Schalm and Theilen, 1970) has been published. Platelet maturation defects (idiopathic thrombocythemia) and acellular bone marrow (aplastic anemia or normoresponsive anemia) are some non-neoplastic entities associated with this disease complex. The bone marrow may become fibrotic (myelofibrosis or myelosclerosis), and as a result blood cells will be

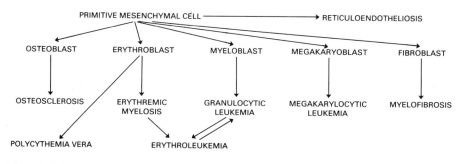

FIGURE 1. Scheme of feline myeloproliferative disease. Modified from Sodikoff and Schalm (1968).

produced in the liver, spleen, or lymph nodes (extramedullary hematopoiesis), a condition referred to as myeloid metaplasia. Abnormally large red blood cells with defects in hemoglobin maturation (megakaryocytic myelosis) may be another nonneoplastic myeloproliferative response. A striking pathological feature of these diseases during the clinical course is transition of one cell type to another, especially the dynamic changes seen between granulocytic leukemia and erythroleukemia. Such changes are detected by sequential peripheral blood and bone marrow studies conducted over a period of weeks or months (Fig. 1).

183

FELINE
LEUKEMIA–
SARCOMA
COMPLEX:
A MODEL FOR
RNA VIRAL
TUMORIGENESIS

a. Gross Pathology. Hepatomegaly and splenomegaly and occasionally lymphadenopathy are the main postmortem changes.

b. Histopathology. Specific abnormal cell types in bone marrow or spleen can be recognized much more easily and accurately when fresh cells are used rather than formalin-fixed tissues. A detailed histological study of these conditions is done by comparing blood, bone marrow, and tissue cells by light and electron microscopy (Herz *et al.*, 1970). Occasionally the liver and kidneys may have foci of involvement, while extramedullary hematopoiesis is common in spleen, liver, and lymph nodes. At times, bone marrow becomes fibrotic, which is thought to be a cellular change that occurs late in the course of myeloproliferative disease.

4.2.2. Differential Diagnosis

A variety of conditions must be considered in differential diagnosis, including:

1. Lymphoreticular neoplasms
2. FIP
3. FIA
4. Other diseases that cause or are associated with anemia
5. Hypoplastic or aplastic bone marrow resulting from drug toxicity

4.3. Multiple Myeloma

Plasma cell dyscrasia is a rare disease in cats, having been reported only a few times (Holzworth and Meier, 1957; Farrow and Penny, 1971).

4.4 Mast Cell Sarcoma

Mast cell sarcoma is a relatively rare neoplasm of cats, and few epidemiological or etiological data are available (Meier and Gourley, 1957). There are solitary or multiple circumscribed lesions in the subcutis or dermis that arise from mast cells in connective tissues of the body. Mast cells are particularly abundant surrounding small blood vessels in the skin and liver. The mast cell is a mononuclear cell and characteristically contains cytoplasmic granules that stain metachromatically with toluidine blue and Giemsa.

4.4.1. Diagnosis

Giemsa-stained preparations of tumor material obtained by needle aspiration or biopsy touch preparations reveal characteristic metachromatically stained granules within pleomorphic cells (mast cells). Some animals may have evidence of internal masses in the abdominal cavity, with an enlarged liver. Occasionally a mast cell leukemia and/or infiltration of bone marrow is the only diagnostic sign and is reason enough to consider this disease along with other conditions included in the leukemia–sarcoma complex. However, the cause has not been established.

a. Gross Pathology. Tumors range in size from one to several centimeters in diameter. They are usually nonencapsulated and often ulcerated. Their consistency is ordinarily hard, and on a cut surface they are fibrotic and whitish in color.

b. Histopathology. The inflammatory reaction may be slight to pronounced around and within the neoplasm. Tumor cells are pleomorphic, being either fusiform, spherical, or stellate in appearance. The nucleus is round or ovoid and, unlike that in the basophilic granulocyte, not lobulated. The architectural pattern is similar to that of fibromas or fibrosarcomas, which makes them difficult to distinguish in sections stained with hematoxylin and eosin. Therefore, whenever a mast cell tumor is suspected, Giemsa stain should be employed.

4.4.2. Differential Diagnosis

Tumors of connective tissue origin within the skin and subcutaneous tissue, particularly fibrosarcomas and neurofibromas, must be considered in differential diagnosis.

4.5. Fibrosarcoma

Fibrosarcoma is a relatively uncommon neoplastic disease of cats compared to other feline neoplasms (Cotchin, 1957; Mulligan, 1951; Schmidt and Langham, 1967). It is more common among aged animals; however, little information is available as to occurrence by sex or breed.

4.5.1. Diagnosis

Feline fibrosarcoma is usually characterized by single and sometimes multiple circumscribed lesions that have a hard consistency. They are found in the dermis or subcutaneous tissue and grow slowly. Metastasis to internal organs may be found in some animals, and in such cases internal masses can be palpated or delineated on X-ray films. Cats with metastasis are debilitated, and anorexia is a common sign. A history of slow-growing subcutaneous masses coupled with the clinical findings is helpful in making a presumptive diagnosis. Tumors often recur following surgical removal.

a. Peripheral Blood and Bone Marrow. Peripheral blood and bone marrow are usually free of tumor cells. Needle aspirations or touch smears are often helpful in substantiating a presumptive clinical diagnosis of cancer, although a definitive diagnosis is dependent on histopathology since exfoliative cytology is difficult to interpret.

185

FELINE
LEUKEMIA–
SARCOMA
COMPLEX:
A MODEL FOR
RNA VIRAL
TUMORIGENESIS

b. Gross Pathology. Moulton (1961) described the pathology of this neoplasm, and Snyder *et al.* (1970) reported clinicopathological changes. Tumors are variable in size and are usually irregular in shape, being poorly demarcated and nonencapsulated. The consistency is firm, with soft friable areas present in the larger neoplasms. In cross-section, the neoplasm is lobulated grayish-white; areas of hemorrhage and necrosis may be seen in larger tumors.

c. Histopathology. The basic pattern of fibrosarcoma consists of whorls and interwoven bundles of immature fibroblasts with moderate amounts of collagen. Cells are pleomorphic, spindled, fusiform, or polygonal in shape.

4.5.2. Differential Diagnosis

Enlargements that are firm, locally invasive, and follow lymphatic chains in metastasis must be differentiated from fibrosarcomas, including:

1. Lymphoreticular neoplasms
2. Neurofibromas
3. Fibromas
4. Mast cell sarcomas

5. Treatment and Prognosis of Leukemia–Sarcoma Complex

5.1. Lymphoreticular Neoplasms

Complete clinical remissions of lymphoreticular neoplasms may be obtained by employing a combination of anticancer drugs (Carpenter and Holzworth, 1971). We have found the following drugs given for 8–12 wk to be satisfactory for induction of partial or complete clinical remission in an adult cat weighing 8–10 lb (Theilen, 1971*b*):

1. Prednisone or prednisolone, 10 mg orally B.I.D. every other day.
2. Cytoxan (Mead Johnson), 12.5 mg orally every other day.
3. Vincristine (Eli Lilly, Oncovin), 0.1 mg intravenously weekly. This drug is very irritating to tissues when given perivascularly.
4. Cytosine arabinoside (Upjohn Cytosar), 25 mg intravenously or subcutaneously daily for 4 days.

Squire and Bush (1971) recommended caution in using anticancer drugs because they are cytotoxic and immunosuppressive. It is recommended that before initiation of treatment each animal be given a thorough physical examination that includes a CBC, platelet count, and BUN. The animal should be checked for a febrile response each day during the course of therapy, and if the temperature goes above 103.5°F it should be placed on broad-spectrum antibiotics. If the white cell count drops below 2500 per milliliter of blood or the platelet count below 50,000 per milliliter of blood, the anticancer drugs should temporarily be stopped.

Supportive therapy includes hematinics and vitamins, while whole blood and fluids are often indicated, particularly in those cases where anemia and bone marrow infiltration are complicating factors.

A maintenance chemotherapy schedule includes a combination of drugs and is followed according to clinical interpretations and progress of the animal for approximately 4 to 6 months.

1. Prednisone, 5 mg orally B.I.D. every other day for the course of the treatment.
2. Cytoxan, 12.5 mg orally every other day for 1 wk, then off for 2–3 wk.
3. Vincristine, 0.1 mg intravenously once at 2- to 3-wk intervals.
4. Cytosine arabinoside, 25 mg intravenously or subcutaneously for 4 days at 2- to 3-wk intervals.

Chemotherapy during clinical relapse consists of discontinuation of cytosine arabinoside and prednisone and switching to methotrexate and vinblastine in place of cytoxan and vincristine as follows:

1. Methotrexate (Lederle, Amethopterin), 0.5 mg orally S.I.D. for 3 days. It is given weekly until tumors disappear or until the animal shows improvement. Folinic acid (calcium leucovorin, Lederle) should be given within 2–3 h to reduce methotrexate toxicity, 1 mg intramuscularly after each administration of methotrexate.
2. Vinblastine (Eli Lilly, Velban), 0.3 mg intravenously at weekly intervals. This drug is also irritating to perivascular tissues.

Lymphoreticular neoplasms are terminally fatal diseases always having an unfavorable prognosis. Treatment will prolong the course of the disease (Theilen, 1971b) (Table 14). It is anticipated that the course may be prolonged much longer

TABLE 14
Results of Treatment of Cats with Lymphoreticular Neoplasms and Myeloproliferative Diseases

Number	Diagnosis	Type of treatment	Average clinical duration (days)
3	Lymphoreticular	Surgery only	14
9	Lymphoreticular	Chemotherapy only	102
32	Lymphoreticular	No treatment	5
6	Myeloproliferative	Blood transfusions and chemotherapy	316
22	Myeloproliferative	No treatment	9

with employment of newer anticancer drugs such as L-asparaginase and utiliza-tion of immunotherapeutic methods (Chirigos, 1971). Two cats in our series lived 2 and 3 yr, respectively, after initiation of treatment, but this should be viewed with cautious optimism because it is known that some cats with lymphoreticular neoplasia have spontaneous remissions without treatment. Following treatment, it should be determined whether cats in complete remission are still shedding virus, which, of course, may have considerable consequences in light of recent evidence of horizontal transmission of feline lymphosarcoma to uninfected adult cats (Hardy *et al.*, 1973; W. F. H. Jarrett *et al.*, 1973*a*). Cats with the generalized and thoracic types respond better to therapy and have a more favorable prognosis than do those with diffuse abdominal involvement.

187

FELINE
LEUKEMIA–
SARCOMA
COMPLEX:
A MODEL FOR
RNA VIRAL
TUMORIGENESIS

5.2. Myeloproliferative Diseases

Supportive therapy in myeloproliferative diseases includes hematinics, vitamins, whole blood transfusions, and administration of fluids. The average clinical response to therapy is usually longer than in cats treated for lymphoreticular neoplasms (Theilen, 1971*b*).

Induction therapy for an 8- to 10-lb cat consists of the following:

1. 10 mg prednisone orally B.I.D. each day for 1 wk, thereafter every other day for 2–4 wk.
2. 12.5 mg cytoxan orally every other day for 2–4 wk.

Remission therapy is as follows:

1. 5 mg prednisone orally every other day for 5 months.
2. 12.5 mg cytoxan given in sequences of 1 wk on and 2 wk off for 5 months. If there are no signs of disease after 6 months of therapy, treatment is stopped. If clinical signs reappear, treatment should be resumed. If recurrence occurs during remission therapy, the following therapeutic change is recommended: Cytoxan is replaced by 0.5 mg of methotrexate orally S.I.D. for 3 days and repeated weekly until clinical improvement is evident. Calcium leucovorin, 1 mg intramuscularly, is used as directed for metho-trexate therapy in treatment of lymphoreticular neoplasms.

We have experienced on the average longer remissions for myeloproliferative diseases than for lymphoreticular neoplasms, so the prognosis is better. It should be noted that compared to lymphoreticular neoplasms nontreated myelo-proliferative diseases are generally chronic, which, of course, might explain the better results of treatment. It should be remembered that although some myeloproliferative disorders are nonmalignant death is the expected outcome without therapy.

5.3 Mast Cell Sarcoma

Mast cell tumors are treated by surgical removal and administration of 3500–4500 rads in fractions of 400–450 rads three times a week. We suggest in cases of generalized mast cell sarcoma that 0.5 mg of vinblastine be administered intravenously at weekly intervals in combination with 12.5 mg cytoxan orally three times a week for 8–12 wk. Prednisolone, 5 mg orally, should be given daily or every other day for 8–12 wk. Thereafter, the dosage schedule should follow an alternating program of treatment for 1 wk and no treatment for 2–3 wk. This maintenance therapeutic regime should continue for 3–4 months before treatment is stopped. Recurrence of generalized mast cell sarcoma is a frequent sequela despite therapy.

5.4. Fibrosarcoma

Surgical removal of fibrosarcoma is the treatment of choice, followed by radiotherapy using 3500–4500 rads. If a radiotherapy machine is used, treatment should consist of 350–500 rads per therapy every other day until the required exposure has been administered. The outcome following treatment must be viewed with skepticism since recurrences are frequent.

6. Other Diseases Associated with Feline Oncornavirus Infection

Several nonneoplastic conditions are associated with FOV infection. These include feline infectious peritonitis (FIP), which causes a generalized vasculitis leading to acute disease accompanied by pleural effusion and ascites or a chronic granulomatous form often mistaken for lymphosarcoma. Thymus atrophy has also been reported, which leads to immunological deficiencies including runting disease in the young and increased susceptibility to bacterial viral infections. Membranous glomerulonephritis, hypoplastic, aplastic or nonresponsive anemia, and infectious anemia caused by *Hemobartanella felis* have also been reported to be associated with FeLV infections.

Many cats with FIP are from households with multiple cases of leukemia, and they are frequently concurrently infected with FeLV type C virus (Theilen *et al.*, 1970*a*; Hardy and Hurvitz, 1971). The causal agent of FIP has not been isolated in the cell-free state; however, it is believed to be a donut-shaped virion having a diameter of 70–75 nm that is found in the endoplastic reticulum of the Golgi zone of the cell (Ward, 1970; Zook *et al.*, 1968). The association between FIP and feline leukemia may be merely coincidental, or there may, in fact, be a real cause-and-effect relation between FeLV infection and the putative FIP agent.

Thymus atrophy in kittens infected neonatally with FeLV was reported by Anderson *et al.* (1971). At approximately 3 months of age, a series of 29 kittens developed signs of retarded growth rate and a tendency toward overwhelming intercurrent infections. Histologically, the thymuses showed severe depletion of lymphocytes, loss of corticomedullary differentiation, and degeneration of the epithelial framework. Lymph nodes were depleted, mainly in the paracortical areas. The other hematopoietic cell distribution was normal. We found a similar syndrome in kittens inoculated intrathymically with FeLV, but they succumbed to intercurrent infections much sooner than 3 months of age (Theilen and Harrold, 1968). We also recorded that kittens inoculated with FeLV at birth did not respond immunologically as efficiently to vaccination with feline infectious enteritis vaccine as did uninoculated controls.

Ward *et al.* (1969) described membranous glomerulonephritis in a cat with myeloid leukemia, and Anderson and Jarrett (1971) reported an association between membranous glomerulonephritis and feline leukemia. The pathogenesis of this condition is probably a result of autoimmune disease caused by concurrent formation of antigen–antibody complexes.

Anemia is a striking feature in most cats with spontaneous and experimentally induced leukemia. The basis of the anemia, which is usually macrocytic in type, is probably a maturation defect of the erythroblast series of cells resulting from FeLV infection. Cats that recover from infectious anemia (FIA) may develop leukemia. It is not known whether this is a reflection of the initial FeLV infection leading to immunosuppression and subsequent clinical expression of concomitant FIA or whether initial *H. felis* infection causes alteration of stem cells such that subsequent FeLV infections quickly result in cell transformation and leukemia. Many cats are known to be silent carriers of the erythrocytic cell parasite *H. felis*, and these carriers will have clinically detectable *H. felis* infection and anemia following splenectomy or during various kinds of stress.

Another logical hypothesis is that FIA leads to biological interaction between an altered reticuloendothelial system and bone marrow stem cell population, allowing for greater expression of FeLV and cell transformation. A similar explanation for a possible association between malaria and Burkitt's lymphoma in equatorial Africa has been proposed by Burkitt (1969).

7. Etiology of Feline Leukemia, Sarcoma, and Myeloproliferative Diseases

The presence of feline type C oncornaviruses in spontaneous feline leukemia has been demonstrated by a number of investigators (Laird *et al.*, 1968; Kawakami *et al.*, 1967; Rickard, 1969). These viruses cause feline leukemia when inoculated into kittens, and type C virus can be isolated from plasma and induced tumors (Kawakami *et al.*, 1967).

A similar virus was found in the tissues of a cat with spontaneous fibrosarcoma (Snyder and Theilen, 1969), and the presence of type C oncornaviruses in spontaneous fibrosarcomas has subsequently also been reported by Gardner *et al.* (1970), McDonough *et al.* (1971), and Snyder (1971).

Herz *et al.* (1970) found type C virus in bone marrow cells in five cats with a variety of myeloproliferative diseases including myelofibrosis, erythroleukemia, and erythremic myelosis. We were not successful in transmitting myeloproliferative diseases or any other neoplastic conditions by inoculating kittens with cell-free filtrates prepared from these cats. W. F. H. Jarrett (1971) reported induction of myeloid leukemia with FeLV. It has been clearly demonstrated that type C virus is associated with various spontaneous hematological and connective tissue neoplasms.

7.1. Transmission Studies

The first transmission studies of feline leukemia were reported by W. F. H. Jarrett *et al.* (1964). Both immature and mature type C particles were present extracellularly in vacuoles and budding from membranes of tumor cells in kittens inoculated with cell-free feline lymphosarcoma material (Jarrett *et al.*, 1964). Cells from the donor cat were not examined electron microscopically, but presumably they contained excessive amounts of FeLV. Jarrett's transmission studies were quickly confirmed by Rickard *et al.* (1968), Kawakami *et al.* (1967), and Theilen *et al.* (1968, 1970a). Lymphoid neoplasms were produced in Jarrett's laboratory and by our group, while Rickard and coworkers demonstrated induction of lymphoid, and perhaps myeloid leukemia as well as liposarcoma. Virus isolated from the liposarcoma produced leukemia (Rickard, 1969).

The first transmission of feline fibrosarcoma was reported by Snyder and Theilen (1969), using tissue from a 2-yr-old cat with multiple subcutaneous fibrosarcoma and internal tumors. The tissue had been frozen at −70°C for 6 months. A tumor-inducing inoculum could be obtained from tissue homogenates prepared by low-speed centrifugation (2000 rpm for 15 min) and 0.45-μm Millipore filtration or from pelletized virus prepared by differential centrifugation (Theilen *et al.*, 1970b). Gardner *et al.* (1970) and McDonough *et al.* (1971) reported the isolation of other feline sarcoma viruses, and Snyder *et al.* (1970) published a detailed report of the clinicopathological aspects of experimentally induced feline fibrosarcoma.

7.2. Viral Structure

FeLV and FeSV are morphologically similar (Laird *et al.*, 1968; Theilen *et al.*, 1970a). Mature particles have an outer diameter of 115 nm, with an electron-dense nucleoid measuring 90 nm. The unit membrane of the envelope may have spikes on its outer surface. Immature particles consist of an outer unit membrane envelope that measures 115 nm in diameter, an intermediate shell that measures 90 nm, and an electron-dense inner ring that measures 65 nm, with an electron-lucent center that measures 45 nm in diameter. Mature and immature particles are found in extracellular spaces and in cytoplasmic vacuoles and can be concentrated from the plasma (Kawakami *et al.*, 1967). Budding from the plasma membrane or from vacuolar cytoplasmic membranes has been observed in tumor cells, in a variety of bone marrow cells and platelets, and, indeed, in almost every cell of the body. Virus has also been seen budding from bladder mucosal cells and salivary secretory cells. It has been demonstrated in the milk of lactating mother cats by Herz and Theilen (1968), and recently type C virus was reported in laryngeal mucosal cells (W. F. H. Jarrett *et al.*, 1973a).

7.3. *Nucleic Acid*

191
FELINE
LEUKEMIA–
SARCOMA
COMPLEX:
A MODEL FOR
RNA VIRAL
TUMORIGENESIS

Burger and Noronha (1970) reported that a minimum of 100 μg of nucleic acid per 1.5 liters of cell culture supernatants was recoverable by their technique. O. Jarrett *et al.* (1971) showed two major species of RNA, a fast-sedimenting 75S component and a slower-sedimenting 4S component that was demonstrated by zonal centrifugation in 5–20% sucrose gradients of virus disrupted with 1% SDS and phenol. A third component of 35S was present in much smaller amounts. Denaturation of the 75S RNA results in establishment of a 37S component, which may be either a subunit or a collapsed form of a previously coiled molecule. Avian and murine viruses have similar nucleic acid components, but feline viral RNA differs in having an unusually high content of adenine in the base composition of the 75S material. Recently, Whalley (1973) demonstrated by electrophoretic analysis of native and denatured RNA that there are small but significant size differences in the RNAs of a number of FeLV isolates. The molecular weight of denatured or subunit RNA was estimated to range from 2.2 to 2.6 $\times$ 10^6 daltons in the different isolates, each of which belonged to one or more FeLV subgroups (A, B, and C) as described by Sarma and Log (1973). Size differences were, however, also found between RNAs of FeLV isolates of a single subgroup (A).

7.4. *Buoyant Density*

The buoyant density of the virion is approximately 1.15 g/ml in linear sucrose gradients (Kawakami *et al.*, 1967). The buoyant density of cores of disrupted virions is 1.25 g/ml (W. F. H. Jarrett, 1971).

7.5. *Proteins*

Oroszlan *et al.* (1971*a*) demonstrated group-specific feline leukemia viruses by isoelectric focusing. The protein had a molecular weight of 25,000, calculated by sodium dodecylsulfate electrophoresis and contained both species-specific antigenic determinants and interspecies specific cross-reactive determinants. O. Jarrett *et al.* (1971) also reported the electrophoretic patterns of FeLV proteins

TABLE 15
Structural Proteins of Feline Leukemia Viruses[a]

Symbol[b]	Approximate mol wt	Site	Antigenicity
p10	10,000	Core RNP	Species gsa
p12	12,000	Virion surface	Species gsa
p15	15,000	Extra-gsa	Species gsa
p30	30,000	Extra-core	Species and interspecies gsa
gp35	35,000	Surface of membrane	Antibodies to these glycoproteins are neutralizing, cytotoxic, and protective

[a] Compliments of W. F. H. Jarrett.
[b] p, Polypeptide; gp, glycoprotein; gsa, group-specific antigen.

using polyacrylamide gels of purified FeLV disrupted with sodium dodecylsulfate (SDS). An international group of feline leukemia research workers assembled at Sloan Kettering Institute in New York in June 1973 to discuss the antigenic significance of FeLV structural proteins. This group developed guidelines for a standard international nomenclature (Table 15) based on what is presently known about gs and subgroup antigens.

8. Natural Transmission

The interest of some investigators in the natural transmission and etiology of feline leukemia has been motivated by its importance as a model for studying the etiology of leukemia in other outbred animals and in man. The modes of transmission of avian and murine leukemia led to the hypothesia that feline leukemia is naturally transmitted both from parent to offspring (vertical), which can be of two types, genetic and congenital, and from animal to animal of the same generation by contact (horizontal). The probable and known modes of transmission of feline leukemia are presented in Table 16.

Both vertical and horizontal infection play a role in avian leukosis, while in mice the vertical route is the major one. Evidence for horizontal transmission of feline leukemia has been building up since Brodey et al. (1970) found convincing but circumstantial evidence for it when infected breeding cats were transferred to supposedly noninfected households. Household clusters were reported by W. F. H. Jarrett (1971) and by a number of other workers, which added to the stronger evidence of horizontal transmission that had been earlier reported by Schneider et al. (1967) and Theilen et al. (1970a). Gardner et al. (1971) found FeLV budding from salivary secretory cells, and mature virus was found in saliva. The best evidence has been accumulated in the laboratory, where leukemia was found to occur in control kittens housed with virus-injected littermates (Rickard, 1969). Leukemia can occur in control kittens housed in a completely separate cage but in

TABLE 16

Probable and Known Modes of Natural Transmission of Feline Leukemia

Vertical	Horizontal
A. Genetic	A. Contact
1. Via male chromosomes	1. Saliva
2. Via female chromosomes	2. Urine
	3. Feces
B. Epigenetic	4. Airborne—sneezing,
1. Prenatal	coughing
a. Preplacental	B. Vectors
b. Placental	1. Fleas, mosquitoes, etc.
2. Postnatal	
a. Milk borne	

close enough proximity so that airborne infection is possible (W. F. H. Jarrett, 1973), and leukemia has been induced by intranasal exposure to the virus in laboratory experiments (Hoover *et al.*, 1972).

193

FELINE
LEUKEMIA–
SARCOMA
COMPLEX:
A MODEL FOR
RNA VIRAL
TUMORIGENESIS

Evidence of horizontal transmission of FeLV now makes it almost certain that feline leukemia is an infectious disease. Hardy *et al.* (1973) have shown that approximately 90% of cats with feline lymphosarcoma are positive for gs antigen detected by immunofluorescence tests. Furthermore, most of the cluster cases occur in unrelated cats, additional evidence supporting horizontal transmission.

Epidemiological studies on feline lymphosarcoma gave no evidence of horizontal transmission of FeLV (Schneider, 1972a), and Gardner *et al.* (1971) demonstrated the presence of type C virus in feline fetuses from apparently normal mothers. Herz and Theilen (1968) observed the presence of type C virus in infected milk, which suggests the possibility of vertical transmission by nursing.

As in avian leukosis, recent experimentation has also demonstrated the presence of an endogenous or genetically transmitted type C virus, designated the RD114 type because of the cells (human rhabdomyosarcoma) from which it was originally believed to have originated (McAllister *et al.*, 1969). The human rhabdomyosarcoma cell line was inoculated into the brain of fetal kittens, and the resulting tumors contained replicating type C virus that had gs antigens and reverse transcriptase immunologically unrelated to the previously described feline leukemia viruses (McAllister *et al.*, 1971, 1972). The virus was expressed (replicated) in human cells and not in cat cells, and it was antigenically unrelated to type C viruses of woolly monkey fibrosarcoma and gibbon leukemia. Hence it was believed to be a human tumor virus.

Subsequently, a virus was isolated from cat cells that was indistinguishable from RD114 virus (Sarma *et al.*, 1973a; Livingston and Todaro, 1973). The virus was spontaneously produced by an established feline cell line of kidney fibroblasts (CCC), and some sublines of CCC did not spontaneously release virus. Normal feline cells could be induced to produce the virus after treatment with 5-iododeoxyuridine. It is now established that RD114 virus represents an endogenous genetically transmitted virus, and once activated by mutagens such as 5-iododeoxyuridine it replicates better in heterologous primate cells (McAllister *et al.*, 1973). Oroszlan *et al.* (1972), Sarma *et al.* (1973a), and Neiman (1973) have shown that feline cells and not human cells contain nucleic acid sequences that are homologous to the RNA of RD114 virus.

There is little doubt that the natural transmission of the feline oncornaviruses is as complex as the natural transmission of avian and murine leukosis viruses. It can be readily appreciated that the horizontally transmitted virus may be the sole cause of feline leukemia, or it may initiate a chain of events which result in "turning on" the endogenous virus. To date, however, no one has shown that the endogenous virus is biologically active in the causation of leukemia in cats or in other species. The last point needs considerable attention: since the endogenous virus replicates best in heterospecific cells *in vitro*, it could be a reservoir of infection for other animals.

Presumably, FeSV is transmitted in a similar fashion to FeLV, but little research has been done on the natural transmission of FeSV, mainly because it is a relatively rare disease.

9. Immunological Aspects

9.1. Antigenic Components of Feline Oncornaviruses

The natural history of feline oncornaviruses in domestic cat populations is a subject of major interest, augmented by development of several seroepidemiology tests. In the extensively studied avian and murine systems and now the feline oncornaviruses, there are two main antigenic complexes, type-specific (ts) and group-specific (gs) antigens.

9.1.1. Immunodiffusion

Immunodiffusion is the best test system on which to base qualitative judgment of the number and kind of reactive antigen–antibody systems within a given mixture and the only test in which cross-reacting components can be delineated.

Several antigenic components of avian and murine oncornaviruses have been reported using the Ouchterlony double-diffusion method of detection (Eckert *et al.*, 1964; Geering *et al.*, 1966). It has been established that the gs antigens are common to all oncornaviruses within a species but not the ts antigens. Antibodies are formed to ts antigens within a species but not gs antigens. Antibodies to gs antigens are prepared in heterologous species, e.g., rabbits, guinea pigs, rats, dogs, goats, and cattle.

Geering *et al.* (1968) identified in immunodiffusion tests with anti-murine leukemia virus (MuLV) serum, a common antigen with FeLV. Schafer and Noronha (1971) confirmed the finding of interspecies antigen in MuLV and FeLV. This antigen has been referred to as the gs-3 or the interspecies gs antigen. Hardy *et al.* (1969) reported that antisera to feline gs antigen could be prepared in rabbits repeatedly inoculated with ether-disrupted virions and Freund's adjuvant but not with intact virions. They could not produce antibody in cats, which is similar to the lack of response in the mouse to disrupted MuLV. Antisera could not be produced in heterospecies using the intact FeLV. It has also been demonstrated that FeLV antigen, like the gs antigen of MuLV, is found in the free state in normal or leukemic cells infected with FeLV.

Sarma *et al.* (1973*a*) and Livingston and Todaro (1973) have demonstrated that in cats there are at least two different oncornavirus gs antigens that do not cross-react with each other, one being the endogenous RD114 prototype and the other the epigenetic horizontally transmitted FeLV. Cats are unique in this regard.

9.1.2. Complement Fixation Test

Sarma *et al.* (1971*a*) developed a successful complement fixation (CF) test for the detection of feline leukemia and sarcoma test viruses (the COCAL test). This test is analogous to the COFAL test for avian leukosis viruses and the COMUL test for murine leukemia viruses and has been used to detect gs antigen of the virions *in vivo* and *in vitro* under natural and experimental conditions. CF viral antibodies used in the COCAL test were prepared by immunizing rabbits, guinea pigs, and goats with ether-disrupted feline leukemia virus and by inducing fibrosarcoma in beagles with the GA strain of the feline fibrosarcoma virus. The dog CF antibodies contained viral envelope antibodies as well as antibodies to the ether-resistant nonsedimentable antigens (gs antigens) of the virus. A tissue culture CF viral antigen induction test was devised for the detection and assay of infectious virus and viral-neutralizing antibodies. The test was useful and sensitive for the routine detection and assay of various field strains of feline leukemia virus. It proved to be more sensitive than the Ouchterlony test (Hardy *et al.*, 1969; Hardy, 1971*b*) for the measurement of viral antigen in tissues of cats with or without leukemia. High titers of infectious virus and/or viral antigen were found in various cells inoculated with the virus. A hundred- to a thousand-fold excess of noncytopathogenic feline leukemia virus was detected in feline sarcoma virus stocks by Sarma *et al.* (1971*b*).

9.1.3. Tanned Red Cell Technique in Hemagglutination and Hemagglutination Inhibition Tests

Sibel *et al.* (1970) and Fink *et al.* (1971) used the tanned red cell technique in hemagglutination (HA) and hemagglutination inhibition (HAI) tests. Sera were prepared in heterospecies, i.e., goats, rabbits, and monkeys. Agglutination of tanned virus-coated sheep red cells was well correlated with immunodiffusion. Normal cat tissue gave no reaction, while nearly all the cats tested with spontaneous leukemia were positive. These authors concluded that the HA reaction is more sensitive than complement fixation for detection of viral antigen. Despite the fact that it does not have the problem of anticomplementary reactivity of the antigens in serum, this test has not been extensively used as a diagnostic tool.

9.1.4. Mixed Hemabsorption Test

Maruyama *et al.* (1970) applied the mixed hemabsorption test to a variety of heterospecific cell cultures infected with murine leukemia–sarcoma viruses and FeLV. Common antigens were detected which appeared to be proteins of the viral coat incorporated into the plasma membrane of infected cells. This test, like the HA and HAI tests, has not been extensively used to detect FeLV antigens.

9.1.5. Indirect Immunofluorescence

Hardy *et al.* (1972) described an indirect immunofluorescent antibody test for the detection of FeLV gs antigen in FeLV-infected cats, in heterospecific tissue

195

FELINE
LEUKEMIA–
SARCOMA
COMPLEX:
A MODEL FOR
RNA VIRAL
TUMORIGENESIS

culture cells, in cells obtained from cats with naturally occurring feline leukemia and other neoplastic diseases, and in normal cats. Antiserum to feline leukemia virus gs antigen was prepared in a female New Zealand rabbit according to methods reported for immunodiffusion (Hardy *et al.*, 1969), and the rabbit anti-FeLV gs serum was absorbed *in vivo* in a kitten to eliminate nonspecific staining reactions. Antiserum has also been produced in goats (W. F. H. Jarrett, 1973), guinea pigs, and other animals (Oroszlan *et al.*, 1972).

Hardy *et al.* (1972) also demonstrated by immunofluorescence the shared gs antigen (gs-3, interspecies) of FeLV, MuLV, hamster sarcoma virus, and rat virus associated with the Novikoff hepatoma.

9.1.6. Tritiated Uridine Labeling

The quantity of FeLV produced in cell cultures can be determined by growing cells in the presence of ^{3}H-uridine and determining the amount of radioactivity incorporated into viral particles (Sarma *et al.*, 1970; O. Jarrett *et al.*, 1972).

9.1.7. Type-Specific Antigens

As in avian leukosis, there are numerous strains of feline leukemia and sarcoma viruses, each capable of eliciting a characteristic or subgroup response in the feline host (Sarma and Log, 1971, 1973; O. Jarrett *et al.*, 1973). The subgroups are characteristically different on the basis of variations in virion envelope antigens that are glycoproteins. Sarma and Log (1972) detected three envelope antigens, which enabled them to classify the feline oncornaviruses into three subgroups—A, B, and C. Antigenic typing is done by viral interference and virus neutralization.

Productive *in vitro* infection of tissue cultures by noncytopathogenic type C viruses is usually accompanied by the development of viral resistance of interference with the cell-transforming effects of closely related focus-forming and sarcomagenic viruses (Rubin, 1960; Sarma *et al.*, 1967; Sarma and Log, 1971). In the avian system, this viral interference is a property of the viral envelopes of the interfering and challenge viruses, occurs at an early step of challenge virus contact with cells (Steck and Rubin, 1965), and is type specific (subgroup specific) and operates only against antigenically related viruses of the same subgroup.

Serum neutralizing antibodies are produced in heterospecies by inoculation of fully intact virus test stocks. Sarma and Log (1973) produced specific serum neutralizing antibodies in weanling beagles.

The presently known strains of FeSV are all antigenic mixtures of A and B viruses. The FeLV derived from the FL74 cell line is a mixture of A, B, and C viruses. Pure subgroups can be cloned and purified into specific strains. Antibodies prepared against BA and ST FeSV strains neutralize A and B leukemia viruses, which verifies that they are mixtures of A and B subgroups.

It has been demonstrated that subgroup A will not infect human cells, while subgroups B and C will multiply in human and canine cells (Sarma *et al.*, 1973*b*). This host range restriction is determined by the virus envelope and operates at the level of virus entry into the cell. Subgroup A virus can be introduced into human 197

FELINE
LEUKEMIA–
SARCOMA
COMPLEX:
A MODEL FOR
RNA VIRAL
TUMORIGENESIS cells by phenotypic mixing with subgroup B viral envelope. When introduced into human cells in this manner, the subgroup A virus replicates (O. Jarrett *et al.*, 1973; Sarma *et al.*, 1973*b*).

9.1.8. Reverse Transcriptase

Temin and Baltimore (1972) have written detailed descriptions of RNA-directed DNA synthesis and RNA tumor viruses. Temin and Mizutani (1970) and Baltimore (1970) reported that RNA tumor viruses contain an enzyme (reverse transcriptase) which utilizes viral RNA as a template for synthesis of DNA. Temin (1972) postulated that viral RNA is transcribed into a "DNA provirus" that is integrated into the DNA of the chromosomes of the host cells. The "provirus" carries information responsible for oncogenic transformation. Experiments by Spiegleman *et al.* (1970) also demonstrated RNA-dependent DNA polymerases in many different RNA tumor viruses, including feline oncornaviruses. The RNA tumor virus polymerases are specific for each species of RNA tumor virus, and indeed with few exceptions are characteristic of RNA tumor viruses (Lin and Thormar, 1972; Schlom *et al.*, 1971), which has provided another means of detecting and classifying these RNA tumor viruses.

Roy-Burman *et al.* (1972) demonstrated an inhibitor of the RNA-dependent DNA polymerases of feline and murine type C viruses in the sera of cats inoculated *in utero* and/or postnatally with the Gardner–Arnstein strain of feline sarcoma virus and in the sera of cats bearing spontaneous sarcomas, lymphomas, or carcinomas. Their results showed inefficiency of the inhibitor against avian virus and a similar efficiency against feline and murine virus polymerases, which implies a high degree of relatedness of feline and murine viral DNA-dependent DNA polymerase structures and activities. Oroszlan *et al.* (1971*b*) demonstrated that serum from a rat immunized with DNA polymerase of FeLV purified by isoelectric focusing inhibits DNA-dependent but not RNA dependent DNA polymerase activity of mammalian oncornaviruses.

9.2. Antibody Response to Feline Oncornavirus Infection

9.2.1. Indirect Membrane Immunofluorescence Test

Essex *et al.* (1971*a*) and Riggs (1971) demonstrated humoral antibodies in sera of cats infected with or exposed to FeLV and FeSV. These antibodies react with the membrane of cells infected with FeLV. Commonly used test cells are FeLV-infected lymphoid cells grown in suspension cultures (Theilen *et al.*, 1969). The presence of antibody in neonatal kittens and their ability to resist the development of tumors or the progression of tumors following inoculation with FeSV have been reported by Essex *et al.* (1971*b*). Passive antibody is passed from mothers that have positive indirect membrane immunofluorescent antibody to their offspring.

Riggs *et al.* (1973) reported the prevalence of type C virus and antibody in normal cats and cats with neoplasia. The sera from 41% of the cats with nonneoplastic diseases were positive, as were the sera from 33% of the cats with neoplastic diseases, but only 5% of "normal" cat sera were positive. Examination of tissues by electron microscopy showed type C virus in 58% of the cats with neoplasia and in 44% of those with nonneoplastic diseases, while none of the "normal" cats examined were positive.

9.2.2. Complement Fixation Inhibition Test

Olsen and Yohn (1972) successfully employed the complement fixation inhibition (CFI) test in evaluating means to detect antibodies in cat sera to feline oncornavirus antigens. Antibody titers ranging from 1:4 to 1:256 were found in sera of both neoplastic and normal cats, but not in sera of clinically normal cats raised in germfree isolation. The specificity of the CFI test was confirmed by demonstrating that the serum titers were inversely proportional to FeLV antigen concentration. It was not determined whether the antibodies detected in the CFI test were to a single FeLV antigen or to multiple ones.

9.2.3. Ferritin-Labeled Antibody

Oshiro *et al.* (1971) described the application of the indirectly labeled antibody method to tissue culture lines established from cats with lymphosarcoma, erythroleukemia, or a bone marrow granulocytic cell aplasia. Dog anti-feline sarcoma and cat anti-feline sarcoma sera were used as intermediates on oncornavirus-positive and -negative cell lines. The tagging of viruses and membranes was similar regardless of the type of disease from which the type C virus had been isolated, indicating a similarity of sharing of antigenic components. Furthermore, fluorescent antibody studies of the same infected cell lines (Riggs, 1971) suggested that ferritin tagging is closely correlated with fluorescent staining. It was demonstrated that membrane antigen was infection mediated, which excluded the possibility that membrane tagging was characteristic of transformed cells unrelated to viral infection.

10. Host Range

10.1. Feline Leukemia Viruses

The experimental *in vivo* host range of FeLV seems to be largely limited to cats, with one report of its tumorigenicity in dogs (Rickard *et al.*, 1969), while O. Jarrett *et al.* (1969, 1970) showed that FeLV could replicate in cell monolayers of feline, canine, porcine, and human origin. Subsequently, Sarma *et al.* (1970, 1973b) and Ubertini (1972) also demonstrated that FeLV can infect human cells. The list of *in vitro* species susceptibility now includes, in addition to those mentioned above, bovine, sheep, and nonhuman primate cells.

199

FELINE
LEUKEMIA–
SARCOMA
COMPLEX:
A MODEL FOR
RNA VIRAL
TUMORIGENESIS

W. F. H. Jarrett (1971) was unable to demonstrate infectivity in rats and mice of various inbred lines and could not demonstrate replication in mouse and rat tissue culture systems. Our group was unable to demonstrate infectivity or replication in embryonating chicken eggs and infectivity in laboratory rodents (unpublished results), which corroborates the observations made by Jarrett's group.

10.2. Feline Sarcoma Viruses

As with the avian and murine sarcoma viruses, feline sarcoma viruses readily produce sarcomas in the host of origin. There are other biological similarities, but, unlike the avian and murine sarcoma viruses, the feline sarcoma viruses have a much wider host range of infectivity *in vivo* with induction of tumors. We have demonstrated that—in addition to cats—dogs, rabbits, marmosets (*Saquinus fuscicollis*), three species of macaques (*Macaca radiata, M. mulatta,* and *M. fasicularis*), squirrel monkeys (*Saimiri sciureus*), and sheep are susceptible to tumor induction (Theilen *et al.*, 1970*b*, 1973; Rabin *et al.*, 1972). Detailed accounts have been published of FeSV-induced tumors in marmosets (Deinhardt *et al.*, 1970) and in sheep (Theilen, 1971*a*; Theilen *et al.*, 1973, 1974). A very striking feature about the FeSV-induced tumors in heterospecies such as dogs, sheep, and macaques is regression of tumors. In dogs, the immune response to regression is overcome by inoculation of fetuses (Gardner *et al.*, 1970). Tumors in sheep fetuses regress *in utero* (Theilen, 1971*a*), and newborn lambs are resistant to tumor induction with FeSV derived from cat tissues or cells; however, tumors can be induced in newborn lambs if the virus is first adapted to sheep cells *in vitro* (Theilen *et al.*, 1973). Sarcoma induction in sheep with sheep cell–adapted FeSV can serve as an excellent model for study of cell-mediated and humoral immunity in larger outbred animals and should give better insights into how a host reacts to progressive as well as regressive tumors (Theilen *et al.*, 1974).

Feline sarcoma viruses will infect a variety of cells in culture and cause foci or microtumors, as avian and murine sarcoma viruses do. They have caused *in vitro* transformations of feline, canine, porcine, rabbit, bovine, sheep, and nonhuman primate cells. McDonald *et al.* (1972) have described a plaque assay for FeSV in marmoset cell cultures. All the known FeSV isolates are mixtures of virus subgroups A and B (Sarma *et al.*, 1971*b, c*, 1972). The B subgroup can be purified by serial passage of FeSV in cells selectively resistant to subgroup viruses such as human cells (Sarma *et al.*, 1973*b*).

11. Prevention and Control

Cats naturally exposed to the horizontal spread of feline oncornavirus infection may develop neoplasms, or some may develop antibodies and become immune to virus challenge (Essex *et al.*, 1973). Females may transfer immunity to their developing or newborn kittens (Essex *et al.*, 1971*b*). These observations make it

theoretically possible to develop a vaccine that will protect against feline oncornavirus infections. By use of the indirect immunofluorescence test (Hardy *et al.*,
1972), it would be possible to detect infection and, depending on the accuracy of
the test, set up control measures to prevent the spread of infection in cat
populations. Some now recommend that all IF-positive cats be killed because they
are potential carriers of FOV and it appears that FOV infections may be
horizontally transmitted in certain situations (Hardy *et al.*, 1973; W. F. H. Jarrett *et
al.*, 1973*a*). However, Essex *et al.* (1973) and W. F. H. Jarrett *et al.* (1973*b*) have
demonstrated by the indirect membrane immunofluorescence (FOCMA) test that
many FOV-infected cats develop antibody titers. High FOCMA titers seem to be
protective, and such cats do not develop leukemia or related diseases as frequently
as those with low FOCMA titers. However, to confuse the issue, cats with leukemia
as well as other neoplastic conditions may also have FOCMA titers (Jarrett *et al.*,
1973*b*; Riggs *et al.*, 1973). Therefore, veterinarians should realize that a positive IF
test for FOV gs antigen is not synonymous with overt clinical signs of leukemia nor
is a positive FOCMA antibody titer synonymous with consistent protection from
tumor development. It is difficult to recommend sound control measures,
particularly in light of the recent discovery of the RD114 endogenous virus
(Livingston and Todaro, 1973; Sarma *et al.*, 1973*a*).

12. References

ANDERSON, L. J., AND JARRETT, W. F. H., 1971, Membranous glomerulonephritis associated with
leukaemia in cats, *Res. Vet. Sci.* **12**:179.

ANDERSON, L. J., JARRETT, W. F. H., JARRETT, O., AND LAIRD, H. M., 1971, Feline leukemia-virus
infection of kittens: Mortality associated with atrophy of the thymus and lymphoid depletion, *J. Natl.
Cancer Inst.* **47**:807.

BALTIMORE, D., 1970, Viral RNA-dependent DNA polymerase, *Nature (Lond.)* **226**:1209.

BOSS, I., AND GIBSON, R., 1970, Cats and Childhood Leukemia, *J. Med.* **1**:180.

BRODEY, R. S., MCDONOUGH, S. K., FRYE, F. L., AND HARDY, W. D., 1970, Epidemiology of feline
leukemia (lymphosarcoma), in: *Fourth International Symposium on Comparative Leukemia
Research, Cherry Hill, N.J., 1969, Bibl. Haematol.* **36**:333.

BURGER, C. L., AND NORONHA, F., 1970, Feline leukemia virus: Purification from tissue culture fluids, *J.
Natl. Cancer Inst.* **45**:499.

BURKITT, D. P., 1969, Etiology of Burkitt's lymphoma—An alternative hypothesis to a vectored virus,
J. Natl. Cancer Inst. **42**:19.

CARPENTER, J. L., AND HOLZWORTH, J., 1971, Treatment of leukemia in the cat, *J. Am. Vet. Med. Assoc.*
158:1130.

CHIRIGOS, M. A., 1971, Comments on treatment of feline leukemia, *J. Am. Vet. Med. Assoc.* **158**:1137.

COTCHIN, E., 1957, Neoplasia in the cat, *Vet. Rec.* **69**:425.

CRIGHTON, G. W., 1969, Feline leukaemia (lymphosarcoma) symposium: The diagnosis of leukaemia
in the cat, *J. Small Anim. Pract.* **10**:571.

DEINHARDT, F., WOLFE, L. G., THEILEN, G., AND SNYDER, S. P., 1970, ST-feline fibrosarcoma virus:
Induction of tumors in marmoset monkeys, *Science* **167**:881.

DORN, C. R., TAYLOR, D. O. N., AND HIBBARD, H. H., 1967, Epizootiologic characteristics of canine and
feline leukemia and lymphosarcoma, *Am. J. Vet. Res.* **28**:993.

DORN, C. R., TAYLOR, D. O. N., FRYE, F. L., AND HIBBARD, H. H., 1968, Survey of animal neoplasms in
Alameda and Contra Costa Countries, California: Methodology and description of cases, *J. Natl.
Cancer Inst.* **40**:295.

ECKERT, E. A., ROTT, R., AND SCHAFER, W., 1964, Studies on the BAI strain A (avian myeloblastosis)
viruses, *Virology* **24**:426.

201

FELINE
LEUKEMIA–
SARCOMA
COMPLEX:
A MODEL FOR
RNA VIRAL
TUMORIGENESIS

ESSEX, M., KLEIN, G., SNYDER, S. P., AND HARROLD, J. B., 1971a, Antibody to feline oncorna-virus associated cell membrane antigen in neonatal cats, *Int. J. Cancer* **8**:384.

ESSEX, M., KLEIN, G., SNYDER, S. P., AND HARROLD, J. B., 1971b, Feline sarcoma virus induced tumors: Correlation between humoral antibody and tumour regression, *Nature (Lond.)* **233**:195.

ESSEX, M., COTTER, S. M., AND CARPENTER, J. L., 1973, Feline virus-induced tumors and the immune response: Recent developments, *Am. J. Vet. Res.* **34**:809.

FARROW, B. R. H., AND PENNY, R., 1971, Multiple myeloma in a cat, *J. Am. Vet. Med. Assoc.* **158**:606.

FINK, M. A., SIBAL, L. R., AND PLATA, E. J., 1971, Serologic detection of feline leukemia virus antigens or antibodies, *J. Am. Vet. Med. Assoc.* **158**:1070.

FISCHINGER, P. J., PEEBLES, P. T., NOMURA, S., AND HAAPALA, D. K., 1973, Isolation of an RD114-like oncornavirus from a cat cell line, *J. Virol.* **11**:978.

GARDNER, M. B., 1971, Current information on feline and canine cancer, *J. Natl. Cancer Inst.* **46**:281.

GARDNER, M. B., RONGEY, R. W., ARNSTEIN, P., ESTES, J. D., SARMA, P., HUEBNER, R. J., AND RICKARD, C. G., 1970, Experimental transmission of feline fibrosarcoma to cats and dogs, *Nature (Lond.)* **226**:807.

GARDNER, M. B., RONGEY, R. W., JOHNSON, E. Y., DEJOURNETT, R., AND HUEBNER, R. J., 1971, C-type tumor virus particles in salivary tissue of domestic cats, *J. Natl. Cancer Inst.* **47**:561.

GARDNER, M. B., HENDERSON, B. E., OFFICER, J. E., RONGEY, R. W., PARKER, J. C., OLIVER, C., ESTES, J. D., HUEBNER, R. J., 1973, A spontaneous lower motor neuron disease apparently caused by indigenous type-C RNA virus in a population of wild mice, *J. Natl. Cancer and Inst.* **51**:1243.

GEERING, G., OLD, L. J., AND BOYSE, E. A., 1966, Antigens of leukemias induced by naturally occurring murine leukemia virus: Their relation to the antigens of Gross virus and other murine leukemia viruses, *J. Exp. Med.* **124**:753.

GEERING, G., HARDY, W. D., OLD, L. J., DEHARVEN, E., AND BRODEY, R. S., 1968, Shared group-specific antigen of murine and feline leukemia viruses, *Virology* **36**:678.

GILMORE, C. E., GILMORE, V. H., AND JONES, T. C., 1964, Reticuloendotheliosis, a myeloproliferative disorder of cats: A comparison with lymphocytic leukemia, *Pathol. Vet.* **1**:161.

HANES, G., GARDNER, M. B., LOOSLI, C. G., HEIDBREDER, G., KOGAN, B., MARYLANDER, H., AND HUEBNER, R., 1970, Pet association with selected human cancers: A household questionnaire survey, *J. Natl. Cancer Inst.* **45**:1155.

HARDY, W. D., JR., 1971a, Feline lymphosarcoma: A model of viral carcinogenesis and significance related to human neoplasia in: *Animal Models of Biomedical Research*, Vol. IV, pp. 11–26, National Academy of Sciences, Washington, D.C.

HARDY, W. D., JR., 1971b, Immunodiffusion studies of feline leukemia and sarcoma, *J. Am. Vet. Med. Assoc.* **158**:1060.

HARDY, W. D., JR., AND HURVITZ, A. I., 1971, Feline infectious peritonitis: Experimental studies, *J. Am. Vet. Med. Assoc.* **158**:994.

HARDY, W. D., JR., GEERING, G., OLD, L. J., DEHARVEN, E., BRODEY, R. S., AND MCDONOUGH, S., 1969, Feline leukemia virus: Occurrence of viral antigen in the tissues of cats with lymphosarcoma and other diseases, *Science* **166**:1019.

HARDY, W. D., JR., HIRSHAUT, Y., AND HESS, P., 1972, Detection of the feline leukemia virus and other mammalian oncornaviruses by immunofluorescence, in: Fifth International Symposium on Comparative Leukemia Research, Padova, Italy, 1971, *Bibl. Haematol.* **39**:778.

HARDY, W. D., JR., OLD, L. J., HESS, P. W., ESSEX, M., AND COTTER, S., 1973, Horizontal transmission of feline leukaemia virus, *Nature (Lond.)* **244**:266.

HERZ, A., AND THEILEN, G. H., 1968, Demonstration of C-type virus in milk of lactating queens, unpublished results.

HERZ, A., THEILEN, G. H., SCHALM, O. W., AND MUNN, R. J., 1970, C-type virus in bone marrow cells of cats with myeloproliferative disorders, *J. Natl. Cancer Inst.* **44**:339.

HOLZWORTH, J., 1960a, Leukemia and related neoplasms in the cat. I. Lymphoid malignancies, *J. Am. Vet. Med. Assoc.* **136**:47.

HOLZWORTH, J., 1960b, Leukemia and related neoplasms in the cat. II. Malignancies other than lymphoid, *J. Am. Vet. Med. Assoc.* **136**:107.

HOLZWORTH, J., AND MEIER, H., 1957, Reticulum cell myeloma in a cat, *Cornell Vet.* **47**:302.

HOOVER, E. A., MCCULLOUGH, C. B., AND GRIESMER, R. A., 1972, Intranasal transmission of feline leukemia, *J. Natl. Cancer Inst.* **48**:973.

JARRETT, O., LAIRD, H. M., CRIGHTON, G. W., JARRETT, W. F. H., AND HAY, D., 1968, Advances in feline leukemia, in: Third International Symposium on Comparative Leukemia Research, Paris, 1967, *Bibl. Haematol.* **30**:244.

JARRETT, O., LAIRD, H. M., AND HAY, D., 1969, Growth of feline leukaemia virus in human cells, *Nature (Lond.)* **224**:1208.

JARRETT, O., LAIRD, H. M., AND HAY, D., 1970, Growth of feline leukemia virus in human canine and porcine cells, in: Fourth International Symposium on Comparative Leukemia Research, Cherry Hill, N. J., 1969, *Bibl. Haematol.* **36**:387.

JARRETT, O., PITTS, J. D., WHALLEY, J. M., CLASON, A. E., AND HAY, J., 1971, Isolation of the nucleic acid of feline leukemia virus, *Virology* **43**:317.

JARRETT, O., LAIRD, H. M., AND HAY, D., 1972, Restricted host range of a feline leukaemia virus, *Nature (Lond.)* **238**:220.

JARRETT, O., LAIRD, H. M., AND HAY, D., 1973, Determinants of the host range of feline leukaemia viruses, *J. Gen. Virol.* **20**:1.

JARRETT, W. F. H., 1966, Recent research in leukaemia in the cat, in: *Symposia of the Zoological Society of London No. 17*, p. 295, Academic Press, London.

JARRETT, W. F. H., 1971, Feline leukemia, *Int. Rev. Exp. Pathol.* **10**:243.

JARRETT, W. F. H., 1973, Viral envelope antigen of the viruses of feline leukemia–sarcoma complex, personal communication.

JARRETT, W. F. H., MARTIN, W. B., CRIGHTON, G. W., DALTON, R. G., AND STEWART, M. F., 1964, Leukaemia in the cat: Transmission experiments with leukaemia (lymphosarcoma), *Nature (Lond.)* **202**:566.

JARRETT, W. F. H., CRIGHTON, G. W., AND DALTON, R. G., 1966, Leukaemia and lymphosarcoma in animals and man. I. Lymphosarcoma or leukaemia in the domestic animal, *Vet. Rec.* **79**:693.

JARRETT, W. F. H., JARRETT, O., MACKEY, L., LAIRD, H., HARDY, W. D., JR., AND ESSEX, M., 1973a, Horizontal transmission of leukemia virus and leukemia in the cat, *J. Natl. Cancer Inst.* **51**:833.

JARRETT, W. F. H., ESSEX, M., MACKEY, L., JARRETT, O., AND LAIRD, H., 1973b, Antibodies in normal and leukemic cats to feline oncornavirus–associated cell membrane antigens, *J. Natl. Cancer Inst.* **51**:261.

KAWAKAMI, T. G., THEILEN, G. H., DUNGWORTH, D. L., MUNN, R. J., AND BEALL, S. G., 1967, C-type viral particles in plasma of cats with leukemia, *Science* **158**:1049.

KAWAKAMI, T. G., HUFF, S. D., BUCKLEY, P. M., DUNGWORTH, D. L., AND SNYDER, S. P., 1972, C-type virus associated with gibbon lymphosarcoma, *Nature (Lond.)* **235**:170.

LAIRD, H. M., JARRETT, O., CRIGHTON, G. W., AND JARRETT, W. F. H., 1968, An electron microscopic study of virus particles in spontaneous leukemia in the cat, *J. Natl. Cancer Inst.* **41**:867.

LIN, F. H., AND THORMAR, H., 1972, Properties of maedi nucleic acid and the presence of ribonucleic acid– and deoxyribonucleic acid–dependent deoxyribonucleic acid polymerase in the virions, *J. Virol.* **10**:228.

LIVINGSTON, D. M., AND TODARO, G. J., 1973, Endogenous type C virus from a cat clone with properties distinct from previously described feline type C viruses, *Virology* **53**:142.

MARUYAMA, K., DMOCHOWSKI, L., AND RICKARD, C. G., 1970, Comparative studies of feline and human leukemia by mixed hemabsorption reaction, in: Fourth International Symposium on Comparative Leukemia Research, Cherry Hill, N.J., 1969, *Bibl. Haematol.* **36**:355.

McALLISTER, R. M., MELNYK, J., FINKLESTEIN, J. Z., ADAMS, E. C., AND GARDNER, M. B., 1969, Cultivation *in vitro* of cells derived from a human rhabdomyosarcoma, *Cancer* **24**:520.

McALLISTER, R. M., NELSON-REES, W. A., JOHNSON, E. Y., RONGEY, R. W., AND GARDNER, M. B., 1971, Disseminated rhabdomyosarcoma formed in kittens by cultivated human rhabdomyosarcoma cells, *J. Natl. Cancer Inst.* **47**:603.

McALLISTER, R. M., NICOLSON, M., GARDNER, M. B., RONGEY, R. W., RASHEED, S., SARMA, P. S., HUEBNER, R. J., HATANAKA, M., OROSZLAN, S., GILDEN, R. V., KABIGTING, A., AND VERNON, L., 1972, C-type virus released from cultured rhabdomyosarcoma cells, *Nature New Biol. (London)* **235**:3.

McALLISTER, R. M., NICOLSON, M., GARDNER, M. B., RASHEED, S., RONGEY, R. W., HARDY, W. D., JR., AND GILDEN, R. V., 1973, RD–114 virus compared with feline and murine type-C viruses released from RD cells, *Nature New Biol. (London)* **242**:75.

McDONALD, R., WOLFE, L. G., AND DEINHARDT, F., 1972, Feline fibrosarcoma virus: Quantitative focus assay, focus monolayer and evidence for a "helper virus," *Int. J. Cancer* **9**:57.

McDONOUGH, S. K., LARSEN, S., BRODEY, R. S., STOCK, N. D., AND HARDY, W. D., JR., 1971, A transmissible feline fibrosarcoma of viral origin, *Cancer Res.* **31**:953.

MEIER, H., AND GOURLEY, G., 1957, Basophilic (myelocyte) or mast cell leukemia in a cat, *J. Am. Vet. Med. Assoc.* **130**:33.

203

FELINE
LEUKEMIA–
SARCOMA
COMPLEX:
A MODEL FOR
RNA VIRAL
TUMORIGENESIS

MOULTON, J. E., 1961, Fibrosarcoma, in: *Tumors in Domestic Animals*, p. 24, University of California Press, Berkeley.

MULLIGAN, R. M., 1951, Spontaneous cat tumors, *Cancer Res.* **11**:271.

NEIMAN, P. E., 1973, Measurement of RD-114 virus nucleotide sequences in feline cellular DNA, in: *Biohazards in Biological Research* (A. Hellman, M. N. Oxman, and R. Pollack, eds.), pp. 114–130, Cold Spring Harbor Laboratory, Cold Spring Harbor, N.Y.

NIELSEN, S. W., 1964, *Neoplastic Diseases in Feline Medicine and Surgery* (E. J. Catcott, ed.), p. 156, American Veterinary Publications, Santa Barbara, Calif.

NIELSEN, S. W., 1969, Spontaneous hematopoietic neoplasms of the domestic cat, in: *Comparative Morphology of Hematopoietic Neoplasms*, p. 73, National Cancer Institute Monograph No. 32.

OLSEN, R. G., AND YOHN, D. S., 1972, Demonstration of antibody in cat sera to feline oncornaviruses by complement fixation inhibition, *J. Natl. Cancer Inst.* **49**:395.

OROSZLAN, S., HUEBNER, R. J., AND GILDEN, R. V., 1971*a*, Species-specific and interspecific antigenic determinants associated with the structural protein of feline C-type virus, *Proc. Natl. Acad. Sci.* **68**:901.

OROSZLAN, S., HATANAKA, M., GILDEN, R. V., AND HUEBNER, R. J., 1971*b*, Specific inhibition of mammalian ribonucleic acid C-type virus deoxyribonucleic acid polymerase by rat antisera, *J. Virol.* **8**:816.

OROSZLAN, S., BOVA, D., MARTINWHITE, M. H., TONI, R., FOREMAN, C., AND GILDEN, R. V., 1972, Purification and immunological characterization of the major internal protein of the RD–114 virus, *Proc. Natl. Acad. Sci.* **69**:1211.

OSHIRO, L. S., RIGGS, J. L., TAYLOR, D. O., LENNETTE, E. H., AND HUEBNER, R. J., 1971, Ferritin labeled antibody studies of feline C-type particles, *Cancer Res.* **31**:1100.

PRIESTER, W. A., 1971, Tumors in domestic animals, *J. Natl. Cancer Inst.* **47**:1333.

PURCHASE, H. G., LUDFORD, C., NAZERIAN, K., AND COX, H. W., 1973, A new group of oncogenic viruses: Reticuloendotheliosis, chick syncytial, duck infectious anemia, and spleen necrosis viruses, *J. Natl. Cancer Inst.* **51**:489.

RABIN, H., THEILEN, G. H., SARMA, P. S., DUNGWORTH, D. L., NELSON-REES, W. A., AND COOPER, R. W., 1972, Tumor induction in squirrel monkeys by the ST strain of feline sarcoma virus, *J. Natl. Cancer Inst.* **49**:441.

RICKARD, C. G., 1969, Feline leukemia (lymphosarcoma) symposium 4. Discussion, *J. Small Anim. Pract.* **10**:615.

RICKARD, C. G., GILLESPIE, J. H., LEE, K. M., NORONHA, F., POST, J. E., AND SAVAGE, E. L., 1968, Transmission and electron microscopy of lymphocytic leukemia in the cat, in: Third International Symposium on Comparative Leukemia Research, Paris, 1967, *Bibl. Haematol.* **30**:282.

RICKARD, C. G., POST, J. E., NORONHA, F., AND BARR, L. M., 1969, A transmissible virus induced lymphocytic leukemia of the cat, *J. Natl. Cancer Inst.* **42**:987.

RIGGS, L. J., 1971, An immunofluorescent test for feline leukemia and sarcoma virus antigens and antibodies, *J. Am. Vet. Med. Assoc.* **158**:1085.

RIGGS, L. J., OSHIRO, L. S., TAYLOR, D. O. N., AND LENNETTE, E. H., 1973, Prevalence of type-C virus and antibodies in normal cats and cats with neoplasia, *J. Natl. Cancer Inst.* **51**:449.

ROY-BURMAN, P., PAL, B. K., AND GARDNER, M. B., 1972, Inhibition of the DNA-dependent DNA polymerase of some RNA tumor viruses in feline sera, *Nature New Biol. (London)* **237**:45.

RUBIN, H., 1960, A virus in chick embryos which induces resistance *in vitro* to infection with Rous sarcoma virus, *Proc. Natl. Acad. Sci.* **46**:1105.

SARMA, P. S., AND LOG, T., 1971, Viral interference in feline leukemia–sarcoma complex, *Virology* **44**:352.

SARMA, P. S., AND LOG, T., 1972, Viral envelope antigens of the viruses of feline leukemia–sarcoma complex, in: Proceedings of the Fifth International Symposium on Comparative Leukemia Research, Padova, Italy, 1971, *Bibl. Haematol.* **39**:113.

SARMA, P. S., AND LOG, T., 1973, Subgroup classification of feline leukemia and sarcoma viruses by viral interference and neutralization tests, *Virology* **54**:160.

SARMA, P. S., CHEONG, M. P., HARTLEY, H. W., AND HUEBNER, R. J., 1967, A viral interference test for mouse leukemia viruses, *Virology* **33**:180.

SARMA, P. S., HUEBNER, R. J., BASKAR, J. F., VERNON, L., AND GILDEN, R. V., 1970, Feline leukemia and sarcoma viruses: Susceptibility of human cells to infection, *Science* **168**:1098.

SARMA, P. S., GILDEN, R. V., AND HUEBNER, R. J., 1971*a*, Complement-fixation for feline leukemia and sarcoma viruses (the COCAL test), *Virology* **44**:137.

SARMA, P. S., LOG, T., AND THEILEN, G. H., 1971b, ST feline sarcoma virus: Biological characteristics and *in vitro* propagation, *Proc. Soc. Exp. Biol. Med.* **137**:1444.

SARMA, P. S., BASKAR, S. F., GILDEN, R. V., GARDNER, M. B., AND HUEBNER, R. J., 1971c, Isolation and characterization of the GA strain of feline virus, *Proc. Soc. Exp. Biol. Med.* **137**:1333.

SARMA, P. S., SHARAR, A. L., AND MCDONOUGH, S., 1972, The SM strain of feline sarcoma virus: Biologic and antigenic characterization of virus, *Proc. Soc. Exp. Biol. Med.* **140**:1365.

SARMA, P. S., TSENG, J., LEE, Y. K., AND GILDEN, R. V., 1973a, Virus similar to RD114 virus in cat cells, *Nature New Biol.* **244**:56

SARMA, P. S., JAIN, D., AND HILL, P. R., 1973b, *In vitro* host range of feline leukemia virus, in: Sixth International Symposium on Comparative Leukemia Research, Nagoya, Japan, 1973.

SARMA, P. S., SHARAR, A., WALTERS, V., AND GARDNER, M., 1974, A survey of cats and humans for prevalence of feline leukemia–sarcoma virus neutralizing serum antibodies, *Proc. Soc. Exp. Biol. Med.* **145**:560.

SCHAFER, W., AND NORONHA, F., 1971, A text system for identification of the antigen shared by leukemia viruses of the cat and other mammalian SPECIES, *J. Am. Vet. Med. Assoc.* **158**:1092.

SCHALM, O. W., 1971, Comments on feline leukemia: clinical and pathologic features, differential diagnosis, *J. Am. Vet. Med. Assoc.* **158**:1025.

SCHALM, O. W., AND THEILEN, G. H., 1970, Myeloproliferative disease in the cat associated with C-type leukovirus particles in bone marrow, *J. Am. Vet. Med. Assoc.* **157**:1686.

SCHOLM, S., HARTER, D. H., BURNY, A., AND SPIEGELMAN, S., 1971, DNA polymerase activities in virions of visna virus, a causative agent of a "slow" neurological disease, *Proc. Natl. Acad. Sci.* **68**:182.

SCHMIDT, R. E., AND LANGHAM, R. F., 1967, A survey of cat neoplasms, *J. Am. Vet. Med. Assoc.* **151**:1325.

SCHNEIDER, R., 1970, The natural history of feline malignant lymphoma and sarcoma and their associations with cancer in man and dog, *J. Am. Vet. Med. Assoc.* **157**:1753.

SCHNEIDER, R., 1972a, Feline malignant lymphoma: Environmental factors and the occurrence of this viral cancer in cats, *Int. J. Cancer* **10**:345.

SCHNEIDER, R., 1972b, Human cancer in households containing cats with malignant lymphoma, *Int. J. Cancer* **10**:338.

SCHNEIDER, R., FRYE, F. L., TAYLOR, D. O. N., AND DORN, C. R., 1967, A household cluster of feline malignant lymphoma, *Cancer Res.* **27**:1316.

SIBEL, L. S., FINK, M. A., PLATA, E. J., KOHLER, B. A., NORONHA, F., AND LEE, K. M., 1970, Methods for the detection of viral antigen and antibody to a feline virus (a preliminary report), *J. Natl. Cancer Inst.* **45**:607.

SNYDER, S. P., 1971, Spontaneous feline fibrosarcoma: Transmissibility and ultrastructure of associated virus-like particles, *J. Natl. Cancer Inst.* **47**:1079.

SNYDER, S. P., AND THEILEN, G. H., 1969, Transmissible feline fibrosarcoma, *Nature (Lond.)* **221**:1074.

SNYDER, S. P., THEILEN, G. H., AND RICHARDS, W. P. C., 1970, Morphological studies on transmissible feline fibrosarcoma, *Cancer Res.* **30**:1658.

SODIKOFF, D. H., AND SCHALM, O. W., 1968, Primary bone marrow disease in the cat. III. Erythremic myelosis and myelofibrosis, a myeloproliferative disorder, *Calif. Vet. Lab. Notes*, December.

SPIEGELMAN, S., BURNEY, A., DAS, M. R., KEYDAR, I., SCHLOM, J., TRAVNICEK, M., AND WATSON, K., 1970, Characterization of the products of RNA directed DNA polymerases in oncogenic RNA viruses, *Nature (Lond.)* **227**:563.

SQUIRE, R. A., 1966, Feline lymphoma: A comparison with Burkitt's tumor of children, *Cancer* **19**:447.

SQUIRE, R. A., AND BUSH, M., 1971, Comments on treatment of leukemia in the cat, *J. Am. Vet. Med. Assoc.* **158**:1134.

STECK, F. T., AND RUBIN, H. S., 1965, The mechanism of interference between an avian leukosis virus and rous sarcoma virus. I. Establishment of interference, *Virology* **28**:628.

SWITZER, J. W., AND SCHALM, O. W., 1968, Bone marrow disorders in cats: Bone marrow sampling techniques, *Calif. Vet. Lab. Notes*, August.

TEMIN, H. M., 1972, The RNA tumor viruses—Background and foreground, *Proc. Natl. Acad. Sci.* **69**:1016.

TEMIN, H. M., AND BALTIMORE, D., 1972, RNA-directed DNA synthesis and RNA tumor viruses, in: *Advances in Virus Research* (K. M. Smith, M. A. Lauffer, and F. B. Bang, eds.), p. 129, Academic Press, New York.

TEMIN, H. M., AND MIZUTANI, S., 1970, RNA-dependent DNA polymerase in virions of Rous sarcoma virus, *Nature (Lond.)* **226**:1211.

205

FELINE
LEUKEMIA–
SARCOMA
COMPLEX:
A MODEL FOR
RNA VIRAL
TUMORIGENESIS

THEILEN, G. H., 1970, The present status of the leukemia–sarcoma complex in man and lower animals, *J. Am. Vet. Med. Assoc.* **157**:1742.

THEILEN, G. H., 1971a, Continuing studies with transmissible feline fibrosarcoma virus in fetal and newborn sheep, *J. Am. Vet. Med. Assoc.* **158**:1040.

THEILEN, G. H., 1971b, Feline leukemia–sarcoma complex; cause and treatment, in: *Proceedings of the International Veterinary Congress*, Mexico City, p. 264.

THEILEN, G. H., AND HARROLD, B., 1968, Intrathymic FeLV injections in newborn kittens with intercurrent infections, unpublished data.

THEILEN, G. H., ZEIGEL, R. F., AND TWIEHAUS, M. J., 1966, Biological studies with RE virus (strain T) that induces reticuloendotheliosis in turkeys, chickens and Japanese quail, *J. Natl. Cancer Inst.* **37**:731.

THEILEN, G. H., KAWAKAMI, T. G., DUNGWORTH, D. L., SWITZER, J. W., MUNN, R. J., AND HARROLD, J. B., 1968, Current status of transmissible agents in feline leukemia, *J. Am. Vet. Med. Assoc.* **153**:1864.

THEILEN, G. H., KAWAKAMI, T. G., RUSH, J. D., AND MUNN, R. J., 1969, Replication of cat leukemia virus in cell suspension cultures, *Nature (Lond.)* **222**:589.

THEILEN, G. H., DUNGWORTH, D. L., KAWAKAMI, T. G., MUNN, R. J., WARD, J. M., AND HARROLD, J. B., 1970a, Experimental induction of lymphosarcoma in the cat with "C"-type virus, *Cancer Res.* **30**:401.

THEILEN, G. H., SNYDER, S. P., WOLFE, L. G., AND LANDON, J. C., 1970b, Biological studies with viral induced fibrosarcomas in cats, dogs, rabbits, and non-human primates, in: Fourth International Symposium on Comparative Leukemia Research, Cherry Hill, N.J., 1969, *Bibl. Haematol.* **36**:393.

THEILEN, G. H., GOULD, D., FOWLER, M., AND DUNGSWORTH, D. L., 1971, C-type virus in tumor tissue of a wooly monkey (*Lagothrix* spp.) with fibrosarcoma, *J. Natl. Cancer Inst.* **47**:881.

THEILEN, G. H., HOKAMA, Y., MANNING, J. S., AND CALLAWAY, E., 1973, Heterospecies infectivity of FeSV: Neoplasms in sheep fetuses and lambs by inoculation of FeSV transformed sheep-cells, in: *Possible Episomes in Eukaryotes* (Fourth Lepetit Colloquium, L. Silvestri, ed.), p. 109, North-Holland, Amsterdam.

THEILEN, G. H., HALL, J., PENDRY, A., GLOVER, D. J., AND REEVES, B. R., 1974, Tumours induced in sheep by injecting cells transformed *in vitro* with feline sarcoma virus (FeSV) transplantation, *Transplantation* **17**:152.

UBERTINI, T. R., 1972, Location of feline leukemia–sarcoma group-specific antigen in infected human tissue culture cells, *Infection Immunity* **5**:400.

WARD, J. M., 1970, Feline infectious peritonitis, thesis, University of California, Davis.

WARD, J. M., SODIKOFF, C. H., AND SCHALM, O. W., 1969, Myeloproliferative disease and abnormal erythrogenesis in the cat, *J. Am. Vet. Med. Assoc.* **155**:879.

WHALLEY, J. M., 1973, Size differences in the ribonucleic acids of feline leukaemia viruses, *J. Gen. Virol.* **21**:39.

WILKINSON, G. T., 1966, *Diseases of the Cat*, Pergamon Press, Oxford.

WOLFE, L. G., DEINHARDT, F., THEILEN, G. H., RABIN, H., KAWAKAMI, T., AND BUSTAD, L. K., 1971, Induction of tumors in marmoset monkeys by simian sarcoma virus, type 1 (*Lagothrix*): A preliminary report, *J. Natl. Cancer Inst.* **47**:1115.

ZAWIDZKA, Z. Z., ZANZEN, E., AND GRICE, H. C., 1964, Erythremic myelosis in a cat: A case resembling Di Guglielmo's syndrome in man, *Pathol. Vet.* **1**:530.

ZEIGEL, R. F., THEILEN, G. H., AND TWIEHAUS, M. J., 1966, Electron microscopic observations on RE virus (strain T) that induces reticuloendotheliosis in turkeys, chickens and Japanese quail, *J. Natl. Cancer Inst.* **37**:709.

ZOOK, B. C., KING, N. W., ROBINSON, R. L., AND McCOMBS, H. L., 1968, Ultrastructural evidence for the viral etiology of feline infectious peritonitis, *Pathol. Vet.* **5**:91.

DNA Viruses

6

DNA Viruses: Molecular Biology

F. RAPP AND M. A. JERKOFSKY

1. Introduction

There is no longer any doubt that viruses are associated with a number of malignant states both under natural conditions in animal populations and after certain defined experimental manipulations in the laboratory. However, there still remains some question as to whether viruses play the principal role in the etiology of the majority of malignant conditions, especially those of human origin. At the present time, work continues in many laboratories in the attempt to find the definitive answer to this question.

Gross (1970) has chronicled the development of the early studies with tumor viruses. This chapter will attempt to present and to examine various factors concerned with the replication of the DNA viruses classified as tumor viruses. Since all of these viruses contain DNA as the source of their genetic capability, they share certain common pathways in their replicative cycle. And yet each group has evolved unique and specialized solutions to the basic problems of replication and maintenance as an evolutionary competent entity. Attempts to understand the oncogenic potential of these viruses and the properties of the transformed cells require consideration of the genetic capabilities that each group possesses. Thus a basic understanding of the molecular biology of the DNA tumor viruses is essential to our understanding of their tumor-producing ability.

F. RAPP and M. A. JERKOFSKY ● Department of Microbiology, College of Medicine, The Milton S. Hershey Medical Center of The Pennsylvania State University, Hershey, Pennsylvania.

No attempt has been made in the following pages to evaluate all of the studies attempted with these agents; other chapters in this volume will consider each of the groups of viruses. Instead, we have tried to concentrate on those areas of current research which seem most promising in enlarging our understanding of the basic mechanisms involved in virus replication and in the transformation of normal cells into cells with malignant potential.

2. Molecular Parameters

The replicative cycle of DNA viruses is usually divided into early and late events separated by the initiation of synthesis of the virus DNA. Thus early events occur prior to the initiation of virus DNA synthesis and can take place in the absence of any DNA synthesis. Late events require either the initiation of virus DNA synthesis or the production of actual progeny virus DNA molecules. In general terms, early events are associated with cell transformation whereas late events are repressed. This distinction is quite useful with the smaller DNA viruses, such as the papovaviruses and the adenoviruses; the distinction is somewhat blurred with the herpesviruses. However, we will use this as a general outline and discuss exceptions as they occur.

In discussing papovaviruses, we will include the simian virus SV40 and the mouse polyoma virus. Studies with adenoviruses include various members of the 31 human serotypes. Most work with the herpesviruses will concentrate on herpes simplex virus, although other members of the group will be mentioned as appropriate. Since very little is known about the mechanisms of adsorption, penetration, and uncoating of these tumor viruses, readers are referred to the excellent review by Dales (1973).

2.1. State of the Virion DNA

2.1.1. Papovaviruses

The DNA found in the virions of SV40 and polyoma viruses is double stranded, circular, and superhelical, with a molecular weight of about 3×10^6 daltons. The guanine plus cytosine (G + C) content of SV40 is 41%, while that of polyoma is 49%.

The double-stranded superhelical circular form of the DNA is called form I DNA. A break or nick in one of the strands results in the formation of open relaxed circles called form II DNA. A double-strand break produces a linear form III molecule.

Papovavirus preparations also contain other types of particles. One is a lighter particle containing less DNA, produced during passage at high multiplicities of infection (Uchida *et al.*, 1966, 1968). The properties of this type of particle will be discussed in the next section. Under certain conditions of cell culture, linear cellular DNA can become encapsidated by both polyoma (Michel *et al.*, 1967; Winocour, 1968) and SV40 (Levine and Teresky, 1970); these pseudovirions then are present in the virus populations. Sambrook (1972) presents a good review of the various particles found in papovavirus preparations.

2.1.2. Adenoviruses

The DNA of the human adenoviruses consists of an uninterrupted linear double-stranded molecule with a molecular weight of $20–25 \times 10^6$ daltons. The G+C content of the 31 human serotypes varies from 48 to 61%. The DNA is neither circularly permutated nor terminally redundant (Green *et al.*, 1970; Van der Eb *et al.*, 1969; Doerfler, 1970*a*).

2.1.3. Herpesviruses

The DNA of the herpesviruses is a double-stranded linear molecule with a molecular weight of about 100×10^6 daltons. The G + C content of the human herpesviruses is 67% for herpes simplex type 1 and 69% for type 2.

The virion DNA of herpes simplex types 1 and 2 consists of one intact strand and one strand in which alkali-labile regions yield six fragments of nonrandom size and unique nucleotide sequence when the DNA is sedimented in alkali (Kieff *et al.*, 1971; Frenkel and Roizman, 1972*a*). The six fragments can be arranged to form three types of the one strand which contains the alkali-labile regions; the same strand in all molecules is intact and the other strand is in one of three possible configurations. Thus the DNA consists of an intact single strand and a single strand interrupted at unique and preferred sites by alkali-labile linkages. Although these linkages are labile to heat and alkali, they are stable to formamide treatment, suggesting that alkali-sensitive phosphodiester bonds may be involved (Gordin *et al.*, 1973) and even possibly ribonucleotides. Similar fragments have been detected in the virion DNA of Marek's disease virus (Lee *et al.*, 1971) and EB virus (Nonoyama and Pagano, 1972). Though no repetitive sequences have been detected in the DNA of herpes simplex virus type 1 (Frenkel and Roizman, 1971), 16% of the DNA of type 2 virus consists of repetitive sequences (Roizman and Frenkel, 1973).

2.2. Integration of Virus DNA

2.2.1. Papovaviruses

It was demonstrated early that both SV40 and polyoma viruses could transform cells *in vitro* and produce tumors when injected into experimental animals. Since the resulting cells retained various new properties, it was assumed that virus DNA remained in the cells and maintained the transformed or changed state of the cell.

Investigators immediately began to look for traces of virus DNA in transformed cells. There was a problem with polyoma virus: complementary RNA prepared from polyoma virus DNA would react with uninfected cell DNA and there was no increase in the reaction if transformed cells were used (Winocour, 1965*a*). In the reciprocal experiment, RNA complementary to mouse DNA would react with purified polyoma virus DNA (Winocour, 1965*b*). There was one report that transformed cells showed an increased reaction and that, therefore, polyoma virus DNA was present in transformed cells (Axelrod *et al.*, 1964). Many of these problems were alleviated with the discovery of cell DNA in pseudovirion particles in the polyoma virus stocks (Michel *et al.*, 1967; Winocour, 1967, 1968).

Although pseudovirions can be produced under certain conditions by SV40 (Levine and Teresky, 1970), they did not present a real problem. However, small amounts of homology were detected between SV40 DNA and normal cell DNA (Reich *et al.*, 1966; Gelb *et al.*, 1971); it was thought that these could be short sequences in the cell DNA that would facilitate integration of the virus DNA. Many workers reported varying amounts of SV40 DNA present in transformed cells; many of the values varied with the sensitivity of the technique used (Reich *et al.*, 1966; Sambrook *et al.*, 1968; Westphal and Dulbecco, 1968; Tai and O'Brien, 1969; Levine *et al.*, 1970; Gelb *et al.*, 1971; Siegel and Levine, 1972). The DNA detected was integrated with the cell DNA by alkali-stable covalent bonds (Sambrook *et al.*, 1968); the techniques were not sensitive enough to determine whether all of the DNA was integrated at a single site or there were multiple sites of integration in transformed cells.

No one was particularly suprised to find papovavirus DNA remaining in cells transformed by the virus. However, it was then discovered that SV40 DNA could form an alkali-stable association with high molecular weight cell nuclear DNA during a lytic infection (Hirai *et al.*, 1971; Hirai and Defendi, 1972). Cell DNA synthesis was not required for this integration (Hirai *et al.*, 1971; Hirai and Defendi, 1972), although DNA synthesis followed by mitotic division enhanced the amount of integration, perhaps by providing more sites for integration to occur (Collins and Sauer, 1972). Polyoma virus has also been shown to integrate into cell DNA during lytic replication (Ralph and Colter, 1972).

One study (Collins and Sauer, 1972) has attempted to detect early structural changes in the incoming SV40 DNA prior to integration. It appears that the incoming form I DNA is nicked prior to insertion as a linear molecule; a slower-sedimenting molecule can be detected prior to the linkage with cell DNA. However, much more work will be required before the mechanism of integration is understood.

At the present time, the importance of virus integration during a lytic replicative cycle is not known; the fact that it can be detected does not mean that it is required. As we will see in a later section, replication of the virus DNA appears to require a circular configuration. However, in studies with the production of messenger RNA it was found that transcription may occur from an integrated genome. Recent studies have also demonstrated that virions can be produced which contain hybrid DNA molecules: SV40 DNA linked to cell DNA in a closed superhelical form. Such particles could be produced by excision of an integrated genome.

It had been known for a long time that if serial undiluted passages of SV40 were performed the yield of infectious virus would decrease but the total yield of particles would remain fairly constant (Uchida *et al.*, 1966). The explanation for this phenomenon was that incomplete, defective particles were produced which interfered with the replication of infectious virus (Uchida *et al.*, 1968). When the DNA from the lighter defective particles was examined, it was found to be shorter than the infectious SV40 DNA although still in the superhelical circular configuration (Yoshiike, 1968).

DNA–DNA hybridization studies demonstrated that the closed circular DNA extracted from the lighter virions shared sequences in common with normal cellular DNA as well as with SV40 (Aloni *et al.*, 1969). However, the production of such particles depended on the conditions of culture (Lavi and Winocour, 1972). Few if any host DNA sequences could be detected in virus populations passed at low multiplicities of infection. However, as the multiplicity of infection was increased, large amounts of hybrid molecules could be detected. These hybrid molecules could not be detected if plaque-purified virus was used to set up the infection. However, after several serial undiluted passages of plaque-purified virus, extensive homology could again be detected with cell DNA. This suggested that during the lytic replicative cycle a recombination event occurred between SV40 and the host cell DNA which permitted SV40 to pick up host information; the excision of an integrated SV40 DNA molecule could be such an event. The substituted molecules did not contain sufficient genetic information for self-replication and could be perpetuated only if an intact infectious SV40 molecule were present, as one would obtain in passage at high multiplicities of infection.

This recombination appeared to be a general phenomenon since it was observed to occur with several separately isolated plaque-purified preparations derived from two different strains of SV40 virus (Lavi *et al.*, 1973). However, the relative yields of such virus progeny varied with passage, including passage of the same virus clone; one could not predict what information the virus would pick up or when. Another study (Gelb and Martin, 1973) showed that the proportion of reiterated or unique cell DNA picked up by SV40 varied with passage in different cell lines.

Heteroduplex mapping techniques showed that more substitutions and deletions could be detected in the shorter molecules as the number of high multiplicity passages increased (Tai *et al.*, 1972). Two of nine fragments obtained from digestion with *Hemophilus influenzae* restriction endonuclease readily hybridized with cell DNA and therefore contained reiterated host cell DNA (Rozenblatt *et al.*, 1973). The hybridization techniques used are only sensitive enough to detect regions of homology in the amplified or reiterated regions of cellular DNA; they cannot detect homology with the unique regions of cellular DNA. One fragment would hybridize only with other serially passaged SV40 molecules, suggesting that it contained a unique cell sequence (Rozenblatt *et al.*, 1973). There is evidence that the substituted host fragments replicate along with the SV40 DNA (Lavi *et al.*,

1973), so a unique cell fragment picked up would become reiterated through passage.

There is also some evidence that a portion of the virus genome becomes amplified during serial undiluted passage. By use of DNA reassociation kinetics, a fraction (about 20%) of the closed circular SV40 DNA was found to reassociate to unsubstituted SV40 DNA 5–7 times faster than the unsubstituted DNA did to itself (Martin *et al.*, 1973). This suggests that certain SV40 sequences are preferentially conserved, amplified, or both. This study also detected both reiterated and unique host sequences inserted at many sites on the superhelical molecules. Further studies with fragments obtained from digestion with *H. influenzae* endonuclease have shown alterations at many sites, although certain changes seem more frequent (Brockman *et al.*, 1973). There are reduced yields of some fragments and the appearance of new fragments. With continued passage at high multiplicities of infection, the digest pattern becomes simpler, with a few dominant pieces. All the molecules retain some SV40 sequences, although these can be reduced to less than 30% in late-passage material. Reiterated cell DNA is present in a high percentage of late-passage molecules but accounts for less than 20% of the total sequences. Therefore, the majority of host sequences must be from the nonreiterated cell DNA.

One study has attempted to determine how such molecules arise (Waldeck *et al.*, 1973). By use of low multiplicity passage virus, so that no host sequences are present, the covalent linkage of host DNA with SV40 DNA has been detected in newly replicated linear double-stranded DNA that is found in the Hirt supernatant fluid. These molecules are 1.5–2 times the contour length of SV40. This model suggests the preferential excision of host DNA sequences rich in integrated virus DNA.

2.2.2. Adenoviruses

Few studies have been carried out to detect adenovirus DNA in transformed cells, although many studies have been done with virus-specific mRNA produced in transformed cells. One study (Dunn *et al.*, 1973) has used *in situ* molecular hybridization to detect adenovirus DNA in the nucleus of transformed and tumor cells and probably associated with the chromosomes.

Adenovirus DNA has also been shown to integrate into cell DNA during the replicative cycle. In baby hamster kidney cells inoculated with labeled adenovirus type 12, the labeled material shifts from the density of virus DNA to that of cell DNA (Doerfler, 1968). The inhibition of DNA synthesis does not affect the shift of virus DNA to covalent linkage with cell DNA and there is only a slight change if RNA or protein synthesis is inhibited (Doerfler, 1970*b*). Other workers (zur Hausen and Sokol, 1969) have found that most of the input virus DNA is degraded and reutilized in the formation of cell DNA. However, they detect a small fraction of the original labeled virus, probably fragments, integrated into both strands of the host cell DNA.

There is no evidence to suggest that the DNA of the herpesviruses integrates into the cellular DNA during the replicative cycle. However, cells transformed by members of the herpesviruses have been shown to retain virus DNA.

Many lines of EB virus-transformed cells continually produced virus, but virus DNA (zur Hausen and Schulte-Holthausen, 1970; Nonoyama and Pagano, 1971) and virus-specific RNA (zur Hausen and Schulte-Holthausen, 1970) are also detected in "virus-free" cells. Some workers (Nonoyama and Pagano, 1972) have suggested that the EB virus DNA is not covalently linked to the large cellular chromosomal DNA, although the number of viral genomes per cell remains constant, and have proposed a plasmid-like mechanism to account for the conservation of the DNA in transformed cells. Other workers (Adams *et al.*, 1973) have suggested that the EB virus DNA is linked to cell DNA, but by alkali-labile bonds.

Virus DNA has been detected in tumors produced by Marek's disease virus, although whether the DNA was free or integrated was not determined (Nazerian *et al.*, 1973). In cells from one human cervical tumor, 42% of the genome of herpes simplex virus type 2 appears to be present and at least part is covalently linked to cellular DNA (Roizman and Frenkel, 1973). The production of virus-specific mRNA is also detected in cells transformed *in vitro* by herpes simplex virus type 2, suggesting the retention of at least some virus DNA (Collard *et al.*, 1973).

2.3. Transcription of Early Virus Messenger RNA

2.3.1. Papovaviruses

As was mentioned previously, little is known of how the infecting virus particle enters the nucleus and is uncoated. Isolated DNA from both SV40 and polyoma viruses is infectious in the absence of any capsid proteins. Therefore, it appears that both of these viruses use cellular enzymes already present for the initial stages of the transcription of mRNA.

The first virus gene products to be detected are mRNA molecules. Benjamin (1966) demonstrated that RNA produced in infected cells would hybridize with polyoma virion DNA. Only small amounts of hybridizable material were detected early after infection, whereas there was a sharp increase in the amount of hybridizable material late in the infection. He was also able to show that similar mRNA could be detected in cells transformed by polyoma virus. Later studies (Martin and Axelrod, 1969a) demonstrated that 50% of the polyoma virus DNA was transcribed in the lytic cycle of infection but that only 10–20% of this mRNA was produced in transformed cells.

Similar studies have been done with SV40 virus. In hybridization studies with SV40 DNA and RNA extracted from infected cells, it was demonstrated that the early mRNA transcribes 28% of the SV40 DNA (Sauer and Kidwai, 1968). Late mRNA has some sequences in common with early mRNA (about 40%) but also some unique sequences (Oda and Dulbecco, 1968a). Transformed cells contain mRNA that will hybridize with some late sequences; it is similar but not always identical to early mRNA (Oda and Dulbecco, 1968a; Sauer and Kidwai, 1968). In competition hybridization experiments (Martin and Axelrod, 1969b; Martin, 1970), 50% of the virus DNA would react with saturating amounts of RNA from lytically infected cells, suggesting that the entire virus genome was transcribed during lytic infection. When similar experiments were done with various lines of transformed cells, the amount of hybridizable mRNA varied from 30 to almost 100% (from transformed cells yielding virus) of the mRNA produced during lytic infection (Aloni et al., 1968; Martin and Axelrod, 1969b; Martin, 1970).

Early mRNA could be distinguished from late mRNA by competition hybridization experiments and by base ratio analysis: early mRNA and RNA from transformed cells were richer in purines and poorer in uridine than late mRNA (Aloni et al., 1968). Small amounts of actinomycin D (0.5 μg/ml) were found to inhibit the production of SV40 DNA, late virus mRNA, and infectious virus progeny but did not inhibit the production of early mRNA (Carp et al., 1969). This demonstrated that only the incoming parental molecules of SV40 DNA were required for the production of early mRNA.

Studies of the transcription of mRNA by SV40 became more selective when it was discovered that the *Escherichia coli* RNA polymerase would transcribe only one strand, now called the (–) strand, of SV40 DNA under *in vitro* conditions (Westphal, 1970). This finding gave investigators a tool to use to separate transcription products derived from each strand of the virus DNA.

A surprising finding was that early mRNA sequences made prior to virus DNA synthesis had the same polarity as mRNA made *in vitro* with the E. *coli* polymerase, whereas late mRNA had complementary sequences (Lindstrom and Dulbecco, 1972). Therefore, it appeared that in the infected cell, early and late mRNA products were transcribed from different strands of the SV40 DNA. Quantitative studies were immediately undertaken to determine how much of each strand was transcribed. It was found that early mRNA was transcribed from 30–40% of the (−) strand and there was no transcription from the (+) strand (Sambrook et al., 1972; Khoury et al., 1972; Khoury and Martin, 1972). In late mRNA, transcription occurred from 30–40% of the (−) strand and from 60–70% of the (+) strand (Sambrook et al., 1972; Khoury et al., 1972; Khoury and Martin, 1972). Therefore, late mRNA contained sequences transcribed from both strands whereas all the early mRNA was transcribed from the (−) strand. In transformed cells, mRNA was transcribed from 30–80% of the (−) strand and from 0–20% of the (+) strand (Khoury et al., 1972; Khoury and Martin, 1972; Ozanne et al., 1973). The actual amounts varied with the cell line tested, but it appeared that transformed cells transcribed more of the (−) strand than was found in early mRNA and that no transcription from the late (+) strand was required since it was not found in all transformed cell lines. In a detailed study comparing 11 lines of transformed cells, Khoury et al. (1973) demonstrated that no transcription occurred from the (+) strand and that 37–50% of the (−) strand was transcribed in nine cell lines. Less than 8% of the (+) strand and 65–75% of the (−) strand were transcribed in the other two lines. All of these studies suggest that overlapping regions of the early or (−) strand of SV40 are transcribed in transformed cells. The actual amount of transcription may be determined by how the SV40 is integrated into the DNA of each cell and which strand of cell DNA is transcribed at that integration site.

Astrin (1973) has taken these studies one step further by studying the *in vitro* transcription of chromatin obtained from SV40-transformed cells (SV 3T3). Only that part of the early (−) strand of SV40 which is transcribed *in vitro* in these cells is transcribed in the *in vitro* system. However, if the protein is removed from the chromatin the entire (−) strand is transcribed. These experiments suggest that the template restriction of chromatin is due to the presence of protein associated with the DNA and that there is, therefore, no need to postulate post-transcriptional control.

Early mRNA appears to have a molecular size smaller than one-half of the SV40 genome (Martin and Byrne, 1970; Tonegawa *et al.*, 1970; Sokol and Carp, 1971). This will be of importance in later discussions of possible processing of late mRNA.

2.3.2. *Adenoviruses*

During productive infection with adenoviruses, the transcription of virus-specific mRNA and the replication of virus DNA occur in the nucleus of the infected cell. Again, little is known of the mechanisms of transport of the virus DNA to the nucleus prior to these events. However, it appears that transcription of the adenovirus DNA, at both early and late times, occurs by means of host cell enzymes. One study (Price and Penman, 1972) has suggested that RNA polymerase II of the host cell is involved since the properties of the enzyme which transcribes adenovirus DNA resemble those of this host enzyme: its activity is inhibited by α-amanitin and stimulated by ammonium sulfate. An earlier study (Parsons and Green, 1971) had shown that the presence of cycloheximide stimulates the production of early adenovirus mRNA. Therefore, the transcription of early adenovirus mRNA does not require protein synthesis, further evidence for the use of preexisting cellular enzymes.

Lucas and Ginsberg (1971) have determined that three classes of adenovirus-specific mRNA are produced during lytic infection. The synthesis of early class I mRNA begins prior to but is terminated at some time after the initiation of virus DNA synthesis. The synthesis of early class II mRNA also begins prior to the initiation of virus DNA synthesis but it continues at an enhanced rate afterward. The synthesis of class III mRNA is typical of that of late mRNA; it is initiated only after the beginning of the replication of virus DNA.

Previous DNA–RNA competition hybridization experiments had suggested that from 8–20% of the adenovirus genome was transcribed early but that this early mRNA species was also present at late times (Fujinaga and Green, 1970). When it was discovered that adenovirus DNA could be separated into a heavy (H) and a light (L) strand, it could be determined which strand served as a template for the production of the various mRNA species. It was demonstrated that 40% of the transcription of early adenovirus mRNA occurs from the H strand and 60% from the L strand; 80% of late mRNA is transcribed from the L strand and 20% from the H strand (Green et al., 1970). The entire adenovirus genome (80–100%) appears to be transcribed during productive infections. Therefore, strand-switching also occurs in the transcription of adenovirus mRNA, a phenomenon seen previously with the papovaviruses.

Adenovirus DNA is also transcribed asymmetrically in vitro by the E. coli RNA polymerase (Green et al., 1970). Strand selection in vitro seems to be identical to that seen in vivo with the KB cell RNA polymerase; transcription in vitro occurs predominantly with the early virus sequences. Thus both the bacterial and mammalian enzymes may recognize the same initiation site for the transcription of mRNA.

Adenovirus-specific RNA has been detected in cells transformed by adenoviruses classified as highly oncogenic (Fujinaga and Green, 1966), weakly oncogenic (Fujinaga and Green, 1967a), and nononcogenic (Fujinaga et al., 1969). However, competition hybridization experiments between RNA species produced in cells transformed by highly and weakly oncogenic adenoviruses have failed to detect common nucleotide sequences (Fujinaga and Green, 1968); thus the virus-coded information appears to be different in these two classes of adenovirus-transformed cells. Since actinomycin D will inhibit the production of adenovirus-specific mRNA in transformed cells, the production of this mRNA appears to be similar to that of normal cellular mRNA (Fujinaga and Green, 1967b). Quantitative studies suggest that the mRNA in transformed cells is homologous to about 50% of the early mRNA produced in lytically infected cells and that no late mRNA is produced in the transformed cells (Fujinaga and Green, 1970).

In normal, uninfected cells, the transcription products of the cellular DNA are a heterogeneous species of high molecular weight nuclear RNA. Cellular enzymes then add between 150 and 250 nucleotides of poly(A) to the heterogeneous nuclear RNA. Most of the heterogeneous nuclear RNA will never leave the nucleus; that which does is transported to the cytoplasm of the cell to serve as cellular mRNA. It has been suggested that the addition of the poly(A) sequences could serve as a mechanism of selection of those RNA sequences which will be conserved to form mRNA (Darnell et al., 1971).

It has been demonstrated that adenovirus-specific RNAs, both nuclear and cytoplasmic, and those produced at both early and late times, contain segments of poly(A) (Philipson et al., 1971). Hybridization experiments have determined that there is no region on the adenovirus DNA molecule to code for the production of such poly(A) sequences (Philipson et al., 1971). Analogues of adenosine such as cordycepin and toyocamycin block the synthesis of poly(A) and prevent the accumulation of adenovirus mRNA on cytoplasmic polyribosomes (Philipson et al., 1971; McGuire et al., 1972). Therefore, the addition of poly(A) sequences to already transcribed adenovirus mRNA appears to involve a host control mechanism to regulate the processing and transport of virus mRNA from its site of transcription in the nucleus to its site of translation in the cytoplasm; a higher proportion of the RNA molecules on the polyribosomes than nuclear RNA molecules contain poly(A) sequences.

It has also been demonstrated that adenovirus RNA begins as a high molecular weight molecule in the nucleus (Wall *et al.*, 1972). This high molecular weight product accumulates in the presence of toyocamycin, which inhibits the addition of poly(A) sequences (McGuire *et al.*, 1972). Following the addition of poly(A), the high molecular weight RNA is cleaved to form adenovirus-specific mRNA. However, 25–30% of the high molecular weight adenovirus-specific nuclear RNA never leaves the nucleus (Wall *et al.*, 1972); this is true at both early and late times. The high molecular weight RNA has been shown to be precursor to the adenovirus mRNA because 70% of the sequences are identical; the other sequences are those lost during the cleavage process (McGuire *et al.*, 1972). As a final result, at least 65% of the early adenovirus mRNA and 85% of the late mRNA have sequences of poly(A) (Lindberg *et al.*, 1972).

Previous studies (Parsons and Green, 1971) had suggested that there might be a difference in the size of nuclear and cytoplasmic adenovirus-specific RNA in transformed cells. More definitive studies (Wall *et al.*, 1973) have shown that adenovirus-specific sequences are covalently linked to cellular sequences in the heterogeneous nuclear RNA of transformed cells but that mRNA from the polysomes of the same cells contains only virus-specific sequences. Therefore, it appears that there is uninterrupted transcription of host sequences and integrated virus sequences in nuclear RNA but that post-transcriptional cleavage removes the host sequences to produce only adenovirus-specific cytoplasmic mRNA.

2.3.3. Herpesviruses

Most of the studies dealing with the transcription of herpes simplex virus DNA have not been separated into early and late stages of mRNA production. As we shall discuss in a moment, early mRNA appears to code for some structural proteins. Therefore, the usual distinction of late events being responsible for the formation of structural proteins does not hold. Most of the studies of herpesvirus transcriptions will be discussed in this section; those specifically concerned with late events will be considered in Section 2.7.3.

As with other DNA viruses, virus-specific nuclear RNA is larger than that found in the cytoplasm and there appears to be a cleavage of large nuclear RNA to produce cytoplasmic mRNA (Wagner and Roizman, 1969*a*, *b*). There are two known forms of transcriptional control with herpes simplex virus. The first, off–on, is the transcription of some sequences early and others only late. The other form of control is the number of copies of each mRNA which are made. Thus, there are abundant and scarce classes of herpes simplex virus–specific mRNA. In infections with herpes simplex virus type 1 (HSV-1), both abundant and scarce classes of mRNA are produced prior to the initiation of virus DNA synthesis (Frenkel and Roizman, 1972*b*). The abundant species account for 99.3% of the total virus-specific mRNA and are transcribed from 14–16% of the virus DNA. The scarce species account for 0.7% of the total virus-specific mRNA and are transcribed from 28–30% of the virus DNA. In infections with herpes simplex virus type 2 (HSV-2), only abundant mRNA species are produced early and these are transcribed from only 21% of the virus DNA (Frenkel *et al.*, 1973). If infected cells are treated with cycloheximide to prevent protein synthesis, HSV-1 still transcribes a total of 44% of the DNA (abundant species plus scarce species) and HSV-2 now transcribes 48% of its DNA (Frenkel *et al.*, 1973). Thus, with both HSV-1 and HSV-2, protein synthesis is not required for early transcription, suggesting that preexisting cellular enzymes are used. The smaller extent of HSV-2 early transcription in a normal cycle of replication may be controlled by proteins to block the full transcription which then occurs if protein synthesis is inhibited.

Frenkel and Roizman (1972*b*) have suggested that abundant mRNA species code for structural proteins. This is based on estimates of the amount of DNA required for the formation of structural proteins and the fact that 19 of 24 structural proteins (or 68% of the genetic information for structural proteins) are made early.

Herpesvirus mRNA contains regions of poly(A) which appear to be added as a post-transcriptional event (Bachenheimer and Roizman, 1972). Abundant species of mRNA contain poly(A), whereas scarce species do not (Silverstein *et al.*, 1973). HSV-1 and HSV-2 share about 50% common DNA sequences and these are transcribed about evenly into abundant and scarce mRNA molecules (Roizman and Frenkel, 1973; Frenkel *et al.*, 1973).

Virus-specific mRNA has been detected in cells transformed by herpesviruses. Such RNA is present in EB virus-transformed cells (zur Hausen and Schulte-Holthausen, 1970), and 10–13% of the sequences transcribed during a productive cycle of replication of HSV-2 are detected in cells transformed by HSV-2 *in vitro* (Collard *et al.*, 1973); these sequences are transcribed from the part of the virus genome shared by HSV-1 and HSV-2. In one cervical tumor, RNA complementary to 50% of the HSV-2 DNA has been detected (Roizman and Frenkel, 1973); these RNA species are similar to those detected at both early and late times during a productive cycle of replication.

2.4. Translation of Early Virus Proteins

2.4.1. Papovaviruses

Although there are many studies of the transcription of early papovavirus mRNA, both in the lytic cycle and in transformed cells, little is known of the functions of the proteins translated from the RNA. The SV40 tumor or T antigen was one of the first to be associated with transformation by DNA viruses. It has been shown to be an early gene product since it is produced in the absence of virus DNA synthesis whereas the virus structural capsid proteins are not (Rapp *et al.*, 1965). It is produced in large quantities in infected and in transformed cells (Hoggan *et al.*, 1965). Yet its function is unknown. The attempts to isolate, purify, and characterize this antigen have failed to assign any specific function to it. Therefore, although its presence is the hallmark of a functioning virus genome in a transformed cell, the vexing problem of its role remains.

U antigen has also been shown to be an early protein produced during infection with SV40 virus (Lewis *et al.*, 1969); again, its function is not known. The production of the SV40 tumor-specific transplantation antigen (TSTA) has also been shown to be independent of virus DNA synthesis (Girardi and Defendi, 1970). Although this antigen, present in transformed cells, appears to take part in the rejection of transformed cells, its function in a normal lytic cycle of virus replication is not known.

Butel *et al.* (1972) present a good discussion of the immunology of these and other antigens present in virus-transformed cells.

2.4.2. Adenoviruses

Adenovirus DNA is known to be present in the nucleus of infected cells, and in all of the early tests the first detection of adenovirus gene products was also in the nucleus. However, Thomas and Green (1966) demonstrated that, like in the cell system, adenovirus mRNA is transported to the cytoplasm for translation into protein on cellular polyribosomes. Early experiments demonstrated that RNA synthesis was required for the production of virus DNA, virus antigens, and infectious virus particles (Flanagan and Ginsberg, 1964) and that the inhibition of protein synthesis at early times interfered with the replication of virus DNA and later virus development (Wilcox and Ginsberg, 1963; Polasa and Green, 1965). Concurrent protein synthesis was required for the continued production of virus DNA (Polasa and Green, 1965).

However, as we have seen previously with the papovavirus system, the function of these essential proteins has not been defined. An adenovirus tumor or T antigen, similar to that of SV40, was discovered in both infected and transformed cells (Huebner *et al.*, 1962; Hoggan *et al.*, 1965; Gilead and Ginsberg, 1968). The production of T antigen did not require virus DNA synthesis, which was required for the production of late capsid antigens (Gilead and Ginsberg, 1965; Feldman and Rapp, 1966). By immunofluorescence techniques, the T antigen appeared as nuclear or cytoplasmic flecks (Pope and Rowe, 1964; Feldman and Rapp, 1966), and with the electron microscope these areas appeared to be bundles of fibers and patches of fibrogranular material (Kalnins *et al.*, 1966). Again, the function of this material is not known.

Another antigen, called P, was discovered whose production did not require the synthesis of virus DNA (Russell *et al.*, 1967; Russell and Skehel, 1972). Since this antigen appears to be the core protein of the virus capsid, its properties will be discussed with those of the other late capsid proteins.

Vasconcelos-Costa *et al.* (1973) reported that early in adenovirus infection a new surface antigen similar to those detected on transformed cells is synthesized. Whether this antigen is similar to the previously detected transplantation rejection antigens (Trentin and Bryan, 1966; Sjögren *et al.*, 1967; Berman, 1967) is not known; the nature, site, and time of synthesis of these antigens are not known.

Therefore, as with the papovaviruses, early in the adenovirus replicative cycle new proteins are made which are required for the replication of the virus DNA and the production of infectious progeny virus. Again, isolation and characterization of these proteins have not yet been accomplished.

2.4.3. Herpesviruses

Most studies on protein synthesis with herpes simplex virus have not been separated into early and late stages. Since 19 of the 24 structural proteins are made from early mRNA (Frenkel and Roizman, 1972b), all of the studies of protein synthesis will be described in this section.

Early in herpesvirus infection, protein synthesis is inhibited. This is followed by a burst of virus-specific protein synthesis and then a decline as the cell dies. The early and late inhibition of protein synthesis is correlated with the breakdown of cell polyribosomes (Sydiskis and Roizman, 1966). Protein synthesis occurs in the cytoplasm, but the structural proteins are rapidly transferred into the nucleus, where they first appear in the soluble fraction and then are incorporated into virus capsids (Olshevsky et al., 1967). Although the first studies detected nine coat proteins (Olshevsky and Becker, 1970), more recent studies with polyacrylamide gels have detected at least 24 bands (Spear and Roizman, 1972). These polypeptide bands are produced in the cytoplasm and are selectively transported to the nucleus; three bands are restricted to the cytoplasm (Spear and Roizman, 1968). The proteins which remain in the cytoplasm bind to the cytoplasmic membranes and become glycosylated in situ (Spear and Roizman, 1970; Heine et al., 1972). These proteins eventually form part of the virus envelope.

Herpes simplex virus also appears to code for some enzymes involved in DNA synthesis, especially thymidine kinase and DNA polymerase (Roizman, 1969; Wildy, 1973).

2.5. Virus Control of Host Functions

2.5.1. Papovaviruses

Papovaviruses have been shown to stimulate rather than to depress host cell functions. SV40 stimulates the production of cellular mRNA but not ribosomal or transfer RNA (Oda and Dulbecco, 1968b). Various enzymes required in the synthesis of DNA are stimulated (Kit, 1968), as is cellular DNA synthesis (Tooze, 1973). This cellular DNA synthesis appears to be out of phase with normal synthesis (Smith, 1970; Tooze, 1973) and has led Levine and Burger (1972) to postulate that this asynchrony may be what maintains transformation of normal cells by papovaviruses. There is also a report that an early virus-specific function that parallels the appearance of T antigen activates or deinhibits the cellular regulatory element that governs chromosomal replication and mitosis; thus SV40 may act as a mitogen (May et al., 1973).

2.5.2. Adenoviruses

Although there are certain conditions in which adenoviruses induce cell DNA synthesis (Shimojo and Yamashita, 1968; Takahashi et al., 1969), the capsid antigens, especially fiber antigen and to a lesser extent hexon antigen, inhibit the function of DNA-dependent RNA polymerase and DNA polymerase (Levine and Ginsberg, 1968). Inhibition of host protein synthesis occurs shortly after initiation of synthesis of these virus capsid antigens (Bello and Ginsberg, 1967). Therefore, the late adenovirus gene products appear to depress cell metabolism.

2.5.3. Herpesviruses

Infection with herpes simplex virus produces an inhibition of cell macromolecular synthesis (Kaplan, 1973). There is a decreased rate of gross RNA synthesis as well as a decrease in the rate of synthesis and processing of ribosomal RNA (Wagner and Roizman, 1969b). Cellular polyribosomes are disaggregated and there is an inhibition of host protein synthesis (Sydiskis and Roizman, 1967). There may be a difference in the mechanisms of transcription in infected cells since cycloheximide will inhibit the production of virus mRNA but not host mRNA (Roizman et al., 1970).

2.6. Replication of Virus DNA

2.6.1. Papovaviruses

The DNA of the papovaviruses replicates in free, circular configurations in the nucleus of the infected cells and not as integrated units with the cell DNA. The replicative intermediates (RI) are circular molecules with two branch points and three branches (Hirt, 1969; Bourgaux et al., 1969; Levine et al., 1970). The earlier forms of the RI sediment faster than the later forms because the unreplicated region has enhanced tertiary structure due to supercoiling; the newly replicated regions increase in size as replication proceeds but are always equal in length (Jaenisch et al., 1971). During the process of DNA replication, the newly replicated strands are never covalently linked to the parental strands, thus excluding the rolling-circle model for DNA replication (Sebring et al., 1971). Since the parental strands are isolated as closed circles, there is no permanent nick introduced as a swivel point. Thus as replication proceeds the unreplicated parental region increases in the number of superhelical turns it possesses until it is impossible to unwind for replication. Therefore, Sebring et al. (1971) postulate that a temporary nick or single-strand break would be introduced as a swivel point to allow further replication to occur; since such nicked forms are not readily isolated, the time in this configuration would be very short.

From the digestion pattern produced with H. influenzae endonuclease on replicating SV40 DNA, Nathans and Danna (1972) have suggested that there is a single point of origin for the replication of SV40 DNA (at or near digest fragment C) and a single terminus (at or near digest fragments G and B). Thoren et al. (1972) have also determined that a single origin of replication exists for SV40 DNA because of the increase in the genetic complexity of the newly replicated DNA. Newly replicated single strands of SV40 DNA 10% and 85% replicated were isolated from replicative intermediates. DNA–DNA reassociation kinetics experiments were then performed based on the fact that the rate of reassociation is determined by the genetic complexity of the DNA. If there were random or at least several sites of initiation of replication on the DNA molecule, there would be no increase in genetic complexity with time and the rate of reassociation would be constant. If there were only one site of initiation, the genetic complexity of the replicating DNA would increase with time, causing a decrease in the rate of reassociation. The results were that as DNA replication proceeded from 10% to 85% the time required for 50% renaturation of the newly synthesized strands increased at a proportional rate. Therefore, the initiation occurred at a single unique site which generated new DNA segments as it replicated more DNA.

These results did not determine whether the replication was unidirectional or bidirectional. Experiments to determine this used the R_1 restriction endonuclease of *E. coli*, which makes one double-strand break in the SV40 DNA. This site was used to study the position of the origin and the two branch points. The R_1 cleavage site is near the terminus of DNA replication. If the replication is unidirectional, the origin and terminus of replication should be adjacent. If one proposes that the branch point nearest the cleavage site is stationary and the other branch moves as replication occurs, the cleavage site should be passed after about 83% of the molecule is replicated. If bidirectional replication occurs, both branches are growing in opposite directions and the cleavage site should be passed when 33% of the molecule is replicated. The results (Fareed *et al.*, 1972) showed that the R_1 cleavage site was 33% of the distance around the molecule and that both branches were growing points. Therefore, the replication of SV40 DNA begins at a unique site and proceeds in a bidirectional manner to a unique terminus.

Other experiments have shown that chain growth occurs in a discontinuous manner. SV40 DNA is made in short chains which are later joined together; these 4S fragments self-anneal so that both strands are involved (Fareed and Salzman, 1972). Similar 4S fragments are found when hydroxyurea is used to block the synthesis of polyoma virus DNA (Magnusson, 1973).

2.6.2. Adenoviruses

During the replication of adenovirus DNA, there are no circular forms. There are reports that adenovirus DNA may be replicated in a DNA–protein complex that may also include some RNA (Pearson and Hanawalt, 1971; Doerfler *et al.*, 1972). However, the replicative intermediates which have been isolated appear to be branched linear structures (Horwitz, 1971; van der Eb, 1973). There are no small fragments less than 10S in size (Horwitz, 1971) and no strands greater than genome length (Horwitz, 1971; van der Eb, 1973). However, peaks of various sizes of newly replicated fragments can be detected in sedimentation analysis studies, suggesting that certain-size intermediates accumulate at certain stages of the replication process (van der Eb, 1973). Studies with the electron microscope (van der Eb, 1973) have demonstrated two types of figures: branched Y-shaped linear structures which contain single-stranded DNA at the branching point, and sometimes one or more single-stranded regions on one of the arms, and also totally linear molecules which are double stranded, single stranded, or double stranded with single strand gaps. Further studies will be required to determine the exact mechanism of replication of this virus DNA.

2.6.3. Herpesviruses

There have been few studies on the molecular mechanisms involved in the replication of the herpesvirus DNA. Protein synthesis must precede the initiation of the replication of virus DNA, but after initiation it is not required for the continued production of progeny virus DNA (Roizman *et al.*, 1963; Roizman and Roane, 1965).

The most recent studies have concerned the possible uses for the alkali-labile regions of the herpesvirus DNA. These studies (Frenkel and Roizman, 1972*a*) have found that newly synthesized virus DNA produces more fragments than virion DNA and that the size of the fragments increases with time. These authors suggest that there are numerous sites for the initiation of virus DNA synthesis along each DNA strand and that the DNA is elongated by the addition of deoxyribonucleotides to the segments between the initiation sites. The adjacent segments are then linked together by some process which could involve ligation alone or ligation with the excision of some nucleotides to generate the limited number of unique fragments present in virion DNA; only maximally processed DNA is put into capsids to form the virions.

2.7. Transcription of Late Virus Messenger RNA

2.7.1. Papovaviruses

Late mRNA is that made after the initiation of synthesis of virus DNA. It is present in greater abundance than early mRNA because newly replicated progeny DNA molecules can take part in its production. Early studies had suggested that progeny virus DNA molecules were required for the production of the late mRNA and that perhaps late mRNA was transcribed only from the newly replicated molecules. However, the results obtained in a recent study (Cowan *et al.*, 1973) with a temperature-sensitive mutant of SV40 modify our understanding of the control of the synthesis of late mRNA. The SV40 temperature-sensitive mutant tsA30 has a mutation in the gene product which regulates the synthesis of virus DNA. Thus no virus DNA synthesis occurs at nonpermissive temperatures, although early mRNA is produced. If the mutant is kept at a permissive temperature so that the initiation of virus DNA synthesis and the production of late mRNA occur and is then shifted to nonpermissive temperature, the continued synthesis of virus DNA is rapidly shut off but late mRNA continues to be transcribed. Thus the function of the gene A product is required for the synthesis of late mRNA, but once this transcription is initiated it can continue without the further expression of the gene A product or the replication of virus DNA. These studies have not been able to determine whether some virus DNA synthesis is required for the initiation of late mRNA production or some modification of the DNA is all that is required.

Another study (Sauer, 1971) has shown that the control of the production of late mRNA differs in cells lytically infected with SV40 and in transformed cells. Although virus DNA synthesis is required for the production of late mRNA in lytically infected cells, late mRNA sequences are transcribed in transformed cells even when DNA synthesis is inhibited. This could reflect a difference in transcriptional control in the two systems or a difference in the physical state of the SV40 DNA.

In Section 2.3.1, it was noted that although early mRNA is produced only from the (−) strand of SV40, late mRNA has components transcribed from both the (+) and the (−) strands. It also appears that there is a difference in the size and processing of late mRNA as compared to the production of early mRNA.

If short pulses with a labeled marker are used late in the lytic infection of SV40 (Aloni, 1972; Fried, 1972) or polyoma (Aloni and Locker, 1973) virus, a double-stranded, self-annealing RNA can be detected. If the short pulse is followed by a chase, the amount of material resistant to RNase because of a double-stranded configuration decreases. Therefore, it appears that late in the infectious cycle of SV40 and polyoma virus the virus DNA is transcribed from both strands. Then some sequences from one or both strands are degraded for the production of late mRNA. There also seems to be a control mechanism to determine the stability of the primary double-stranded gene product, for some sequences have a shorter half-life in this configuration than other sequences. If one looks only for stable forms of virus-specific mRNA, the double-stranded intermediate is not detected.

From study of RNA made late in the infectious cycle, it appears that there is a difference in size between virus-specific RNA present in the nucleus and in that isolated from polyribosomes. Lindberg and Darnell (1970) showed that in transformed cells the nuclear virus-specific RNA was in a molecule larger than the entire SV40 genome, whereas the size of the virus-specific RNA isolated from polyribosomes was less than half the length of the SV40 genome. These investigators suggested that perhaps the larger nuclear form was precursor to the smaller polysomal form and that the nuclear species might have cell sequences attached. Other workers were able to demonstrate that in transformed cells the nuclear RNA contained both SV40 and host sequences while the polysomal molecules contained only SV40 sequences (Tonegawa et al., 1970; Wall and Darnell, 1971) and suggested that a selective cleavage mechanism may be used to produce SV40-specific mRNA.

Larger than genome length molecules were also found in the nuclei of infected cells late in the infectious cycle, whereas only smaller species were present in the cytoplasm (Martin and Byrne, 1970; Hudson et al., 1970; Tonegawa et al., 1970; Sokol and Carp, 1971; Acheson et al., 1971). Again, the larger nuclear species were shown to contain both host and SV40 sequences (Jaenisch, 1972; Rozenblatt and Winocour, 1972). Since SV40 particles containing both SV40 and host genetic material can be readily produced (see Section 2.2.1), plaque-purified virus in which no such substituted molecules could be detected were used to produce the infection. Again, RNA molecules containing both SV40 and host genetic information could readily be detected (Rozenblatt and Winocour, 1972). Therefore, it appears that such molecules arise from the cotranscription of integrated SV40 virus DNA and adjacent cell DNA. Since the size of early mRNA is much smaller than the genome length of SV40 (Martin and Byrne, 1970; Tonegawa *et al.*, 1970; Sokol and Carp, 1971), either early mRNA is made prior to integration of the virus DNA into the cell genome or the amounts of early mRNA are too small for detection of such a precursor form.

Sequences of poly(A) attached to SV40-specific RNA isolated from transformed cells and from lytically infected cells have also been detected (Weinberg *et al.*, 1972; Warnaar and de Mol, 1973). Since poly(A) sequences are not present on *in vitro* transcripts of SV40 DNA and no sequences of poly(T) are detected in the SV40 virion DNA when poly(U) is used as a probe, it is suggested that host cell enzymes add poly(A) to SV40 RNA as a post-transcriptional modification (Weinberg *et al.*, 1972).

2.7.2. Adenoviruses

There does not appear to be much difference in the production of early and late adenovirus mRNA except that more sites are available for transcription late in the infectious cycle; from 80 to 100% of the adenovirus genome is transcribed following the initiation of virus DNA replication (Fujinaga *et al.*, 1968). The expression of late virus genes thus appears to be controlled at two levels: the binding of RNA polymerase to new specific initiation sites not transcribed early and the formation of large precursor RNA molecules which are cleaved after transcription to produce the actual mRNA molecules. During a short pulse late in the infectious cycle, four species of virus RNA can be detected in the nucleus with sedimentation values between 36 and 43S (Parsons *et al.*, 1971). Following a chase, six to eight virus RNA species appear in the cytoplasm with sedimentation values of 10–29S. Hybridization experiments have shown that the smaller molecules arise from the larger by a process of cleavage.

There have been a number of interesting studies using *in vitro* techniques to study the transcription of late adenovirus mRNA. In one study (Brunner and Raskas, 1972), nuclei were isolated from infected cells late in the infectious cycle. Most of the adenovirus-specific RNA occurred as high molecular weight molecules. When the nuclei were incubated in the presence of ATP and an ATP-generating system, adenovirus-specific RNA the size of virus mRNA was released. The processing of the RNA did not appear to require exogenous ATP, but the subsequent release of the processed RNA did.

Another study (Wallace and Kates, 1972) isolated newly replicated adenovirus DNA from the nuclei of infected cells and found it to be slightly active in producing RNA *in vitro*. The RNA products were of high molecular weight and were adenovirus specific. The *in vitro* system required manganese ions and high salt concentrations and was inhibited by α-amanitin, features similar to those found in infected cells. There is also a report (Doerfler *et al.*, 1973) that late mRNA may be transcribed in a DNA–RNA complex which can be isolated from infected cells; both parental and newly replicated progeny virus DNA can be detected in such complexes.

2.7.3. Herpesviruses

The same types of transcriptional controls exist for late herpesvirus mRNA as for early mRNA: on–off control and abundance control. At times late in HSV-1 infection, 93.5% of the total virus-specific RNA transcribes 19–22% of the virus DNA and 6.5% transcribes 28–30% of the virus genome (Frenkel and Roizman, 1972*b*); thus a total of 48% of the HSV-1 genome is transcribed at late times and the abundant species at late times appear to contain all of the abundant species produced at early times, with transcription of some new species. In HSV-2 infection, 50% of the virus DNA is transcribed and this represents both abundant and scarce mRNA species (Frenkel *et al.*, 1973).

2.8. Translation of Late Virus Proteins

2.8.1. Papovaviruses

As with early protein synthesis, there is more known about the production of late mRNA with papovaviruses than about the translation products. The late proteins are first detected in the cell nucleus, although they are synthesized in the cytoplasm and transported to the nucleus. Since SV40 does not shut off cell protein synthesis, one must look for SV40-specific proteins while the cell continues to produce its own proteins. However, by use of polyacrylamide gels various components of the SV40 capsid have been detected as late proteins (Fischer and Sauer, 1972; Anderson and Gesteland, 1972; Walter *et al.*, 1972); their production is dependent on virus DNA synthesis. Other apparently virus-specific but nonvirion polypeptides have been detected but not characterized (Fischer and Sauer, 1972; Anderson and Gesteland, 1972; Walter *et al.*, 1972).

Other workers (Ozer and Tegtmeyer, 1972) have found that with short pulses of labeled amino acids, labeled material is incorporated into empty particles and then can be chased into full, mature particles. The inhibition of DNA synthesis late in the infection does not affect the continued synthesis of the empty particles, although it does inhibit formation of mature virions (Ozer, 1972). Thus the empty particles appear to serve as precursors to the intact full particles.

There is also some evidence that papovaviruses may pick up and carry cellular histones (Frearson and Crawford, 1972).

2.8.2. Adenoviruses

As mentioned previously, the production of late virus capsid antigens is dependent on the synthesis of virus DNA (Flanagan and Ginsberg, 1962). The morphological and structural units of the adenovirus capsid have been defined as hexon, penton, and fiber (Ginsberg *et al.*, 1966). Philipson and Pettersson (1973) have written a very good review of the structure and function of the various adenovirus virion proteins.

Adenovirus proteins are formed on 200S polyribosomes in the cytoplasm of the cell and the majority of these newly made polypeptide chains are transported into the nucleus within 6 min of their release and formed into the various virion morphological units (Velicer and Ginsberg, 1970). The various polypeptides are synthesized at different rates, rates which do not reflect the ratio in which they are found in the completed virion (White *et al.*, 1969); the penton base and fiber are made in considerable excess while the inner core is made in relatively short supply.

There are two species of arginine-rich proteins which make up the core protein (Prage *et al.*, 1968). These are detected if frozen and thawed virions are extracted with acid (Prage *et al.*, 1968) or if virions are allowed to "age" at 4°C (Russell and Knight, 1967). These form the P antigen mentioned previously (Russell *et al.*, 1967). If an infected cell is deprived of arginine, no infectious adenovirus progeny are produced (Rouse and Schlesinger, 1967). If arginine is added, there is no lag in the production of infectious virus. If DNA synthesis is inhibited as the arginine is added, infectious virus is still produced, suggesting that virus DNA synthesis occurs in the absence of arginine (Rouse and Schlesinger, 1967). There is an arginine-requiring step in the production of P antigen (Russell and Becker, 1968). Since virus DNA is made in the absence of arginine (Rouse and Schlesinger, 1967), it appears that P antigen is required for a step in virus maturation, perhaps to interact with virus DNA to facilitate its folding into the capsid.

Some recent studies suggest that there may be a processing step in the formation of the adenovirus virion. In one study (Anderson *et al.*, 1973), 22 virus-induced polypeptide components could be detected. Although most virion components were readily detected, several were absent. In a pulse-chase experiment, there was an increase in the production of two virion components parallel to a decrease in two nonvirion polypeptides. This suggests that a precursor–product relationship may exist and that at least two virion components are derived by cleavage of higher molecular weight precursor polypeptides; the change in molecular weight is not very great, so the cleavage process results in a conformational change, perhaps to control virus assembly, rather than in the separation of polypeptide products.

Sundquist *et al.* (1973) suggest that purified incomplete adenovirus particles contain some polypeptides not present in complete particles and lack some of the polypeptides associated with the core. These authors believe that the complete particles are assembled from the incomplete particles by a process of modification that requires active protein synthesis. Thus, with the adenoviruses, processing may occur both with the production of mRNA and with the assembly of mature virions.

2.8.3. Herpesviruses

Most (19 to 24) structural proteins of herpes simplex virus are made early in the infectious cycle (Frenkel and Roizman, 1972*b*), and very few studies of herpesvirus proteins have differentiated between early and late production. Therefore, herpesvirus protein synthesis is discussed in Section 2.4.3.

2.9. Induction of Virus

2.9.1. Papovaviruses

During the initial stages of cell transformation with SV40, the virus can frequently be isolated from cell cultures. However, as the cultures are passed it becomes progressively harder to isolate infectious virus (Black and Rowe, 1963). Thus it is generally impossible to isolate infectious virus from cells transformed with SV40, although there are a few lines which consistently produce small amounts of virus.

Various techniques have been used to try to induce virus from seemingly "virus-free" transformed cells. Inducers of lysogenic phage such as ultraviolet irradiation, mitomycin C, and 5-bromodeoxyuridine have been tried with varying success in a number of transformed cell lines (Rothschild and Black, 1970). The techniques that seemed to give the best result was cocultivation of transformed cells with cells permissive for the growth of the virus (Gerber and Kirschstein, 1962; Sabin and Koch, 1963; Black et al., 1963; Black and Rowe, 1963). It was then discovered that the intranuclear SV40 T antigen present in the transformed cell could be transferred to the susceptible cell but direct cell-to-cell contact was required (Gerber, 1966). By use of inactivated Sendai virus, heterokaryocytes could be produced from the transformed and permissive cells; this greatly increased the rate of recovery of infectious SV40 virus (Koprowski et al., 1967; Watkins and Dulbecco, 1967). In the heterokaryocytes, transmission of the SV40 T antigen could also be detected (Steplewski et al., 1968). The transfer of the SV40 T antigen was not sensitive to the inhibition of DNA synthesis but was inhibited if protein or RNA synthesis was blocked (Steplewski et al., 1968). Therefore, a simple process of diffusion could not explain the appearance of SV40 T antigen in the nuclei of susceptible cells. Weaver et al. (1970) performed detailed studies and found that newly formed SV40 virus was first detected in the nucleus of the transformed cell and then spread to the nucleus of the susceptible cell. Therefore, the nucleus of the transformed cell was the principal site of virus production and the induction process did not require the transfer of SV40 into the nucleus of the susceptible cell. In fact, the cytoplasm of the susceptible cell was enough to permit the induction of SV40 virus since infectious virus could be rescued from heterokaryon cultures made with transformed cells and enucleated permissive cells (Croce and Koprowski, 1973).

Other workers (Boyd and Butel, 1972) have shown that SV40 virus can be released from some previously nonyielder lines of transformed cells by isolating the DNA of the transformed cell and using it to infect permissive cells. The infectivity is recovered only with the high molecular weight cell DNA and thus no free SV40 DNA is detected. The mechanism to explain this transfer has not been found.

Studies with induction of polyoma virus have not yielded as much information because most polyoma virus–transformed lines produce small amounts of virus. Therefore, these studies show enhanced yields of virus rather than release of virus from previously "virus-free" cultures.

2.9.2. Adenoviruses

Use of techniques that work for the papovaviruses has not routinely accomplished the rescue of infectious adenovirus from adenovirus-transformed cells.

2.9.3. Herpesviruses

EB virus can readily be induced from "virus-free" cells by treating them with 5-bromodeoxyuridine (Gerber, 1972; Hampar *et al.*, 1972). Similar treatment causes the induction of virus antigens and particles in "virus-free" heterokaryons produced by fusion of EB virus–transformed cells and sternal marrow cells (Glaser and Rapp, 1972).

Changes in temperature have been shown to induce herpesvirus production in frog adenocarcinoma cells. Tumors found in frogs in late spring and summer produce no virus particles, whereas herpesvirus particles are readily detected in tumor cells of frogs during winter months (Rafferty, 1964). Frogs maintained in the laboratory at 20–25°C have tumors with no virus particles while frogs maintained at 7°C yield virus-producing tumors (Mizell *et al.*, 1969). Virus-free tumor cells maintained *in vitro* at 7.5°C begin to produce virus particles (Breidenbach *et al.*, 1971). Thus it appears that incubation at low temperatures is the principal factor in stimulating virus production. However, the actual mechanism of induction in this and the other virus systems remains unknown at this time.

3. Summary and Conclusions

The diverse DNA viruses discussed in this chapter have one thing in common: each is capable of changing a normal cell into a cell with neoplastic potential. Whether a common mechanism exists is yet unknown. Apparently, in each instance the incoming virus DNA is either integrated into or associated with the cellular DNA. With the smaller papovaviruses, the entire circular genome appears to be inserted. From the present studies with adenoviruses and herpesviruses, it appears that only fragments of virus DNA are inserted or associated with the cell genome and perhaps with different cell chromosomes. If this pattern of insertion is the correct one, it may explain the lower frequency of transformation by the larger DNA tumor viruses.

In all cells transformed by DNA tumor viruses, at least part of the virus genome is transcribed into mRNA. This mRNA is most often associated with early functions of the virus genome. At least a portion of the mRNA is transcribed into virus-specific proteins such as T antigens. Changes at the surface of the transformed cell are also detected, but more work is needed to determine whether these represent new proteins coded for by the virus genome or cellular proteins whose synthesis has been depressed. One of the large unresolved problems is the role, if any, that these newly detected proteins play in the transformation process.

The actual underlying mechanisms which control cell transformation are not understood. Does the strand-switching mechanism for the production of various mRNA species by the papovaviruses play a role in controlling which mRNA molecules will be produced? Do the alkali-labile regions of herpesvirus DNA have a role in cell transformation? Is the actual site of integration of virus genetic material important? All of these questions remain unanswered. However, it now appears that all DNA viruses which replicate in the nucleus are capable of inducing cell transformation under certain conditions. Whether this occurs under natural conditions will be the subject of much investigation in the next decade.

4. References

ACHESON, N. H., BUETTI, E., SCHERRER, K., AND WEIL, R., 1971, Transcription of the polyoma virus genome: Synthesis and cleavage of giant late polyoma–specific RNA, Proc. Natl. Acad. Sci. 68:2231

ADAMS, A., LINDAHL, T., AND KLEIN, G., 1973, Linear association between cellular DNA and Epstein–Barr virus DNA in a human lymphoblastoid cell line, Proc. Natl. Acad. Sci. 70:2888.

ALONI, Y., 1972, Extensive symmetrical transcription of simian virus 40 DNA in virus-yielding cells, Proc. Natl. Acad. Sci. 69:2404.

ALONI, Y., AND LOCKER, H., 1973, Symmetrical in vitro transcription of polyoma DNA and the separation of self-complementary viral and cell RNA, Virology 54:495.

ALONI, Y., WINOCOUR, E., AND SACHS, L., 1968, Characterization of the simian virus 40-specific RNA in virus-yielding and transformed cells, J. Mol. Biol. 31:415.

ALONI, Y., WINOCOUR, E., SACHS, L., AND TORTEN, J., 1969, Hybridization between SV40 DNA and cellular DNA's, J. Mol. Biol. 44:333.

ANDERSON, C. W., AND GESTELAND, R. F., 1972, Pattern of protein synthesis in monkey cells infected by simian virus 40, J. Virol. 9:758.

ANDERSON, C. W., BAUM, P. R., AND GESTELAND, R. F., 1973, Processing of adenovirus 2–induced proteins, J. Virol. 12:241.

ASTRIN, S. M., 1973, In vitro transcription of simian virus 40 sequences in SV3T3 chromatin, Proc. Natl. Acad. Sci. 70:2304.

AXELROD, D., HABEL, K., AND BOLTON, E. T., 1964, Polyoma virus genetic material in a virus-free polyoma-induced tumor, Science 146:1466.

BACHENHEIMER, S. L., AND ROIZMAN, B., 1972, Ribonucleic acid synthesis in cells infected with herpes simplex virus. VI. Polyadenylic acid sequences in viral messenger ribonucleic acid, J. Virol. 10:875.

BELLO, L. J., AND GINSBERG, H. S., 1967, Inhibition of host protein synthesis in type 5 adenovirus–infected cells, J. Virol. 1:843.

BENJAMIN, T. L., 1966, Virus-specific RNA in cells productively infected or transformed by polyoma virus, J. Mol. Biol. 16:359.

BERMAN, L. D., 1967, On the nature of transplantation immunity in the adenovirus tumor system, J. Exp. Med. 125:983.

BLACK, P. H., AND ROWE, W. P., 1963, An analysis of SV40-induced transformation of hamster kidney tissue in vitro. I. General characteristics, Proc. Natl. Acad. Sci. 50:606.

BLACK, P. H., ROWE, W. P., AND COOPER, H. L., 1963, An analysis of SV40-induced transformation of hamster kidney tissue in vitro. II. Studies of three clones derived from a continuous line of transformed cells, Proc. Natl. Acad. Sci. 50:847.

BOURGAUX, P., BOURGAUX-RAMOISY, D., AND DULBECCO, R., 1969, The replication of the ring-shaped DNA of polyoma virus. I. Identification of the replicative intermediate, Proc. Natl. Acad. Sci. 64:701.

BOYD, V. A. L., AND BUTEL, J. S., 1972, Demonstration of infectious deoxyribonucleic acid in transformed cells. I. Recovery of simian virus 40 from yielder and nonyielder transformed cells, *J. Virol.* **10**:399.

BREIDENBACH, G. P., SKINNER, N. S., WALLACE, J. H., AND MIZELL, M., 1971, *In vitro* induction of a herpes-type virus in "summer phase" Lucké tumor explants, *J. Virol.* **7**:679.

BROCKMAN, W. W., LEE, T. N. H., AND NATHANS, D., 1973, The evolution of new species of viral DNA during serial passage of simian virus 40 at high multiplicity, *Virology* **54**:384.

BRUNNER, M., AND RASKAS, H. J., 1972, Processing of adenovirus RNA before release from isolated nuclei, *Proc. Natl. Acad. Sci.* **69**:3101.

BUTEL, J. S., TEVETHIA, S. S., AND MELNICK, J. L., 1972, Oncogenicity and cell transformation by papovavirus SV40: The role of the viral genome, *Advan. Cancer Res.* **15**:1.

CARP, R. I., SAUER, G., AND SOKOL, F., 1969, The effect of actinomycin D on the transcription and replication of simian virus 40 deoxyribonucleic acid, *Virology* **37**:214.

COLLARD, W., THORNTON, H., AND GREEN, M., 1973, Cells transformed by human herpesvirus type 2 transcribe virus-specific RNA sequences shared by herpesvirus types 1 and 2, *Nature New Biol.* **243**:264.

COLLINS, C. J., AND SAUER, G., 1972, Fate of infecting simian virus 40–deoxyribonucleic acid in nonpermissive cells: Integration into host deoxyribonucleic acid, *J. Virol.* **10**:425.

COWAN, K., TEGTMEYER, P., AND ANTHONY, D. D., 1973, Relationship of replication and transcription of simian virus 40 DNA, *Proc. Natl. Acad. Sci.* **70**:1927.

CROCE, C. M., AND KAPROWSKI, H., 1973, Enucleation of cells made simple and rescue of SV40 by enucleated cells made even simpler, *Virology* **51**:227.

DALES, S., 1973, Early events in cell–animal virus interactions, *Bacteriol. Rev.* **37**:103.

DARNELL, J. E., PHILIPSON, L., WALL, R., AND ADESNIK, M., 1971, Polyadenylic acid sequences: Role in conversion of nuclear RNA into messenger RNA, *Science* **174**:507.

DOERFLER, W., 1968, The fate of the DNA of adenovirus type 12 in baby hamster kidney cells, *Proc. Natl. Acad. Sci.* **60**:636.

DOERFLER, W., 1970a, Denaturation pattern of the DNA of adenovirus type 2 as determined by electron microscopy, *J. Mol. Biol.* **50**:579.

DOERFLER, W., 1970b, Integration of the deoxyribonucleic acid of adenovirus type 12 into the deoxyribonucleic acid of baby hamster kidney cells, *J. Virol.* **6**:652.

DOERFLER, W., LUNDHOLM, U., AND HIRSCH-KAUFFMANN, M., 1972, Intracellular forms of adenovirus deoxyribonucleic acid. I. Evidence for a deoxyribonucleic acid–protein complex in baby hamster kidney cells infected with adenovirus type 12, *J. Virol.* **9**:297.

DOERFLER, W., LUNDHOLM, U., RENSING, U., AND PHILIPSON, L., 1973, Intracellular forms of adenovirus DNA. II. Isolation in dye–buoyant density gradients of a DNA–RNA complex from KB cells infected with adenovirus type 2, *J. Virol.* **12**:793.

DUNN, A. R., GALLIMORE, P. H., JONES, K. W., AND MCDOUGALL, J. K., 1973, *In situ* hybridization of adenovirus RNA and DNA. II. Detection of adenovirus-specific DNA in transformed and tumor cells, *Int. J. Cancer* **11**:628.

FAREED, G. C., AND SALZMAN, N. P., 1972, Intermediate in SV40 DNA chain growth, *Nature New Biol.* **238**:274.

FAREED, G. C., GARON, C. F., AND SALZMAN, N. P., 1972, Origin and direction of simian virus 40 deoxyribonucleic acid replication, *J. Virol.* **10**:484.

FELDMAN, L. A., AND RAPP, F., 1966, Inhibition of adenovirus replication by 1-β-D-arabinofuranosylcytosine, *Proc. Soc. Exp. Biol. Med.* **122**:243.

FISCHER, H., AND SAUER, G., 1972, Identification of virus-induced proteins in cells productively infected with simian virus 40, *J. Virol.* **9**:1.

FLANAGAN, J. F., AND GINSBERG, H. S., 1962, Synthesis of virus-specific polymers in adenovirus-infected cells: Effect of 5-fluorodeoxyuridine, *J. Exp. Med.* **116**:157.

FLANAGAN, J. F., AND GINSBERG, H. S., 1964, Role of ribonucleic acid biosynthesis in multiplication of type 5 adenovirus, *J. Bacteriol.* **87**:987.

FREARSON, P. M., AND CRAWFORD, L. V., 1972, Polyoma virus basic proteins, *J. Gen. Virol.* **14**:141.

FRENKEL, N., AND ROIZMAN, B., 1971, Herpes simplex virus: Genome size and redundancy studied by renaturation kinetics, *J. Virol.* **8**:591.

FRENKEL, N., AND ROIZMAN, B., 1972a, Separation of the herpesvirus deoxyribonucleic acid duplex into unique fragments and intact strand on sedimentation in alkaline gradients, *J. Virol.* **10**:565.

FRENKEL, N., AND ROIZMAN, B., 1972b, Ribonucleic acid synthesis in cells infected with herpes simplex virus: Control of transcription and of RNA abundance, *Proc. Natl. Acad. Sci.* **69:**2654.

FRENKEL, N., SILVERSTEIN, S., CASSAI, E., AND ROIZMAN, B., 1973, RNA synthesis in cells infected with herpes simplex virus. VII. Control of transcription and of transcript abundances of unique and common sequences of herpes simplex virus 1 and 2, *J. Virol.* **11:**886.

FRIED, A. H., 1972, Density heterogeneity of simian virus 40 ribonucleic acid late after infection of permissive cells, *J. Virol.* **10:**1236.

FUJINAGA, K., AND GREEN, M., 1966, The mechanism of viral carcinogenesis by DNA mammalian viruses: Viral-specific RNA in polyribosomes of adenovirus tumor and transformed cells, *Proc. Natl. Acad. Sci.* **55:**1567.

FUJINAGA, K., AND GREEN, M., 1967a, Mechanism of viral carcinogenesis by DNA mammalian viruses. II. Viral-specific RNA in tumor cells induced by "weakly oncogenic" human adenoviruses, *Proc. Natl. Acad. Sci.* **57:**806.

FUJINAGA, K., AND GREEN, M., 1967b, Mechanism of viral carcinogenesis by deoxyribonucleic acid mammalian viruses. IV. Related virus-specific ribonucleic acids in human cells induced by "highly" oncogenic adenovirus types 12, 18, and 31, *J. Virol.* **1:**576.

FUJINAGA, K., AND GREEN, M., 1968, Mechanism of viral carcinogenesis by DNA mammalian viruses. V. Properties of purified viral-specific RNA from human adenovirus-induced tumor cells, *J. Mol. Biol.* **31:**63.

FUJINAGA, K., AND GREEN, M., 1970, Mechanism of viral carcinogenesis by DNA mammalian viruses. VII. Viral genes transcribed in adenovirus type 2 infected and transformed cells, *Proc. Natl. Acad. Sci.* **65:**375.

FUJINAGA, K., MAK, S., AND GREEN, M., 1968, A method for determining the fraction of the viral genome transcribed during infection and its application to adenovirus-infected cells, *Proc. Natl. Acad. Sci.* **60:**959.

FUJINAGA, K., PIÑA, M., AND GREEN, M., 1969, The mechanism of viral carcinogenesis by DNA mammalian viruses. VI. A new class of virus-specific RNA molecules in cells transformed by group C human adenoviruses, *Proc. Natl. Acad. Sci.* **64:**255.

GELB, L. D., AND MARTIN, M. A., 1973, Simian virus 40 DNA integration within the genome of virus-transformed mammalian cells, *Virology* **51:**351.

GELB, L. D., KOHNE, D. E., AND MARTIN, M. A., 1971, Quantitation of simian virus 40 sequences in African green monkey, mouse, and virus-transformed cell genomes, *J. Mol. Biol.* **57:**129.

GERBER, P., 1966, Studies on the transfer of subviral infectivity from SV40-induced hamster tumor cells to indicator cells, *Virology* **28:**501.

GERBER, P., 1972, Activation of Epstein–Barr virus by 5-bromodeoxyuridine in "virus-free" human cells, *Proc. Natl. Acad. Sci.* **69:**83.

GERBER, P., AND KIRSCHSTEIN, R. L., 1962, SV40-induced ependymomas in newborn hamsters. I. Virus–tumor relationships, *Virology* **18:**582.

GILEAD, Z., AND GINSBERG, H. S., 1965, Characterization of a tumorlike antigen in type 12 and type 18 adenovirus–infected cells, *J. Bacteriol.* **90:**120.

GILEAD, Z., AND GINSBERG, H. S., 1968, Characterization of the tumorlike (T) antigen induced by type 12 adenovirus. I. Purification of the antigen from infected KB cells and a hamster tumor cell line, *J. Virol.* **2:**7.

GINSBERG, H. S., PEREIRA, H. G., VALENTINE, R. C., AND WILCOX, W. C., 1966, A proposed terminology for the adenovirus antigens and virion morphological subunits, *Virology* **28:**782.

GIRARDI, A. J., AND DEFENDI, V., 1970, Induction of SV40 transplantation antigen (TrAg) during the lytic cycle, *Virology* **42:**688.

GLASER, R., AND RAPP, F., 1972, Rescue of Epstein–Barr virus from somatic cell hybrids of Burkitt lymphoblastoid cells, *J. Virol.* **10:**288.

GORDIN, M., OLSHEVSKY, U., ROSENKRANZ, H. S., AND BECKER, Y., 1973, Studies on herpes simplex virus DNA: Denaturation properties, *Virology* **55:**280.

GREEN, M., PARSONS, J. T., PIÑA, M., FUJINAGA, K., CAFFIER, H., AND LANDGRAF-LEURS, I., 1970, Transcription of adenovirus genes in productively infected and in transformed cells, *Cold Spring Harbor Symp. Quant. Biol.* **35:**803.

GROSS, L., 1970, *Oncogenic Viruses*, 2nd ed., Pergamon Press, New York.

HAMPAR, B., DERGE, J. G., MARTOS, L. M., AND WALKER, J. L., 1972, Synthesis of Epstein–Barr virus after activation of the viral genome in a "virus-negative" human lymphoblastoid cell (Raji) made resistant to 5-bromodeoxyuridine, *Proc. Natl. Acad. Sci.* **69:**78.

HEINE, J. W., SPEAR, P. G., AND ROIZMAN, B., 1972, Proteins specified by herpes simplex virus. VI. Viral proteins in the plasma membrane, *J. Virol.* **9**:431.

HIRAI, K., AND DEFENDI, V., 1972, Integration of simian virus 40 deoxyribonucleic acid into the deoxyribonucleic acid of permissive monkey kidney cells, *J. Virol.* **9**:705.

HIRAI, K., LEHMAN, J., AND DEFENDI, V., 1971, Integration of simian virus 40 deoxyribonucleic acid into the deoxyribonucleic acid of primary infected Chinese hamster cells, *J. Virol.* **8**:708.

HIRT, B., 1969, Replicating molecules of polyoma virus DNA, *J. Mol. Biol.* **40**:141.

HOGGAN, M. D., ROWE, W. P., BLACK, P. H., AND HUEBNER, R. J., 1965, Production of "tumor-specific" antigens by oncogenic viruses during acute cytolytic infections, *Proc. Natl. Acad. Sci.* **53**:12.

HORWITZ, M. S., 1971, Intermediates in the synthesis of type 2 adenovirus deoxyribonucleic acid, *J. Virol.* **8**:675.

HUDSON, J., GOLDSTEIN, D., AND WEIL, R., 1970, A study on the transcription of the polyoma viral genome, *Proc. Natl. Acad. Sci.* **65**:226.

HUEBNER, R. J., ROWE, W. P., AND LANE, W. T., 1962, Oncogenic effects in hamsters of human adenovirus types 12 and 18, *Proc. Natl. Acad. Sci.* **48**:2051.

HUEBNER, R. J., ROWE, W. P., TUTNER, H. C., AND LANE, W. T., 1963, Specific adenovirus complement-fixing antigens in virus-free hamster and rat tumors, *Proc. Natl. Acad. Sci.* **50**:379.

JAENISCH, R., 1972, Evidence for SV40 specific RNA containing virus and host specific sequences, *Nature New Biol.* **235**:46.

JAENISCH, R., MAYER, A., AND LEVINE, A., 1971, Replicating SV40 molecules containing closed circular template DNA strands, *Nature New Biol.* **233**:72.

KALNINS, V. I., STICH, H. F., AND YOHN, D. S., 1966, Electron microscopic localization of virus-associated antigens in human amnion cells (AV-3) infected with human adenovirus, type 12, *Virology* **28**:751.

KAPLAN, A. S., 1973, A brief review of the biochemistry of herpesvirus–host cell interaction, *Cancer Res.* **33**:1393.

KHOURY, G., AND MARTIN, M. M., 1972, Comparison of SV40 DNA transcription *in vivo* and *in vitro*, *Nature New Biol.* **238**:4.

KHOURY, G., BYRNE, J. C., AND MARTIN, M. A., 1972, Patterns of simian virus 40 DNA transcription after acute infection of permissive and nonpermissive cells, *Proc. Natl. Acad. Sci.* **69**:1925.

KHOURY, G., BYRNE, J. C., TAKEMOTA, K. K., AND MARTIN, M. A., 1973, Patterns of simian virus 40 deoxyribonucleic acid transcription II in transformed cells, *J. Virol.* **11**:54.

KIEFF, E. D., BACHENHEIMER, S. L., AND ROIZMAN, B., 1971, Size, composition, and structure of the deoxyribonucleic acid of herpes simplex virus subtypes 1 and 2, *J. Virol.* **8**:125.

KIT, S., 1968, Viral-induced enzymes and the problem of viral oncogenesis, *Advan. Cancer Res.* **11**:73.

KOPROWSKI, H., JENSON, F. C., AND STEPLEWSKI, Z., 1967, Activation of production of infectious tumor virus SV40 in heterokaryon cultures, *Proc. Natl. Acad. Sci.* **58**:127.

LAVI, S., AND WINOCOUR, E., 1972, Acquisition of sequences homologous to host deoxyribonucleic acid by closed circular simian virus 40 deoxyribonucleic acid, *J. Virol.* **9**:309.

LAVI, S., ROZENBLATT, S., SINGER, M. F., AND WINOCOUR, E., 1973, Acquisition of sequences homologous to host DNA by closed circular simian virus 40 DNA. II. Further studies on the serial passage of virus clones, *J. Virol.* **12**:492.

LEE, L. F., KIEFF, E. D., BACHENHEIMER, S. L., ROIZMAN, B., SPEAR, P. G., BURMESTER, B. R., AND NAZERIAN, K., 1971, Size and composition of Marek's disease virus deoxyribonucleic acid, *J. Virol.* **7**:289.

LEVINE, A. J., AND BURGER, M. M., 1972, A working hypothesis explaining the maintenance of the transformed state by SV40 and polyoma, *J. Theoret. Biol.* **37**:435.

LEVINE, A. J., AND GINSBERG, H. S., 1968, Role of adenovirus structural proteins in the cessation of host-cell biosynthetic functions, *J. Virol.* **2**:430.

LEVINE, A. J., AND TERESKY, A. K., 1970, Deoxyribonucleic acid replication in simian virus 40–infected cells. II. Detection and characterization of simian virus 40 pseudovirions, *J. Virol.* **5**:451.

LEVINE, A. J., KANG, H. S., AND BILLHEIMER, F. E., 1970, DNA replication in SV40 infected cells. I. Analysis of replicating SV40 DNA, *J. Mol. Biol.* **50**:549.

LEWIS, A. M., JR., LEVIN, M. J., WIESE, W. H., CRUMPACKER, C. S., AND HENRY, P. H., 1969, A nondefective (competent) adenovirus–SV40 hybrid isolated from the Ad. 2–SV40 hybrid population, *Proc. Natl. Acad. Sci.* **63**:1128.

LINDBERG, U., AND DARNELL, J. E., 1970, SV40-specific RNA in the nucleus and polyribosomes of transformed cells, *Proc. Natl. Acad. Sci.* **65**:1089.

LINDBERG, U., PERSSON, T., AND PHILIPSON, L., 1972, Isolation and characterization of adenovirus messenger ribonucleic acid in productive infection, *J. Virol.* **10**:909.

LINDSTROM D. M., AND DULBECCO, R., 1972, Strand orientation of simian virus 40 transcription in productively infected cells, *Proc. Natl. Acad. Sci.* **69**:1517.

LUCAS, J. J., AND GINSBERG, H. S., 1971, Synthesis of virus-specific ribonucleic acid in KB cells infected with type 2 adenovirus, *J. Virol.* **8**:203.

MAGNUSSON, G., 1973, Hydroxyurea-induced accumulation of short fragments during polyoma DNA replication. I. Characterization of fragments, *J. Virol.* **12**:600.

MARTIN, M. A., 1970, Characteristics of SV40 DNA transcription during lytic infection, abortive infection and in transformed mouse cells, *Cold Spring Harbor Symp. Quant. Biol.* **35**:833.

MARTIN, M. A., AND AXELROD, D., 1969a, Polyoma virus gene activity during lytic infection and in transformed animal cells, *Science* **164**:68.

MARTIN, M. A., AND AXELROD, D., 1969b, SV40 gene activity during lytic infection and in a series of SV40 transformed mouse cells, *Proc. Natl. Acad. Sci.* **64**:1203.

MARTIN, M. A., AND BYRNE, J. C., 1970, Sedimentation properties of simian virus 40–specific ribonucleic acid present in green monkey cells during productive infection and in mouse cells undergoing abortive infection, *J. Virol.* **6**:463.

MARTIN, M. A., GELB, L. D., FAREED, G. C., AND MILSTIEN, J. B., 1973, Reassortment of simian virus 40 DNA during serial undiluted passage, *J. Virol.* **12**:748.

MAY, E., MAY, P., AND WEIL, R., 1973, "Early" virus-specific RNA may contain information necessary for chromosome replication and mitosis induced by simian virus 40, *Proc. Natl. Acad. Sci.* **70**:1654.

McGUIRE, P. M., SWART, C., AND HODGE, L. D., 1972, Adenovirus messenger RNA in mammalian cells: Failure of polyribosome association in the absence of nuclear cleavage, *Proc. Natl. Acad. Sci.* **69**:1578.

MICHEL, M. R., HIRT, B., AND WEIL, R., 1967, Mouse cellular DNA enclosed in polyoma viral capsids (pseudovirions), *Proc. Natl. Acad. Sci.* **58**:1381.

MIZELL, M., STACKPOLE, C. W., AND ISAACS, J. J., 1969, Herpestype virus latency in the Lucké tumor, in: *Biology of Amphibian Tumors* (M. Mizell, ed.), pp. 337–347, special supplement to *Recent Results in Cancer Research*, Springer, New York.

NATHANS, D., AND DANNA, K. J., 1972, Specific origin in SV40 DNA replication, *Nature New Biol.* **236**:200.

NAZERIAN, K., LINDAHL, T., KLEIN, G., AND LEE, L. F., 1973, Deoxyribonucleic acid of Marek's disease virus in virus-induced tumors, *J. Virol.* **12**:841.

NONOYAMA, M., AND PAGANO, J. S., 1971, Detection of Epstein–Barr viral genome in nonproductive cells, *Nature New Biol.* **233**:103.

NONOYAMA, M., AND PAGANO, J. S., 1972, Separation of Epstein–Barr virus DNA from large chromosomal DNA in non-virus-producing cells, *Nature New Biol.* **238**:169.

ODA, K., AND DULBECCO, R., 1968a, Regulation of transcription of the SV40 DNA in productively infected and in transformed cells, *Proc. Natl. Acad. Sci.* **60**:525.

ODA, K., AND DULBECCO, R., 1968b, Induction of cellular mRNA synthesis in BSC-1 cells infected by SV40, *Virology* **35**:439.

OLSHEVSKY, U., AND BECKER, Y., 1970, Herpes simplex virus structural proteins, *Virology* **40**:948.

OLSHEVSKY, U., LEVITT, J., AND BECKER, Y., 1967, Studies on the synthesis of herpes simplex virions, *Virology* **33**:323.

OZANNE, B., SHARP, P. A., AND SAMBROOK, J., 1973, Transcription of simian virus 40. II. Hybridization of RNA extracted from different lines of transformed cells to the separated strands of simian virus 40 DNA, *J. Virol.* **12**:90.

OZER, H. L., 1972, Synthesis and assembly of simian virus 40. I. Differential synthesis of intact virions and empty shells, *J. Virol.* **9**:41.

OZER, H. L., AND TEGTMEYER, P., 1972, Synthesis and assembly of simian virus 40. II. Synthesis of the major capsid protein and its incorporation into viral particles, *J. Virol.* **9**:52.

PARSONS, J. T., AND GREEN, M., 1971, Biochemical studies on adenovirus multiplication. XVIII. Resolution of early virus-specific RNA species in ad 2 infected and transformed cells, *Virology* **45**:154.

PARSONS, J. T., GARDNER, J., AND GREEN, M., 1971, Biochemical studies of adenovirus multiplication. XIX. Resolution of late viral RNA species in the nucleus and cytoplasm, *Proc. Natl. Acad. Sci.* **68**:557.

PEARSON, G. D., AND HANAWALT, P. C., 1971, Isolation of DNA replication complexes from uninfected and adenovirus-infected HeLa cells, *J. Mol. Biol.* **62**:65.

PHILIPSON, L., AND PETTERSSON, U., 1973, Structure and function of virion proteins of adenoviruses, *Prog. Exp. Tumor Res.* **18**:1.

PHILIPSON, L., WALL, R., GLICKMAN, G., AND DARNELL, J. E., 1971, Addition of polyadenylate sequences to virus-specific RNA during adenovirus replication, *Proc. Natl. Acad. Sci.* **68**:2806.

POLASA, H., AND GREEN, M., 1965, Biochemical studies on adenovirus multiplication. VIII. Analysis of protein synthesis, *Virology* **25**:68.

POPE, J. H., AND ROWE, W. P., 1964, Immunofluorescent studies of adenovirus 12 tumors and of cells transformed or infected by adenoviruses, *J. Exp. Med.* **120**:577.

PRAGE, L., PETTERSSON, U., AND PHILIPSON, L., 1968, Internal basic proteins in adenovirus, *Virology* **36**:508.

PRICE, R., AND PENMAN, S., 1972, Transcription of the adenovirus genome by an α-amanitine-sensitive ribonucleic acid polymerase in HeLa cells, *J. Virol.* **9**:621.

RAFFERTY, K. A., JR., 1964, Kidney tumors of the leopard frog: A review, *Cancer Res.* **24**:169.

RALPH, R. K., AND COLTER, J. S., 1972, Evidence for the integration of polyoma virus DNA in a lytic system, *Virology* **48**:49.

RAPP, F., MELNICK, J. L., AND KITAHARA, T., 1965, Tumor and virus antigens of simian virus 40: Differential inhibition of synthesis by cytosine arabinoside, *Science* **147**:625.

REICH, P. R., BLACK, P. H., AND WEISSMAN, S. M., 1966, Nucleic acid homology studies of SV40 virus–transformed and normal hamster cells, *Proc. Natl. Acad. Sci.* **56**:78.

ROIZMAN, B., 1969, The herpesviruses—A biochemical definition of the group, *Curr. Topics Micros. Immunol.* **49**:1.

ROIZMAN, B., AND FRENKEL, N., 1973, The transcription and state of herpes simplex virus DNA in productive infection and in human cervical cancer tissue, *Cancer Res.* **33**:1402.

ROIZMAN, B., AND ROANE, P. R., JR., 1965, The multiplication of herpes simplex virus. II. The relation between protein synthesis and the duplication of viral DNA in infected HEp-2 cells, *Virology* **22**:262.

ROIZMAN, B., AURELIAN, L., AND ROANE, P. R., JR., 1963, The multiplication of herpes simplex virus. I. The programming of viral DNA duplication in HEp-2 cells, *Virology* **21**:482.

ROIZMAN, B., BACHENHEIMER, S., WAGNER, E. K., AND SAVAGE, T., 1970, Synthesis and transport of RNA in herpesvirus-infected mammalian cells, *Cold Spring Harbor Symp. Quant. Biol.* **35**:753.

ROTHSCHILD, H., AND BLACK, P. H., 1970, Analysis of SV40-induced transformation of hamster kidney tissue *in vitro*. VII. Induction of SV40 virus from transformed hamster cell clones by various agents, *Virology* **42**:251.

ROUSE, H. C., AND SCHLESINGER, R. W., 1967, An arginine-dependent step in the maturation of type 2 adenovirus, *Virology* **33**:513.

ROZENBLATT, S., AND WINOCOUR, E., 1972, Covalently linked cell and SV40-specific sequences in an RNA from productively infected cells, *Virology* **50**:558.

ROZENBLATT, S., LAVI, S., SINGER, M. F., AND WINOCOUR, E., 1973, Acquisition of sequences homologous to host DNA by closed circular simian virus 40 DNA. III. Host sequences, *J. Virol.* **12**:501.

RUSSELL, W. C., AND BECKER, Y., 1968, A maturation factor for adenovirus, *Virology* **35**:18.

RUSSELL, W. C., AND KNIGHT, B. E., 1967, Evidence for a new antigen within the adenovirus capsid, *J. Gen. Virol.* **1**:523.

RUSSELL, W. C., AND SKEHEL, J. J., 1972, The polypeptides of adenovirus-infected cells, *J. Gen. Virol.* **15**:45.

RUSSELL, W. C., HAYASHI, K., SANDERSON, P. J., AND PEREIRA, H. G., 1967, Adenovirus antigens—A study of their properties and sequential development in infection, *J. Gen. Virol.* **1**:495.

SABIN, A. B., AND KOCH, M. A., 1963, Behavior of noninfectious SV40 viral genome in hamster tumor cells: Induction of synthesis of infectious virus, *Proc. Natl. Acad. Sci.* **50**:407.

SAMBROOK, J., 1972, Transformation by polyoma virus and simian virus 40, *Advan. Cancer Res.* **16**:141.

SAMBROOK, J., WESTPHAL, H., SRINIVASAN, P. R., AND DULBECCO, R., 1968, The integrated state of viral DNA in SV40-transformed cells, *Proc. Natl. Acad. Sci.* **60**:1288.

SAMBROOK, J., SHARP, P. A., AND KELLER, W., 1972, Transcription of simian virus 40. I. Separation of the strands of SV40 DNA and hybridization of the separated strands to RNA extracted from lytically infected and transformed cells, *J. Mol. Biol.* **70**:57.

SAUER, G., 1971, Apparent differences in transcriptional control in cells productively infected and transformed by SV40, *Nature New Biol.* **22**:135.

SAUER, G., AND KIDWAI, J. R., 1968, The transcription of the SV40 genome in productively infected and transformed cells, *Proc. Natl. Acad. Sci.* **61**:1256.

SEBRING, E. D., KELLY, T. J., JR., THOREN, M. M., AND SALZMAN, N. P., 1971, Structure of replicating simian virus 40 deoxyribonucleic acid molecules, *J. Virol.* **8:**478.

SHIMOJO, H., AND YAMASHITA, T., 1968, Introduction of DNA synthesis by adenoviruses in contact inhibited hamster cells, *Virology* **36:**422.

SIEGEL, S. E., AND LEVINE, A. S., 1972, Virus-specific nucleic acids in simian virus 40–transformed hamster cell clones varying in oncogenic potential, *J. Natl. Cancer Inst.* **49:**1667.

SILVERSTEIN, S., BACHENHEIMER, S. L., FRENKEL, N., AND ROIZMAN, B., 1973, Relationship between post-transcriptional adenylation of herpesvirus RNA and messenger RNA abundance, *Proc. Natl. Acad. Sci.* **70:**2101.

SJÖGREN, H. O., MINOWADA, J., AND ANKERST, J., 1967, Specific transplantation antigens of mouse sarcomas induced by adenovirus type 12, *J. Exp. Med.* **125:**689.

SMITH, B. J., 1970, Light satellite-band DNA in mouse cells infected with polyoma virus, *J. Mol. Biol.* **47:**101.

SOKOL, F., AND CARP, R. I., 1971, Molecular size of simian virus 40–specific RNA synthesized in productively infected cells, *J. Gen. Virol.* **11:**177.

SPEAR, P. G., AND ROIZMAN, B., 1968, The proteins specified by herpes simplex virus. I. Time of synthesis, transfer into nuclei, and properties of proteins made in productively infected cells, *Virology* **36:**545.

SPEAR, P. G., AND ROIZMAN, B., 1970, Proteins specified by herpes simplex virus. IV. Site of glycosylation and accumulation of viral membrane proteins, *Proc. Natl. Acad. Sci.* **66:**730.

SPEAR, P. G., AND ROIZMAN, B., 1972, Proteins specified by herpes simplex virus. V. Purification and structural proteins of the herpesvirion, *J. Virol.* **9:**143.

STEPLEWSKI, Z., KNOWLES, B. B., AND KOPROWSKI, H., 1968, The mechanism of intranuclear transmission of SV40-induced complement fixation antigen in heterokaryocytes, *Proc. Natl. Acad. Sci.* **59:**769.

SUNDQUIST, B., EVERITT, E., PHILIPSON, L., AND HOGLUND, S., 1973, Assembly of adenoviruses, *J. Virol.* **11:**449.

SYDISKIS, R. J., AND ROIZMAN, B., 1966, Polysomes and protein synthesis in cells infected with a DNA virus, *Science* **153:**76.

SYDISKIS, R. J., AND ROIZMAN, B., 1967, The disaggregation of host polyribosomes in productive and abortive infection with herpes simplex virus, *Virology* **32:**678.

TAI, H. T., AND O'BRIEN, R. L., 1969, Multiplicity of viral genomes in an SV40 transformed hamster cell line, *Virology* **38:**698.

TAI, H. T., SMITH, C. A., SHARP, P. A., AND VINOGRAD, J., 1972, Sequence heterogeneity is closed simian virus 40 deoxyribonucleic acid, *J. Virol.* **9:**317.

TAKAHASHI, M., OGINO, T., BABA, K., AND ONAKA, M., 1969, Synthesis of deoxyribonucleic acid in human and hamster kidney cells infected with human adenovirus type 5 and 12, *Virology* **37:**513.

THOMAS, D. C., AND GREEN, M., 1966, Biochemical studies on adenovirus multiplication. XI. Evidence of a cytoplasmic site for the synthesis of viral-coded proteins, *Proc. Natl. Acad. Sci.* **56:**243.

THOREN, M. M., SEBRING, E. D., AND SALZMAN, N. P., 1972, Specific initiation site for simian virus 40 deoxyribonucleic acid replication, *J. Virol.* **10:**462.

TONEGAWA, S., WALTER, G., BERNARDINI, A., AND DULBECCO, R., 1970, Transcription of the SV40 genome in transformed cells and during lytic infection, *Cold Spring Harbor Symp. Quant. Biol.* **35:**823.

TOOZE, J. (ed.), 1973, *The Molecular Biology of Tumour Viruses*, Cold Spring Harbor Laboratory, New York.

TRENTIN, J. J., AND BRYAN, E., 1966, Virus-induced transplantation immunity to human adenovirus type 12 tumors of the hamster and mouse, *Proc. Soc. Exp. Biol. Med.* **121:**1216.

UCHIDA, S., WATANABE, S., AND KATO, M., 1966, Incomplete growth of simian virus 40 in African green monkey kidney culture induced by serial undiluted passages, *Virology* **28:**135.

UCHIDA, S., YOSHIIKE, K., WATANABE, S., AND FURUNO, A., 1968, Antigen-forming defective viruses of simian virus 40, *Virology* **34:**1.

VAN DER EB, A. J., 1973, Intermediates in type 5 adenovirus DNA replication, *Virology* **51:**11.

VAN DER EB, A. J., VAN KESTEREN, L. W., AND VAN BRUGGEN, E. F. J., 1969, Structural properties of adenovirus DNA's, *Biochim. Biophys. Acta* **182:**530.

VASCONCELOS-COSTA, J., GERALDES, A., AND CARVALHO, Z. G., 1973, Adenovirus type 12 surface antigen detected by immunofluorescence in infected KB cells, *Virology* **52:**337.

VELICER, L. F., AND GINSBERG, H. S., 1970, Synthesis, transport, and morphogenesis of type 5 adenovirus capsid proteins, *J. Virol.* **5**:338.

WAGNER, E. K., AND ROIZMAN, B., 1969a, Ribonucleic acid synthesis in cells infected with herpes simplex virus. I. Patterns of ribonucleic acid synthesis in productively infected cells, *J. Virol.* **4**:36.

WAGNER, E. K., AND ROIZMAN, B., 1969b, RNA synthesis in cells infected with herpes simplex virus. II. Evidence that a class of viral mRNA is derived from a high molecular weight precursor synthesized in the nucleus, *Proc. Natl. Acad. Sci.* **64**:626.

WALDECK, W., KAMMER, K., AND SAUER, G., 1973, Preferential integration of simian virus 40 deoxyribonucleic acid into a particular size class of CV-1 cell deoxyribonucleic acid, *Virology* **54**:452.

WALL, R., AND DARNELL, J. E., 1971, Presence of cell and virus specific sequences in the same molecules of nuclear RNA from virus transformed cells, *Nature New Biol.* **232**:73.

WALL, R., PHILIPSON, L., AND DARNELL, J. E., 1972, Processing of adenovirus specific nuclear RNA during virus replication, *Virology* **50**:27.

WALL, R., WEBER, J., GAGE, Z., AND DARNELL, J. E., 1973, Production of viral mRNA in adenovirus-transformed cells by the post-transcriptional processing of heterogeneous nuclear RNA containing viral and cell sequences, *J. Virol.* **11**:953.

WALLACE, R. D., AND KATES, J., 1972, State of adenovirus 2 deoxyribonucleic acid in the nucleus and its mode of transcription: Studies with isolated viral deoxyribonucleic acid–protein complexes and isolated nuclei, *J. Virol.* **9**:627.

WALTER, G., ROBLIN, R., AND DULBECCO, R., 1972, Protein synthesis in simian virus 40–infected monkey cells, *Proc. Natl. Acad. Sci.* **69**:921.

WARNAAR, S. O., AND DE MOL, A. W., 1973, Characterization of two simian virus 40–specific RNA molecules from infected BS-C-1 cells, *J. Virol.* **12**:124.

WATKINS, J. F., AND DULBECCO, R., 1967, Production of SV40 virus in heterokaryons of transformed and susceptible cells, *Proc. Natl. Acad. Sci.* **58**:1396.

WEAVER, G. H., KIT, S., AND DUBBS, D. R., 1970, Initial site of synthesis of virus during rescue of simian virus 40 from heterokaryons of simian virus 40–transformed and susceptible cells, *J. Virol.* **5**:578.

WEINBERG, R. A., BEN-ISHAI, Z., AND NEWBOLD, J. E., 1972, Poly A associated with SV40 messenger RNA, *Nature New Biol.* **238**:111.

WESTPHAL, H., 1970, SV40 DNA strand selection by *Escherichia coli* RNA polymerase, *J. Mol. Biol.* **50**:407.

WESTPHAL, H., AND DULBECCO, R., 1968, Viral DNA in Polyoma- and SV40-transformed cell lines, *Proc. Natl. Acad. Sci. USA* **59**:1158.

WHITE, D. O., SCHARFF, M. D., AND MAIZEL, J. V., JR., 1969, The polypeptides of adenovirus. III. Synthesis in infected cells, *Virology* **38**:395.

WILCOX, W. C., AND GINSBERG, H. S., 1963, Protein synthesis in type 5 adenovirus–infected cells: Effect of *p*-fluorophenylalanine on synthesis of protein, nucleic acids, and infectious virus, *Virology* **20**:269.

WILDY, P., 1973, Antigens of herpes simplex virus of oral and genital origin, *Cancer Res.* **33**:1465.

WINOCOUR, E., 1965a, Attempts to detect an integrated polyoma genome by nucleic acid hybridization. I. "Reconstruction" experiments and complementarity tests between synthetic polyoma RNA and polyoma tumor DNA, *Virology* **25**:276.

WINOCOUR, E., 1965b, Attempts to detect an integrated polyoma genome by nucleic acid hybridization. II. Complementarity between polyoma virus DNA and normal mouse synthetic RNA, *Virology* **27**:520.

WINOCOUR, E., 1967, On the apparent homology between DNA from polyoma virus and normal mouse synthetic RNA, *Virology* **31**:15.

WINOCOUR, E., 1968, Further studies on the incorporation of cell DNA into polyoma related particles, *Virology* **34**:571.

YOSHIIKE, K., 1968, Studies on DNA from low-density particles of SV40. I. Heterogeneous defective virions produced by successive undiluted passages, *Virology* **34**:391.

ZUR HAUSEN, H., AND SCHULTE-HOLTHAUSEN, H., 1970, Presence of EB virus nucleic acid homology in a "virus-free" line of Burkitt tumour cells, *Nature (Lord.)* **227**:245.

ZUR HAUSEN, H., AND SOKOL, F., 1969, Rate of adenovirus type 12 genomes in nonpermissive cells, *J. Virol.* **4**:256.

7

Herpes Simplex and Epstein–Barr Viruses in Human Cells and Tissues: A Study in Contrasts

BERNARD ROIZMAN AND ELLIOTT D. KIEFF

1. Introduction

Humans are blessed with at least five herpesviruses, i.e., herpes simplex 1 (human herpesvirus 1, HSV-1), herpes simplex 2 (human herpesvirus 2, HSV-2), herpes zoster virus (human herpesvirus 3, HZV), Epstein–Barr virus (human herpesvirus 4, EBV), and cytomegalovirus (human herpesvirus 5, CMV). In recent years three of these viruses, EBV, HSV-1, and HSV-2, have become prominently associated with human cancer. The purpose of this chapter is to describe briefly the biology of these three herpesviruses in human cells and tissues. The chapter is organized into four sections dealing respectively with the virion and its components, the replication of herpesviruses in permissive cells, the infection of restrictive and nonpermissive cells, and with the acute diseases, latency, and neoplastic diseases associated with these herpesviruses.

It should be emphasized that although herpesviruses are classified primarily on the basis of the structure of the virion, they also share numerous biological properties. Specifically, at the cellular level, all herpesviruses utilize the nucleus of

BERNARD ROIZMAN and ELLIOTT D. KIEFF • Division of Biological Sciences, The University of Chicago, Chicago, Illinois.

the cell for transcription and replication of viral DNA, and for the assembly of the nucleocapsids. The virus matures by budding through the inner lamella of the nuclear membrane. At the level of the organism, the herpesviruses characteristically remain intimately associated with specific cells and tissues, sometimes for the life of the host. However, the three herpesviruses differ in several significant details. HSV-1 and HSV-2 readily multiply not only in a variety of human cells but also in cells derived from many animal species. We have no information on the cells which sustain EBV replication in natural infections of humans. In the laboratory, EBV multiplies only in lymphoblastoid cell lines, and poorly at that.

Our information regarding the three herpesviruses is not even. The available data on the structure and replication of herpesviruses are derived chiefly from studies on HSV-1. On the other hand, much of our information regarding nonlethal interactions of herpesviruses with cells is derived from studies of EBV.

We would like to add that herpesviruses are not recently discovered infectious entities: they have been known for many years but largely ignored. The recent upsurge of interest in herpesviruses is related to their possible involvement in cancers of humans, nonhuman primates, other mammals, and even vertebrates in general.

2. The Herpesvirion

2.1. Structure and Composition

Herpesviruses are defined on the basis of their structure. The virion consists of four architectural elements, the core, capsid, tegument, and envelope, arranged concentrically (Roizman and Spear, 1973; Roizman and Furlong, 1974).

The innermost architectural component is the core, which in HSV-1 and HSV-2 appears to consist of DNA coiled around a protein bar (Furlong et al., 1972) so as to give the appearance of a toroid or doughnut. Similar structures have been seen in electron micrographs of EBV (Schidlovsky and Toplin, 1966). The failure to detect these structures in CMV might be due to poor fixation (Smith and de Harven, 1973).

The core is surrounded by protein layers known collectively as the capsid. The capsid of the HSV virion is approximately 105 nm in diameter and has a characteristic icosadeltahedral shape with five capsomeres along the sides of the triangular faces. The calculated number of capsomeres per virion is 162 (Wildy et al., 1960). The characteristic arrangement of the capsomeres made possible the identification of EBV as herpes-like in spite of early data which suggested that the EBV capsid was 20% smaller than that of HSV (Epstein et al., 1964). Subsequent studies of EBV derived from Africa and North America could not differentiate between the capsid structure of EBV and that of HSV (O'Connor and Rabson, 1965; Rabson et al., 1966). The hexameric capsomeres are commonly seen in negatively stained preparations of HSV, CMV, and EBV (Wildy et al., 1960; Hummeler et al., 1966; Schidlovsky and Toplin, 1966; Yamaguchi et al., 1967).

Each capsomere appears to be 12.5 nm long by 8.0–9.0 nm wide at the end projecting outside. A hole, 4.0 nm in diameter, runs through the long axis of the capsomere. Pentagonal capsomeres have been predicted (Wildy *et al.*, 1960), but pictures showing clearly resolved pentameres have not been published.

The space between the outermost structure of the herpesvirion—the envelope—and the capsid is frequently filled with an amorphous, fibrillar material (Furlong and Roizman, unpublished data) designated the tegument. The thickness and structure of the tegument seem to vary according to the virus and the cells in which it was grown (Roizman and Furlong, 1974).

The envelope of the herpesvirion is a trilaminar membrane bearing short spikes on its outer surface. The envelope, like most membranes, is less rigid and confers on the complete virus particle a diameter ranging from 150 to as much as 200 nm.

The major chemical components of the herpesvirion are DNA, proteins including glycoproteins, polyamines, and lipids.

243

HERPES
SIMPLEX AND
EPSTEIN–BARR
VIRUSES IN
HUMAN CELLS
AND TISSUES:
A STUDY IN
CONTRASTS

2.2. Herpesvirus DNAs

The DNAs of a number of herpesviruses have now been studied extensively. The base composition of herpesvirus DNAs has been found to range from 32 to 74 guanine plus cytosine moles percent. The base compositions of HSV-1 and HSV-2 DNAs are 67 and 69 guanine plus cytosine moles percent (Goodheart *et al.*, 1968; Kieff *et al.*, 1971). In contrast to earlier estimates of the molecular weight of HSV DNA at from 5×10^6 to approximately 60×10^6, recent studies by a number of techniques have narrowed the range to $82–100 \times 10^6$. The DNAs of both HSV-1 and HSV-2, as determined from electron microscopic, thermal denaturation, and renaturation studies (Roizman *et al.*, 1973), are linear double-stranded molecules. The sedimentation constant of HSV-1 and HSV-2 DNAs in neutral pH solutions has been estimated at from 54 to 56S (Kieff *et al.*, 1971; Wagner *et al.*, 1974). Studies of the renaturation kinetics of HSV DNA yield an estimate of the kinetic complexity of the DNA very close to that calculated from sedimentation studies and from electron microscopic measurements. This finding indicates that the genome of HSV is not segmented—i.e., the entire informational content of the infectious particle is contained in one molecule of viral DNA—in agreement with the calculation that the core of the virion contains sufficient space for one molecule of DNA only (Furlong *et al.*, 1972).

Studies published from this laboratory (Frenkel and Roizman, 1971; Frenkel *et al.*, 1972) have shown that HSV-1 DNA reassociates with a single rate constant whereas HSV-2 DNA contains a more rapidly reassociating component consisting of approximately 16% of the DNA. Recent studies (Frenkel and Roizman, unpublished data) indicate that the rapidly reassociating fraction might be due to DNA contained in defective particles arising during virus multiplication since HSV-2 DNA extracted from plaque-purified virus and virus passaged at low multiplicity of infection reassociates with a single rate constant.

Moreover, analyses of DNA extracted from virus deliberately passaged at high multiplicity consisted of a mixture of two kinds of molecules. One type was identical to that found in virions passaged at low multiplicity. The second had a higher buoyant density similar to that described by Bronson *et al.* (1973). Analyses of this DNA with restriction endonucleases indicated that it consists of tandem repeats of a DNA fragment approximately 6.0 million in molecular weight, which account for the rapidly reassociating fraction (Roizman *et al.*, 1975).

A peculiar characteristic of HSV-1 and HSV-2 DNA is the presence of breaks in the DNA strands following denaturation at alkaline pH (Kieff *et al.*, 1971). The single-strand fragments thus produced are situated at nonrandom (Wilkie, 1973) and possibly unique (Frenkel and Roizman, 1972a) sites. It is not certain whether the fragments arise from alkali-labile bonds or single-strand interruptions.

Probably the most interesting findings relate to the architecture of HSV DNA. Analytical studies involving several techniques have produced convincing evidence that HSV-1 and HSV-2 DNA molecules consist of two palindromes. The first, beginning at the left end of the molecule, consists of regions A–B–L–B–A. The second, continuing from left to right, consists of regions A–C–S–C–A. The left end of the palindrome, A–B, is inverted and complementary to the internal region B–A. Similarly, the right end, C–A, of the second palindrome is inverted and complementary relative to the internal sequence A–C. Terminal sequences A amounting to 1–2% of the DNA appear to be identical, indicating that HSV-1 DNA, like the DNA of most viruses, is terminally redundant (Grafstrom *et al.*, 1974). The regions A–B, B–A, A–C, and C–A together form 20% of the molecule. L and S comprise 71 and 9%, respectively. The anatomy of the DNA becomes immediately apparent when the DNA is denatured and the intact strand allowed to self-anneal. Under those conditions, the DNA forms a barbell structure in which the bar consists of double-stranded DNA formed by annealing of the right and left ends of the DNA to the internal regions B–A–A–C. The bells consist of single-stranded regions L and S (Sheldrick and Berthelot, 1974; Roizman *et al.*, 1975). The architecture of the DNA predicts that L and S regions might rapidly become inverted. Indeed, studies of the DNA by restriction endonucleases and electron microscopy indicate that such is the case and that molecules containing inversions of L and S regions occur independently and equilibrate in the population of DNA molecules (Hayward, Wadsworth, Jacob, and Roizman, manuscript in preparation, Roizman *et al.*, 1975).

Current knowledge of the physical structure of EBV DNA can be summarized as follows: (1) Estimates of the relative sedimentation value of native DNA in sucrose gradients range from 44–45S relative to 28S RNA in low salt (zur Hausen and Schulte-Holthausen, 1970; Nonoyama and Pagano, 1971) to $59 \pm 2S$ relative to T4 or PM 2 DNA (data and conditions not published, Jehn *et al.*, 1972). The size of the DNA of EBV purified from HR1 and B95-8 lymphoblast cell lines has recently been determined by two independent methods (Pritchett *et al.*, 1975). The S value of EBV DNA relative to T4 DNA (57S) in neutral, high-salt, sucrose velocity gradients was 55S, indicating a molecular weight of $101 \pm 3 \times 10^6$ daltons. This value agreed well with the value of $105 \pm 3 \times 10^6$ daltons obtained by measurement of the length of EBV DNA relative to form II DNA of phage PM2. (2) The buoyant density of EBV DNA in CsCl solution is reported to range from

1.716 to 1.723 (Wagner *et al.*, 1970; Schulte-Holthausen and zur Hausen, 1970; Nonoyama and Pagano, 1971; Jehn *et al.*, 1972; Weinberg and Becker, 1969; Ludwig *et al.*, 1971; Pritchett *et al.*, 1975). Assuming that EBV DNA contains no unusual bases, the buoyant density of EBV DNA corresponds to 57–59 guanine plus cytosine moles percent. The DNA of EBV purified from B95-8 cells differs from the DNA of EBV purified from HR-1 cells in being relatively rich in sequences having a guanine plus cytosine content of 60–61 moles percent (Pritchett *et al.*, 1975). (3) Sedimentation of EBV DNA in alkaline sucrose gradients indicates that less than 50% of the DNA molecules form a discrete band sedimenting more slowly than T4 DNA and corresponding to intact single strands of approximately 50×10^6 daltons (Pritchett *et al.*, 1975). The remainder of the single-stranded DNA sediments as molecules of smaller size. The sedimentation pattern of the molecules of smaller size varies, suggesting that there is no specificity to the single-strand breaks as was suggested by the analysis of HSV DNA (Kieff *et al.*, 1971).

2.3. Structural Proteins

Analyses of viral structural proteins require purified preparations of virions as well as high-resolution separation of virion polypeptides. Most of the problems associated with purification of virions stem from the lability of the viral envelope and from the similarity of the physicochemical properties of the virion to those of the membrane vesicles generated in the course of extraction. The membrane vesicle, however, contains both host and viral proteins (Heine and Roizman, 1973), whereas purified virions contain only variable, trace amounts of host proteins (Spear and Roizman, 1972). At least two techniques for purification of herpesvirions have been extensively documented (Spear and Roizman, 1972; Vahlne and Blomberg, 1974). Both techniques involve banding of the virions in dextran gradients, but one (Spear and Roizman, 1972) involves additional banding in either sucrose density gradients or potassium tartrate, whereas the other involves banding of the virus in colloidal silica prior to the centrifugation on dextran gradients.

To date, all separations of viral polypeptides have been done in polyacrylamide gels containing sodium dodecylsulfate. Earlier studies were based on a gel system with low resolving power; as a consequence, it was reported that herpesvirions contained nine to 11 polypeptides. Current studies (Spear and Roizman, 1972; Heine *et al.*, 1974) based on high-resolution polyacrylamide gels indicate that the purified virions contain at least 33 species of polypeptides ranging in molecular weight from 25,000 to approximately 280,000.

Information regarding HSV-1 virion polypeptides is fragmentary, and may be summarized (Spear and Roizman, 1972; Heine *et al.*, 1974; Gibson and Roizman, 1972, 1974) as follows: (1) It is likely that a substantial number of virion polypeptides are not the primary products of translation. Thus at least 14 polypeptides are extensively glycosylated and several are phosphorylated. An unspecified number of virion polypeptides do not correspond in electrophoretic mobility to the polypeptides detected in infected cells after a short labeling interval. In part, the change in electrophoretic mobility may be due to glycosylation, phosphorylation, etc. However, data derived from pulse-chase experiments (Honess and Roizman, 1973) indicate that at least some of the structural polypeptides result from cleavage of larger, precursor polypeptides. (2) For any given virus strain, the molar ratios of virion polypeptides remain constant from preparation to preparation. The molar concentrations of individual polypeptides per mole of virions range from less than 20 (minor polypeptides) to well over 1000 (major polypeptides). (3) Major differences in the amount and electrophoretic mobility of noncapsid polypeptides have emerged from comparisons between virus strains with a history of few passages outside the human host and laboratory strains characterized by a history of numerous ones. The data have many implications, from two points of view. First, since some of the noncapsid polypeptides determine the immunological specificity of the virion, laboratory strains may not be suitable prototypes for seroepidemiological studies (Ejercito et al., 1968; Roizman et al., 1973). Second, since many of the noncapsid polypeptides become incorporated into cellular membranes biochemical studies employing laboratory strains may not be immediately applicable to understanding the biochemical events in human cells infected with "wild" strains.

The only available studies of the structural proteins of EBV (Weinberg and Becker, 1969; Becker and Weinberg, 1972) were undertaken at a time when the technology of polyacrylamide gel electrophoresis permitted the resolution of eight or nine polypeptides of HSV. These studies indicated that the eight resolvable structural proteins of EBV were similar in molecular weight to the corresponding proteins in HSV.

2.4. Other Constituents

The presence of lipids in the virion has been deduced from experiments involving lipid solvents and enzymes attacking lipids as well as from the finding of lipids in partially purified virus preparations (Roizman and Furlong, 1974). The characterization of the lipid content of virions is far from complete, but indirect evidence suggests that lipid composition is determined at least in part by the cell in which the virus was grown (Spear and Roizman, 1967).

Virions also contain polyamines (Gibson and Roizman, 1971, 1973). When HSV-1 is grown in HEp-2 cells, both spermine and spermidine are found in the virions. Whereas spermidine is readily removed by stripping the envelope off the virion, spermine is not. The function of the polyamine is probably to neutralize the phosphate backbone of the DNA to allow tight packaging of the DNA in the core.

2.5. Distribution of Chemical Components in the Virion

The topology of chemical constituents in the virion is not well defined, but certain elements of the virion structure are already discernible. Briefly:

1. Electron microscopic studies indicate that the DNA is contained in the core (Epstein, 1962; Furlong et al., 1972). The core probably contains proteins as well as polyamines, if the hypothesis concerning their functions proves to be correct. Comparison of the capsids lacking DNA with full capsids suggests that at least one polypeptide (No. 21) functions as a core protein.

2. To date, three kinds of capsids have been isolated (Gibson and Roizman, 1972, 1974). The A and B capsids have been isolated from nuclei of infected cells and represent empty and full capsids, respectively. The C capsids were obtained by stripping the envelope off the virion with nonionic detergents. The A capsids lack DNA, but contain four polypeptides, Nos. 5, 19, 23, and 24. The B capsids contain two additional polypeptides, Nos. 21 and 22A, as well as DNA. The C capsids contain DNA, the same polypeptides as those present in the empty A capsids as well as polypeptides 21 and 1 and 2, and trace amounts of most glycoproteins, but lack polypeptide 22A. Polypeptide 22A is also absent from virions, which suggests that it is a precursor molecule that is cleaved or replaced at the time of envelopment and hence may be situated on the surface of the B capsid.

3. It is likely that all the glycosylated polypeptides are components of the virion envelope (Roizman and Furlong, 1974). Apart from theoretical considerations involving the process of glycosylation of the polypeptides, it has been shown that the glycosylated polypeptides can be labeled in vitro by transfer of tritium from tritiated borohydrate during reduction of the Schiff's base in the presence of pyridoxal phosphate. In addition, the glycosylated polypeptides have been found in purified membranes extracted from infected cells (Heine et al., 1972; Heine and Roizman, 1973).

4. The localization of nonglycosylated polypeptides other than those accounted for in the capsid is not known. We suspect that at least some of these polypeptides are localized in the underside of the envelope and are thus not available for glycosylation whereas others are in the tegument, i.e., the structure between the capsid and envelope.

2.6. Requirements for Infection of Cells

Numerous studies from several laboratories published in recent years indicate the following: (1) To be infectious, the viral nucleocapsids must be enveloped and the enveloped particle is the epidemiologically significant unit. The envelope need not be intact, although an intact envelope probably increases the stability of the particle (Spring and Roizman, 1968; Nii et al., 1968a). (2) Naked nucleocapsids obtained from the nucleus by detergent treatment before envelopment or from virions by stripping of the envelope are not infectious (Smith, 1964; Stein et al., 1970; Rubenstein et al., 1972). (3) Viral DNA rendered free of proteins is infectious (Lando and Ryhiner, 1969; Sheldrick et al., 1973). What is particularly interesting is that both native and alkaline-denatured DNAs are infectious (Sheldrick et al., 1973). (4) It is not known why naked nucleocapsids are not infectious. It is conceivable that the specific infectivity of the virus and its subunits may be determined by the mode of entry into the cell. The observation that DNA is infectious indicates that the virion proteins are not essential for the multiplication of the virus. The infectivity of the virion is especially sensitive to detergent and lipid solvents, lipases and proteases, and protein-denaturing agents (Roizman, 1969; Roizman and Furlong, 1974). The conditions which best preserve the infectivity of the herpesviruses appear to be storage in distilled water at 4°C and storage in various other media at temperatures below −60°C.

Although particle infectivity ratios of 1:10 have been reported (Watson *et al.*, 1964), most preparations used in general laboratory work show a much higher ratio. For HSV-1 and HSV-2, standard virus stocks prepared at 34°C from HEp-2 cells infected at multiplicities less than 1 PFU/cell contain one infectious unit for every 80–400 particles.

2.7. Relatedness Among Herpesviruses

It has been known for many years that certain herpesviruses are immunologically related. Thus antisera against HSV-1 neutralize HSV-2 and *vice versa*, although the homologous reaction is favored. HSV has been reported to be neutralized by antisera to herpes B (Van Hoosier and Melnick, 1961) and to bovine mammillitis virus (Stertz *et al.*, 1974). By tests other than neutralization, several other herpesviruses have been shown to share common antigens (Watson *et al.*, 1967; Plummer, 1964; Evans *et al.*, 1972; Hull *et al.*, 1972). However, existing evidence for a common antigen in all herpesviruses is rather weak (Kirkwood *et al.*, 1972; Ross *et al.*, 1972*b*).

Relatedness may be more precisely estimated from DNA–DNA and even DNA–RNA hybridizations, but this technique is useful only if there are sufficient amounts of homology between the DNAs, i.e., if evolutionary divergence of these viruses was rather recent. DNA–DNA hybridizations indicate that HSV-1 and HSV-2 DNAs show approximately 50% homology, with 85% matching of base pairs of the homologous regions (Kieff *et al.*, 1972). Trace amounts of homology between HSV and several other viruses (Stertz *et al.*, 1974; Bachenheimer *et al.*, 1972; Bronson *et al.*, 1972; Ludwig *et al.*, 1972; Ludwig, 1972; zur Hausen *et al.*, 1970) cannot be evaluated since the extent of base mismatch in the hybrid has not been determined. Thus, little base pairing has yet been demonstrated between the DNAs of heterologous herpesviruses. Liquid-filter DNA–DNA hybridization between HSV-1 or HSV-2 DNA and the DNA of Marek's disease herpesvirus indicated less than 2% homology (Bachenheimer *et al.*, 1972). No homology was detected between HSV-1, HSV-2, Marek's disease herpesvirus, or CMV DNAs and EBV DNA labeled *in vivo* or *in vitro* (zur Hausen and Schulte-Holthausen, 1970; zur Hausen *et al.*, 1970; Huang and Pagano, 1974). HSV-1, HSV-2, EBV, simian, and murine CMV DNAs had no effect on the kinetics of reassociation of *in vitro* labeled human CMV DNA of the AD 169 strain (Huang and Pagano, 1974). Lack of DNA homology does not in general exclude genetic relatedness, because, in principle at least, the synthesis of identical polypeptides could result from completely nonhomologous mRNA.

3. Replication of Herpesviruses

249

HERPES
SIMPLEX AND
EPSTEIN–BARR
VIRUSES IN
HUMAN CELLS
AND TISSUES:
A STUDY IN
CONTRASTS

3.1. Initiation of Infection and General Characteristics of the Reproductive Cycle

3.1.1. Adsorption, Penetration, and Uncoating

Little is known of the receptors on the cell surfaces to which herpesviruses adsorb. Adsorption in general is slow and both volume and cation dependent. Sulfated polyanions, both natural (agar, mucopolysaccharides, heparin) and synthetic, prevent adsorption (see review by Roizman and Furlong, 1974). The events following adsorption are also unclear. On the basis of electron microscopic studies, two mechanisms have been proposed for the mode of events of entry of the virus into the cell. One (Dales and Silverberg, 1969; Siegert and Falke, 1966) suggests that herpesviruses are taken into the cell in phagocytic vesicles in which they are uncoated. The second (Abodeely *et al.*, 1970; Iwasaki, 1973; Morgan *et al.*, 1968; Hummeler *et al.*, 1969) proposes that the entry is effected by fusion of the viral envelope with the plasma membrane followed by passage of the capsid through the fused membranes into the cytoplasm. The critical experiment, i.e., demonstration of viral membrane proteins immediately following penetration either in the plasma membrane or in the cytoplasm, has not been done. It has been reported that the capsid disaggregates in the cytoplasm and that a DNA–protein complex is transported into the nucleus (Hochberg and Becker, 1968).

3.1.2. General Characteristics of the Reproductive Cycle

In general, the duration of the reproductive cycle, the time course of major events, and the yield of viral products are highly reproducible within a given cell host–virus system, but vary considerably from system to system depending on (1) the degree to which the host restricts virus multiplication, (2) the multiplicity of infection, (3) the temperature, and (4) the nutritional properties of the medium (Roizman, 1969; Roizman and Furlong, 1974). Under most optimal conditions, such as encountered in the multiplication of HSV-1 or HSV-2 in HEp-2 cells, the replicative cycle lasts 17–19 h. The progeny virus is detected first by electron microscopy at about 4 h after infection and then by infectivity measurements 1–2 h later. Virus accumulates in the infected cell at exponential rates. Release of virus from infected cells varies from system to system, but is in general temperature dependent. Thus, at 34°C HSV-1 yield in human cells is optimal, but no more than 20% of the virus is released into the extracellular fluid (Hoggan and Roizman, 1959a). Hence it is convenient to harvest the virus from the infected cells and to discard the extracellular fluid.

3.2. Biosynthesis and Assembly of Herpesviruses

3.2.1. General Considerations

This section deals with productive infection of permissive cells. It is convenient to describe the replication of viruses from the point of view of two parallel, interrelated series of events. The first series involves the synthesis of viral macromolecules, i.e., viral mRNA, proteins, and DNA, and virion assembly. The second series of events involves inhibiton of host macromolecular function, alteration in cellular structures, and ultimately cell death, which invariably accompanies productive infection.

3.2.2. RNA Synthesis

Transcription of viral DNA is the first major event in the replication of herpesviruses. Most of the available information on transcription of herpesvirus DNAs emerged from studies of HSV-1 and HSV-2 and may be summarized as follows:

1. It is likely that transcription is at least initiated by a host RNA polymerase. This conclusion is based on the report that deproteinized HSV DNA is infectious (Sheldrick *et al.*, 1973). It is also likely that the host polymerase is capable of transcribing the whole genome of the virus since viral RNA complementary to nearly 50% of viral DNA is made in cells exposed to inhibitors of protein synthesis at the time of infection. However, as discussed later in the text, some of the experimental data suggest that only a fraction of these transcripts are competent to function as mRNA.

2. Although the transcripts accumulating in the nuclei of infected cells are complementary to >50% of viral DNA, the transcripts accumulating in the polyribosomes represent 40–43% of the DNA, and this may well be the only informational RNA specified by HSV. The function of the remainder of the transcripts is not known. There is currently general agreement (Morris *et al.*, 1970; Bell *et al.*, 1971) that HSV does not specify arginyl or seryl RNA as was once claimed (Subak-Sharpe and Hay, 1965; Subak-Sharpe *et al.*, 1966).

3. The transcripts appear first in the nucleus, and only after a lag do they appear in the cytoplasm (Wagner and Roizman, 1966a). In the nucleus, substantial quantities of the transcripts are characterized by a sedimentation constant much larger than that of polyribosomal mRNA. On the basis of hybridization-competition studies showing the presence of nearly identical RNA sequences in both species of RNA, it has been concluded that the high molecular weight transcripts are cleaved and processed before they appear as mRNA in polyribosomes (Wagner and Roizman, 1969b). The processing includes adenylation of a large fraction of the RNA (Bachenheimer and Roizman, 1972). Adenylation has been shown to be a post-transcriptional event and involves the addition of 150–200 adenylic acid residues to the 3'-end of the RNA prior to its transport into the cytoplasm. Pertinent to the overall understanding of the process of transcription is the observation that a small quantity of the stable transcripts arise by symmetrical transcription (Kozak and Roizman, manuscript in preparation).

4. There is evidence for extensive multilevel regulation of transcription, accumulation of transcripts, and transport of the transcripts into the cytoplasm. Briefly, a temporal control of transcription regulating the total amount of DNA transcribed at different times after infection has been reported (Wagner, 1972;

Frenkel and Roizman, 1972b; Frenkel *et al.*, 1973). However, it is not at all clear whether a temporal control actually exists or whether the concentrations of viral RNA are too low to drive all of the DNA template into hybrid (Kozak and Roizman, manuscript in preparation).

251
HERPES
SIMPLEX AND
EPSTEIN–BARR
VIRUSES IN
HUMAN CELLS
AND TISSUES:
A STUDY IN
CONTRASTS

A second control of transcription emerges from studies of the kinetics of reassociation of excess viral RNA to trace amounts of labeled viral DNA. The data indicate that viral RNA sequences fall into at least two classes differing in molar concentration. The nature of the mechanisms regulating viral DNA abundance is not known. Although both abundant and scarce viral RNA species present in the cytoplasm and arising from 21 and 19% of viral DNA, respectively, contain poly(A) chains of identical length, the behavior of the two RNA classes differ. Both classes of RNA anneal to poly(U) bound to filters, but only the abundant RNA binds to nitrocellulose filters in an undenatured state. Scarce species bind to nitrocellulose filters only after denaturation. These data suggest that the abundant and scarce RNA species in the cytoplasm of infected cells differ in secondary structure (Silverstein *et al.*, 1973; Millette and Silverstein, manuscript in preparation). Last, a third regulatory process emerges from comparison of the total viral RNA sequences in nuclei and cytoplasm. Thus although nearly the entire genome is transcribed when protein synthesis is inhibited by puromycin or cycloheximide, transcripts from only 10% of the DNA appear in the cytoplasm during treatment and function on cytoplasmic polyribosomes following withdrawal of the drug (Kozak and Roizman, manuscript in preparation). Furthermore, the remaining nuclear transcripts do not appear in the cytoplasm even after a prolonged chase in the presence of cycloheximide. These and other data cited below suggest not only that the bulk of the transcripts made in the presence of inhibitors of protein synthesis are nonfunctional but also that the transport of the nuclear RNA into cytoplasm is regulated.

3.2.3. Viral Protein Synthesis

Several lines of evidence indicate that viral polypeptides are made in cytoplasm, on both free and bound polyribosomes (Sydiskis and Roizman, 1966, 1967, 1968). In general, analysis of the events governing viral protein synthesis requires identification of the individual viral polypeptides and measurement of their rates of synthesis throughout infection. The most extensive studies have been done in HSV-1-infected HEp-2 cells. It is convenient to summarize the available data as follows:

1. Classification of the polypeptides made in infected cells as virus specific or cell specific at the present state of herpesvirus technology requires somewhat arbitrary criteria. The criteria chosen in this instance (Honess and Roizman, 1973) are based on three observations. First, overall host protein synthesis declines rapidly after infection (Roizman *et al.*, 1965; Sydiskis and Roizman, 1966, 1967). Polypeptides synthesized at increasing rates at the time of decline of host polypeptide synthesis would therefore be expected to be virus specific. Second,

antisera prepared in rabbits against infected rabbit cells grown in rabbit serum precipitate a number of infected human or rabbit cell polypeptides but not uninfected cell polypeptides (Honess and Watson, 1974). Polypeptides reactive with these antisera could be considered virus specific if they also increase in rates of synthesis after infection. Last, it has been observed in cells infected with variants of HSV-1 or with HSV-2 that some polypeptides are either overproduced, underproduced, or replaced with polypeptides differing in electrophoretic mobilities (Honess and Roizman, 1973). The polypeptides whose production is under the genetic control of the virus may also be considered as virus specific provided that they are absent from uninfected cells and show increasing rates of synthesis after infection. On the basis of these criteria, approximately 48 polypeptides separated in high-resolution polyacrylamide gels have been classified as virus specific. They consist of both virion structural components and polypeptides for which a counterpart in the virion has not been found which are therefore nonstructural (Honess and Roizman, 1973).

2. Meaningful analysis of the rates of synthesis of these 48 polypeptides depends on a knowledge of whether they are primary products of translation or of rapid post-translational cleavage. Comparisons of polypeptides accumulating in infected cells in three types of experiments—(a) during short and long labeling intervals, (b) during short pulse followed by prolonged chase, and (c) during treatment of infected cells with inhibitors of proteolytic enzymes known to be involved in post-transcriptional cleavages—produced no evidence that virus-specific polypeptides undergo rapid post-translational cleavage even though cleavages of some polypeptides related to virus assembly were readily demonstrable (Honess and Roizman, 1973). Based on the conclusion that the 48 polypeptides are primary gene products, the size of viral DNA, and the amount of the DNA transcribed, it was estimated that the polypeptides account for at least 70–80% of the maximum amount of genetic information that could be encoded in viral DNA.

3. The rates of synthesis of viral polypeptides were analyzed under two experimental conditions. The first involved measurements of polypeptides in parasynchronously infected cells at various times in the course of the reproductive cycle (Honess and Roizman, 1973). The second involved analyzing the polypeptides and the rates at which they were synthesized after removal of inhibitors of protein synthesis added either at the time of infection or at intervals thereafter (Honess and Roizman, 1974). The two series of experiments revealed that viral protein synthesis is sequentially ordered and coordinately regulated.

Specifically, in parasynchronously infected cells all polypeptides could be fitted into five classes differing in the temporal pattern of their replication. Class E contained polypeptides which could not be identified as virus specific and which were synthesized at decreasing rates throughout infection. Polypeptides in classes C and D reached maximum rates of synthesis early in infection and declined afterward. The two classes differed solely in the time at which maximal rates were attained; however, class C contained only structural polypeptides whereas class D contained both minor structural and nonstructural polypeptides. The rates of synthesis of class B polypeptides reached a maximum level early in infection and remained constant thereafter. The polypeptides in class A were identified as the major structural components of the virion and were synthesized at ever-increasing rates until at least 15 h after infection. Analysis of the rates of polypeptide synthesis in the parasynchronously infected cells also indicated that although the temporal patterns of synthesis of the polypeptides in each class were identical, the absolute rates of synthesis varied, suggesting a polypeptide abundance control superimposed on the temporal control of synthesis. Another interesting finding was that structural polypeptides could not be differentiated from nonstructural polypeptides with respect to their maximal or their average molar rate of synthesis (Honess and Roizman, 1973).

The analysis of polypeptides made after withdrawal of inhibitors of protein synthesis brought into relief four aspects of the regulation of viral protein synthesis. First, the polypeptides could be readily segregated into three groups designated α, β, and γ. Group α consisted of one minor structural polypeptide and several nonstructural ones. The synthesis of these polypeptides required no prior infected cell protein synthesis; i.e., they were made immediately after withdrawal of inhibitors of protein synthesis that had been added to the medium at the time of cell infection. In untreated cells, these polypeptides were made soon after infection and were synthesized thereafter at decreasing rates. The β group also consisted of minor structural and nonstructural polypeptides. In untreated cells, they were synthesized at maximum rates somewhat later than α polypeptides, but, as the latter group, their rates of synthesis subsequently declined. Polypeptides of group β were made immediately after withdrawal of inhibitors of protein synthesis only if the inhibitors were added after 1–3 h post infection, i.e., after α polypeptides had been synthesized. The γ group contained largely the major structural polypeptides. The γ group polypeptides correspond to the A class; i.e., in untreated infected cells they were synthesized at ever-increasing rates. In the treated cells, the γ group polypeptides were synthesized immediately after removal of inhibitors of protein synthesis only if the addition of the drug to the medium was delayed sufficiently to permit both α and β polypeptides to be made (Honess and Roizman, 1974).

The second observation concerns the requirements for β and γ polypeptide synthesis. The data indicate that the presence of α polypeptides alone is insufficient for the synthesis of β polypeptides, which seem also to require new RNA synthesis. This conclusion is based on the observation that addition of actinomycin D at the time of removal of cycloheximide, which had been added at the time of infection, allowed the continued synthesis of α polypeptides but precluded the synthesis of β polypeptides. It is noteworthy that while transcripts arising from 50% of DNA accumulate in nuclei of cells infected and maintained for 7 h in the presence of cycloheximide, transcripts arising from only 10% of the DNA accumulate in the cytoplasm and in the polyribosomes both immediately after removal of the cycloheximide and after a 90-min actinomycin D chase (Kozak and Roizman, manuscript in preparation). Similarly, addition of actinomycin D at the time of maximal rates of synthesis of β polypeptides precludes the synthesis of γ polypeptides (Honess and Roizman, 1974).

The third observation relates to cessation of α and β polypeptide synthesis late in infection. The data indicate that α polypeptide synthesis declined very rapidly when β polypeptides were made and very slowly when β polypeptide synthesis was blocked by actinomycin D. A similar relationship was found between β and γ polypeptide synthesis (Honess and Roizman, 1974).

The last observation is that inhibitors of DNA synthesis do not affect the transition from α to β polypeptide synthesis but do reduce the amounts of γ polypeptides made. The data suggest that parental viral DNA is capable of supplying mRNA for all three groups of polypeptides but that the mRNA for optimal rates of γ polypeptide synthesis arises in untreated infected cells from both parental and progeny DNA. The need for progeny DNA for amplification of mRNA is uncertain. Experiments involving exposure of infected cells to actinomycin D suggest that the half-life of γ mRNA is shorter than that of the other mRNAs (Honess and Roizman, 1974).

The emerging determinants of the cascade regulation of viral protein may be summarized as follows: (1) The only transcripts translatable in infected cells in which no viral mRNA was previously translated are those specifying α polypeptides. (2) The α polypeptides and new RNA synthesis are required for the synthesis of β polypeptides. (3) The β polypeptides effect at a post–transcriptional level the shutoff of α and host polypeptide synthesis and enable γ polypeptides to be made. (4) The γ polypeptides mediate at a post–transcriptional level the shutoff of β polypeptide synthesis. (5) The transcripts made off DNA templates for β and γ polypeptides in the absence of α polypeptides are nonfunctional. (6) The operation of the coordinate "on" and "off" controls which have emerged to date predicts that mRNAs specifying the polypeptides within each group share at least one and possibly several structural features, which may determine synthesis, transport into cytoplasm, and possibly regulation at the level of translation and functional half-life.

3.2.4. Processing and Transport of Herpesvirus Macromolecules Across the Membranes

As pointed out earlier in the text, the bulk of virus-specific mRNA is processed in the nucleus before it is transported into the cytoplasm. From comparison of the mRNA in polyribosomes with RNA contained in the nucleus, we can infer that processing includes cleavage of high molecular weight precursor RNAs (Wagner and Roizman, 1969b). Experimental data do in fact indicate that the processing of the bulk of viral RNA sequences includes adenylation. The interval between the time of synthesis and the appearance of the RNA in the cytoplasm has been estimated at approximately 10–20 min (Bachenheimer and Roizman, 1972). Little is known of the mechanism of actual transport. The discrepancy between viral DNA sequences represented by stable transcripts in the nucleus as opposed to those in the cytoplasm suggests that the transcripts of some sequences are preferentially conserved in the nucleus and that the nucleus retains nontranslatable viral RNA (Kozak and Roizman, 1974).

At least three kinds of post-translational processing of viral polypeptides have been described to date. Comparison of polypeptides made within a short pulse with those present in the infected cells after a long chase suggested that at least some of the polypeptides are cleaved, presumably in the course of virus assembly (Honess and Roizman, 1973). Independent evidence of cleavage emerged from comparison of polypeptides derived from nucleocapsids which had not been enveloped with those derived from nucleocapsids of enveloped virus (Gibson and Roizman, 1972, 1974). These studies suggest that virion polypeptide 22A is cleaved during envelopment and that at least one of the products, virion polypeptide 22, remains associated with the capsid.

Other post-translational modifications involve glycosylation and phosphorylation of viral proteins. As indicated Section 2.3, HSV-1 virions contain several phosphorylated polypeptides (Gibson and Roizman, 1974), and at least 14 glycosylated virion polypeptides have been resolved in high-resolution polyacrylamide gels (Heine *et al.*, 1974). The glycosylation takes place in membranes (Spear and Roizman, 1970).

Transport of polypeptides from cytoplasm to nuclei has been measured and found to be relatively slow (Spear and Roizman, 1968). The mechanisms regulating this transport are not known. Arginine deprivation has been shown to prevent accumulation of viral polypeptides in the nucleus in addition to blocking viral assembly (Courtney *et al.*, 1971). The immunological specificity of the polypeptides or their aggregates in the nucleus might be different from that of those contained in the cytoplasm (Roizman *et al.*, 1967; Ross *et al.*, 1968).

3.2.5. Function of Viral Polypeptides

Of the 48 polypeptides identified in the infected cell as virus specific, 24 have been found to be structural polypeptides and 16 to be nonstructural (Honess and Roizman, 1973). The function of the remainder is not known. It is likely, although direct evidence is lacking, that at least some of the 24 polypeptides have functions in virus multiplication other than as structural components of the virion. This conclusion is based on the observation that some of the structural components, notably exemplified by virus polypeptide No. 4, are very minor yet are produced early in infection in larger quantities than would be required for structural components.

None of the nonstructural polypeptides has been specifically related to a functional viral protein. There is, however, good evidence that the virus specifies a thymidine kinase (Hay *et al.*, 1971; Thouless, 1972) and a DNA polymerase (Keir, 1968). It has been suggested that ribonucleotide reductase, CdR-MP diaminase, and at least one DNase are also specified by the virus, but the available data are inconclusive (Cohen, 1972; Keir, 1968).

3.2.6. DNA Synthesis

Considerably less information is available on viral DNA synthesis than on either viral mRNA or protein synthesis. The available data may be summarized as follows:

1. Viral DNA synthesis takes place in the nucleus (Munk and Sauer, 1964), probably in the space occupied by the Cowdry type A inclusion body, for many years known to be diagnostic of herpesvirus-infected cells (Roizman, 1969).

2. In HSV-infected cells, viral DNA synthesis is first detected around 3 h after infection. An interval of viral protein synthesis is required for the onset of synthesis of viral DNA. Thus viral DNA is not made in cells treated with inhibitors of protein synthesis from the time of infection. Addition of the inhibitors after the onset of DNA synthesis reduces the rate, but does not entirely shut if off (Roizman and Roane, 1964).

3. Alkaline denaturation of viral DNA pulse-labeled for various lengths of time indicates that nascent DNA consists of small fragments which are repaired and/or ligated before it is incorporated into the virion (Frenkel and Roizman, 1972a).

4. It has been reported that the regulation of pseudorabies DNA is semiconservative (Kaplan et al., 1967). However, details of the replication of the DNA are unavailable.

5. At least one published paper, as well as unpublished studies, suggests that the products of viral DNA synthesis depend to some extent on the multiplicity of infection. The fundamental observation is that DNA with a guanine plus cytosine content higher than that of viral DNA is produced in the course of productive infection (Bronson et al., 1973). Studies of the reassociation kinetics of DNA also indicate the emergence of aberrant viral DNA molecules on repeated passage of the virus at high multiplicities of infection (Frenkel and Roizman, unpublished studies).

3.2.7. Replication of EBV in Lymphoblasts

EBV is unique among the herpesviruses in that no cell line fully permits viral reproduction. What is known of the sequence of events in productive infections stems from studies of structural changes, virus morphogenesis, and virus-related antigen production in latently or chronically infected continuous lymphoblastoid cell cultures of human or primate origin. Three points should be made at the outset: (1) not all continuous lymphoblastoid cultures contain subpopulations which produce virus; (2) the percentage of virus-producing cells in a given line varies widely over a matter of weeks in culture; (3) although a number of parameters are known to affect the percentage of cells in a given culture which produce virus, insufficient attention has been drawn to the irregularity with which these defined parameters reproduce their effects on virus production; (4) while in most laboratories only a minority of cells (less than 20%) produce virus under optimal conditions, sublines of lymphoblasts have been reported on occasion to contain as many as 78% virus-producing cells (Hinuma et al., 1967).

Long-term lymphoblast cell lines have been established from Burkitt tumors (Epstein et al., 1964, 1967; Stewart et al., 1965; Rabson et al., 1966), nasopharyngeal carcinoma biopsies (de The et al., 1969, 1970), and peripheral blood of patients with acute and convalescent infectious mononucleosis (Pope, 1967; Glade et al.,

1968) and normal adults who have been previously infected with EBV (Gerber and Monroe, 1968; Nilsson, 1971; Nilsson *et al.*, 1972). The complex media supplemented with 5–10% serum that are required to sustain cell growth have been a serious obstacle to the definition of optimal conditions for virus production.

a. Morphogenesis of EBV. The available studies of the morphology of virus-producing cells (Epstein *et al.*, 1964, 1965; Stewart *et al.*, 1965; O'Connor and Rabson, 1965; Rabson *et al.*, 1966; Hinuma *et al.*, 1967; Pope *et al.*, 1968b; Epstein and Achong, 1970) suffer from the lack of a system in which infection can be synchronized. The fixed frames in virus production have been sequenced by extrapolation from known events in the synthesis and assembly of HSV. With this reservation, studies of thin sections of lymphoblasts which contain identifiable EBV agree in the following ways: (1) Lymphoblasts in which virions are found display cytopathic changes typical of herpesvirus-infected cells. Nucleoli become dispersed, nuclear chromatin is marginated at the nuclear membrane, the nuclear membrane is altered, etc. These changes indicate that virus multiplication results in cell death. (2) Hexagonal nucleocapsids approximately 100 nm in diameter are found in nuclei and cytoplasm of cells which exhibit cytopathic changes. These particles may be empty or they may contain a core. In most cell lines, there are fewer nucleocapsids than would be seen in HSV-infected cells. Nucleocapsids have been observed in juxtaposition with modified nuclear membrane and interpreted as being in the process of envelopment (Epstein *et al.*, 1967). Fully enveloped virions approximately 120 nm in diameter have been seen in the perinuclear space, in cytoplasmic vacuoles, and in the extracellular fluid (Epstein and Achong, 1970).

b. Biochemical Events in Virus Production. Studies of the biochemical events in productively infected cells have relied almost exclusively on immunological techniques for the identification of virus-specific products. The evidence that these antigens are specified by EBV is indirect. In this section, we will consider five aspects of EBV-related antigens made in producing and nonproducing lymphoblasts: (1) the intracellular location of antigens, (2) correlation of antigen production with the presence of morphologically identifiable viral structures, (3) sensitivity of antigen production to inhibitors of DNA synthesis, (4) evidence that the antigen is specified by EBV, and (5) possible function of the antigenic material. It should be kept in mind that at no time do we imply that any one antigen is a single molecular species and not a collection of antigenic molecules.

Complement-Fixing Nuclear Antigen (EBNA): Virus-producing and non-virus-producing continuous lymphoblastoid cells can possess soluble antigens detectable by complement fixation assays employing immune human serum (Armstrong *et al.*, 1966; Vonka *et al.*, 1970a,b; Gerber and Deal, 1970; Pope *et al.*, 1969b; Walters and Pope, 1971; Reedman and Klein, 1973). More recently, with the use of anti-complementary immunofluorescence, a finely granular intranuclear complement-fixing antigen has been demonstrated in Burkitt tumor biopsies and 90%

of cells of both virus-producing and non-virus-producing continuous lympho-blast cell lines (Reedman and Klein, 1973). Evidence that this antigen is EBV specific stems from the observations that (1) no antibody activity against soluble complement-fixing antigen has been found in subjects lacking other antibodies against EBV (Vonka *et al.*, 1970a; Pope *et al.*, 1969b); (2) sera positive in complement fixation tests do not react with a variety of cells and tissues including neuroblastoma cells, Wilm's tumor cells (Armstrong *et al.*, 1966), tissue antigens, and both established and primary cell lines (Pope *et al.*, 1969b; Reedman and Klein, 1973); (3) primate cell lines transformed by EBV react in anticomplemen-tary immunofluorescence tests while lines carrying herpesvirus saimiri and human cord blood leukocytes induced by phytohemagglutinin are negative (Reedman and Klein, 1973).

Cell lines and biopsy material without either morphologically detectable virions or the antigenic determinants associated with purified virus are positive when assayed by anticomplementary immunofluorescence (Reedman and Klein, 1973) or by the soluble complement-fixing antigen test (Vonka *et al.*, 1970a; Pope *et al.*, 1969b; Walters and Pope, 1971). The relationship of the soluble, heat-stable complement-fixing activity to the insoluble, heat-stable activity of sucrose gradient fractions containing virions is not clear (Walters and Pope, 1971).

Early Antigen (EA): Sera from patients with acute, infectious mononucleosis and from some with Burkitt's lymphoma and postnasal carcinoma react with an antigen which can be induced in the cytoplasm of non-virus-producing lymphoblast cultures by superinfection with concentrates of virus-producing (EB3 or HR1) lines (W. Henle *et al.*, 1970a). This antigen is not present in tumor cells or in Raji cells prior to superinfection with EBV (Gergely *et al.*, 1971a,b). The ability of culture supernatants to induce antigen is removed by prior incubation with serum containing antibody to other EBV antigens, but not with nonimmune sera. Several lines of evidence suggest that EA is made in cells in which viral genome expression has proceeded as far as inhibition of host macromolecular synthesis, but does not require viral DNA synthesis: (1) Some non-virus-producing, continuous lymphoblastoid cell cultures superinfected with EBV possess EA but not morphologically detectable virus or viral capsid antigen (W. Henle *et al.*, 1970a; Gergely *et al.* 1971a). (2) EA appears first in the nucleus and spreads later to the cytoplasm (Gergely *et al.*, 1971a,b). (3) The appearance of EA is not prevented by inhibition of DNA synthesis using cytosine arabinoside or iododeoxyuridine (W. Henle *et al.*, 1970a; Gergely *et al.*, 1971a,b). (4) Superin-fected EA-positive Raji cells have an abnormally low level of DNA, RNA, and protein synthesis compared to EA-negative control cells, suggesting that EA production correlates with inhibition of host macromolecular synthesis (Gergely *et al.*, 1971c). (5) EA is made in continuous lymphoblastoid cells which produce virus. If virus capsid antigen (VCA) production and virus formation are inhibited by cytosine arabinoside and iododeoxyuridine, the number of EA-positive cells increases while the number of cells producing virus or VCA decreases. On resumption of DNA synthesis, more VCA appears than in controlled cells Gergely *et al.*, 1971b).

Two distinct early antigenic activities have been detected in superinfected Raji cells using human sera (G. Henle et al., 1971b). These have been associated with two patterns of fluorescent staining: diffuse staining of the nucleus and cytoplasm and restricted staining of cytoplasmic masses. The diffuse antigenic activity is resistant to alcohol fixation.

Membrane Antigen (MA): The first evidence for new antigen in Burkitt tumor cells arose from the observation that the sera of some patients with Burkitt's lymphoma, particularly patients in long-term remission, possess antibody to an antigen termed "membrane antigen" (MA) present on the surface of live tumor biopsy cells, but not normal lymphocytes or bone marrow cells (Klein et al., 1966, 1967a,b). MA was found on continuous lymphoblast cell cultures soon after explantation (Klein et al., 1968; Nadkarni et al., 1969) at a time when virus was not detectable by electron microscopic observation or by a fluorescence test using acetone-fixed smears (VCA assay). In general, cell lines in which virus could not be detected, e.g., Raji, Futi, Ogan, did not possess MA (Klein et al., 1968a,b). MA could be induced in as many as 50–60% of continuous lymphoblastoid cells following superinfection of virus-negative cell lines (W. Henle and G. Henle, 1970; Horosziewicz et al., 1970; Gergely et al., 1971a,b,c) with supernatants of HR1 cells, but not with supernatants of HR1 cells preincubated with serum containing antibody to EBV (Gergely et al., 1971a,b). Accumulated evidence suggests that MA is a component of the viral envelope synthesized prior to inhibition of host macromolecular synthesis or viral DNA synthesis: (1) HR1 virus superinfected Raji cells produce no virus or VCA and induction of MA is not prevented by inhibitors of DNA synthesis such as cytosine arabinoside or iododeoxyuridine (Gergely et al., 1971a,b). Superinfected MA-positive cells continue to synthesize RNA and protein. DNA synthesis is reduced, possibly as an artifact resulting from a decrease in MA synthesis during S phase (Gergely et al., 1971c). (2) The ability of antisera to neutralize virus correlates with MA antibody but not with anti-VCA activity (Pearson et al., 1970a,b). MA appears transiently on the surface of non-virus-producing cells following adsorption of EBV (Gergely et al., 1971a). Adsorption of MA activity from sera removes the neutralizing activity of the sera, despite persistent anti-VCA activity (Gergely et al., 1971a). MA and not VCA titer correlates directly with the ability of serum to coat enveloped virus particles and to bind to localized stretches of cytoplasmic membrane of virus-producing cells (Silvestre et al., 1971). (3) Sera of rabbits immunized with EBV concentrations block MA activity (Bremberg et al., 1969). (4) Studies of human sera differing in their capacity to block the binding of membrane-reactive antisera indicate that there are three components to MA activity. All components of the MA complex seem to appear in lymphoblast membrane at the same time following superinfection of Raji cells (Svedmyr and Demissie, 1971).

Viral Capsid Antigen (VCA): Sera from patients with Burkitt's lymphoma reproducibly contain antibody to an antigen present in large amounts in a minority of cells in acetone-fixed preparations of virus-producing lymphoblast cultures (G. Henle and W. Henle, 1966a,b; W. Henle et al., 1966). Cross-blocking studies suggest that, like MA, VCA is a complex of antigenic activities (Svedmyr

259

HERPES
SIMPLEX AND
EPSTEIN–BARR
VIRUSES IN
HUMAN CELLS
AND TISSUES:
A STUDY IN
CONTRASTS

and Demissie, 1971). A substantial body of evidence exists which suggests that this antigenic activity resides predominantly in structural components of the viral capsid and requires prior viral DNA synthesis for expression: (1) Sera active against other human herpesviruses fail to react (G. Henle and W. Henle, 1966a,b; W. Henle et al., 1966). (2) In general, the number of fluorescence-positive cells correlates well with electron microscopic evaluation of the number of cells containing virus (G. Henle and W. Henle, 1966a; W. Henle et al., 1966). Manipulations which increase fluorescence in acetone-fixed smears increase the number of cells containing virions (G. Henle and W. Henle, 1966a; W. Henle et al., 1966; Hinuma et al., 1967; W. Henle and G. Henle, 1968). Cells containing electron microscopic and immunofluorescent evidence of viral multiplication demonstrate similar cytopathic changes (G. Henle and W. Henle, 1966a). Cells which possess VCA activity can be shown to incorporate ^{3}H-thymidine into cytoplasmic structures (zur Hausen et al., 1967). Individual fluorescence-positive cells contain large numbers of virus particles (zur Hausen et al., 1967; Epstein and Achong, 1968). Human sera (W. Henle et al., 1966) or hyperimmunized rabbit antisera (Mayyasi et al., 1967) containing anti-VCA activity coat virus nucleocapsids and not enveloped virions (Mayyasi et al., 1967; Silvestre et al., 1971). (3) Electron microscopic and immunofluorescent assays indicate that inhibitors of DNA synthesis such as 5-methylaminodexoxyuridine (G. Henle and W. Henle, 1966a), iododeoxyuridine, and cytosine arabinoside block the synthesis of structural components of EBV. Superinfection of non-virus-producing continuous lymphoblastoid cells with virus from HR1 cells results in production of EA and MA but not VCA (W. Henle et al., 1970a; Gergely et al., 1971a). Withdrawal of inhibitors of DNA synthesis in virus-producing cell lines leads to a decrease in EA-positive VCA-negative cells and to a rise in VCA-positive cells (Gergely et al., 1971a,b).

3.2.8. Assembly of Herpesviruses and Egress from Infected Cells

Most of the information concerning the assembly of herpesviruses and their egress from infected cells comes from electron microscopic studies and is supplemented by very few biochemical data. The available information, dealt with in detail elsewhere (Roizman and Furlong, 1974), can be summarized briefly as follows:

1. Electron microscopic observations indicate that both capsids and cores are assembled in the nucleus. It is not clear whether the core contains DNA at the time of assembly or whether the DNA enters the core subsequent to the assembly of the core. Numerous types of cores differing in structure have been observed. Their role in and relevance to assembly are not clear (Roizman and Furlong, 1974).

2. In most cells infected with herpesviruses, envelopment seems to take place at the inner lamella of the nuclear membrane. The characteristic image is that of a

capsid in apposition to or partially surrounded by the inner lamella of the nuclear membrane. Capsids in apposition to or partially surrounded by cytoplasmic membranes have also been noted, but in this instance it is not clear whether the particle is undergoing envelopment, which raises the question of how a naked capsid would arrive at that location, or whether the particle is undergoing development (Roizman and Furlong, 1974). At the site of envelopment, the inner lamella appears to be altered in two respects; on the nuclear side, it is bounded by an electron-opaque, densely staining plaque consisting of fibrillar material which is probably the precursor of the tegument. On the cytoplasmic side, the nuclear lamella appears to be bound by numerous spikes. Plaques of similar appearance can be seen along stretches of the inner lamella of the nuclear membranes as well as on cytoplasmic membranes, but only at sites opposite nucleocapsids.

3. Little is known of the biochemical events preceding assembly. It has been suggested that virion polypeptide 22A attaches to the surfaces of capsids containing DNA only and that in the process of assembly this polypeptide becomes cleaved (Gibson and Roizman, 1972, 1974). Significantly, capsids are found in apposition to modified regions of membranes only and enveloped virions do not contain host polypeptides. The data suggest that the modified regions of membranes enveloping nucleocapsids contain viral polypeptides which have aggregated and displaced host membrane proteins. It is noteworthy that late in infection the modified regions of the nuclear membranes consist of long stretches folded many times upon themselves. These have been described in the old literature as reduplicated membranes.

4. Enveloped particles are usually found in the space between the inner lamellae of the nuclear membrane and in components of the cytoplasmic vascular system bound by membranes. Enveloped particles in the cytoplasm not bound by cytoplasmic membranes generally appear to be degraded.

5. The mode of egress from the sites of accumulation to extracellular space is uncertain and may well be variable. Two mechanisms have been proposed. One, designated as the continuous route (Schwartz and Roizman, 1969a), is from the inner lamella through the vascular system to the extracellular fluid. The other, which may well be designated as the discontinuous route, is by way of excretory vacuoles in a manner similar to that of other exported cellular products. The two proposed mechanisms of release of mature virus may not be mutually exclusive. Tubules containing mature virions and connecting endoplasmic reticulum to extracellular space have been reported; however, cross-sections of these tubules could readily be interpreted as vacuoles containing virions. In general, the efficiency of release varies depending on the cell, the virus strain, the temperature of incubation, and other factors. Thus HSV-1 strains produce by and large higher yields of virus and the release is generally more efficient. The cytoplasm of cells infected with HSV-2 has been shown to contain many partially enveloped or de-enveloped particles possibly due to damage in transit. The release of HSV-1 from infected cells is near optimal at 37°C and very much reduced at 31–33°C (Hoggan and Roizman, 1959a).

3.3. Modification of Host Structure and Function in Productive Infection

3.3.1. General Comments

The preceding section dealt with the synthesis and assembly of the virus. This section deals with the modification of host structures which become prominent during infection. It is convenient to present the available information in the three sections dealing, respectively, with structural changes in cellular organelles exclusive of membranes, modification of host macromolecular metabolism, and alteration in cellular membranes.

3.3.2. Changes in the Structure of Cellular Organelles

In addition to partially assembled capsids and the plaques in the nuclear membrane described in the preceding section and related to virion morphogenesis, the infected cell nucleus exhibits gross changes in the structure of the nucleolus and chromatin. The nucleolus becomes enlarged and is often found displaced toward the nuclear membrane. Late in infection the nucleolus appears disaggregated or fragmented (Nii, 1971a,b; Schwartz and Roizman, 1969b). Although the changes in the structure of the nucleolus seem to correlate with the inhibition of processing of ribosomal precursor RNA (Wagner and Roizman, 1969a), a causal relationship has not been established.

Displacement and condensation of the chromatin at the nuclear membrane is an early sign of infection. Nothing is known of the mechanism of displacement, although it has been suggested that it is not invariant in cells infected with all herpesviruses (Smith and de Harven, 1973). Two phenomena are correlated with the displacement of chromatin. The first has been erroneously labeled amitotic nuclear division (Scott et al., 1953; Kaplan and Ben-Porat, 1959; Reissig and Kaplan, 1960; Nii and Kamahora, 1963) but is probably an extreme consequence of the distortion of the nucleus leading to fragmentation. The second, of which little is known, is chromosome breakage (Hampar and Ellison, 1961, 1963; O'Neill and Rapp, 1971a,b; Huang and Minowada, 1972). Aberrations induced by HSV cannot be differentiated by site or type from those occurring spontaneously or induced by mutagenic agents (Stich et al., 1964; Huang, 1967). O'Neill and Rapp (1971a) have reported, however, that there is more chromosome breakage in cells infected with HSV-2 and treated with cytosine arabinoside than in either uninfected cells so treated or untreated infected cells. Some early products of infection may be responsible for the breakage of the chromosomes (O'Neill and Rapp, 1971b) since it is reduced in cells pretreated with interferon. A problem of interpretation arises, however, in the light of reports (Stoker, 1959; Stoker and Newton, 1959; Vantis and Wildy, 1962) that infection can both prevent and abort mitosis. For chromosome analysis, cells are arrested in mitosis a few hours after infection at a multiplicity of 2–5 PFU/cell. It is possible therefore that the data are derived from a small sample of cells which have been able to proceed into mitosis because for one reason or another they have escaped infection. It is even conceivable that chromosome breakage is causally linked in some cells with resistance to infection. Until these questions are settled, the significance of the chromosome analyses must remain in doubt.

A characteristic of cells late in productive infection is the presence of long stretches of nuclear membranes folded upon themselves (Nii *et al.*, 1968*a*; Schwartz and Roizman, 1969*a*). Their staining properties resemble those of the "plaques" at the nuclear membrane at which capsids become enveloped.

The most striking feature of the infected cell cytoplasm is the increase in the size of polyribosomes. Polyribosome spirals containing 15–23 ribosomes have been seen (Roizman and Furlong, 1974) and probably account for the increased sedimentation rate of infected cell polyribosomes reported by Sydiskis and Roizman (1966, 1968). Both free and bound polyribosomes have been seen in infected cells, but it is not known whether they polymerize the same or different classes of polypeptides.

3.3.3. Alteration in Host Macromolecular Metabolism

The alterations in host macromolecular metabolism investigated to date involve host DNA, protein, and RNA synthesis. The available data can be briefly summarized as follows:

1. Inhibition of host DNA synthesis has been reported in cells infected with HSV-1 (Aurelian and Roizman, 1965; Roizman, 1969; Roizman and Roane, 1964) and EBV (Gergely *et al.*, 1971*a,b*; Nonoyama and Pagano, 1972*b*).

2. Host protein synthesis also declines rapidly after infection. Cessation of host protein synthesis is accompanied by a decrease in the number of polyribosomes and a concurrent drop in the amino acid incorporation rate soon after infection (Sydiskis and Roizman, 1966; Roizman *et al.*, 1965). Cessation of host protein synthesis is accompanied by a cessation of glycosylation of host proteins (Spear *et al.*, 1970; Heine *et al.*, 1972).

3. The effects of viral infection on host RNA metabolism have been studied extensively in HSV-infected cells (Aurelian and Roizman, 1965; Flanagan, 1967; Hay *et al.*, 1966; Rakusanova *et al.*, 1971, 1972; Wagner and Roizman, 1969*a*). The emerging picture is complex and poorly understood. Very briefly, there is an overall decrease in host RNA synthesis, but the decrease is not uniform for all types of RNA. The decrease in the rate of synthesis is least for RNA greater than 28S and more pronounced for 4S RNA. The biosynthesis of new ribosomal RNA is inhibited at a stage after the synthesis and methylation of 45S precursor (Wagner and Roizman, 1969*a*). Nonribosomal RNA made after infection seems to be incapable of directing host protein synthesis (Roizman *et al.*, 1970). The report by Roizman *et al.* (1970) that host RNA is transported from the nucleus to cytoplasm without delay, in contrast to the bulk of viral RNA, which lingers in the nucleus some 10–20 min after it is made, indicates an alteration in processing of host RNA. Just why host RNA synthesis is not inhibited as completely as host DNA or protein synthesis remains a mystery.

4. Little is known of the mechanism by which host macromolecular synthesis is inhibited, but several comments should perhaps be made. First, the inhibitor of

host macromolecular metabolism must discriminate between analogous host and viral processes, interact with host macromolecules, and produce remarkably invariant effects on host macromolecular metabolism in a wide variety of nonhuman cells. Second, the inhibitory effect is due largely if not entirely to polypeptides made after infection since inhibition of viral expression precludes the inhibition of host functions. A further question is whether a single virus-specific inhibitor is responsible for the cessation of all host cell functions or whether entirely different mechanisms are responsible for the inhibition of DNA and protein synthesis and for the gross alteration in host RNA metabolism. Last, some lines of evidence suggest that inhibition of host functions is a requirement for virus multiplication.

3.3.4. Alteration in the Structure and Function of Cellular Membranes

a. Introduction. The alteration of cellular membranes in the course of malignant transformation of cells has now been firmly established. Viruses have been known to alter the cell membranes both in productive infections, in which the virus multiplies, and in abortive infections, which occasionally result in transformation of cells. Herpesviruses produce extensive alterations in cellular membranes, and in the light of their possible role in human cancer it seems desirable to treat this area extensively and separately from the preceding sections on viral replication.

b. General Description. The first inkling that herpesviruses alter the structure of the plasma membrane (Roizman 1962a,b) came from the isolation of mutant variants of HSV, pseudorabies, and herpes B virus strains which differ from the "wild" or parental strains in their effects on cells (Tokumaru, 1957; Gray *et al.*, 1958; Hoggan and Roizman, 1959b; Hinze and Walker, 1961; Falke, 1961; Nii and Kamahora, 1961; Kohlhage and Siegert, 1962; Schneweiss, 1962; Kohlhage, 1964; Wheeler, 1964; Kohlage and Schieferstein, 1965; Ejercito *et al.*, 1968; Schiek, 1967; Schneweiss *et al.*, 1972; Schiek and Schneweiss, 1968). Whereas the parental strains cause the cells to round up and clump, the variants cause cells to fuse. Ejercito *et al.* (1968) classified HSV strains into four groups: (1) strains causing rounding of cells but no adhesion or fusion, (2) strains causing loose aggregation of rounded cells, (3) strains causing tight adhesion of cells, and (4) strains causing polykaryocytosis. The viruses comprising each group may have slightly different effects on cells. Thus polykaryocytes induced by various strains of HSV differ in size and morphology (Roizman and Aurelian, 1965; Kohlhage, 1964; Wheeler, 1964). The term "social behavior of infected cells" was introduced (Roizman, 1962a,b, 1969; Ejercito *et al.*, 1968) to describe the different interactions demonstrable in monolayer cultures of cells infected at very low multiplicities in which the infected cells can easily be differentiated from the surrounding lawn of uninfected cells. So striking is the appearance of the foci of infected cells that the technique is used not only for differentiation of strains but also as a precise and reproducible plaque assay for the infectivity of virus preparations (Hoggan *et al.*, 1960; Roizman and Roane, 1961a, 1963).

The conclusion that viruses alter the structure of the plasma membrane (Roizman, 1971a,b) was based on the reasoning that the shape, adhesiveness, and social behavior of infected cells must reflect membrane properties and the observation that the social behavior of infected cells is genetically determined by the virus. All subsequent studies have been directed toward elucidating the structural, functional, and immunological properties of the infected cell membranes and have yielded four lines of evidence indicating changes in structure and function of plasma membranes. These are presented in a logical rather than the chronological order.

c. Leakage of Macromolecules from Infected Cells. The evidence that macromolecules leak from infected cells emerged from studies (Kamiya *et al.*, 1964, 1965; Zemla *et al.*, 1967) whose objectives were to elucidate the regulation of viral macromolecules and has been reviewed in detail elsewhere (Roizman, 1969). Suffice it to mention that in the first of the papers Kamiya *et al.* (1964) reported an *in vitro* system measuring collectively the enzymes involved in the incorporation of deoxynucleotides into DNA. The authors showed that the limiting enzyme increased in activity during the first 6 h, leveled off between 6 and 10 h and subsequently decreased. However, no leveling off or decrease in enzyme activity was observed in extracts of infected cells grown in a medium containing bromodeoxyuridine. This led to the conclusion that (1) the enzymes are regulated, (2) substitution of bromodeoxyuridine for thymidine interferes with the regulation, and (3) regulation is dependent not on the presence of viral DNA *per se* but on the presence of a newly synthesized complement of viral DNA. In subsequent studies of the regulation of enzyme activity in infected cells, Kamiya *et al.* (1965) and Zemla *et al.* (1967) found significant leakage of proteins beginning 5–8 h after infection. On the basis of experiments with inhibitors, they concluded that the leakage is due to one or more proteins synthesized approximately 4 h after infection. Although the evidence for the involvement of early viral proteins in the leakage is inadequate (Roizman, 1969), leakage of RNA was also manifestly higher in HEp-2 cells infected with HSV-1 than in uninfected cells (Wagner and Roizman, 1969a). It is conceivable that the change in transmembrane potential observed in HSV-infected cells is related to the leakiness of infected cell membranes (Fritz and Nahmias, 1972).

d. Changes in the Surface Structure of Infected Cells. Wilbanks and Campbell (1972) differentiated between uninfected and HSV-infected cells by the number of microvilli. Changes in the reactivity of the cells with concanavalin A following infection were also reported (Tevethia *et al.*, 1972). In this instance, the cells became agglutinable by concanavalin A by 2 h after infection.

e. Incorporation of Viral Proteins into Plasma Membrane. The presence of viral proteins in cellular membranes was reported in several publications (Spear *et al.*, 1970; Keller *et al.*, 1970; Heine *et al.*, 1972; Heine and Roizman, 1973). The pertinent data may be summarized as follows:

1. Purified fractionated cytoplasmic membranes (Spear *et al.*, 1970) and plasma membranes (Heine *et al.*, 1972) extracted from HSV-1 (F) infected cells cosediment with proteins made after infection and absent from uninfected cells. In polyacrylamide gels, these proteins comigrate in polyacrylamide gels with the major noncapsid virion proteins and have a similar glycosylation profile. The studies of the plasma membranes of infected and uninfected cells have not revealed major changes in the composition of the host membrane proteins after infection.

2. The virus-specific proteins cosedimenting with the plasma membranes throughout purification do not constitute either adventitious contaminants adhering to the plasma membranes or fragments of viral envelopes stripped off virions during the preparation of the infected cell plasma membranes. The data are as follows: Mixtures of infected and uninfected plasma membranes are readily separated by isopycnic centrifugation in sucrose gradients following reaction with antiviral antibody, which binds to viral proteins in the membranes and thereby augments the total protein mass relative to that of lipids. Consequently, membranes binding antiviral antibody band at a higher density than those lacking these antigens (Roizman and Spear, 1971). In a series of experiments, Heine and Roizman (1973) have shown that whereas artificial mixtures of labeled infected and uninfected cell membranes are readily separable by isopycnic centrifugation following reaction with antiviral antibody, the host polypeptides labeled before infection band with the infected cell membrane and not with the host proteins contained in the membranes extracted from uninfected cells. Moreover, microcavitation employed for preparation of plasma membranes does not inactivate the infectious virus accumulating in infected cells. The viral proteins are thus bound on the same membrane fragments as host proteins and with sufficient tenacity to withstand hydrodynamic stress augmented by the presence of bound antibody. The fact that not all viral glycoproteins appear in the plasma membrane, as discussed in a subsequent section, suggests that the binding of viral polypeptides is not only tenacious but also specific.

f. Alteration in Immunological Specificity of the Plasma Membrane. The studies on immunological specificity of cells infected with herpesviruses were prompted by the observation that herpesviruses alter the social behavior of cells (Roizman, 1962b), as discussed in the preceding section.

The new immunological specificity of infected cells can be detected by a test based on the observation that viruses fail to multiply in somatic cells injured by antibody and complement (Roizman and Roane, 1961b). Cells infected with HSV-1, suspended, washed, and incubated at 37°C with antibody and complement are seeded after 1 h on monolayer cultures of HEp-2 cells, where uninjured cells can be detected by the formation of plaques. The assay was initially standardized with 2-h infected cells and antibody made against uninfected cells (Roizman and Roane, 1961b), which cannot be differentiated immunologically from 2-h infected cells.

267

HERPES
SIMPLEX AND
EPSTEIN–BARR
VIRUSES IN
HUMAN CELLS
AND TISSUES:
A STUDY IN
CONTRASTS

The alteration of immunological specificity after infection can be seen by exposing 20–24-h infected cells to rabbit sera prepared against HSV-1-infected cells (Roane and Roizman, 1964b). Complement and unabsorbed anti–infected cell serum prevent plaque formation by 2-, 24-, and 48-h infected cells. However, complement with serum absorbed with uninfected cells prevents plaque formation by only 24- and 48-h infected cells. This implies that cells acquire one or more new antigens between 2 and 20 h after infection. Structural alterations in the membranes of infected cells have also been found by Watkins (1964) in HeLa cells infected with the HFEM strain of herpes simplex, which adhere to sheep erythrocytes sensitized with rabbit anti–sheep erythrocyte serum. The adhesion of sensitized erythrocytes to the infected cells could be abolished by exposing the infected HeLa cells to antiviral serum but not to normal rabbit serum or rabbit anti–sheep erythrocyte serum. Virus-specific antigens have since been demonstrated by a variety of techniques in cells infected not only with HSV (Ito and Barron, 1972; Smith et al., 1972a,b; Nahmias et al., 1971; Wildy, 1973; Espmark, 1965; Brier et al., 1971) but also with EBV (Klein et al., 1968a,b) and herpes zoster virus (Ito and Barron, 1973).

The new antigen is probably a structural component of the viral envelope. The evidence is as follows: (1) Absorption of serum with partially purified HSV-1 virions removes both neutralizing and cytolytic antibody (Roane and Roizman, 1964b). However, the significance of this observation is limited by the possibility of contamination of the purified virus preparation by host antigens. There is similar evidence for antigens appearing on the surface of EBV-infected lymphocyte and EB virion antigens (Pearson et al., 1970a,b). (2) The neutralizing and cytolytic titers of hyperimmune sera prepared against a variety of antigens extracted from infected permissive and nonpermissive cells correlate well (Roizman and Spring, 1967). (3) Rabbit hyperimmune sera produced against dog kidney cells abortively infected with HSV-1 (MP) and which make nucleocapsids but not enveloped virus lack both neutralizing and cytolytic antibody (Roizman and Spring, 1967; Spring et al., 1968). (4) Purified plasma membranes from HSV-1-infected cells contain herpesvirus glycoproteins (Heine et al., 1972; Heine and Roizman, 1973). The infected cell membranes readily react with antiviral antibody, as discussed earlier (Roizman and Spear, 1971). Purified infected cell membranes compete with the infectious virus neutralizing antibody (Roizman et al., 1973). (5) Passage of infected cell membranes through columns prepared with immune sera established that glycoproteins are the reactive constituents of the infected membrane (Savage et al., 1972).

g. *Viral Membrane Proteins and the Social Behavior of Infected Cells.* Although it is too early to judge their precise significance, there are suggestive correlations between the polypeptide composition of cellular membranes and the social behavior of cells infected with different strains of herpesvirus. In particular, the number and electrophoretic mobility of the proteins on the smooth membranes of cells infected with HSV-1 (MP), which causes cells to fuse, differ from those of the smooth membrane proteins of cells infected with HSV-1 (mP), which causes cells to clump. In cells doubly infected with HSV-1 (MP) and HSV-1 (mP) and in which both viruses multiply (Roizman, 1963), both the composition of the cellular membrane proteins and the social behavior of the cells are characteristic of HSV-1 (mP) infection (Roizman, 1962b, 1971b). Recent studies using polyacrylamide gels cross-linked with DATD show that the HSV-1 (mP) virion contains a glycoprotein (VP8) absent from HSV-1 (MP) (Heine et al., 1974). Moreover, this difference is reflected in the composition of the plasma membranes of cells infected with the different strains, which also differ in the proportion of polypeptides 7 and 8.5 to 17 and 18. The relative amounts of 7 and 8.5 are less in cells infected with HSV-1 (MP) (Roizman and Furlong, 1974). However, a causal relationship between these differences in the social behavior of the infected cells has yet to be established; and the evaluation of their significance must await the results of studies on temperature-sensitive mutants and perhaps on isolated membrane proteins in vitro.

4. Infection of Restrictive and Nonpermissive Cells

4.1. Definitions

The preceding section dealt with productive infection of herpesviruses, particularly herpes simplex, in permissive cells. Productive infection is easy to synchronize and yields large quantities of infectious virus. But it is infection in restrictive cells giving low virus yields and in nonpermissive cells, in which infection aborts, that is of particular interest to us in connection with the putative role of herpesviruses in human cancer. This is because herpesviruses kill the cells in which they multiply. Transformation by herpesviruses must therefore occur only when for one reason or another the virus cannot replicate.

4.2. Herpes Simplex Viruses

Abortive infections with HSV fall into three classes. In the first, nonpermissive cells fail to support infection with virus capable of reproducing in permissive cells under the same experimental conditions. In this case, the cells are generally derived from species which do not normally become infected with the virus in question, so that abortive infection is due to a shift in host range. Second, abortive infections may result from infection of permissive cells either with damaged virus or with competent virus under nonphysiological conditions such as supraoptimal temperatures. Third, infection may abort in permissive cells infected with temperature-sensitive mutants and incubated at nonpermissive temperatures. Here we shall be concerned with the first two classes. It is too early to derive conclusions from the studies on the temperature-sensitive mutants.

269

HERPES
SIMPLEX AND
EPSTEIN–BARR
VIRUSES IN
HUMAN CELLS
AND TISSUES:
A STUDY IN
CONTRASTS

4.2.1. Abortive Infection of Nonpermissive Cells

Of the many studies on abortive infection of nonpermissive cells reported to date, two detailed ones are worth reporting. The first involved a strain of HSV-1 (HSV-1 MPdk⁻) which would multiply in HEp-2 cells but not in dog kidney (DK) cells (Aurelian and Roizman, 1964, 1965). Mutants derived from this strain multiply in both cell lines (Roizman and Aurelian, 1965). In this instance, the outcome of infection was dependent on the multiplicity of virus to which cells were exposed. At high multiplicities of virus, the DK cells made viral DNA and capsids but not enveloped particles and only one-tenth the surface antigen seen in productive infection of HEp-2 cells (Spring *et al.*, 1968). At low multiplicities, abortively infected DK cells made interferon only and no apparent viral products (Aurelian and Roizman, 1964, 1965). The second study was based on experiments utilizing chick embryo cultures in which HSV-2 isolates produced plaques whereas most HSV-1 isolates did not. Comparison of a HSV-1 strain capable of growing in duck embryo cells with one which can not showed that the abortively infected cells make complement-fixing antigens but fail to make either DNA or detectable amounts of surface antigens (Lowry *et al.*, 1971).

Of potential interest are the reports that a cell line derived from the rat and transformed with Rous sarcoma virus (XC line) is nonpermissive to HSV even though rat cell cultures are permissive. Infected XC cells are reported to produce viral antigen but not infectious progeny and appear to survive infection (Docherty *et al.*, 1973; Garfinkle and McAuslan, 1974).

4.2.2. Abortive Infection of Permissive Cells

There are two types of studies of abortive infection of permissive cells. In the first, the virus is damaged so that it cannot replicate. In the second, the infected cells are incubated at supraoptimal temperatures at which the virus cannot multiply.

a. Abortive Infection and Transformation of Cells with Damaged Virus. For most studies of abortive infection and transformation of cells with damaged virus, virus is inactivated by ultraviolet irradiation (Rapp and Duff, 1972*a,b*, 1973; Duff and Rapp, 1971; Rapp *et al.*, 1972). A study has recently been reported on virus damaged by acridine dye and visible light (Rapp *et al.*, 1973).

Ultraviolet irradiation of HSV prevents replication, presumably through damage to the DNA, as well as all the major manifestations of viral infection: inhibition of host function, alteration in social behavior of cells, and production of appreciable amounts of viral antigen. The fate of the entering viral DNA is not known. Several studies have shown that ultraviolet-damaged DNA can be repaired under certain conditions (Pfefferkorn *et al.*, 1966; Ross *et al.*, 1972*a*). Viral functions have been shown to be expressed in a small fraction of infected cells and have been the subject of two series of studies.

In the first (Munyon *et al.*, 1971, 1972*a,b*; Davidson *et al.*, 1973), mutants of L cells lacking thymidine kinase (LtK⁻ cells) were exposed to ultraviolet-irradiated virus and plated in a medium selective for cells carrying thymidine kinase.

Subsequent studies have demonstrated that the enzyme expressed in cells growing in the selective medium resembles the enzyme made in productively infected cells and differs from the uninfected cell enzyme in electrophoretic mobility and serological reactivity (Munyon et al., 1972b; Wadsworth and Roizman, unpublished studies). Although the cells retain the genetic information for the viral enzyme, expression is lost on continued passage of the cells. The evidence (Davidson et al., 1973) for this conclusion is that some of the cells derived from a single LtK⁺ clone and grown in nonselective media can multiply in medium containing BUdR and must therefore lack thymidine kinase. On the other hand, populations derived from these cells and placed in the selective medium give rise to clones capable of making the enzyme. Very preliminary attempts to recover appreciable amounts of viral transcripts in these cells have failed, so it is not known how much of the viral DNA has been retained and what proportion of viral DNA is expressed under conditions of induction of kinase activity (Wadsworth and Roizman, unpublished studies).

The second series of studies have dealt with hamster embryo fibroblasts exposed to ultraviolet-irradiated HSV-1 and HSV-2 viruses, which cause transformation of the cultured cells. All of these transformed cell lines reported to date multiply continuously, but vary in morphology and ability to induce tumors in hamsters. Thus HSV-2 transformants include lines of fibroblastic cells, giant cells, and primitive mesenchymal cells. HSV-1 transformants include lines of epitheloid cells. The cell lines vary from highly oncogenic and capable of causing metastatic tumors to only nominally oncogenic and nononcogenic lines. Both HSV-1 and HSV-2 strains are capable of transforming cells but the efficiency, even within serotypes, varies considerably. All transformed cell lines demonstrate virus antigen in the cytoplasm and on cell surfaces and a few induce neutralizing antibody on inoculation in the hamster. These observations suggest that viral genetic information is retained in these cells, although how much is present and how much is transcribed is not known.

b. Abortive Infection Resulting from Maintenance of Infected Cells in Nonphysiological Conditions. Darai and Munk (1973) and Munk and Darai (1973) reported on abortive infection and apparent transformation of human embryonic fibroblasts by HSV-1 and HSV-2 in cells maintained at 42°C for several days immediately after infection. Although the cells made viral antigens and at least traces of viral DNA, they were readily passaged continuously and by the sixty-fifth passage were reported not to have reached the senescence characteristic of uninfected cells at these high passages.

4.3. Epstein–Barr Virus

EBV is characterized by two properties of experimental significance. First, it has a very restricted host range. Second, as pointed out earlier in the text, the small fraction of susceptible cells, defined as producer cell lines, are at best restrictive; the bulk of the cells are, in any case, nonpermissive.

271
HERPES
SIMPLEX AND
EPSTEIN–BARR
VIRUSES IN
HUMAN CELLS
AND TISSUES:
A STUDY IN
CONTRASTS

4.3.1. Host Range

Following the initial discovery of EBV in cultured lymphoblasts derived from Burkitt's lymphoma, numerous efforts were made to culture the virus in a wide variety of primary cell cultures and in continuous cell lines of human and animal origin (Epstein *et al.*, 1965; Rabson *et al.*, 1966). To date, EBV antigens have been detected only in lymphoid cells. All efforts to propagate the virus on cells derived from other tissues have been unsuccessful. Little is known of the fate of the virus to which these cells had been exposed. Of particular interest in connection with experimental extension of the host range are the studies of Glaser and O'Neill (1972) in which virus-producing human lymphoblastoid cells were fused with human bone marrow cells or with mouse cells using inactivated Sendai virus. From 1 to 20% of the cells in clones of the human hybrid lines could be induced to produce EBV antigens on exposure to 5-iododeoxyuridine (Glaser and Rapp, 1972). Induction of EBV antigen was enhanced by treatment of the human hybrid cells with dibutyryl cyclic AMP (Zimmerman *et al.*, 1973).

4.3.2. Infection of Lymphocytes with EBV: Transformation of Lymphocytes

The first successful experimental transmission of EBV was in 1967 (W. Henle *et al.*, 1967). Cocultivation of female infant lymphocytes with lethally irradiated virus-producing cells of the male Jijoye line resulted in establishment of long-term lymphoblast cultures with the female karyotype. On the other hand, attempts to establish long-term cultures by cocultivation with nonproducing Raji cells failed. Establishment of long-term lymphoblastoid cultures from fetal and/or peripheral cell suspensions, normally capable of limited life span in culture, is subsequently defined as a "transforming" event. Subsequent studies have confirmed and amplified the report by W. Henle *et al.* (1967): (1) Fetal cord blood lymphocytes and cells from normal EBV-seronegative individuals rarely, if ever, spontaneously give rise to long-term lymphoblast cultures (Nilsson, 1971; Chang, 1971; Miller *et al.*, 1971; Gerber *et al.*, 1969; Pope *et al.*, 1968*b*, 1969*a*). Exposure of lymphocytes from fetal cord blood or from EBV-seronegative adults to cell-free extracts of EBV producer lines in contrast to nonproducer lines results in establishment of long-term continuous lymphoblast cell lines (Pope *et al.*, 1969*a*; Gerber *et al.*, 1969). Throat washings from patients with acute and convalescent infectious mononucleosis have pronounced "transforming capability" (Chang and Golden, 1971). (2) Preincubation of cell-free extracts or throat washings with human sera containing measurable amounts of anti-VCA, but probably containing anti-MA activity as well, prevents transformation; sera lacking antibody had no effect (Miller *et al.*, 1971; Gerber *et al.*, 1969; Pope *et al.*, 1969*a*). (3) Many, but not all, of the long-term lymphoblast cell lines established following exposure to EBV contain subpopulations of VCA-positive cells (W. Henle *et al.*, 1967; Gerber *et al.*, 1969; Miller *et al.*, 1971; Chang, 1971; Chang and Golden, 1971; Pope *et al.*, 1969*a*; Nilsson *et al.*, 1971).

Preliminary observations suggest that cell lines containing more than a few percent VCA-positive cells occur following transformation of adult but not of fetal leukocytes (Gerber, personal communication). Under rigidly controlled conditions, *in vitro* transformation can be exploited to provide a quantitative bioassay for EBV (Morse and Pope, 1972). The leukocyte cultures must be maintained for several weeks to establish a clear end point. Anticomplementary immunofluorescence may detect EBNA within transformed cells within 6 days (Menezes *et al.*, 1974; Leibold *et al.*, 1974).

Long-term lymphoblastoid cell lines have been established following exposure of peripheral leukocytes of two New World primates, the squirrel monkey and the cottontop marmoset, to extracts of lymphoblastoid cells from a patient with transfusion-induced mononucleosis (Miller *et al.*, 1972b). Two resultant simian continuous lymphoblastoid cell lines have been extensively studied. Evidence that the cells were transformed by EBV included (1) visualization of a herpesvirus in thin sections of a small percentage of the cells, (2) identification of EB viral antigens in continuous lymphoblastoid cell lines by immunofluorescence and complement fixation assays, and (3) transformation of human lymphocytes by spent medium cleared of cells. The transforming activity by centrifugation was neutralized by human sera containing antibodies to EBV. Also, (4) the sera of primates used in these studies contained no detectable CF antibody reactive with EBV or with the transformed cell lines, and (5) no cytopathic activity could be demonstrated by cocultivation of the simian continuous lymphoblastoid cell lines with African green or owl monkey kidney or human placental cell lines. The interpretation of these studies is complicated by the report of Gerber and Lorenz (1974) that New World primates, as well as chimpanzees and Old World monkeys, naturally possess CF antibodies reactive with EBV. Until the "EBV"-like agent infecting nonhuman primates is isolated and its properties are defined, we cannot be sure that the agent recovered from experimental infection of New World monkeys is the same as the agent with which they have been inoculated. Analysis of the DNA (Pritchett *et al.*, 1974) of EBV purified from the marmoset cell line (B95-8) of Miller *et al.* (1972b) indicates the following: (1) The DNA is a linear, double-strand molecule with a molecular weight of approximately $1.03 \pm 5 \times 10^6$ daltons. (2) The DNA bands at 1.718 cm/cm^3 in CsCl. If there were no unusual bases in EBV DNA, this would correspond to a guanine plus cytosine content of 58 moles percent. (3) The DNA possesses single-strand nicks. (4) All the sequences of EBV from B95–8 cells hybridize to EBV purified from HR1 cells. The hybrids thus formed have identical thermal stability to homohybrid DNA, indicating that there is less than 1.5% unmatching of base pairs in the heterohybrid DNAs. (5) B95-8 DNA lacks approximately 15% of the sequences of HR1 DNA and is relatively rich in sequences of approximately 60–61% guanine plus cytosine. These data support the biological and immunological data which suggest that the EBV derived from B95–8 cells probably originated from the infectious mononucleosis lymphoblast extracts to which the marmoset leukocytes were exposed.

Of the two populations of human lymphocytes, B, or immunoglobulin producing, and T, or thymus dependent and mediating cellular immunity, EBV seems only to infect the former. Almost all continuous lymphoblastoid cell lines produce immunoglobulin (Nilsson, 1971) and possess surface marker immunoglobulin in detectable amounts (E. Klein *et al.*, 1972; Moore and Minowada, 1973). Direct evidence suggests that EBV cannot adsorb to (Jondal and Klein, 1973) or transform (Pattengale *et al.*, 1973) a pure T-cell population.

Conversely, two continuous lymphoblastoid cell lines established from patients with leukemia lack surface immunoglobulin and form rosettes with sheep erythrocytes, presumptive evidence for identification as T cells. Both of these cell lines lack EB viral intranuclear complement-fixing antigen and EBV DNA detectable by DNA–DNA reassociation kinetics (Kawai *et al.*, 1973; Pagano, 1974). A weakness of this analysis is that distinguishing features applicable to lymphocytes may not differentiate between lymphoblastoid cells in culture, and EBV may influence the surface characteristics of the infected cell.

4.3.3. *Expression of EBV DNA in Transformed Cell Lines*

Continuous lymphoblastoid cell lines, whether isolated from EBV-seropositive patients or transformed *in vitro*, vary in the extent of the EBV genome expressed in these cells. Several points should be made in this regard:

1. Of 20 cell lines established from lymphoid tissue or peripheral blood of EBV-seropositive adults, 19 contained 0.1–5% VCA-positive cells when tested within 2 months of establishment in culture. Eleven of the 19 VCA-positive cell lines became negative within 2–4 months of continuous cultivation (Nilsson *et al.*, 1971). Similar findings have been reported by others (Klein *et al.*, 1968*b*).

2. As stated repeatedly, here at least, continuous lymphoblastoid cell lines are only partially permissive for EBV and only a minority of cells produce virus. Only three cell lines have produced sufficient quantities of virus to permit partial purification of virions for structural or biochemical studies. Two lines, HR1 and EB3, are derived from Burkitt tumors. The EB3 line has ceased to provide adequate quantities of virus. The fraction of VCA-positive cells in the HR1 cell line during several years of cultivation at the University of Chicago has varied from 0.1 to 20%. Single-cell clones have been derived from virus-producing cell lines in the presence of antiviral serum (Miller *et al.*, 1970; Zajac and Kohn, 1970). Each clone contained the same proportion of virus-producing cells as the parent population. These data suggest that all virus-producing cells contain a competent viral genome repressed through a mechanism which permits characteristic frequency of activation. This conclusion is supported by recent data of Hampar *et al.* (1973, 1974) that activation of the viral genome in the virus-producing EB3 line is dependent on a critical event in early S phase. Thus exposure of synchronized EB3 cultures to inhibitors of DNA synthesis for 1–2 h following reversal of a thymidine block resulted in an increase in EA- and VCA-positive cells. Recent studies indicate that a marmoset cell line derived by exposure of cells to the spent medium from cultures of human infectious mononucleosis lymphoblasts produces relatively large amounts of virus; the fraction of producing cells has been estimated to be as high as 10%.

3. Several continuous lymphoblastoid cell lines of infectious mononucleosis, Burkitt's lymphoma, and nasopharyngeal carcinoma origin have never been

shown to express VCA or EA (Klein and Dombos, 1973). The observation that viral antigen production and virion synthesis could be activated in a previously antigen-negative cell line by exposure to IUdR or BUdR (Sugawara *et al.*, 1972; Hampar *et al.*, 1972; Gerber, 1972) has led to a systematic evaluation of the sensitivity of 14 nonproducing cell lines to superinfection with virus extracted from HR1 cells, and to the activation of the presumed latent viral genome by inhibitors of DNA synthesis (Klein and Dombos, 1973). EA appeared following superinfection of six cell lines of the 13 which absorbed virus (G. Klein *et al.*, 1972). Eleven of 14 cell lines showed significant activation of EA fluorescence following exposure to IUdR or BUdR. The percentage of cells of a given culture expressing EA following superinfection tends to correlate with the number of cells producing EA following exposure to IUdR or BUdR. Although additional data may be required to establish the significance of these observations, so far it seems likely that most continuous lymphoblast cell lines which do not express viral antigen possess most, if not all, of the viral genome and that there are at least two blocks in viral replication before EA production but after virus absorption.

4. Recent observations suggest that there are highly significant biological differences between the virus which is released from most continuous lymphoblast cell lines and the HR1 virus (Miller *et al.*, 1974; Menezes *et al.*, 1974). Virus released from HR1 cells is capable of superinfecting non-virus-producing continuous lymphoblastoid cell lines. Infection is followed by the induction of EA and even virion antigen synthesis. Despite the relatively large quantities of virus produced, as determined by superinfection assay (defined by the induction of EA synthesis in non-virus-producing Raji cells) and by the physical and biochemical enumeration of virions, little if any activity is detectable in *in vitro* transformation assays.

The variability in the extent of expression of the EBV genome in different cell lines raises some interesting questions. On one hand, it seems likely that the expression of the viral genome would be determined by the expression of the host genome. This view is compatible with the enhancement of virus expression observed in cells deprived of arginine or treated with halogenated pyrimidines, cyclic nucleotides, or a variety of inhibitors of DNA synthesis. On the other hand, the virus released by HR1 cells, unlike that produced by other lines, does not transform cells. It seems likely, therefore, that the biological properties of EBV contained in lymphoblasts may also be responsible, at least in part, for the extent of expression of viral genome in these cells. It is clear that while differences may be found between viruses contained in various lymphoblast cell lines, in the absence of permissive cells capable of reproducing the virus synchronously and in large amounts it will be difficult to ascertain their relevance to those of the epidemiologically significant "wild" virus transmitted from man to man.

4.3.4. Relationship Between Viral and Cellular Genomes in Nonpermissive Infection

Single-cell clones derived from partially permissive and nonpermissive lymphoblastoid cell lines in the presence of antiviral serum contain viral genetic information, demonstrable by complement-fixing antigen assay and the presence of viral DNA. A mechanism must therefore exist for the transmission of viral genetic information. A potential flaw in this analysis arises from the evidence cited above that the continuous growth of lymphoblastoid cells *in vitro* may require the presence of at least part of the EBV genome. Thus progeny lacking viral DNA may not give rise to clones. Available biochemical data do not permit a choice between chromosomal or extrachromosomal mode of inheritance. In general, three types of data are available which have a direct bearing on this question.

a. Estimates of the Number of Copies of Viral Genome in Lymphoblastoid Cells. A variety of techniques have been employed to detect EBV-specific sequences in biopsy materials and in continuous lymphoblastoid cell lines. All are subject to quantitative errors of one sort or another. Two-phase liquid filter hybridization has for the most part been done without kinetic analysis, and in any event the amount of cellular DNA which can be applied to filters is limited and it is most difficult to control precisely for variability in DNA hybridization sites on the filter. Single-phase hybridizations are amenable to quantitative kinetic analysis (Wetmur and Davidson, 1968), and have been employed more recently. A second problem arises with regard to labeling of EBV DNA for hybridization studies. Attempts to modify media to enhance incorporation of labeled nucleotide precursors have, in general, resulted in markedly decreased virus yields. Most studies have employed *Escherichia coli* DNA-dependent RNA polymerase or DNA polymerase 1 to label EBV nucleic acid *in vitro*. Available data suggest that only the latter procedure results in uniform labeling (Gelb *et al.*, 1971; Petterson and Sambrook, 1973) and is suitable only under conditions in which DNA is nicked in a random fashion and polymerization is carried out at low temperature (Kelly *et al.*, 1970). By use of polymerase 1 labeled nucleic acid, it is possible not only to estimate the number of genome copies but also to determine whether complete copies are present, at least to within 10 or 20%.

A large number of specimens have been examined by cRNA–DNA liquid filter hybridization and a smaller number by DNA–DNA renaturation kinetics. The results may be summarized as follows: Burkitt tumor tissues, with a single exception out of more than 20 samples analyzed, contained between 4 and 113 genome equivalents by cRNA–DNA hybridization (Nonoyama *et al.*, 1973; Lindahl *et al.*, 1974). Three Burkitt tumors have been studied by DNA–DNA renaturation. The single biopsy specimen, negative by cRNA–DNA hybridization, was negative by DNA–DNA renaturation (Kawai *et al.*, 1973). Two other biopsies had 45 (Nonoyama and Pagano, 1973) and 8 genome (Kawai *et al.*, 1973) equivalents per cell. Of 19 continuous lymphoblastoid cell lines studied to date, all contained between 5 and 510 genome equivalents per cell according to cRNA–DNA hybridization (Pagano, 1974; zur Hausen and Schulte-Holthausen, 1972; zur Hausen *et al.*, 1972; Nonoyama and Pagano, 1971). The Raji cell line has been studied most extensively and has been found to have approximately 50 genome equivalents per cell by both cRNA–DNA (zur Hausen and Schulte-Holthausen, 1970; Nonoyama and Pagano, 1971) and DNA–DNA hybridization

(Nonoyama and Pagano, 1973). The estimated genome equivalent content was remarkably consistent in several laboratories during more than a year of continuous cultivation of the Raji cell line. Three continuous lymphoblast cell lines established from human cord blood following exposure to throat washings from patients with mononucleosis were found by DNA–DNA reassociation to contain 5.5–7.5 genome equivalents per cell (Kawai *et al.*, 1973).

The importance of these quantitative estimates is that they suggest that if there is a unique chromosomal insertion site it must be capable of holding tandem repeats of the viral genome or, alternatively, most copies may be episomally situated. Further, there is probably a mechanism which assures the propagation of the same number of genome equivalents over many generations in culture. Whether or not the primary site of preservation of the EBV genome is chromosomal, the question naturally arises of whether the entire genome is invariably conserved—and, if so, why? Nine EBV-positive biopsies or continuous lymphoblastoid cell lines have been examined to date by DNA–DNA renaturation kinetics. All seem to contain more than 80% of the EBV genome when the HR1 virus is used as the reagent probe (Nonoyama and Pagano, 1973; Kawai *et al.*, 1973; Kieff and Levine, 1974).

b. Physical State of Viral DNA in Nonpermissive Cells. Adams *et al.* (1973) have examined the density of EBV complementary sequences in Raji cells following gentle lysis to prevent breakage of the DNA. Most of the EBV complementary sequences are distinctly separable from the cell DNA peak. Following rebanding of the DNA in the region of cell DNA under conditions which preserve the size of DNA at about 10^8 daltons, the small residuum of EBV complementary sequences bands with almost the same isopycnic distribution as the cell DNAs. Shearing of the cell DNA prior to rebanding results in distinctly separable peaks of EBV and cell DNA. Isopycnic banding (Adams *et al.*, 1973) or sucrose velocity sedimentation (Nonoyama and Pagano, 1972*b*) of high molecular weight DNAs under alkaline conditions gives complete separation. Taken together, these data strongly suggest that some, but probably not all, EBV DNA in nonproductively infected cells is linked to cell DNA at an unknown site in an alkali-labile fashion. It is likely that EBV DNA itself possesses alkali-labile linkages much as HSV and MDV DNAs do (Lee *et al.*, 1971; Kieff *et al.*, 1971).

c. Chromosomal Abnormalities and Studies of Chromosomal Localization of EBV. Extensive search has been undertaken for chromosomal abnormalities in Burkitt tumor biopsy specimens and continuous lymphoblastoid cell lines (zur Hausen, 1972; Epstein and Achong, 1973). Most of the early lymphoblastoid cell lines have been found to be diploid or near diploid. The incidence of abnormality increases with time in culture (Cooper *et al.*, 1966) and in productively infected cells. The abnormalities reported have been inconstant, with the exception of a subterminal secondary constriction of chromosome 10 initially reported by Kohn *et al.* (1967) in four of five Burkitt cell lines. The association of this finding with EBV infection is strengthened by its appearance in cell lines transformed *in vitro* on exposure to EBV (W. Henle *et al.*, 1967; Pope *et al.*, 1968*a*). But more recent workers have cast doubt on the generality of the association (Steel *et al.*, 1971; Manolov and Manolova, 1972). Using quinacrine staining and fluorescence microscopy, Manlov and Manlova (1972) have recently reviewed the karyotype of six biopsy specimens and nine continuous lymphoblastoid cell lines. Of the 15 specimens examined, 12 possessed an extra marker band at the end of the long arm of chromosome 14. In the positive cultures, all analyzable cells were found to possess the abnormality.

Attempts made over several years by the zur Hausen laboratory at *in situ* hybridization have recently been reviewed (zur Hausen, 1972). The data are difficult to interpret. Despite the fact that Raji cells contain 60 genome equivalents per cell, the average number of grains exceeded the grain count of control preparations only by a factor of 8. Although the grains seemed to be associated with the chromosomes, the altered morphology of the chromosomes following denaturation has prohibited precise determination of the chromosomal location. It is conceivable that more heavily labeled cRNA or even DNA labeled *in vitro* might improve the resolution of this technique.

Some indirect evidence is provided by the studies of Hampar using synchronized Raji cells. Induction of EA synthesis required exposure of cells to IUdR during an early critical period of S phase as in virus-producing EB3 cells (Hampar *et al.*, 1973). Analysis of the relative number of viral and cell genome equivalents in Raji cells following reversal of a double thymidine block indicated that viral DNA is synthesized during this same critical interval (Hampar *et al.*, 1974*b*). An attractive hypothesis suggested by Hampar to explain this temporal association of activation following induction and normal synthesis of viral DNA is that viral DNA is linked to an early-replicating piece of cell DNA. More direct evidence bearing on this question may come from studies currently in progress correlating the persistence of viral genetic information with the persistence of human chromosomes in hybrid cells (Glaser and Rapp, 1972; Pagano, 1974; Klein *et al.*, 1974*a*).

5. Disease, Latency, and Cancer

5.1. The Infected Cell in Culture and in Multicellular Organism

The preceding sections dealt with the properties and expression of herpesvirus genetic information in permissive and nonpermissive cells grown in culture. This section deals with infection of multicellular organisms and more specifically of humans.

The obvious objective of this transition is to examine the behavior of the virus in multicellular organisms from the vantage point of the studies on infected *in vitro* cell systems described earlier in the text. From this point of view, several

BERNARD
ROIZMAN AND
ELLIOTT
D. KIEFF

comments should be made:

1. There is considerable difference in the function of animal cells in the artificial environment of the cell culture and in the whole animal. In principle, cultured cells act as single entities competing independently for survival. In the animal, they are dependent components of a multicellular organism, perhaps readily expendable if they constitute a threat to the life of the animal. In evolution the selective processes operate only at the level of the entire animal, whereas in cultures they operate at the level of the single cell. It is also likely that regulatory pressures on cells in a multicellular organism and in culture are entirely different. Another and perhaps more relevant issue is that multicellular organisms contain a variety of differentiated cells varying in their capacity to supply the virus with necessary enzymes and precursors. These arguments may be trivial, but they preclude sweeping generalizations on the behavior of the infected cells in humans based on *in vitro* studies.

2. Cells *in vivo* do not become infected under the same conditions as cells in culture. One of the requirements of biochemical studies is that cells in culture be infected synchronously or at least parasynchronously. This requirement is easily satisfied by infecting cells at relatively high multiplicities of infection. However, the multiplicity of infection plays a role in its outcome. The effect is more pronounced in cells which are nonpermissive or which at least reproduce the virus poorly than in cells which are entirely permissive and reproduce the virus very well (Aurelian and Roizman, 1965). Moreover, high multiplicity of infection has been reported to generate particles containing defective viral DNA (Bronson *et al.*, 1973). In general, the measurements of the multiplicity of infection are misleading, because for every infectious virus particle there can be many hundreds of noninfectious or defective particles which also enter the cell. It is very likely that the multiplicity of infection of cells in multicellular organisms under natural conditions is no greater than one virus particle per cell. On the basis of the data available in the preceding sections, we can anticipate that highly permissive cells might reproduce the virus, albeit more slowly, than if they were infected at high multiplicities of infection. We cannot predict the outcome of infection in restrictive cells infected at these low multiplicities nor do we know much about infection of permissive cells with defective virus particles.

3. An additional level of complexity is the immune system operative in the multicellular organism, which can be analyzed in part but not wholly in the *in vitro* system.

4. The extent to which we can extrapolate from the infected *in vitro* cell culture to the *in vivo* situation is at best variable. The only legitimate extrapolation from our point of view is that events taking place in infected permissive cells producing virus in the multicellular organism and in culture are probably similar. This conclusion is based on the fact that electron micrographs of cells producing virions in biopsy materials show nuclear and cytoplasmic changes identical to those seen in infected cells in culture (Luse and Smith, 1959; Patrizi *et al.*, 1968; Swanson *et al.*, 1966).

279

HERPES
SIMPLEX AND
EPSTEIN–BARR
VIRUSES IN
HUMAN CELLS
AND TISSUES:
A STUDY IN
CONTRASTS

5.2. Herpes Simplex Viruses

5.2.1. Range of Clinical Manifestations

Herpes simplex viruses infect a wide variety of tissues and organs and in the past 50 years have been associated with a wide variety of clinical investigations. A thorough discussion of the gamut of infections observed with these viruses is outside the scope of this chapter. For detailed discussions of clinical infection with these viruses, the reader should consult reviews by Rawls (1973) and by Nahmias and Roizman (1973). For the purpose of this chapter, several broad generalizations are necessary:

1. Although the virus infects humans of all ages and although infections of a wide variety of organs and tissues have been reported, the topology of the viral lesions tends to cluster depending on the age and the serotype of the virus. Thus although in the newborn infection is frequently disseminated, in the adult the lesions on the face, particularly in and around the mouth, are predominantly due to HSV-1, whereas the lesions in the urogenital tract and superficially on or near the genitals are due predominantly to HSV-2. The topology of infection in the adult raises interesting questions from the point of view of both the cause for localization of the virus at those sites and the evolution of HSV-1 and HSV-2.

2. An epidemiologically and biologically significant sequela of infection with HSV is the persistence of the virus in the tissues of the host in an inapparent form, sometimes for the life of the host. This phenomenon, designated as latency, becomes readily manifest when the virus is induced to multiply and cause lesions.

3. A considerable body of data has emerged in the past few years on the association of herpesviruses with human malignancy.

In this section, expression of the virus in latent infections will be discussed first, followed by a summary of the present data on the association of HSV with human malignancy. The basis for the topology of HSV in the body and the evolution of HSV, which are far more speculative, will be dealt with at the end of the chapter.

5.2.2. Recurrent HSV Infection

The ability to persist in their natural host is a general property of all herpesviruses of human and nonhuman species studied to date (Roizman, 1965, 1971a; Nahmias, 1972; Paine, 1964). With respect to HSV-1 and HSV-2, the phenomenon itself is deceptively simple. Otherwise healthy individuals with serological evidence of past primary infection may exhibit recurrent infections caused by the same virus and localized on a specific area of the body, such as the face, cornea, or genitals. The state of the virus in the interim between recrudescences of clinically recognized disease has been designated as latent. Latent infections have been recognized not only for HSV but also for herpes zoster, cytomegaloviruses, and EBV. Descriptions and analyses of the phenomenon, as reviewed by several workers (Roizman, 1965, 1971a; Terni, 1971), reveal some very curious facets that are both perplexing and paradoxical.

It is convenient to discuss latency from two points of view: the virological aspect, describing what may occur at the virus–cell level, and the immunological aspect, focusing on possible mechanisms that might render an individual susceptible to recurrent infection or allow him to localize the infection, once it has recurred.

a. *Virological Aspects.* The origin of the virus responsible for a recurrent infection is not usually apparent. Four possible sources of virus can be envisioned: exogenous infection; endogenous infection from another site of the body; chronic, continuous, low-level viral multiplication around the site of involvement; and persistence of the virus in a nonreplicating form at, or near, the site of the recurrent infection.

Evidence for exogenous reinfection is available from studies on animals. For instance, several animals have been shown to be reinfected with their own herpesviruses acquired from an exogenous source (Nahmias, 1972). More specifically, it has been found possible to demonstrate exogenous genital reinfection with HSV-2 in mice or in cebus monkeys which had recovered from prior genital inoculation with the same virus type (London *et al.*, 1971). In man, attempts to terminate labial or genital recrudescences by autoinoculation at a distant site have on occasion produced new lesions, and in some cases new recurrent infections at the inoculated sites. It is therefore not unlikely that some of the genital and nongenital HSV recurrences in man could be due to exogenous reinfection from their infected contacts.

It is unlikely that infection with an exogenous virus would explain most of the nongenital HSV recurrences that affect the same or a very close neighboring site. A major objection to this explanation is the fact that patients with frequent recurrences are able to predict the onset fairly accurately; the recrudescences may be triggered by exposure to sunlight or wind, by fever, menstruation, or certain hormones, or by a severe emotional experience (Roizman, 1965, 1971a; Terni, 1971). It therefore seems unlikely that the exogenous virus is propitiously available at the right moment.

Infection of localized regions of the face or genitals with endogenous virus produced at another location has been documented on occasion—e.g., infections of the genitals with virus from a recurrent oral infection (Nahmias *et al.*, 1968). Moreover, virus has been isolated from oral and lacrimal secretions of apparently healthy persons in the interim between recurrences (Kaufman, 1968; Kaufman *et al.*, 1967, 1968; Brown and Kaufman, 1969; Laibson and Kibrick, 1969). However, the conclusion that the lip, cornea, and other areas of the body become reinfected with endogenous virus only under physical, emotional, or hormonal stress does not seem very satisfactory, for it does not explain either the effect of the stimuli that provoke the recurrences or the corollary conclusion that only one localized area, such as the mucocutaneous junction of the lip, is sufficiently stimulated to become reinfected.

The fact that recrudescent herpes generally occurs in localized areas also argues against low-grade, chronic virus multiplication, particularly in case of skin involvement. Another objection to this hypothesis is the failure of numerous attempts to isolate virus from biopsies removed from the site in the interim between recrudescences (Roizman, 1971a; Terni, 1971). Although negative results should be taken with a grain of salt, we could nevertheless exclude appreciable amounts of infectious virus in the tissues between recrudescences.

The last alternative, the persistence of HSV in noninfectious form at, or close to, the site of the recurrence, is supported by a number of observations in man and in laboratory animals. The earliest pertinent observations relate to the common appearance of facial lesions after section of the trigeminal nerve root (Carton, 1953; Carton and Kilbourne, 1952; Cushing, 1905). More recent reports demonstrating HSV by special culture techniques in trigeminal ganglia obtained from human cadavers (Bastian *et al.*, 1972; Baringer and Swoveland, 1973) suggest that the virus may be harbored in the neurons or supporting cells. Studies in model systems (Plummer *et al.*, 1970; Stevens and Cook, 1971a,b, 1972, 1973) indicate that the virus may persist in the sacrosciatic spinal ganglia of mice and in the trigerminal ganglia of rabbits after inoculation in the food pad and cornea, respectively. In both areas, the virus was demonstrable by cocultivation with susceptible cells, but not if the susceptible cells were inoculated with homogenized ganglion cells. The data suggest that the virus is in the "static state" (Roizman, 1965)—i.e., not in an infectious, replicating form.

The persistence of other herpesviruses in cells of human and animal origin has now been well documented (Nahmias, 1972). As pointed out earlier in the text, EBV is maintained in nonproducing cell lines, some of which can be induced to make viral products by appropriate treatment. Similarly, tumor cells of wild frogs caught during the summer months are usually virus free. Nevertheless, the tumor cells contain herpesvirus-specific nucleic acids, and the virus itself can be induced to multiply by storage of the frogs or tumor explants for several weeks in a cold room (Rafferty, 1964; Breidenbach *et al.*, 1971).

No definite information is yet available regarding the mechanism by which HSV-1 or HSV-2 persists and is triggered to multiply, or regarding the cells that harbor the virus. Two considerations bear on these problems. For the virus to persist, the cell that harbors it must remain alive, so that in the interim between recurrences the virus should not express any of its productive functions, which could lead to the death of the cell. Second, we have already called attention to the induction of recurrent HSV infection by physical provocation (heat), hormones, emotional provocation (hormones again?), and physical damage to the sensory nerve. The factor common to the various stimuli may well be their effect on nerve cells, cells associated with nerve trunks and nerve endings.

b. Immunological Aspects. We are concerned here with two questions: the role of immune factors in determining the frequency and the severity of the recurrences and the mechanisms involved in curtailing the virus from unimpeded spread in the infected person. These issues might best be discussed from the point of view of the three possible effects of immune factors on the outcome of a herpesvirus infection: virus neutralization, lysis of the virus-infected cell, and immunopathological disease (bearing in mind the well-appreciated fact that recurrent

HSV infections develop in the face of circulating neutralizing antibodies; Burnet and Williams, 1939).

Analyses of the neutralization of HSV and of the antibodies participating in the reaction have yielded interesting information that may be summarized as follows: It has been found, in certain laboratory animals, that maintenance of elevated neutralizing antibody titers is dependent on persistent antigenic stimulation (Nahmias et al., 1969a; London et al., 1971). However, the titers of neutralizing antibody in patients only occasionally fluctuate before, during, or after the recrudescences (Cesario et al., 1969). We are therefore faced with at least three possible alternatives: that there is a continuous antigenic stimulation as a consequence of chronic infection related or unrelated to the antigens produced at the site of recurrences; that the antigenic stimulation arises from recurrent infections, which are more frequent than the clinical manifestations lead us to believe; and that the quality of the antibody, which requires more precise serological assays, actually varies from person to person and in the interim between recurrences. We cannot at present differentiate between the first two alternatives. The third alternative, however, has been studied more extensively.

A characteristic of the *in vitro* neutralization test is that in antibody excess a residual fraction, ranging from 0.01 to 1% of the input virus, remains unneutralized (Ashe and Notkins, 1966). The size of the residual unneutralized fraction can be diminished substantially by the addition of antispecies globulins or of complement (Notkins, 1971). The importance of these *in vitro* phenomena, particularly in relation to *in vivo* situations, is not clear, since complement may be responsible *in vitro* for enhancement of immunoaggregation of the herpesvirus or may actually be involved in virolysis (Wallis and Melnick, 1971). It has also been shown *in vivo* that complement boosts the neutralizing activity of early HSV antibody (Taniguchi and Yoshino, 1965; Yoshino and Taniguchi, 1965). Although complement-requiring neutralizing antibody assays have been used by some workers (Yoshino and Taniguchi, 1965; Lerner et al., 1970) for the early diagnosis of primary HSV infection, no correlation has been found in cases of recurrent infections (Heineman, 1967).

A depression in IgA antibodies in patients with HSV recurrences has been suggested (Tokumaru, 1966), but not confirmed (Deforest and Klein, 1968; Centifanto et al., 1970; Douglas and Couch, 1970).

It has been known for many years that neutralizing antibodies by themselves are not effective in curtailing cell-to-cell spread of virus (Hoggan et al., 1960). However, antibodies may have a role in conjunction with other host factors. Thus it has been well demonstrated *in vitro* that the addition of complement to specific HSV antibodies will cause lysis of viral-infected cells (Roane and Roizman, 1964b; Roizman and Spring, 1967; Brier et al., 1971; Smith et al., 1972a). The new cell-surface antigens are the same virus-specified glycoproteins as those appearing on the surface of enveloped virus particles, and purified membranes of infected cells compete with enveloped virus for neutralizing antibody (Roizman and Spring, 1967; Roizman et al., 1973). Since the surface antigens are produced early after infection, one possibility would be that cell lysis occurs before progeny virus can spread to neighboring cells. However, an *in vitro* study has suggested that virus cell-to-cell spread can occur before the cells become damaged by complement and antibody cell lysis (Lodmell *et al.*, 1973). Antibodies with or without complement were found to be effective in eliminating virus only if rabbit peritoneal leukocytes (presumably macrophages) had first been added to the rabbit-kidney tissue culture system used for these assays.

283
HERPES
SIMPLEX AND
EPSTEIN–BARR
VIRUSES IN
HUMAN CELLS
AND TISSUES:
A STUDY IN
CONTRASTS

The importance of macrophages in host resistance to HSV infection has been corroborated by several workers in experimental mouse systems (Johnson, 1964; Zisman *et al.*, 1970; Hirsch *et al.*, 1970; Stevens and Cook, 1971b). These studies, stimulated by earlier observations on increased susceptibility to HSV infection of newborn mice as compared to adult animals, have demonstrated a deficiency in the ability of newborn macrophages to eliminate the virus. The increased resistance of rabbits to HSV-2 genital infection after administration of BCG might also support a role of macrophages (Larson *et al.*, 1972).

Immune mouse lymphocytes have been shown to be involved in HSV infection. *In vitro*, these cells have been reported to cause a reduction in plaque size, further accentuated by the presence of antibody (Ennis, 1973a). Passively transferred sensitized syngeneic cells also increased the survival of mice inoculated with HSV-1 (Ennis, 1973b). It had been noted earlier that more frequent fatal infections develop in mice given antithymocyte serum or those neonatally thymectomized than in control animals (Zisman *et al.*, 1970; Nahmias *et al.*, 1969b; Mori *et al.*, 1967).

Several workers have shown that a tuberculin-like delayed skin test could be elicited in guinea pigs (Rogers *et al.*, 1972) and in human beings with prior HSV infection (Yamamoto, 1966; Bubola and Olivetti, 1968). However, no correlation with frequency or time of human recurrent infections was noted. Similarly, even though there is no apparent correlation between frequency of recrudescences and the ability of lymphocytes to respond to HSV antigens *in vitro*, the lymphocytes collected from patients at the onset of recrudescences behaved sluggishly in cytotoxicity and macrophage migratory inhibition tests (Wilton *et al.*, 1972). It is of interest, parenthetically, that lymphocytes from rabbits immunized with HSV-1 react more vigorously in culture to the homologous virus than to HSV-2 and *vice versa* (Rosenberg *et al.*, 1972). Improved quantitation of such lymphocyte assays should permit a better evaluation of the behavior of lymphocytes in *in vitro* tests and of the immune status of the patient suffering from recurrent HSV infections. Such evaluations would be particularly valuable in those with various immunological defects (e.g., the Wiskott–Aldrich syndrome), those with certain cancers (e.g., Hodgkin's disease), and those on immunosuppressive therapy, in whom recurrent HSV infections tend to be more persistent and severe (Nahmias, 1970; Logan *et al.*, 1971; Muller *et al.*, 1972).

The role of interferon in host resistance to HSV infection also remains to be elucidated. High interferon levels have been detected in the blood and spinal fluid of a newborn with a severe HSV infection (Bellanti *et al.*, 1971). Interferon has been found to be effective in preventing infection in mice when a very low amount of virus is administered (Catalano and Baron, 1970). In addition, interferon stimulants, such as polyriboinosinic-polyribocytidylic acid, appear to be effective in preventing ocular herpes in laboratory animals (Park and Baron, 1968).

Lodmell *et al.* (1973) have proposed a complex unifying hypothesis, involving both nonspecific and specific mechanisms, to explain how the immune responses stop cell-to-cell spread of HSV infections. It seems clear, however, that many of the recent data merely underscore how little we know about the immune response in primary and recurrent infections and how far we are from understanding all of the immunological phenomena operative in individuals infected with these viruses.

5.2.3. HSV and Cancer

In recent years, several lines of investigation have sought to link herpes simplex viruses with human tumors. The accumulated evidence is not conclusive by any means, but impressive in its totality. Initially the studies on possible involvement of HSV dealt primarily with HSV-2 and cervical carcinoma. Currently, several more types of cancers have been associated with HSV.

The bulk of the evidence concerns the relationships between HSV-2 and cervical carcinoma. We may summarize the evidence as follows:

1. Epidemiological studies have suggested that women with cervical carcinoma possess characteristics which predict that they run a higher probability of acquiring venerally transmitted infections than other women (Rotkin, 1967, 1973; Martin, 1967; Priden and Littlefield, 1971). Translated, this simply means that acquisition of venereal infections and development of cervical carcinoma are covariant properties. Clearly, a causal relationship requires at the very minimum that infection invariably precede the evolution of cervical carcinoma. All of the studies on the involvement of HSV-1 and HSV-2 have addressed themselves specifically to at least one of the two aspects of this requirement, i.e., the association of HSV infection with cervical carcinoma and the relationship between the onset of infection and the detection of neoplastic lesions.

2. From a virological point of view, HSV-2 is an optimal candidate as a causative agent for cervical carcinoma for two reasons. First, it is transmitted venereally. Second, because of its topological distribution, recurrent genital infections satisfy the requirement of adequate contact with the tissues in which malignancy appears.

3. The association of HSV with cervical carcinoma is based on seroepidemiological studies whose main thrust is assays for antibody to HSV in patients with malignancy as compared with suitable control populations of similar age, sexual experience, socioeconomic group, etc. Since neutralizing antibody is the most unequivocal evidence of infection, most epidemiological studies have been based on measurements of this activity. The results are impressive. Numerous studies (Royston and Aurelian, 1970a; Nahmias *et al.*, 1970a,b; Rawls *et al.*, 1969, 1970, 1973; Catalano and Johnson, 1971) have shown a higher incidence of neutralizing antibody in patients with cervical carcinoma than in control populations. At this point, a digression is necessary. While in the study of Royston and

Aurelian (1970a) 100% (32/32) of women with cervical carcinoma had antibody to HSV-2 compared to 57% (17/32) of women in the control group, only 32% (14/44) of women with malignancy were positive in the study of Rawls *et al.* (1970). A lesser incidence of antibody in women with malignancy was also noted in the studies of Catalano and Johnson (1971), Rawls *et al.* (1969), Plummer and Masterson (1970), and Priden and Lilienfeld (1971), although again the incidence was higher in women with malignancy than in the control group. *A priori*, the finding of women with cervical carcinoma lacking demonstrable neutralizing antibody would seem to violate our requirement that infection precede development of cervical carcinoma. Mitigating factors, however, abound. To begin with, HSV-2 is neutralized by antibody to HSV-1 and *vice versa*. Although the homologous reaction is always stronger, it is difficult to measure low levels of anti-HSV-2 antibody in the face of high anti-HSV-1 antibody titers. Second, the antibody response to HSV-2 may be diminished or absent in an individual who had responded well to a previous HSV-1 infection (Smith *et al.*, 1972a,b). Furthermore, to interject a purely theoretical note, since a tumor could arise only from an abortively infected cell, it would be fallacious to expect that every abortive infection is invariably proceeded by virus multiplication extensive enough to stimulate virus-specific neutralizing antibody. Herein lies the major pitfall of using neutralizing antibody as an indicator of past infection. Nevertheless, the existing data do show that the neutralizing antibody patterns in women with cervical carcinoma differ from those of the control population in at least two respects. First, the antibody titers are higher in women with malignancy (Skinner *et al.*, 1971; Adam *et al.*, 1972, 1973). Second, the presence of neutralizing antibody to HSV-2 is age dependent in women in the control population but not in women with malignancy (Royston and Aurelian, 1970a; Adam *et al.*, 1972). This suggests that women with cancer are infected earlier in life than women in the control population. Again we must point out that the incidence of cervical carcinoma is higher in women who engage in sexual activity early in life. According to Rotkin (1973), "onset of sexuality before age 17 is the most powerful discriminating variable in virtually all studies where this has been investigated."

Before we leave seroepidemiological studies based on surveys of neutralizing antibody for greener fields, several more points should be made. Coincident with expectations, a higher incidence of neutralizing antibody was also found in women with preinvasive lesions (Royston and Aurelian, 1970a; Nahmias *et al.*, 1970b). Other studies reported that infection precedes cervical lesions (Catalano and Johnson, 1971) or at least predisposes women with genital herpetic infections to develop cervical dysplasias and *in situ* carcinoma (Naib *et al.*, 1969; Nahmias *et al.*, 1973).

4. As pointed out above, the seroepidemiological studies based on the presence of neutralizing antibody as evidence of past infection take advantage of the specificity of the reaction but make the unnecessary assumption that the virus multiplied to an extent sufficient to induce large amounts of neutralizing antibody which persisted to the date of the test. Another approach is based on the assumption that, by analogy with the experimentally induced viral tumors, cells

transformed into invasive, malignant cells by HSV will continue to express a portion of the viral genome coding for specific polypeptides which could be identified immunologically. In many instances, these antigens are nonstructural viral proteins. Sabin and Tarro set out to look for the nonstructural antigens, with rather interesting results. In a series of publications, they (Tarro and Sabin, 1970, 1973; Sabin and Tarro, 1973) described the preparation, properties, and, ultimately, the reactivity of such an antigen with sera from cancer patients. Briefly, the Sabin–Tarro antigen designated by them as "nonvirion antigen" possesses three fundamental properties which permit its utilization in serological tests. First, its antigenic reactivity is probably due to the state of an aggregation of several components. The antigenic reactivity is unstable on storage even at low temperatures. Second, the rate of accumulation varies from one type of infected cells to another. In HEp-2 cells, the antigen accumulates throughout infection. In guinea pigs, the antigen accumulates early (3 h after infection). Third, although the HSV-1 nonvirion antigen appears to be serotype specific, HSV-2 produces nonvirion antigens which react with antisera to both HSV-1 and HSV-2. Furthermore, virus strains differ in the amounts of the antigen they produce. Antibody to the nonvirion antigen was detected by absorbing from hyperimmune sera and from test sera antibody to stable antigens with infected cell lysates stored until all nonvirion antigen reactivity disappeared. The absorbed sera were then tested in complement fixation tests with freshly prepared cell lysates. In the initial studies (Sabin and Tarro, 1973) antibody to the nonvirion antigens was detected in patients with cancer of the lip, mouth, nasopharynx, oropharynx, kidney, bladder, prostate, cervix uteri, and vulva, but not in a variety of other cancers. Alas, subsequent analyses by Sabin (1974) failed to confirm the initial observations.

Of the variety of other immunological tests not involving virus neutralization, mention should be made of the complement fixation tests of Aurelian et al. (1973a,b) employing an antigen accumulating in HEp-2 cells 4 h after infection with HSV-2 and of the complement fixation tests of Hollinshead et al. (1972) with an antigen which defies comprehension. Aurelian et al. (1973a,b) reported a high-incidence of antibody to their antigen in women with malignancy and at least a decrease in the antibody levels following treatment of the cancers. Hollinshead et al. (1972, 1973) reported finding antibody to their HSV-1 and HSV-2 antigens in sera of patients with cancer of the head and neck, larnyx, and cervix uteri. Again, the major problem with tests which do not involve virus neutralization is the lack of evidence that the antigen is virus specific.

5. It could be expected, by analogy with experimental virus-induced tumors, that if HSV causes cervical carcinoma, at least some portion of the viral genome is expressed in the cancer cells. The search for the presence of viral products of viral nucleic acids in cancer cells has produced interesting data. In the order of their appearance, Royston and Aurelian (1970b) reported the detection by immunofluorescence of HSV antigens in atypical cells from women with preinvasive or invasive lesions. This antigen has not been characterized further. Subsequently, the same laboratory (Aurelian et al., 1971; Aurelian 1972, 1973) reported the

"induction" of HSV-2 in a cell line derived from a lesion of carcinoma *in situ* and maintained at high pH. However, since the induction was limited to a few passages of the cells and could not be reproduced in parallel cultures of the same line, chance contamination of the culture with virus being passaged in the laboratory cannot be excluded, although a valiant attempt based on electron microscopic studies was made (Aurelian and Stranberg, 1974). In other studies, Frenkel *et al.* (1972) reported the detection of viral DNA corresponding to only a fragment of the HSV-2 genome and transcripts arising from approximately 4% of the DNA in a cervical carcinoma specimen consisting largely of cancer cells. The kinetics of hybridization of the viral DNA sequences in unsheared DNA suggested that they were covalently linked to host DNA regions in the proximity to reiterated regions. More recently, Nahmias and his colleagues (personal communication) found by means of a complement-dependent immunofluorescence test an antigen in cervical cancer cells, in cells derived from experimental tumors in hamsters, and in *in vitro* transformed hamster cells.

As pointed out once before, the finding of viral antigens, DNA, and RNA in cancer cells would be expected if HSV caused the transformation of the cells, but does not exclude the possibility that malignancy induced a latent virus or that the cells were infected after they became transformed.

5.3. Epstein–Barr Virus

5.3.1. Primary, Latent, and Recurrent Infection

The growth of Burkitt tumor cells in culture (Epstein and Barr, 1964; Pulvertaft, 1964) and the isolation of continuous lymphoblastoid cell lines which produce EBV (Epstein *et al.*, 1964) made possible the development of techniques for detection of antibody to EBV-related antigens (G. Henle and W. Henle, 1966a; Armstrong *et al.*, 1966; Old *et al.*, 1966). The prevalence of antibody to EBV antigens has been determined for several human subpopulations (Demissie and Svedmyr, 1969; Gerber and Birch, 1967; Gerber and Rosenblum, 1968; Goldman *et al.*, 1968a; G. Henle and W. Henle, 1966a,b, 1967; Moore *et al.*, 1966; Pereira *et al.*, 1969; Svedmyr and Demissie, 1968; G. Henle *et al.*, 1969; W. Henle *et al.*, 1970a; Kafuko *et al.*, 1972; Klein *et al.*, 1968b; Niederman *et al.*, 1970; Porter *et al.*, 1969; Hirshaut *et al.*, 1969) and among subhuman primates (Gerber and Birch, 1967; Landon *et al.*, 1968; Goldman *et al.*, 1968b; Dunkel *et al.*, 1972; Kalter *et al.*, 1972; Gerber and Lorenz, 1974). The picture that emerges from these studies is that infection with EBV is an almost inevitable accompaniment of societal life. Eighty-five to ninety percent of adults in most populations surveyed possess antibody to EBV-related antigens. Infection of Old and New World subhuman primates with an EBV-like agent is, on the other hand, a much less constant event. Current knowledge of the natural history of primary human infection with EBV has been dealt with in several reviews (Klein, 1971, 1973; Epstein and Achong, 1973) and is summarized as follows: (1) Congenital infection with EBV is apparently an exceedingly rare event since long-term lymphoblastoid cell lines have been established from fetal cord blood leukocytes only following exposure to

EBV *in vitro*. More than 80% of newborn infants possess antibody to EBV, but titers fall in parallel with other passively transferred antibody activities. (2) The rate of acquisition of antibody through childhood varies among different socioeconomic groups. In underdeveloped countries and among lower socioeconomic groups in developed countries, antibody acquisition is greater than 80% by adolescence. (3) Infection in childhood has not been clearly associated with disease (G. Henle and W. Henle, 1970). In contrast, acquisition of antibody during adolescence is usually associated with heterophil-positive infectious mononucleosis (G. Henle *et al.*, 1968; Sawyer *et al.*, 1971). Retrospective and prospective studies have indicated that infectious mononucleosis occurs only in EBV-seronegative individuals and is accompanied by seroconversion (Evans *et al.*, 1968; Niederman *et al.*, 1968, 1970; University Health Physicians, 1971; Sawyer *et al.*, 1971). The pattern of IgM and IgG immunoglobulin response to EBV-related antigens during acute infectious mononucleosis suggests primary antigenic exposure (Hampar *et al.*, 1971; Banatvala *et al.*, 1972). VCA, MA (Klein *et al.*, 1968*b*; Miller *et al.*, 1972*a*; Hewetson *et al.*, 1973), and neutralizing antibody activities appear over the course of acute illness and persist for years thereafter. Seventy-five percent of patients develop anti-EA activity of the diffuse type (W. Henle *et al.*, 1971). Anti-EA titers fall within several months of the acute illness. (4) Epidemiological data suggest that oral contact favors transmission of infectious mononucleosis (Hoagland, 1967). EBV can be readily recovered from the throat washings of patients with acute infectious mononucleosis (Chang and Golden, 1971; Pereira *et al.*, 1972; Gerber *et al.*, 1972). Virus has been demonstrated in oropharyngeal secretions years after acute illness (Miller *et al.*, 1973). (5) The spectrum of diseases associated with primary EBV infection is burgeoning. Thus several workers have associated EBV infection with the postperfusion (W. Henle *et al.*, 1970*b*) and Guillain–Barré syndromes (Grose and Feorino, 1972).

Despite the clear evidence that EBV is the causative agent of classical heterophil-positive infectious mononucleosis, several key aspects of the pathophysiology of this disease remain inexplicable: (1) Heterophil antibodies of the Paul Bunnel–Davidson type appear regularly during acute infectious mononucleosis and tend to correlate with disease activity. Attempts to associate heterophil antigen with EBV have been unsuccessful (Springer *et al.*, 1974). Immunization of squirrel monkeys with autologous EBV-transformed lymphoblasts produced heterophil antibody in small amounts (Shope and Miller, 1973). Heterophil activity was reduced following absorption with guinea pig kidney, indicating a difference in specificity with the antibody seen during acute infectious mononucleosis. (2) The atypical lymphocyte which appears in the peripheral blood during acute infectious mononucleosis is probably not an EBV-transformed lymphocyte. The percentage of atypical lymphocytes in the peripheral blood of eight patients with acute infectious mononucleosis correlated with the percentage of cells capable of forming rosettes with sheep erythrocytes, a characteristic of T cells, and not with cells possessing immunoglobulin surface markers, a characteristic of B cells (Sheldon *et al.*, 1973). Evidence cited previously suggests that EBV can infect only B lymphocytes. Atypical lymphocytes may be T

289

HERPES
SIMPLEX AND
EPSTEIN–BARR
VIRUSES IN
HUMAN CELLS
AND TISSUES:
A STUDY IN
CONTRASTS

cells responding to new antigens in EBV-infected B cells. Mitogenic response to EBV-transformed lymphocytes has been demonstrated *in vitro*. Thus autologous mitomycin C–treated continuous lymphoblastoid cell lines isolated from patients with acute infectious mononucleosis have been demonstrated to stimulate convalescent lymphocytes in a mixed lymphocyte reaction (Junge *et al.*, 1971). (3) Evidence cited above suggests that EBV infection produces infectious mononucleosis with a high frequency only in adolescents. We cannot differentiate between the possibility that adolescents are exposed to higher doses of virus and the possibility that they are more prone to develop infectious mononucleosis rather than asymptomatic infections. We prefer the latter hypothesis since the outcome of primary herpesvirus infection, particularly with HSV-1 and varicella zoster, varies depending on the age of the individual. (4) EBV exhibits remarkably restricted tissue specificity *in vitro*. Infectious mononucleosis is a systemic disease. Visceral organ involvement, particularly hepatitis, is a frequent, though usually asymptomatic, accompaniment (Stern, 1972). Furthermore, the possibility that EBV can infect nonlymphoid cells must be entertained in view of the large amounts of virus found in convalescent nasopharyngeal secretions.

There is excellent evidence that EBV can remain latent in lymphocytes both *in vitro* and *in vivo*, although the precise definition of latency at the level of interaction of virus and cell is more difficult than with HSV. Long-term lymphoblastoid lines can be recovered from EBV-seropositive normal adults, probably for life, although this has not been systematically studied. Whether individual lymphocytes *in vivo* have the capability for long-term growth *in vitro* or acquire this capability following explantation is not clear. All continuous lymphoblastoid cell lines containing EBV seem to possess the intranuclear complement-fixing antigen. Whether this antigen is,produced in latently infected cells *in vivo* is not yet known. *In vitro*, production of EBNA does not appear to be detrimental to the cell. The source of genetic information and the function of EBNA are unclear. If EBNA is viral specified, the question arises as to why it alone is expressed in nearly all cells grown *in vitro* and carrying EBV. The simplest hypothesis would relate EBNA to control of EBV-induced cell proliferation.

Very little is known about recurrent infection with EBV. Specifically, it is not known whether cellular or humoral immunity plays a dominant role in surveillance of single-cell reactivation, whether recurrences occur at the single-cell level *in vivo*, or what factor(s) affect the frequency of recurrences. Preliminary observations suggest that productive infection can occur in latently infected lymphocytes *in vivo* and that cell-mediated immunity plays a dominant role in ongoing surveillance. Thus a patient undergoing immunosuppressive therapy for prevention of renal homograft rejection has been found to excrete EBV (Lipman *et al.*, 1974). Whether any clinical illness is associated with reactivation of EBV *in vivo* remains to be determined.

5.3.2. Association with Cancer

The impetus for the discovery of EBV arose from two observations of Denis Burkitt (1961, 1962; Burkitt and Davies, 1961): first, that there was lymphomatous disease in Africa which was unusual elsewhere and yet was a distinct clinical entity, and, second, that this tumor occurred with a high incidence in certain climatically similar regions of Africa. The geographic clustering suggested an infectious etiology. A substantial body of circumstantial evidence suggests that EBV is the putative infectious agent or at least a key part to a more complex etiology. In addition, seroepidemiological data suggested that EBV may be implicated as an etiological agent in nasopharyngeal carcinoma (Old *et al.*, 1966; W. Henle *et al.*, 1970*a*; de Schryver *et al.*, 1969), in sarcomatous Hodgkin's disease (Johansson *et al.*, 1970; Levine *et al.*, 1971), and with less significant evidence in a number of other disease states (Wahren *et al.*, 1971). Our analysis will be concerned primarily with virus–cell interaction in Burkitt's lymphoma and will touch only briefly on nasopharyngeal carcinoma. The pathology, clinical spectrum (Burkitt and Wright, 1970; Wright, 1972; Shanmugaratnan, 1972), and epidemiology (Burkitt, 1972; Ho, 1972; Muir, 1972; Geser and de Thé, 1972) of Burkitt's lymphoma and nasopharyngeal carcinoma have been reviewed and will not be dealt with here.

Data bearing on the association of EBV with Burkitt's lymphoma can be summarized as follows: (1) EBV homologous nucleic acid or EBNA has been detected in all but two of approximately 100 African Burkitt tumor biopsies tested (Pagano, 1974). EBNA can be detected in more than 80% of tumor cells in a biopsy specimen (Reedman and Klein, 1973). A smaller percentage of biopsy cells have MA activity (Klein *et al.*, 1966, 1967*a,b*). (2) Continuous lymphoblastoid cell lines can be readily established from Burkitt tumor tissue. Comparative studies of cytogenetic (Gripenberg *et al.*, 1969; Rabson *et al.*, 1966; Stewart *et al.*, 1965; Manolov and Manolova, 1972), immunoglobulin (Levin *et al.*, 1969; Nadkarni *et al.*, 1969), and isoenzyme markers (Fialkow *et al.*, 1970, 1973) indicate that lymphoblastoid cells grown in culture are representative of the tumor biopsies from which the cultures were established. After explantation to culture, VCA regularly appears in a small percentage of cells (Nadkarni *et al.*, 1970). All Burkitt-derived lymphoblastoid clones isolated in the presence (Hinuma and Grace, 1967; Zajac and Kohn, 1970; Maurer *et al.*, 1970) or absence of EBV antisera (Pope *et al.*, 1969*b*; Vonka *et al.*, 1970*a*; Gerber and Deal, 1970; zur Hausen and Schulte-Holthausen, 1970*a*; Nonoyama and Pagano, 1971; Walters and Pope, 1971; Sugawara *et al.*, 1972) contain EBV related antigens or viral DNA. (3) The more than 80% prevalence of anti-EBV antibody in normal African control populations precludes judgment of causality on the basis of seroepidemiological data despite the fact that 100% of African patients with Burkitt's lymphoma have antibodies to EBV (G. Henle *et al.*, 1969; G. Henle and W. Henle, 1966*a*; Levy and Henle, 1966; Moore *et al.*, 1966; Gunven *et al.*, 1970; Armstrong *et al.*, 1966). Similarly the higher titer of VCA activity in Burkitt patients must be cautiously interpreted. High titers to "opportunistic pathogens" are common in lymphomatous processes. Of interest in this regard is the observation that titers of Burkitt's lymphoma patients were substantially higher than those of a group of controls with lymphoreticular malignancies (G. Henle *et* *al.*, 1969). Of greater significance are the associations of antibody activity with clinical state. Thus the antibody titer to EA tends to be lower in patients during tumor regression, and, conversely, recurrences are more frequent in patients with EA antibody (G. Henle *et al.*, 1971*a,b*; W. Henle *et al.*, 1973*a,b*). An unusual feature of the EA activity associated with Burkitt's lymphoma was the restricted cytoplasmic fluorescence characteristically but not exclusively seen with the sera of patients (G. Henle *et al.*, 1971*b*; W. Henle *et al.*, 1973*a,b*). Clinical correlations have been described for MA. Antibody titers tend to correlate directly with a favorable outcome following chemotherapy (Klein *et al.*, 1966, 1967*b*). In one case, a fall in MA activity preceded clinical recurrence by 6 months, suggesting cause and effect (Klein *et al.*, 1969; Gunven *et al.*, 1974). The data suggest that, despite the lack of direct evidence for EA and VCA in biopsy tissue, these antigens are produced in tumorous patients, although possibly not in tumor cells themselves. (4) Finally, evidence cited above that EBV is a potent transforming agent of lymphocytes *in vitro* must be given some weight.

291

HERPES
SIMPLEX AND
EPSTEIN–BARR
VIRUSES IN
HUMAN CELLS
AND TISSUES:
A STUDY IN
CONTRASTS

A large number of studies have documented the regular association of anti-VCA (W. Henle *et al.*, 1970*a*), anti-MA (de Schryver *et al.*, 1969, 1972), and precipitating (Old *et al.*, 1966; Oettgen *et al.*, 1967) antibodies with postnasal carcinoma. Sera from 75% of patients contained antibody to EAd antigen (G. Henle *et al.*, 1971*b*). Antibody titers in a control patient population were substantially less in all cases. Although nasopharyngeal carcinoma is an epithelial tumor, there is frequently a rich admixture of lymphocytes (Shanmugaratnan, 1972). Proof of the association of EBV with the malignant epithelial cells is difficult in the presence of lymphoid elements which may themselves contain EBV. Growth of the malignant epithelial cells in culture has not been possible (de Thé, 1972). DNA homologous to EBV cRNA has been demonstrated in most, but not all, tumor biopsies tested (zur Hausen *et al.*, 1970*b*; Wolf *et al.*, 1973; Pagano, 1974; Kawai *et al.*, 1973). Of particular interest are the observations (Wolf *et al.*, 1973) that (1) tumors binding the largest quantity of EBV cRNA are predominantly epithelial; (2) cRNA tends to localize in the nuclei of epithelial cells, as opposed to lymphocytes, as determined by autoradiography following *in situ* hybridization; and (3) epithelial tumor cells contain an intranuclear antigen stainable with test serum containing antibody to EBV using anticomplementary immunofluorescence. The major question in evaluating this study is whether unequivocal differentiation of lymphoid from epithelial cells can be made on morphological grounds using refrigerated material. DNA extracted from two nasopharyngeal carcinoma biopsies failed to increase the rate of renaturation of labeled EBV DNA, suggesting that these tumors contain much less than one EBV genome equivalent per cell (Kawai *et al.*, 1973).

Recent data (Klein *et al.*, 1974*b*) indicate that human nasopharyngeal carcinoma biopsies can be grown in "nude" mice deficient in thymus-dependent immunity. The carcinoma cells maintain their histologic appearance but the infiltrating lymphocytes are replaced by mouse cells. A well-differentiated squamous tumor passaged in nude mice contained neither EBV DNA nor EBNA. Three anaplastic nasopharyngeal tumors passaged in nude mice lost their lymphocytic elements and were found to contain EBV DNA and EBNA.

The evidence associating EBV with Burkitt's lymphoma, though circumstantial, is compelling by virtue of its consistency. Nevertheless, a key question necessarily arises. How can a ubiquitous agent be implicated in the etiology of a disease entity of constricted locale? Several alternative hypotheses need to be seriously considered:

1. EBV is the single etiological agent of Burkitt's lymphoma and the incidence of disease is either genetically determined or requires a unique phenotypic alteration of host functions, or there exist more than one EB virus.
2. EBV is a necessary but not sufficient factor for malignant transformation; i.e., another infectious agent is also required.
3. EBV is a passenger virus, whose presence is merely amplified by the malignant cells.

Although we cannot come to a definitive conclusion, the hypotheses are not equally tenable:

1. Observations on the incidence of tumors among migrating tribes indicate that genetic factors do not alone account for the high tumor incidence in endemic areas.

2. The Burkitt endemic region is characterized by a multiplicity of arthropod-vectored diseases. The hypothesis has been put forward that immunosuppression resulting from holoendemic malaria leads to emergence of malignant clones and lymphomatous disease. Several lines of evidence are opposed to a simple immunosuppressive model. An important expectation of the immunosuppression hypothesis is that Burkitt-like lymphoma would occur in the western world in patients naturally or iatrogenically immunosuppressed since the vast majority of adults harbor EBU. The most common tumor in immunosuppressed patients in nonendemic areas is reticulum cell sarcoma (Hoover and Fraumeni, 1973). Conversely, if Burkitt's lymphoma arises only in immunosuppressed individuals, other kinds of tumors associated with immunologically compromised individuals should also be quite frequent in endemic areas. Immunosuppression could, but probably does not, account for development of a tumor from a cell which became transformed. It cannot account for the transformation unless immunosuppression generates a cell type in which transformation is more likely to occur. If this were the case, we would have to postulate that holoendemic malaria among all other infectious diseases uniquely causes specific transformation-susceptible cells to arise.

3. The existence of many EBV subtypes must be considered at several levels. At the first level, we might consider that these approximate the difference which exists between HSV-1 and HSV-2. Available data from several laboratories exclude this possibility. Thus DNA–DNA renaturation kinetics using HR1 virus derived from a Burkitt tumor as a probe have demonstrated that lymphoid cells from patients with mononucleosis contain sequences homologous to at least 90%

of the DNA used as a probe (Kieff and Levine, 1974; Kawai *et al.*, 1973). Hybrid DNA molecules formed by annealing HR1 viral DNA with the homologous DNA of infectious mononucleosis lymphoblasts had identical thermostability to native EBV DNA, indicating less than 1.5% unmatched base pairs in heterohybrid DNAs (Kieff and Levine, 1974). At another level we might consider the possibility that EBV generates variants which differ in a small number of genes which would be more difficult to detail by DNA reassociation studies utilizing whole molecules as the probe. Variant viruses could be expected to be more efficient in transformation. A characteristic of herpesviruses is that they kill the cells in which they multiply. There is ample evidence that experimental manipulations which alter herpes simplex virus or adenoviruses so that they are incapable of replication may produce an agent which possesses enhanced ability to transform cells *in vitro* (Duff and Rapp, 1971; Graham *et al.*, 1974; Sharp *et al.*, 1974). Variants of EBV have been described. Thus, EBV derived from the HR-1 cell line causes EA induction and kills cells when used to superinfect the antigen negative Raji cell line but lacks the ability to transform leukocytes of EBV seronegative donors; while EBV derived from the B95-8 cell line lacks the ability to induce EA and kill cells but possesses the ability to transform. Recent evidence indicates that the virus purified from B95-8 cells lacks 15% of the genetic complexity of the HR-1 virus (Pritchett *et al.*, 1975). However, there are two problems. First, it is difficult to explain without invoking numerous hypotheses why these variants would arise or would be effective solely in geographically separated endemic regions in the light of the fact that virus from infectious mononucleosis does transform cells. Second, if the variant were infectious, it should have spread elsewhere. One simple and at least partially testable hypothesis arises from the assumption that variants arise in susceptible infected individuals or in unusual vectors.

4. Burkitt tumor biopsies have been reported to contain a trace of RNA in the polysome fraction homologous to murine leukemia virus (Kufe *et al.*, 1973). However, these data must be considered with caution. These RNA sequences are far less defined than the EBV DNA, and in the final analysis any other putative agent impugned in the causation of this disease must also account for all of its vagaries.

5. The "passenger" hypothesis is a necessary accompaniment of any situation in which the role of a putative agent in a disease cannot be established experimentally. In this instance, we are confronted with two alternatives; i.e., either Burkitt's lymphoma arises only from cells infected with EBV or EBV almost invariably infects Burkitt's lymphoma cells. Although the first alternative implicitly states that EBV infection is a requirement for malignancy, there is no simple way to establish the role of the virus in the etiology of the tumor. The second alternative is more difficult to deal with. The argument that EBV does not regularly infect cells of other lymphoid malignancies even in seropositive individuals is weak. In the final analysis, proof of the role of EBV in Burkitt's lymphoma will rest on a direct operational test of the hypothesis—"Will eradication of EBV infection preclude development of lymphoma?"

5.4. Herpesvirus Latency and Cancer—A Unifying Hypothesis

5.4.1. The Problems

From review of the pathogenesis of the herpesviruses discussed in this chapter, it seems clear that the distributions of cells infected with the various herpesviruses in the human body rarely overlap. Thus although HSV-1 and HSV-2 are both capable of causing disseminated infection which might be difficult to differentiate without laboratory tests, each virus does have its own topological niche in which it is more commonly found. The topological niche of EBV is probably even more restricted. The problem we are focusing on is the significance of the distribution of the infected cells in the human body. Is the topology a consequence of the mode of transmission? Can we deduce from the available data that the evolution of human herpesvirus involved the acquisition of affinity (defined in terms of relative ability to multiply) for different kinds of cells?

A second problem arises from considerations of another set of biological properties of herpesviruses. Without exception, herpesviruses destroy the cells in which they multiply. Yet without apparent exception herpesviruses are notorious for their ability to remain latent in the host without causing clinically obvious disease. The problem confronting us is the biochemical basis for latency, or, to phrase it in the form of a question, is there a biochemical basis for reconciling the observation that herpesviruses are invariably lethal to the cells in which they multiply and the rather common observation that the virus can remain latent for the lifetime of the host?

Last, herpesviruses have also been associated with human cancer, albeit proof that they are oncogenic in man remains elusive. Assuming for heuristic reasons that herpesviruses are etiological agents for certain human cancers, the question arises of whether the ability to cause latent infections plays a major role in human cancer.

The purpose of this section is not to provide "solutions" to these problems since none currently exist but rather to discuss them in the light of current studies on these viruses and to point to the eventual avenues of biochemical research which might furnish answers to at least some of the questions which effusively punctuate this text.

5.4.2. Acquisition of Affinity of Herpesviruses for Specific Cells

For heuristic reasons, it is convenient to approach the problem of the acquisition by herpesviruses of affinity for specific cells from the point of view of evolution. In the specific instance of herpesviruses infecting man, two points should be made. First, on morphological grounds alone it is virtually impossible to differentiate among the electron micrograph images of herpes zoster, HSV-1, HSV-2, cytomegalovirus and Epstein–Barr virus. Second, with the possible exception of cells infected with HSV-2 which contain peculiar tubular structures that could be diagnostic and the perinuclear inclusions which occur in some cells infected with cytomegalovirus (Couch and Nahmias, 1969; Schwartz and Roizman, 1969a; Roizman and Furlong, 1974), it is virtually impossible to differentiate between the morphogenesis of these viruses in productively infected cells. Yet all five viruses do differ widely in base composition (Roizman and Furlong, 1974), and measurable homology has been detected between HSV-1 and HSV-2 DNAs only (Kieff *et al.*, 1972). It is therefore very likely that HSV-1 and HSV-2 are derived from a common parent. With respect to the other herpesviruses infecting man, while we cannot differentiate between "convergent" and "divergent" evolution, the former is not really a viable hypothesis. Considering the great variation in the structure and modes of replication of viruses infecting man and the many permutations which are possible, it seems rather naive to consider the hypothesis of convergent evolution for very long. However, even if we confine ourselves to HSV-1 and HSV-2, whose relatedness is now well established, could we ascribe their divergence to selection of viruses having higher affinity for certain cells? If the answer is yes, what is its significance with respect to the overall theme of this section? The answer to the first question may be many years in coming, and perhaps only a few points should suffice. Herpesviruses are not particularly known for their stability in the physical environments inhabited by man. Studies of the epidemiology of herpesvirus infections support the notion that they are transmitted by close personal contact. Infectious mononucleosis associated with EBV has been termed the "kissing" disease. Herpes gladiatorum is a recognized affliction of wrestlers resulting from transmission of HSV-1 by close body contact as well as by the biting indulged in in that sport. Chickenpox is transmitted not only from one child to the next but also by adults suffering from herpes zoster to the susceptible population around them. It seems reasonable to postulate that HSV-1 infection of the susceptible young population is the consequence of close personal contact between susceptible children and adults suffering recrudescences of herpetic lesions. Among adults, the closest common personal contact is sexual intercourse. It is perhaps not surprising that the herpesviruses are transmitted by this contact, also. But if sexual contact is just another close personal contact and if HSV-1 and HSV-2 are derived from a common parent, why the genetic difference between the two? There may be more than one answer to this question. First, infections with HSV-1 and HSV-2 do not occur at the same age. HSV-2 generally follows HSV-1 infection, and conceivably the immunological status of the host plays a role in selection. A mutant with altered antigenic specificity may have a better chance of surviving and being perpetuated. Although this hypothesis explains the difference in the antigenic specificity of structural components of HSV-1 and HSV-2, it does not fully explain the differences in nonstructural polypeptides or the extent of divergence of the DNAs of these viruses. Another possibility arises from laboratory observations which suggest that the cell is not an inert body in which the virus replicates but rather that it acts as a filtering agent selecting the mutants best suited for multiplication in that cell. A specific example is the study of Roizman and Aurelian (1965) showing that dog kidney cells abortively infected with HSV-1 (MP) and passaged serially ultimately succumbed to a mutant capable of multiplying in those cells whereas the parent virus could not. Evidence that the mutation resulted in major changes in the proteins specified by the virus could be deduced from the altered antigenic specificity, thermal stability, and other phenotypic properties of the mutants. Directly bearing on this issue is the observation by Heine *et al.* (1974) that the polypeptide compositions of the virions of two HSV-1 isolates passaged a limited time in culture were identical, whereas several strains with a long history of laboratory passages differed not only from each other but also from the two isolates with respect to the number and electrophoretic mobility of their structural polypeptides. Are the differences between HSV-1 and HSV-2 the consequences of the mode of transmission into different topological niches containing different kinds of cells? It is noteworthy that the cells forming the topological niches of HSV-1 and HSV-2 are distinctly different, not so much, perhaps, in morphology as in their physiological responses to hormones and in membrane structure (Jensen and de Sombre, 1972). Ultimate proof that HSV-1 and HSV-2 arose as a consequence of selection of viruses best able to grow in the topological niche associated with the mode of transmission is lacking. It should not, however, be too difficult to stimulate such a "selection" in the laboratory by serial passages of virus either in partially restrictive cells in culture or in experimental animals.

The issues pursued here have very obvious implications. Since we are dealing with different parts of the same body, and since HSV-1 can be transmitted venereally and can multiply in the urogenital tract (Nahmias and Roizman, 1973), it is not necessary to postulate that HSV-1 genetic information cannot be expressed in cells of the urogenital tract. A more likely explanation for the role of the cells as a selective milieu is that viral and cellular products must necessarily interact. As indicated in the preceding sections, viral DNA is probably transcribed by a host transcriptase and viral polypeptides must enter into host membranes for viral maturation. More complex interactions between viral and cellular macromolecules have to account for the inhibition of host macromolecular synthesis which accompanies productive infection. If host proteins, membranes, etc., differ as a consequence of differentiation in different parts of the body, it could be expected that the effectiveness of some of the virus–host macromolecular complexes might vary. Hence any mutation which results in a more effective complex is likely to give that mutant a selective advantage. The purpose of the discussion is not to stress that oral and vaginal mucosa differ but rather to stress that virologists working with animal viruses have not yet come to grips with the wide spectrum of host–viral macromolecular complexes which play a crucial role in viral development and necessarily determine the pathogenesis of human disease.

5.4.3. Biochemical Basis of Latency

The key question with respect to the biochemical basis of latency is the mechanism by which the herpesviruses remain latent in the body. As pointed out earlier in the text, CMV, EBV, and both herpes simplex viruses remain latent in the body. Little is known about the mechanism of survival of EBV, although it is clear that

EBV-infected lymphoid cells may be recovered from peripheral blood cultures long after an episode of infectious mononucleosis. Much more is known about latent HSV infections. With respect to HSV, two hypotheses have been offered to explain the state of the virus (Roizman, 1965): The "dynamic-state hypothesis" predicts that the virus multiplies in "pockets" of chronically infected tissue at the same or distant sites and that the stimuli responsible for the recrudescence "heighten" the susceptibility of the tissues. The alternative or "static-state hypothesis" states that the viral genome is conserved in a nonproductively infected cell and that the infection becomes productive when the cell is "induced" to make virus as a consequence of physical or emotional provocations to the host. Two points should be made here. The first concerns the tissue in which the virus is maintained in the interim between recrudescences. No virus has ever been isolated from biopsy material removed from the sites of recurrent lesions and either inoculated into susceptible cultures or grown in cell culture (see reviews by Roizman, 1965, 1971a, 1972; Terni, 1971). However, several lines of evidence suggest that the virus is capable of being maintained in sensory neurons. The involvement of nerve tissue has been suspected for many years (Goodpasture, 1929), but only recently has there been good evidence suggesting that it harbors the virus. Thus Stevens' laboratory (Stevens and Cook 1971a,b, 1972, 1973) has been able to establish latent infections in rabbits and mice. The pertinent observation is that although the viruses could not be induced to multiply in the animal and no infectious virus could be detected in any of the tissues removed surgically and inoculated into susceptible cell cultures, the viruses could be induced to multiply by maintaining the surgically removed ganglia in *in vitro* cultures or by implanting them into virgin animals. The studies on human material are equally relevant. Thus Gasserian ganglia removed from cadavers at random yielded virus on prolonged cultivation in culture (Bastian *et al.*, 1972; Baringer and Swoveland, 1973). The second and key point concerns the mechanism by which the virus survives in tissues in the interim between recrudescences. Both the dynamic and static hypotheses present paradoxes, but the weight of the evidence does not seem entirely equal. The dynamic hypothesis is unsatisfactory from two points of view. First, a characteristic of productive infection in animal cells is the appearance of viral antigens, presumably viral glycoproteins (Roane and Roizman, 1964b; Roizman and Spring, 1967; Roizman *et al.*, 1973). In cell culture, these cells readily react and are lysed by convalescent human serum and complement. It is difficult to imagine that chronically infected nerve cells continuously shedding virus particles could persist without provoking a foreign body reaction, inflammatory responses, etc., of the kind seen in herpes encephalitis. The hypothesis that such patients suffer from an immune deficiency is not fully compatible with the fact that they do react to the fever blisters and ultimately recover. Second, if the virus is continuously produced in the Gasserian ganglion, or even some other tissue, the question arises as to the mechanism by which the tissues in which recrudescences occur become more susceptible or accessible to the virus as a result of the physical or emotional provocations which induce the recurrence of herpetic lesions. Although a variety of *ad hoc* hypotheses could be proposed, none satisfactorily explains why one site, and no other, becomes reinfected from these putative pockets of chronically infected tissue during recrudescence. The static-state hypothesis creates a different paradox. In cell culture, at least, human cells including nerve cells are invariably susceptible and rapidly succumb to infection (Roizman, 1972). The static-state hypothesis, on the other hand, requires that the cells maintain the virus without reproducing it and without being killed.

Although no rigorous differentiation between these two hypotheses is possible at present, there is merit in discussing the requirements and predictions of the static-state hypothesis. To restate its essence, the hypothesis requires that the viral genomes present in the cells should express only as much information as is compatible with the survival of the cell. Two questions therefore arise. First, what is the relationship of cell death as a consequence of infection to the reproductive cycle of the virus, and, second, what controls expression of the viral genetic information?

Cell death is an anthropomorphic expression difficult to define in biochemical terms. In terms of cell functions as described earlier in the text, we see cessation of DNA and protein synthesis, decrease and modification of RNA synthesis, extensive alterations in the structure of chromatin and membranes, and, perhaps superficially significant, inhibition of mitosis. We do not know which of these events strikes the lethal blow; probably any one would suffice. The measurable events, i.e., inhibition of host macromolecular functions, appear to be initiated very early in the reproductive cycle of HSV (Roizman, 1972; Kaplan, 1973). The only events which could precede it are the transcription of the HSV DNA and the translation of the transcript, if the inhibition is the consequence of action of proteins specified by the virus. The present evidence indicates the existence of several controls operating at the level of transcription, transport, and processing of RNA and possibly at the level of translation of mRNA. We have no data as to how the controls operate, but several points should be made. First, no transcriptase has so far been reported in the virion itself. This is reinforced by the finding that deproteinated DNA is infectious (Sheldrick et al., 1973; Lando and Ryhiner, 1969). Second, the HSV genome is almost totally transcribed in the absence of protein synthesis but only a fraction of the genome transcribed under these conditions yields transcripts capable of functioning as mRNA. These data necessarily imply that the HSV is at least capable of utilizing a host polymerase, and possibly this is the only enzyme which transcribes the DNA early in infection. Although it is not known which of the several host enzymes transcribes HSV DNA, the prediction of the static-state hypothesis is that in the cells harboring HSV this transcriptase is either absent or unable to transcribe viral DNA. Since the phenomenon has not been reproduced with cells in culture, the question that arises is, if the static hypothesis is the correct one, what could be the difference between cells in culture and those in the tissues themselves? We obviously do not have an answer, but the most striking difference is that cells in culture are stimulated to grow and generally they are dividing cells. The neuron in situ is not a replicating cell and even when put into culture, in which it generally does not divide, it may be biochemically different. It is conceivable that *in situ* it lacks the specific transcriptase capable of reproducing the virus except after stimulation by the factors associated with physical and emotional provocations to the host.

299

HERPES
SIMPLEX AND
EPSTEIN–BARR
VIRUSES IN
HUMAN CELLS
AND TISSUES:
A STUDY IN
CONTRASTS

The objective of this discussion is to stress three significant points. First, we have no definitive biochemical description of HSV latency. We are confronted with the fact that neurons, which lack the capacity to replicate, are probably harboring the virus. It remains to be seen whether this is a trivial or significant observation. If the virus does not replicate between recrudescences of the disease, as the static-state hypothesis predicts, the fact that neurons do not replicate could account for both the maintenance of the virus for the lifetime of the host and the failure to transcribe the virus beyond the point where it would kill the cell.

Second, while we can suppress virus multiplication in cell culture by damaging the virus (Duff and Rapp, 1971), by elevating the temperature of incubation (Darai and Munk, 1973), or by using drugs, we do not have in cell culture a model mimicking the condition of maintenance of the viral genome defined by the static-state hypothesis. It is possible that the static-state hypothesis is incorrect. A more plausible hypothesis is that the type of maintenance of the HSV genome required by the static-state hypothesis cannot take place in dividing cells because of the availability of all the host factors necessary for virus multiplication and that even neurons maintained in cell culture undergo the type of stimulation which makes all necessary host factors available. Clearly the crucial test of the static-state hypothesis rests on finding in cell culture the conditions for rendering Gasserian ganglion neurons permissive and nonpermissive at will, and defining the host factors, operative and inoperative, in each instance.

The last point is that this discussion of HSV latency is, superficially at least, not directly applicable to EBV. It is not clear, for example, whether EBV survives in peripheral lymphocytes as a result of chronic, low-grade multiplication or whether EBV in peripheral leukocytes arises from transmission of the genome during morphogenesis of the leukocytes from infected stem cells. If the first hypothesis turns out to be correct, it would imply that the mechanism of maintenance of EBV is inherently different from that of HSV. If the second hypothesis is correct, it would imply that the factors necessary for EBV multiplication are absent from the infected cells even during cell division. This conclusion may also be reached from the fact that the bulk of rapidly dividing human lymphoblastoid cells in culture, while containing the viral genome, do not make EBV.

5.4.4. Latency and Human Cancer

The difficulty in establishing the etiological role of herpesvirus in human cancer arises from three considerations. First, herpesviruses are ubiquitous. It is difficult to relate rather common infection with relatively rare malignancies. Second, unlike acute infectious diseases in which the onset of infection and disease can be reasonably well established and may be monitored independently, the long interval which exists between infection and malignancy renders prospective epidemiological studies not only costly but difficult to perform. The last, and perhaps most significant, consideration is that because of the nature of the disease, human experimentation is inadmissible. A reasonable conclusion for the purpose of this presentation is that the evidence that humans are infected either before or immediately after malignancy develops is quite good whereas the etiological role of the virus is by no means established.

Let us assume for heuristic reasons that herpesviruses are etiological agents of human cancer. If this be the case, two pertinent questions arise. First, is the virus ever latent in the cells it transforms? Second, when the cell is induced to multiply, why does the virus not also multiply and destroy the cell? Again, analyses of EBV and HSV infections indicate that no simple answer is applicable to both viruses. With respect to HSV, the question regarding precancerous "latency" is not answerable at present. It is clear that at least with HSV-2 an interval of time, measurable in years, elapses between primary infection with that virus and the appearance of cervical carcinoma (Nahmias and Roizman, 1973).

With regard to EBV, the interval of time between primary infection and childhood Burkitt's lymphoma must be frequently less than 5 yr. Prospective studies to precisely establish the sequence of virus infection and malignant eventuality will be difficult (Geser and de Thé, 1972). Regions of high tumor endemicity are plagued by an extraordinarily high incidence of primary infection during the first decade of life. Use of populations outside the Burkitt endemic area, even for retrospective studies, presents difficulties for two reasons: First, although the clinical and pathological features of Burkitt's lymphoma are sufficiently distinctive to serve as an adequate basis for broad epidemiological studies, the features are not sufficiently specific or unique to assure that the Burkitt-like cases occurring in nonendemic areas do not represent the end of the spectrum of more common lymphoid malignancy. Second, the bulk of available evidence favors dissimilarity between endemic and nonendemic cases. Seroepidemiological data on cases in nonendemic areas are not consistent (Klein, 1973). Although Levine et al., (1972) feel that the seronegative cases can be discounted, more recent data have indicated that tumor biopsies from four patients from nonendemic areas lacked EBV DNA (Pagano et al., 1973).

If we pursue our heuristic approach, it is conceivable that either herpesviruses stay dormant for a length of time or the cell ultimately destined to become malignant becomes infected immediately before transformation with virus from an exogenous source. The first alternative implies that not only nerve cells but also other cells in the body are capable of maintaining the virus in a static state and therefore the same considerations and predictions might apply as those discussed in the case of virus maintained in neurons. However, regardless of when the cell becomes infected, if the analysis of the events occurring in the case of virus maintained in the Gasserian ganglion is correct, once the cell becomes infected and begins to multiply, all necessary host factors for viral multiplication should become available and the host should be destroyed. The paradox could be resolved in several ways. One admittedly likely hypothesis is that the foregoing analysis of latent neural infection is incorrect. One alternative is that host or viral factors which we may designate as "repressors" block virus multiplication. The fact is that cervical carcinoma cells are susceptible to infection with HSV. This is not what would be predicted if they contain a repressor. While we cannot reject the hypothesis on the basis of this observation alone, its chief demerit is that it is not readily testable. Another hypothesis, whose chief merit is that it is in part defensible at present and testable in the future, is that virus multiplication does not occur, even though all remaining host factors are available, because the genome is defective. The hypothesis envisions that some cells other than neurons can be latently infected with HSV, that induction of virus multiplication cells containing the functional viral genome are destroyed, and that cells maintaining the appropriate defective genome become transformed. This hypothesis predicts (1) that both functional and defective viral genomes can be maintained in a latent state by cells other than neurons, (2) that defective genomes are produced during productive infection, and (3) that defective genomes can indeed transform cells.

301
HERPES
SIMPLEX AND
EPSTEIN–BARR
VIRUSES IN
HUMAN CELLS
AND TISSUES:
A STUDY IN
CONTRASTS

With respect to the first prediction, as pointed out earlier in the text, there is no evidence that cells other than neurons are capable of maintaining the virus in a latent state. The crucial experiments which need to be done are to determine the site of maintenance of HSV-2 responsible for recurrent infections on genitals. It would be extraordinarily interesting if the virus were maintained not in the ganglia innervating urogenital organs but in other cells of these tissues. The second prediction has been fulfilled only in part. Bronson *et al.* (1973) published evidence which could be interpreted as indicating that defective DNA is produced and incorporated into virions in cells infected at a high multiplicity of infection. Definitive evidence consisting of the isolation of the DNA and demonstration that it contains only a part of the HSV-2 sequences remains to be obtained. The last prediction is the only one which at the moment is promising. First, the studies of Rapp and Duff (1972a,b, 1973) clearly show that the virus must be damaged by ultraviolet light or other treatments capable of altering the structure of the DNA in order for the cell to become transformed rather than productively infected. The necessary corollary that the transformed cell contain only a part of the genome also appears to be fulfilled. Apart from the analysis of the one cervical carcinoma shown to contain a fragment of HSV-2 DNA (Frenkel *et al.*, 1972), only a fragment was found in one of the transformed lines of Duff and Rapp (M. Green, personal communication). Preliminary studies in several laboratories including ours indicate that the L cells which acquired and perpetuated the viral thymidine kinase following exposure to ultraviolet-irradiated HSV-1 (Munyon *et al.*, 1972a,b; Davidson *et al.*, 1973) lack a complete viral genome or very little of it is transcribed.

It should be pointed out that the fulfillment of one or even all three predictions does not prove the hypothesis. What remains to be done, if this work is to have any meaning, is to determine whether the transformation requires the presence and maintenance of a unique set of sequences of viral DNA. Even then we might not fully escape the possibility that it is a laboratory phenomenon unless the same set of DNA sequences is also found in all cancers suspected to be caused by HSV.

The foregoing arguments are not directly applicable to EBV. For heuristic purposes, it is necessary to define the wild-type virus as the epidemiologically significant agent present in throat washings. One unsettled question is the property of EBV in lymphoblastoid cell cultures. In the absence of a susceptible cell population in which the virus multiplies well, it is difficult to determine whether the virus isolated from throats of patients with infectious mononucleosis and that trickling out in lymphoblastoid cell cultures are identical. We are therefore confronted with the possibility that the viruses carried in the lympho-blastoid cell lines may be defective. The biological and biochemical differences between the virus produced in the HR1 and in the other virus-producing Burkitt and infectious mononucleosis cell lines suggest that at least some of these viruses are defective, but which and to what extent? The B95-8 virus is clearly defective but capable of replication and of transformation, at least in experimental systems. The observation that multiplying lymphoblastoid cells must be "induced" to express viral functions suggests that the virus involved in these cells is capable of function and that the factors required for viral multiplication are absent in the cells and become available only on treatment with chemical agents which are themselves deleterious to host functions. Finally, the malignancies EBV appears to be associated with occur in very limited populations characterized by genetic traits or bounded by specific geographic constraints. It seems reasonable to postulate that in the case of EBV the cells giving rise to malignancies are nonpermissive and that expression of viral functions is regulated at three levels. The first probably is expressed in peripheral leukocytes of patients with infectious mononucleosis and does not result in malignant transformation of cells. The second occurs in specific cell populations, and may result in malignant transfor-mation. This hypothesis is supported by the observation that infectious mononuc-leosis is a multiclonal disease whereas Burkitt's lymphoma is uniclonal (Fialkow *et al.*, 1970, 1973). If multiclonal infection could be shown to precede a uniclonal tumor, it would clearly imply not only that malignant transformation is rare but also that it follows a specific event in a single infected cell.

Last, complete expression of the viral genome occurs in very few cells and only under very special conditions determined either by the topology of the cell (oropharynx?) or by specific physiological states resulting from suppression of undefined host functions by chemical inducers. Although the fundamental principle that not all viral functions are expressed in herpesvirus-transformed cells seems to hold for EBV as well, the available data indicate that the mechanisms by which this principle is upheld in EBV-and HSV-infected cells differ. In HSV-transformed cells, the failure of expression of all viral functions is probably the result of infection with defective virus. In the case of EBV, the failure may well be due to very tight regulation of host factors necessary for viral expression.

5.4.5. Conclusions

303

HERPES
SIMPLEX AND
EPSTEIN–BARR
VIRUSES IN
HUMAN CELLS
AND TISSUES:
A STUDY IN
CONTRASTS

The central theme of this discussion has been the interaction of HSV and EBV with their host. In addition to the productive infection, whose analysis at least in the artificial milieu of cultured cells is well under way, we are confronted with latency, for which herpesviruses are noted, and cancer, for which they are at least suspect. We cannot account for either latency or cancer on the basis of what we know about productive infection except in a most restricted way by pointing out what is likely not to happen. Analysis of productive infections does indeed point a way to elucidation of latency and cancer. It seems reasonable that if virus is to coexist with its host, a defined level of molecular interaction between host and viral gene products must exist, and both the biochemical basis of latency and the etiological role of herpesviruses in human cancer may emerge from a broad analysis of these interactions at the molecular level.

ACKNOWLEDGMENTS

When we are not engaged in writing reviews, our work is supported by the United States Public Health Service (CA 08494), the American Cancer Society (VC 103I and VC 113), the Chicago Cancer Research Center Project (CA-14599), and the Leukemia Research Foundation. E. Kieff is a Research Career Development Awardee of the Schweppe Foundation. We thank Dr. Andre Nahmias for useful discussions on the immunology of herpesvirus infections and Dr. George Klein for helpful discussions of Epstein–Barr virus.

6. References

ABODEELY, R. A., LAWSON, L. A., AND RANDALL, C. C., 1970, Morphology and entry of enveloped and de-enveloped equine abortion (herpes) virus, *J. Virol.* 5:513–523.

ADAM, E., KAUFMAN, R. H., MELNICK, J. L., LEVY, A. H., AND RAWLS, W. E., 1972, Seroepidemiologic studies of herpesvirus type 2 and carcinoma of the cervix. III. Houston, Texas, *AM. J. Epidemiol.* 96:427–442.

ADAM, E., KAUFMAN, R. H., MELNICK, J. L., LEVY, A., AND RAWLS, E., 1973, Seroepidemiologic studies of herpesvirus type 2 and carcinoma of the cervix. IV. Dysplasia and carcinoma *in situ, Am. J. Epidemiol.* 98:77–87.

ADAMS, A., LINDAHL, T., AND KLEIN, G., 1973, Linear association between cellular DNA and Epstein–Barr virus DNA in a human lymphoblastoid cell line, *Proc. Natl. Acad. Sci.* 70:2888–2892.

ARMSTRONG, D., HENLE, G., AND HENLE, W., 1966, Complement fixation tests with cell lines derived from Burkitt's lymphoma and acute leukemias, *J. Bacteriol.* 91:1257–1262.

ASHE, W. K., AND NOTKINS, A. L., 1966, Neutralization of an infectious herpes simplex virus–antibody complex by anti-gamma-globulin, *Proc. Natl. Acad. Sci.* 56:447–451.

AURELIAN, L., 1972, Possible role of herpesvirus hominis, type 2, in human cervical cancer, *Fed. Proc.* 21:1651–1659.

AURELIAN, L., 1973, Virions and antigens of herpes virus type 2 in cervical carcinoma, *Cancer Res.* 33:1539–1547.

AURELIAN, L., AND ROIZMAN, B., 1964, The host range of herpes simplex virus: Interferon, viral DNA and antigen synthesis in abortive infection of dog kidney cells, *Virology* 22:452–461.

AURELIAN, L., AND ROIZMAN, B., 1965, Abortive infection of canine cells by herpes simplex virus. II. The alternative suppression of synthesis of interferon and viral constituents, *J. Mol. Biol.* **11**:539–548.

AURELIAN, L., AND STRANDBERG, J. D., 1974, Biologic and immunologic comparison of two HSV-2 variants, one an isolate from cervical tumor cells, *Arch. Ges. Virusforsch.* (in press).

AURELIAN, L., STRANDBERG, J. D., MELENDEZ, L. V., AND JOHNSON, L. A., 1971, Herpesvirus type 2 isolated from cervical tumor cells grown in tissue culture, *Science* **174**:704–707.

AURELIAN, L., SCHUMANN, B., MARCUS, R. L., AND DAVIS, H. J., 1973a, Antibody to HSV-2 induced tumor specific antigens in serums from patients with cervical carcinoma, *Science* **181**:161–164.

AURELIAN, L., DAVIS, H. G., AND JULIAN, C. G., 1973b, Herpesvirus type 2 induced, tumor-specific antigen in cervical carcinoma, *Am. J. Epidemiol.* **98**:1–9.

BACHENHEIMER, S. L., AND ROIZMAN, B., 1972, Ribonucleic acid synthesis in cells infected with herpes simplex virus. VI. Polyadenylic acid sequences in viral messenger ribonucleic acid, *J. Virol.* **10**:875–879.

BACHENHEIMER, S. L., KIEFF, E. D., LEE, L., AND ROIZMAN, B., 1972, Comparative studies on DNAs of Marek's disease and herpes simplex virus, in: *Oncogenesis and Herpesviruses* (P. M. Biggs, G. de Thé, and L. N. Payne, eds.), pp. 74–81, International Agency for Research on Cancer, Lyon.

BANATVALA, J. E., BEST, J. M., AND WALKER, D. K., 1972, Epstein–Barr virus-specific IgM in infectious mononucleosis, Burkitt lymphoma, and nasopharyngeal carcinoma, *Lancet* **1**:1205–1208.

BARINGER, J. R., AND SWOVELAND, M. A., 1973, Recovery of herpes simplex virus from human trigeminal ganglia, *New Engl. J. Med.* **288**:648–650.

BASTIAN, F. O., RABSON, A. S., LEE, C. L., AND TRALKA, T. S., 1972, Herpesvirus hominis: Isolation from human trigeminal ganglion, *Science* **178**:206–207.

BECKER, Y., AND WEINBERG, A., 1972, Molecular events in the biosynthesis of Epstein–Barr virus in Burkitt lymphoblasts, in: *Oncogenesis and Herpesviruses* (P. M. Biggs, G. de Thé, and L. N. Payne, eds.), pp. 326–335, International Agency for Research on Cancer, Lyon.

BELL, D., WILKIE, N. M., AND SUBAK-SHARPE, J. H., 1971, Studies on arginyl transfer ribonucleic acid in herpesvirus infected baby hamster kidney cells, *J. Gen. Virol.* **13**:463–475.

BELLANTI, J. A., CATALANO, L. W., AND CHAMBERS, R. W., 1971, Herpes simplex encephalitis: Virologic and serologic study of a patient treated with an interferon inducer, *J. Pediat.* **78**:136–145.

BREIDENBACH, G. P., SKINNER, M. S., WALLACE, J. H., AND MIZELL, M., 1971, *In vitro* induction of a herpes-type virus in "summer-phase" Lucké tumor explants, *J. Virol.* **7**:679–682.

BREMBERG, S., KLEIN, G., AND EPSTEIN, M., 1969, Direct membrane fluorescence reaction of EBV carrying human lymphoblastoid cells blocking tests with xenogenic antisera, *Int. J. Cancer* **4**:761–766.

BRIER, A. M., WOHLENBERG, C., ROSENTHAL, J., MAGE, M., AND NOTKIUS, A. L., 1971, Inhibition or enhancement of immunological injury of virus-infected cells, *Proc. Natl. Acad. Sci.* **68**:3073–3077.

BRONSON, D. L., GRAHAM, B. J., LUDWIG, H., BENYESH-MELNICK, M., AND BISWAL, N., 1972, Studies on the relatedness of herpes viruses through DNA–RNA hybridization, *Biochim. Biophys. Acta* **259**:24–34.

BRONSON, D. L., DREESMAN, G. R., BISWAL, N., AND BENYESH-MELNICK, M. T., 1973, Defective virions of herpes simplex viruses, *Intervirology* **1**:141–153.

BROWN, D. C., AND KAUFMAN, H. E., 1969, Chronic herpes simplex infection of the ocular adnexa, *Arch. Ophthalmol.* **81**:837–839.

BUBOLA, D., AND OLIVETTI, L., 1968, L'Intradermoreazione con virus erpetico inattivato. I. Analisi dei fattori che influenzano la reazione, *G. Ital. Dermatol.* **109**:363–376.

BURKITT, D. P., 1961, Observations on the geography of malignant lymphoma, *E. Afr. Med. J.* **38**:511–514.

BURKITT, D. P., 1962, A tumour safari in east and central Africa, *Brit. J. Cancer* **16**:379–386.

BURKITT, D. P., 1972, The trail to a virus, in: *Oncogenesis and Herpesvirus* (P. M. Biggs, G. de Thé, and L. N. Payne, eds.), pp. 345–348, International Agency for Research on Cancer, Lyon.

BURKITT, D. P., AND DAVIES, J., 1961, Lymphoma syndrome in Uganda and tropical Africa, *Med. Press* **245**:367–369.

BURKITT, D. P., AND WRIGHT, D., eds., 1970, *Burkitt Lymphoma*, Livingstone, Edinburgh.

BURNET, F. M., AND WILLIAMS, S. W., 1939, Herpes simplex: A new point of view, *Med. J. Austral.* **1**:637–642.

CARTON, C. A., 1953, Effect of previous sensory loss on the appearance of herpes simplex following trigeminal sensory root section, *J. Neurosurg.* **10**:463–468.

305

HERPES
SIMPLEX AND
EPSTEIN–BARR
VIRUSES IN
HUMAN CELLS
AND TISSUES:
A STUDY IN
CONTRASTS

CARTON, C. A., AND KILBOURNE, E. D., 1952, Activation of latent herpes simplex by trigeminal sensory-root section, New Engl. J. Med. 246:172–176.

CATALANO, L. W., AND BARON, S., 1970, Protection against herpes virus and encephalomyocarditis virus encephalitis with a double-stranded RNA inducer of interferon, Proc. Soc. Exp. Biol. Med. 133:684–687.

CATALANO, L. W., AND JOHNSON, L. D., 1971, Herpesvirus antibody and carcinoma in situ of the cervix, J. Am. Med. Assoc. 217:447–450.

CENTIFANTO, Y. M., LITTLE, J. M., AND KAUFMAN, H. E., 1970, The relationship between virus chemotherapy, secretory antibody formation and recurrent herpetic disease, Ann. N.Y. Acad. Sci. 173:649–656.

CESARIO, T. C., POLAND, J. D., WULF, H., CHIN, Y., AND WERMER, H., 1969, Six years experience with herpes simplex virus in a children's home, Am. J. Epidemiol. 90:416–422.

CHANG, R. S., 1971, Umbilical cord leukocytes transformed by lymphoid cell filtrates from healthy people, Nature New Biol. 233:124.

CHANG, R. S., AND GOLDEN, H. D., 1971, Transformation of human leukocytes by throat washing from infectious mononucleosis patients, Nature (Lond.) 234:359–360.

COHEN, G. H., 1972, Ribonucleotide reductase activity of synchronized KB cells infected with herpes simplex virus, J. Virol. 9:408–418.

COOPER, E. H., HUGHES, D. T., AND TOPPING, N. E., 1966, Kinetics and chromosome analyses of tissue culture lines derived from Burkitt lymphomata, Brit. J. Cancer 20:102–113.

COURTNEY, R. J., McCOMBS, R. M., AND BENYESH-MELNICK, M., 1971, Antigens specified by herpesviruses. II. Effect of arginine deprivation on the synthesis of cytoplasmic and nuclear proteins, Virology 43:356–365.

COUCH, E. F., AND NAHMIAS, A. J., 1969, Filamentous structures of type 2 herpesvirus hominis infection of the chorioallantoic membrane, J. Virol. 3:228–232.

CUSHING, H., 1905. The surgical aspects of major neuralgia of trigeminal nerve; a report of twenty cases of operation on Gasserian ganglion with anatomic and physiologic notes on consequence of its removal, J. Am. Med. Assoc. 44:773–779, 860–865, 920–929, 1002–1008, 1088–1093.

DALES, S., AND SILVERBERG, H., 1969, Viropexis of herpes simplex virus by HeLa cells, Virology 37:475–480.

DARAI, G., AND MUNK, K., 1973, Human embryonic lung cells abortively infected with herpes virus hominis type 2 shows some properties of cell transformation, Nature New Biol. 241:268–269.

DAVIDSON, R. L., ADELSTEIN, S. J., AND OXMAN, M. N., 1973, Herpes simplex virus as a source of thymidine kinase for thymidine kinase deficient mouse cells: Suppression and reactivation of viral enzyme DNAs, Proc. Natl. Acad. Sci. 70:1912–1916.

DEFOREST, A., AND KLEIN, M., 1968, The immunoglobulin response in recurrent herpes simplex infection in man, Fed. Proc. 27:734.

DEMISSIE, A., AND SVEDMYR, A., 1969, Age distribution of antibodies to EB virus in Swedish females as studied by indirect immunofluorescence on Burkitt cells, Acta Pathol. Microbiol. Scand. 75:457–465.

DE SCHRYVER, A., FRIBERG, S., JR., KLEIN, G., HENLE, W., HENLE, G., DE THE, G., CLIFFORD, P., AND HO, H. C., 1969, Epstein–Barr virus (EBV)–associated antibody patterns in carcinoma of the post-nasal space, Clin. Exp. Immunol. 5:443–459.

DE SCHRYVER, A., KLEIN, G., HENLE, G., HENLE, W., CAMERON, H. M., SANTESSON, L., AND CLIFFORD, P., 1972, EB-virus associated serology in malignant disease: Antibody levels to viral capsid antigens (VCA), membrane antigens (MA) and early antigens (EA) in patients with various neoplastic conditions, Int. J. Cancer 9:353–364.

DE THÉ, G., 1972, Virology and immunology of nasopharyngeal carcinoma: Present situation and outlook—A review, in: Oncogenesis and Herpesvirus (P. M. Biggs, G. de The, and L. N. Payne, eds.), pp. 275–284, International Agency for Research on Cancer, Lyon.

DE THÉ, G., AMBROSIONI, J., HO, H., AND KWAN, H., 1969, Lymphoblastoid transformation and presence of herpes type particles in Chinese nasopharyngeal tumor culture in vitro, Nature (Lond.) 221:770.

DE THÉ, G., HO, H., KWAN, H., DESRANGES, C., AND FARRE, M., 1970, Nasopharyngeal carcinoma. I. Types of cultures derived from tumor biopsies and non tumorous tissues of Chinese patients with special reference to lymphoblastoid transformation, Int. J. Cancer 6:189–206.

DOCHERTY, J. J., MITCHELL, W. R., AND THOMPSON, C. J., 1973, Abortive herpes simplex virus replication in Rous sarcoma virus transformed cells, Proc. Soc. Exp. Biol. Med. 144:697–704.

DOUGLAS, R. G., JR., AND COUCH, R. B., 1970, A prospective study of chronic herpes simplex virus infection and recurrent herpes labialis in humans, J. Immunol. 104:289–295.

DUFF, R., AND RAPP, F., 1971, Properties of hamster embryo fibroblasts transformed *in vitro* after exposure to ultraviolet-irradiated herpes simplex virus type 2, *J. Virol.* **8:**469–477.

DUNKEL, V., PRY, T., HENLE, G., AND HENLE, W., 1972, Immunofluorescence tests for antibodies to Epstein–Barr virus with sera of lower primates, *J. Natl. Cancer Inst.* **49:**435–440.

EJERCITO, P. M., KIEFF, E. D., AND ROIZMAN, B., 1968, Characterization of herpes simplex virus strains differing in their effect on social behavior of infected cells, *J. Gen. Virol.* **3:**357–364.

ENNIS, F. A., 1973a, Host defense mechanisms against herpes simplex virus. I. Control of infection *in vitro* by sensitized spleen cells and antibody, *Infect. Immunol.* **7:**898–904.

ENNIS, F. A., 1973b, Host defense mechanisms against herpes simplex virus. II. Protection conferred by sensitized spleen cells, *J. Infect. Dis.* **127:**632–638.

EPSTEIN, M. A., 1962, Observations on the fine structure of mature herpes simplex virus and on the composition of its nucleoid, *J. Exp. Med.* **115:**1–11.

EPSTEIN, M. A., AND ACHONG, B. G., Specific immunofluorescence test for the herpes type EB virus of Burkitt lymphoblasts, authenticated by electron microscopy, *J. Natl. Cancer Inst.* **40:**593–607.

EPSTEIN, M. A., AND ACHONG, B. G., 1970, The EB virus, in: *Burkitt's Lymphoma* (D. P. Burkitt and D. H. Wright, eds.), pp. 231–248, Livingstone, Edinburgh.

EPSTEIN, M. A., AND ACHONG, B. G., 1973, The EB virus, *Ann. Rev. Microbiol.* pp. 413–436.

EPSTEIN, M. A., AND BARR, Y. M., 1964, Cultivation *in vitro* of human lymphoblasts from Burkitt's malignant lymphoma, *Lancet* **1:**252–253.

EPSTEIN, M. A., ACHONG, B. G., AND BARR, Y., 1964, Virus particles in cultured lymphoblasts from Burkitt's lymphoma, *Lancet* **1:**702–703.

EPSTEIN, M. A., ACHONG, B. G., AND BARR, Y., 1965, Morphological and biological studies on a virus in cultured lymphoblasts from Burkitt's lymphoma, *J. Exp. Med.* **121:**761–770.

EPSTEIN, M. A., ACHONG, B. G., AND POPE, J., 1967, Virus in cultured lymphoblasts from a New Guinea Burkitt lymphoma, *Brit. Med. J.* **21:**290–291.

ESPMARK, J. A., 1965, Rapid serological typing of herpes simplex virus and titration of herpes simplex antibody by the use of mixed hemadsorption, a mixed antiglobulin reaction applied to virus infected tissue cultures. *Arch. Ges. Virusforsch.* **17:**89–97.

EVANS, A. S., NIEDERMAN, J. C., AND MCCOLLUM, R. W., 1968, Seroepidemiologic studies of infectious mononucleosis with EB virus, *New Engl. J. Med.* **279:**1121–1127.

EVANS, D. L., BARNETT, J. W., BOWEN, J. M., AND DMOCHOWSKI, L., 1972, Antigenic relationship between the herpesviruses of infectious bovine rhinotracheitis, Marek's disease, and Burkitt's lymphoma, *J. Virol.* **10:**277–287.

FALKE, D., 1961, Isolation of two variants with different cytopathic properties from a strain of herpes B virus, *Virology* **14:**492–495.

FIALKOW, P. J., KLEIN, G., GARTLER, S. M., AND CLIFFORD, P., 1970, Clonal origin for individual Burkitt tumors, *Lancet* **1:**384–386.

FIALKOW, P., KLEIN, E., KLEIN, G., CLIFFORD, P., AND SINGH, S., 1973, Immunoglobulin and glucose 6 phosphate dehydrogenase as markers of cellular origin in Burkitt lymphoma, *J. Exp. Med.* **138:**89–102.

FLANAGAN, J. F., 1967, Virus-specified ribonucleic acid synthesis in KB cells infected with herpes simplex virus, *J. Virol.* **1:**583–590.

FRENKEL, N., AND ROIZMAN, B., 1971, Herpes simplex virus: Studies of the genome size and redundancy by renaturation kinetics, *J. Virol.* **8:**591–593.

FRENKEL, N., AND ROIZMAN, B., 1972a, Separation of the herpesvirus deoxyribonucleic acid on sedimentation in alkaline gradients, *J. Virol.* **10:**565–572.

FRENKEL, N., AND ROIZMAN, B., 1972b, Ribonucleic acid synthesis in cells infected with herpes simplex virus: Control of transcription and of RNA abundance, *Proc. Natl. Acad. Sci.* **69:**2654–2658.

FRENKEL, N., ROIZMAN, B., CASSAI, E., AND NAHMIAS, A., 1972, A herpes simplex 2 DNA fragment and its transcription in human cervical cancer tissue, *Proc. Natl. Acad. Sci.* **69:**3784–3789.

FRENKEL, N., SILVERSTEIN, S., CASSAI, E., AND ROIZMAN, B., 1973, RNA synthesis in cells infected with herpes simplex virus. VII. Control of transcription and of transcript abundancies of unique and common sequences of herpes simplex 1 and 2, *J. Virol.* **11:**886–892.

FRITZ, M. E., AND NAHMIAS, A. J., 1972, Reversed polarity in transmembrane potentials of cells infected with herpesviruses, *Proc. Soc. Exp. Biol. Med.* **139:**1159–1161.

FURLONG, D., SWIFT, H., AND ROIZMAN, B., 1972, Arrangement of herpesvirus deoxyribonucleic acid in the core, *J. Virol.* **10:**1071–1074.

GARFINKLE, B., AND MCAUSLAN, B. R., 1974, Transformation of cultured mammalian cells by viable herpes simplex virus subtypes 1 and 2, *Proc. Natl. Acad. Sci.* **71:**220–224.

GELB, L., KOHNE, D., AND MARTIN, M., 1971, Quantitation of simian virus 40 sequences in African green monkey, mouse and virus transformed cell genomes, *J. Mol. Biol.* **57:**119.

GERBER, P., 1972, Activation of Epstein–Barr virus by 5′-bromodeoxyuridine in virus free human cells, *Proc. Natl. Acad. Sci.* **69:**83–85.

GERBER, P., AND BIRCH, S. M., 1967, Complement-fixing antibodies in sera of human and nonhuman primates to viral antigens derived from Burkitt's lymphoma cells, *Proc. Natl. Acad. Sci.* **58:**478–484.

GERBER, P., AND DEAL, D. R., 1970, Epstein–Barr virus-induced viral and soluble complement-fixing antigens in Burkitt lymphoma cell cultures, *Proc. Soc. Exp. Biol. Med.* **134:**748–751.

GERBER, P., AND LORENZ, D., 1974, Complement-fixing antibodies reactive with EBV in sera of marmosets and prosimians, *Proc. Soc. Exp. Biol. Med.* **145:**654–657.

GERBER, P., AND MONROE, J., 1968, Studies in leukocytes growing in continuous culture derived from normal human donors, *J. Natl. Cancer Inst.* **40:**855–866.

GERBER, P., AND ROSENBLUM, E. N., 1968, The incidence of complement-fixing antibodies to herpes simplex and herpes-like viruses in man and rhesus monkeys, *Proc. Soc. Exp. Biol. Med.* **128:**541–546.

GERBER, P., WHANG-PENG, J., AND MONROE, J. H., 1969, Transformation and chromosome changes induced by Epstein–Barr virus in normal human leukocyte cultures, *Proc. Natl. Acad. Sci.* **63:**740–747.

GERBER, P., NONOYAMA, M., LUCAS, S., PERLIN, E., AND GOLDSTEIN, L. I., 1972, Oral excretion of Epstein–Barr virus by healthy subjects and patients with infectious mononucleosis, *Lancet* **2:**988–989.

GERGELY, L., KLEIN, G., AND ERNBERG, I., 1971a, The action of DNA antagonists on Epstein–Barr virus (EBV)–associated early antigen (EA) in Burkitt lymphoma lines, *Int. J. Cancer* **7:**293–302.

GERGELY, L., KLEIN, G., AND ERNBERG, I., 1971b, Appearance of Epstein–Barr virus–associated antigens in infected Raji cells, *Virology* **45:**10–21.

GERGELY, L., KLEIN, G., AND ERNBERG, I., 1971c, Host cell macromolecular synthesis in cells containing EBV-induced early antigens, studied by combined immunofluorescence and radioautography, *Virology* **45:**22–29.

GESER, A., AND DE THÉ, G., 1972, Does the Epstein–Barr virus play an aetiological role in Burkitt's lymphoma? in: *Oncogenesis and Herpesvirus* (P. M. Biggs, G. de Thé, and L. N. Payne, eds.), pp. 372–375, International Agency for Research on Cancer, Lyon.

GIBSON, W., AND ROIZMAN, B., 1971, Compartmentalization of spermine and spermidine in herpes simplex virion, *Proc. Natl. Acad. Sci.* **68:**2818–2821.

GIBSON, W., AND ROIZMAN, B., 1972, Proteins specified by herpes simplex virus. VIII. Characterization and composition of multiple capsid forms of subtypes 1 and 2, *J. Virol.* **10:**1044–1052.

GIBSON, W., AND ROIZMAN, B., 1973, The structural and metabolic involvement of polyamines with herpes simplex virus, in: *Polyamines in Normal and Neoplastic Growth* (D. H. Russell, ed.), pp. 123–135, Raven Press, New York.

GIBSON, W., AND ROIZMAN, B., 1974, Proteins specified by herpes simplex virus. X. Staining and radiolabeling properties of B-capsid and virion proteins in polyacrylamide gels, *J. Virol.* **13:**155–165.

GLADE, P., KAREL, J., MORSE, H., WHANG PENG, J., HOFFMAN, P., KAMMERMEYER, J., AND CHENIN, L., 1968, Infectious mononucleosis continuous suspension cultures of peripheral leukocytes, *Nature (Lond.)* **217:**564–565.

GLASER, R., AND O'NEILL, F. J., 1972, Hybridization of Burkitt lymphoblastoid cells, *Science* **176:**1245–1247.

GLASER, R., AND RAPP, F., 1972, Rescue of Epstein–Barr virus from somatic cell hybrids of Burkitt lymphoblastoid cells, *J. Virol.* **10:**288–296.

GOLDMAN, M., REISKER, J. I., AND BUSHAR, H. F., 1968a, Serum antibodies to Burkitt cell virus, *Lancet* **1:**1156.

GOLDMAN, M., LANDON, H. C., AND REISHER, J. I., 1968b, Fluorescent antibody and gel diffusion reactions of human and chimpanzee sera with cells cultured from Burkitt tumors and normal chimpanzee blood, *Cancer Res.* **28:**2489–2495.

GOODHEART, C. R., PLUMMER, G., AND WANER, J. L., 1968, Density difference of DNA of human herpes simplex viruses types I and II, *Virology* **35:**473–475.

GOODPASTURE, E. W., 1929, Herpetic infection with especial reference to involvement of the nervous system, *Medicine* **8:**223–243.

GRAFSTROM, R. H., ALWINE, J. C., STEINHART, W. L., AND HILL, C. W., 1974, Terminal redundancy of herpes simplex virus type 1 DNA, *Cold Spring Harbor Symp. Quant. Biol.* **36,** in press.

307

HERPES
SIMPLEX AND
EPSTEIN–BARR
VIRUSES IN
HUMAN CELLS
AND TISSUES:
A STUDY IN
CONTRASTS

GRAHAM, F., VAN DER EB, A., AND HEIJNEKER, H., 1974, Size and location of the transforming region in human adenovirus type 5 DNA, *Nature (Lond.)* **251**:687–691.

GRAY, A., TOKUMARU, T., AND SCOTT, T. F. MCN., 1958, Different cytopathogenic effects observed in HeLa cells infected with herpes simplex virus., *Arch. Ges. Virusforsch.* **8**:60–76.

GRIPENBERG, U., LEVAN, A., AND CLIFFORD, P., 1969, Chromosomes in Burkitt lymphomas. I. Serial studies in a case with bilateral tumors showing different chromosomal stemlines, *Int. J. Cancer* **4**:334–349.

GROSE, C., AND FEORINO, P. M., 1972, Epstein–Barr virus and Guillain–Barré syndrome, *Lancet* **2**:1285–1287.

GUNVEN, P., KLEIN, G., HENLE, G., HENLE, W., AND CLIFFORD, P., 1970, Antibodies to EBV associated membrane and viral capsid antigens in Burkitt lymphoma patients, *Nature (Lond.)* **228**:1053–1056.

GUNVEN, P., KLEIN, G., CLIFFORD, P., AND SINGH, S., 1974, EBV associated membrane reactive antibodies during long term survival after Burkitt's lymphoma, *Proc. Natl. Acad. Sci.* **71**:1422–1426.

HAMPAR, B., AND ELLISON, S. A., 1961, Chromosomal aberrations induced by an animal virus, *Nature (Lond.)* **192**:145–147.

HAMPAR, B., AND ELLISON, S. A., 1963, Cellular alterations in the MCH line of Chinese hamster cells following infection with herpes simplex virus, *Proc. Natl. Acad. Sci.* **49**:474–480.

HAMPAR, B., HSU, K. C., MARTOS, L. M., AND WALKER, J. L., 1971, Serologic evidence that a herpes-type virus is the etiologic agent of heterophile-positive infectious mononucleosis, *Proc. Natl. Acad. Sci.* **68**:1407–1411.

HAMPAR, B., DERGE, J. G., MARTOS, L. M., AND WALKER, J. L., 1972, Synthesis of Epstein–Barr virus after activation of the viral genome in a "virus-negative" human lymphoblastoid cell (Raji) made resistant to 5-bromodeoxyuridine, *Proc. Natl. Acad. Sci.* **69**:78–82.

HAMPAR, B., DERGE, J. G., MARTOS, L. M., TAGAMETS, M. A., CHANG, S. Y., AND CHAKRABARTY, A., 1973, Identification of a critical period during the S phase for activation of the Epstein–Barr virus by 5-iododeoxyuridine, *Nature New Biol.* **244**:214–217.

HAMPAR, B., DERGE, J. G., AND SHOWALTER, S. D., 1974a, Enhanced activation of the repressed Epstein–Barr viral genome by inhibitors of DNA synthesis, *Virology* **58**:298–301.

HAMPAR, B., TANAKA, A., NONOYAMA, M., AND DERGE, J., 1974b, Replication of the resident repressed EBV genome during early S phase (S-1 period) of nonproducer Raji cells, *Proc. Natl. Acad. Sci.* **71**:631–633.

HAY, J., ICOTELES, G. J., KEIR, H. M., AND SUBAK-SHARPE, H., 1966, Herpesvirus specified ribonucleic acids, *Nature (Lond.)* **210**:387–390.

HAY, J., PERERA, P. A. J., MORRISON, J. M., GENTRY, G. A., AND SUBAK-SHARPE, J. H., 1971, Herpes virus specified proteins, in: *Ciba Symposium on Strategy of the Viral Genome* (G. E. W. Wolstenholme and M. O'Connor, eds.), pp. 355–372, Churchill Livingstone, London.

HEINE, J. W., AND ROIZMAN, B., 1973, Proteins specified by herpes simplex virus. IX. Contiguity of host and viral proteins in the plasma membrane of infected cells, *J. Virol.* **11**:810–813.

HEINE, J. W., SPEAR, P. G., AND ROIZMAN, B., 1972, The proteins specified by herpes simplex virus. VI. Viral protein in the plasma membrane, *J. Virol.* **9**:431–437.

HEINE, J. W., HONESS, R. W., CASSAI, E., AND ROIZMAN, B., 1974, Proteins specified by herpes simplex virus. XII. The virion polypeptides of type 1 strains, *J. Virol.* **14**:640–651.

HEINEMAN, H. S., 1967, Herpes simplex neutralizing antibody—Quantitation of the complement-dependent fraction in different phases of adult human infection, *J. Immunol.* **99**:214–222.

HENLE, G., AND HENLE, W., 1966a, Immunofluorescence in cells derived from Burkitt's lymphoma, *J. Bacteriol.* **91**:1248–1256.

HENLE, G., AND HENLE, W., 1966b, Studies on cell lines derived from Burkitt's lymphoma, *Trans. N.Y. Acad. Sci.* **29**:71.

HENLE, G., AND HENLE, W., 1967, Immunofluorescence, interference, and complement fixation technics in the detection of herpes-type virus in Burkitt tumor cell lines, *Cancer Res.* **27**:2442–2446.

HENLE, G., AND HENLE, W., 1970, Observations on childhood infections with the Epstein–Barr virus, *J. Infect. Dis.* **121**:303–310.

HENLE, G., HENLE, W., AND DIEHL, V., 1968, Relation of Burkitt tumor associated herpes-type virus to infectious mononucleosis, *Proc. Natl. Acad. Sci.* **59**:94–101.

HENLE, G., HENLE, W., CLIFFORD, P., DIEHL, V., KAFUKO, G. W., KIRYA, B. G., KLEIN, G., MORROW, R. H., MUNUBE, G. M. R., PIKE, M. C., TUKEI, P. M., AND ZIEGLER, J. L., 1969, Antibodies to Epstein–Barr virus in Burkitt's lymphoma and control groups, *J. Natl. Cancer Inst.* **43**:1147–1157.

309

HERPES
SIMPLEX AND
EPSTEIN–BARR
VIRUSES IN
HUMAN CELLS
AND TISSUES:
A STUDY IN
CONTRASTS

HENLE, G., HENLE, W., KLEIN, G., GUNVEN, P., CLIFFORD, P., MORROW, R. H., AND ZIEGLER, J. L., 1971a, Antibodies to early Epstein–Barr virus-induced antigens in Burkitt's lymphoma, *J. Natl. Cancer Inst.* **46**:861–871.

HENLE, G., HENLE, W., AND KLEIN, G., 1971b, Demonstration of two distinct components in the early antigen complex of Epstein–Barr virus infected cells, *Int. J. Cancer* **8**:272–282.

HENLE, W., AND HENLE, G., 1968, Effect of arginine-deficient media on the herpes-type virus associated with cultured Burkitt tumor cells, *J. Virol.* **2**:182–191.

HENLE, W., AND HENLE, G., 1970, *Comparative Leukemia Research* (R. M. Dutcher, ed.), pp. 706–713, Karger, New York.

HENLE, W., HUMMELER, K., AND HENLE, G., 1966, Antibody coating and agglutination of virus particles separated from EB3 line of Burkitt lymphoma cells, *J. Bacteriol.* **92**:269–271.

HENLE, W., DIEHL, V., KOHN, G., ZUR HAUSEN, H., AND HENLE, G., 1967, Herpes-type virus and chromosome marker in normal leukocytes after growth with irradiated Burkitt cells, *Science* **157**:1064–1065.

HENLE, W., HENLE, G., HO, H. C., BURTIN, P., CACHIN, Y., CLIFFORD, P., DE SCHRYVER, A., DE THÉ, G., DIEHL, V., AND KLEIN, G., 1970a, Antibodies to Epstein–Barr virus in nasopharyngeal carcinoma, other head and neck neoplasms and control groups, *J. Natl. Cancer Inst.* **44**:225–231.

HENLE, W., HENLE, G., SCRIBA, J., JOYNER, C. R., HARRISON, S., JR., VON ESSEN, R., PALOHEIMO, J., AND KLEMOLA, E., 1970b, Antibody responses to the Epstein–Barr virus and cytomegaloviruses after open-heart and other surgery, *New Engl. J. Med.* **282**:1068–1074.

HENLE, W., HENLE, G., ZAJAC, B., PEARSON, G., WAUBKE, R., AND SCRIBA, M., 1970c, Differential reactivity of human serums with early antigens induced by Epstein–Barr virus, *Science* **169**:188–190.

HENLE, W., HENLE, G., NIEDERMAN, J. C., KLEMOLA, E., AND HALTIA, K., 1971, Antibodies to early antigens induced by Epstein–Barr virus in infectious mononucleosis, *J. Infect. Dis.* **124**:58–67.

HENLE, W., HENLE, G., GUNVEN, P., KLEIN, G., CLIFFORD, P., AND SINGH, S., 1973a, Patterns of antibodies to Epstein–Barr virus-induced early antigens in Burkitt's lymphoma: Comparison of dying patients with long-term survivors, *J. Natl. Cancer Inst.* **50**:1163–1173.

HENLE, W., HO, H.-C., HENLE, G., AND KWAN, H., 1973b, Antibodies to Epstein–Barr virus-related antigens in nasopharyngeal carcinoma: Comparison of active cases with long-term survivors, *J. Natl. Cancer Inst.* **51**:361–369.

HEWETSON, J. F., ROCCHI, G., HENLE, W., AND HENLE, G., 1973, Neutralizing antibodies against Epstein–Barr virus in healthy populations and patients with infectious mononucleosis, *J. Infect. Dis.* **128**:283–289.

HINUMA, Y., AND GRACE, J. T., 1967, Cloning of immunoglobulin-producing human leukemic and lymphoma cells in long-term cultures, *Proc. Soc. Exp. Biol.* **124**:107–111.

HINUMA, Y., KONN, M., YAMAGUCHI, J., WUDARSKI, D., BLAKESLEE, J., AND GRACE, J., 1967, Immunofluorescence and herpes type virus particles in the P3HR-1 Burkitt lymphoma gene, *J. Virol.* **1**:1045–1051.

HINZE, H. C., AND WALKER, D. L., 1961, Variation of herpes simplex virus in persistently infected tissue cultures, *J. Bacteriol.* **82**:498–504.

HIRSCH, M. S., ZISMAN, B., AND ALLISON, A. C., 1970, Macrophages and age-dependent resistance to herpes simplex virus in mice, *J. Immunol.* **104**:1160–1165.

HIRSHAUT, Y., GLADE, P., MOSES, H., MANAHER, B., AND CHESSIN, L., 1969, Association of herpes-like virus infection with infectious mononucleosis, *Am. J. Med.* **47**:520–527.

HO, H., 1972, Current knowledge of the epidemiology of nasopharyngeal carcinoma, in: *Oncogenesis and Herpesvirus* (P. M. Biggs, G. de The, and L. N. Payne, eds.), pp. 357–366, International Agency for Research on Cancer, Lyon.

HOAGLAND, R. J., 1967, *Infectious Mononucleosis*, Grune and Stratton, New York.

HOCHBERG, E., AND BECKER, Y., 1968, Adsorption penetration and uncoating of herpes simplex virus, *J. Gen. Virol.* **2**:231–241.

HOGGAN, M. D., AND ROIZMAN, B., 1959a, The effect of the temperature of incubation on the formation and release of herpes simplex virus in infected FL cells, *Virology* **8**:508–524.

HOGGAN, M. D., AND ROIZMAN, B., 1959b, The isolation and properties of a variant of herpes simplex producing multinucleated giant cells in monolayer cultures in the presence of antibody, *Am. J. Hyg.* **70**:208–219.

HOGGAN, M. D., ROIZMAN, B., AND TURNER, T. B., 1960, The effect of the temperature of incubation on the spread of herpes simplex virus in an immune environment in cell culture, *J. Immunol.* **84**:152–159.

HOLLINSHEAD, A., O'BONG, L., McKELWAY, W., MELNICK, J. L., AND RAWLS, W. E., 1972, Reactivity between herpesvirus type 2 related soluble cervical tumor cell membrane antigens and matched cancer and control sera, *Proc. Soc. Exp. Biol. Med.* **141:**688–693.

HOLLINSHEAD, A. C., O'BONG, L., CHRÉTIEN, P. B., TARPLEY, J. L., RAWLS, W. E., AND ADAM, E., 1973, Antibodies to herpesvirus nonvirion antigens in squamous carcinomas, *Science* **182:**713–715.

HONESS, R. W., AND ROIZMAN, B., 1973, Proteins specified by herpes simplex virus. XI. Identification and relative molar rates of synthesis of structural and nonstructural herpesvirus polypeptides in the infected cell, *J. Virol.* **12:**1347–1365.

HONESS, R. W., AND ROIZMAN, B., 1974, Regulation of herpesvirus macromolecular synthesis. I. Cascade regulation of the synthesis of three groups of viral proteins, *J. Virol.* **14:**8–19.

HONESS, R. W., AND WATSON, D. H., 1974, Herpes simplex virus–specific polypeptides studied by polyacrylamide gel electrophoresis of immune precipitates, *J. Gen. Virol.* **22:**171–185.

HOOVER, R., AND FRAUMENI, J., 1973, Risk of cancers in renal transplant patients, *Lancet* **2:**55–57.

HOROSZIEWICZ, J., DUNKEL, V., AVELA, L., AND GRACE, J., 1970, *Comparative Leukemia Research* (R. M. Dutcher, ed.), pp. 722–730, Karger, New York.

HUANG, C. C., 1967, Induction of a high incidence of damage to X chromosomes of *Rattus* (*Mastomys*) *natalensis* by base analogues, viruses and carcinogens, *Chromosoma* **23:**162–179.

HUANG, C. C., AND MINOWADA, J., 1972, Differential effects of infection with herpes simplex virus on the chromosomes of human hematopoietic cell, *Cancer Res.* **32:**1218–1225.

HUANG, E. S., AND PAGANO, J. S., 1974, Human cytomegalovirus. II. Lack of relatedness to DNA of herpes simplex I and II, Epstein–Barr virus, and nonhuman strains of cytomegalovirus, *J. Virol.* **13:**642–645.

HULL, R. N., DWYER, A. C., HOLMES, A. W., NOWAKOWSKI, E., DEINHARDT, F., LENNETTE, E. H., AND EMMONS, R. W., 1972, Recovery and characterization of a new simian herpesvirus from a fatally infected spider monkey, *J. Natl. Cancer Inst.* **49:**225–231.

HUMMELER, K., HENLE, G., AND HENLE, W., 1966, Fine structure of a virus in cultured lymphoblasts from Burkitt lymphoma, *J. Bacteriol.* **91:**1366–1368.

HUMMELER, K., TOMASSIAN, N., AND ZAJAC, B., 1969, Early events in herpes simplex virus infection: A radioautographic study, *J. Virol.* **4:**67–74.

ITO, M., AND BARRON, A. L., 1972, Surface antigen produced by herpes simplex virus (HSV), *J. Immunol.* **108:**711–718.

ITO, M., AND BARRON, A. L., 1973, Surface antigens produced by herpesviruses: Varicella-zoster virus, *Infect. Immun.* **8:**48–52.

IWASAKI, Y., 1973, Ultrastructural study on the sequence of human cytomegalovirus infection in human diploid cells, *Arch. Ges. Virusforsch.* **40:**311–324.

JEHN, U., LINDAHL, T., AND KLEIN, G., 1972, Fate of virus DNA in the abortive infection of human lymphoid cell lines by Epstein–Barr virus, *J. Gen. Virol.* **16:**409–412.

JENSEN, E., AND DE SOMBRE, E., 1972, Mechanism of action of sex hormones, *Ann. Rev. Biochem.* **41:**203–230.

JOHANSSON, B., KLEIN, G., HENLE, W., AND HENLE, G., 1970, Epstein–Barr virus (EBV)-associated antibody patterns in malignant lymphoma and leukemia. I. Hodgkin's disease, *Int. J. Cancer* **6:**450–462.

JOHNSON, R. T., 1964, The pathogenesis of herpes virus encephalitis. II. A cellular basis for the development of resistance with age, *J. Exp. Med.* **120:**359–374.

JONDAL, M., AND KLEIN, G., 1973, Surface markers on human B and T lymphocytes. II. Presence of Epstein–Barr virus receptors on B lymphocytes, *J. Exp. Med.* **138:**1365–1378.

JUNGE, U., HOEKSTRA, J., AND DEINHARDT, F., 1971, Stimulation of peripheral lymphocytes by allogeneic and antochthonous mononucleosis lymphocyte cell lines, *J. Immunol.* **106:**1306–1315.

KAFUKO, G. W., HENDERSON, B. E., KIRYA, B. G., MUNUBE, G. M. R., TUKEI, P. M., DAY, N. E., HENLE, G., HENLE, W., MORROW, M. H., PIKE, M. C., SMITH, P. G., AND WILLIAMS, E. H., 1972, Epstein–Barr virus antibody levels in children from the West Nile District of Uganda: Report of a field study, *Lancet* **1:**706–709.

KALTER, S. S., HEBERLING, R. L., AND RATNER, J. J., 1972, EBV antibody in sera of nonhuman primates, *Nature (Lond.)* **238:**353–354.

KAMIYA, T., BEN-PORAT, T., AND KAPLAN, A. S., 1964, The role of progeny viral DNA in the regulation of enzyme and DNA synthesis, *Biochem. Biophys. Res. Commun.* **16:**410–415.

KAMIYA, T., BEN-PORAT, T., AND KAPLAN, A. S., 1965, Control of certain aspects of the infective process by progeny viral DNA, *Virology* **26:**577–589.

KAPLAN, A. S., 1973, A brief review of the biochemistry of herpesvirus host cell interaction, *Cancer Res.* **33**:1393–1398.

KAPLAN, A. S., AND BEN-PORAT, T., 1959, The effect of pseudorabies virus on the nucleic acid metabolism and on the nuclei of rabbit kidney cells, *Virology* **8**:352–366.

KAPLAN, A. S., BEN-PORAT, T., AND COTO, C., 1967, Studies on the control of the infective process in cells infected with pseudorabies virus, in: *Molecular Biology of Viruses* (J. Colter, ed.), pp. 527–545, Academic Press, New York.

KAUFMAN, H. E., 1968, Mechanisms of recurrent herpes simplex keratitis, *Am. J. Ophthalmol.* **66**:559.

KAUFMAN, H. E., BROWN, D. C., AND ELLISON, E. D., 1967, Recurrent herpes in the rabbit and man, *Science* **156**:1628–1629.

KAUFMAN, H. E., BROWN, D. C., AND ELLISON, E. D., 1968, Herpes virus in the lacrimal gland, conjunctiva and cornea of man—A chronic infection, *Am. J. Ophthalmol.* **65**:32–35.

KAWAI, Y., NONOYAMA, M., AND PAGANO, J., 1973, Reassociation kinetics for EBV DNA: Non-homology to mammalian DNA and homology of viral DNA in various diseases, *J. Virol.* **12**:1006–1012.

KEIR, H. M., 1968, Virus-induced enzymes in mammalian cells infected with DNA viruses, in: *Molecular Biology of Viruses* Vol. 18, pp. 67–99, Cambridge University Press, Cambridge.

KELLER, J. M., SPEAR, P. G., AND ROIZMAN, B., 1970, The proteins specified by herpes simplex virus. III. Viruses differing in their effects on the social behaviour of infected cells specify different membrane glycoproteins, *Proc. Natl. Acad. Sci.* **65**:865–871.

KELLY, R., COZZARELLI, N., DEUTSCHER, M., LEHMAN, I., AND KORNBERG, A., 1970, Enzymatic synthesis of DNA. XXXII. Replication of duplex DNA by polymerase I a single strand break, *J. Biol. Chem.* **245**:39–45.

KIEFF, E. D., AND LEVINE, J., 1974, Homology between Burkitt herpes viral DNA and DNA in continuous lymphoblastoid cells from patients with infectious mononucleosis, *Proc. Natl. Acad. Sci.* **71**:355–358.

KIEFF, E. D., BACHENHEIMER, S. L., AND ROIZMAN, B., 1971, Size, composition and structure of the DNA of subtypes 1 and 2 herpes simplex virus, *J. Virol.* **8**:125–132.

KIEFF, E. D., HOYER, B., BACHENHEIMER, S. L., AND ROIZMAN, B., 1972. Genetic relatedness of type 1 and type 2 herpes simplex viruses, *J. Virol.* **9**:738–745.

KIRKWOOD, J., GEERING, G., AND OLD, L. J., 1972, Demonstration of group- and type-specific antigens of herpes viruses, in: *Oncogenesis and Herpesvirus* (P. M. Biggs, G. de Thé, and L. N. Payne, eds.), p. 479, International Agency for Research on Cancer, Lyon.

KLEIN, E., VANFURTH, R., JOHANNSEN, B., ERNBERG, I., AND CLIFFORD, T., 1972, Immunoglobulin synthesis as cellular marker of malignant lymphoid cells, in: *Oncogenesis and Herpesvirus* (P. M. Biggs, G. de Thé, and L. N. Payne, eds.), pp. 253–260, International Agency for Research on Cancer, Lyon.

KLEIN, G., 1971, Immunologic aspects of Burkitt's lymphoma, *Advan. Immunol.* **14**:187–250.

KLEIN, G., 1973, The Epstein–Barr virus, in: *The Herpesviruses* (A. S. Kaplan, ed.), pp. 521–555, Academic Press, New York.

KLEIN, G., AND DOMBOS, L., 1973, Relationship between the sensitivity of EBV-carrying lymphoblastoid lines to superinfection and the inducibility of the resident viral genome, *Int. J. Cancer* **11**:327–337.

KLEIN, G., CLIFFORD, P., KLEIN, E., AND STJERNSWÄRD, J., 1966, Search for tumor specific immune reactions in Burkitt lymphoma patients by the membrane immunofluorescence reaction, *Proc. Natl. Acad. Sci.* **55**:1628–1635.

KLEIN, G., CLIFFORD, P., KLEIN, E., AND STJERNSWÄRD, J., 1966, Search for tumor specific immune reactions in Burkitt lymphoma patients by the membrane immunofluorescence reaction, in: Symposium on the Chemotherapy of Burkitt Lymphoma, *Unio Int. Contra Cancrum Monogr. Ser.* **8**:209–232.

KLEIN, G., CLIFFORD, P., HENLE, G., HENLE, W., OLD, L. J., AND GEERING, L., 1969, EBV-associated serological patterns in a Burkitt lymphoma patient during regression and recurrence, *Int. J. Cancer* **4**:416–421.

KLEIN, G., DOMBOS, L., AND GOTHOSHAR, B., 1972, Sensitivity of EBV producer and nonproducer human lymphoblastoid cell lines to superinfection with EBV, *Int. J. Cancer* **10**:44–57.

KLEIN, G., KLEIN, E., AND CLIFFORD, P., 1967*b*, Search for host defenses in Burkitt lymphoma: Membrane immunofluorescence tests on biopsies and tissue culture lines, *Cancer Res.* **27**:2510–2520.

KLEIN, G., PEARSON, G., HENLE, G., HENLE, W., DIEHL, V., AND NIEDERMAN, J. C., 1968*a*, Relation between Epstein–Barr viral and cell membrane immunofluorescence in Burkitt tumor cells. II.

Comparison of cells and sera from patients with Burkitt's lymphoma and infectious mononucleosis, *J. Exp. Med.* **128**:1021–1030.

KLEIN, G., PEARSON, G., NADKARNI, J. S., NADKARNI, J. J., KLEIN, E., HENLE, G., HENLE, W., AND CLIFFORD, P., 1968b, Relation between Epstein–Barr viral and cell membrane immunofluorescence of Burkitt tumor cells. I. Dependence of cell membrane immunofluorescence on presence of EB virus, *J. Exp. Med.* **128**:1011–1020.

KLEIN, G., WIENER, F., ZECH, L., ZUR HAUSEN, H., AND REEDMAN, B., 1974a, Segregation of the EBV-determined nuclear antigen (EBNA) in somatic cell hybrids derived from the fusion of a mouse fibroblast and a human Burkitt lymphoma line, *Int. J. Cancer* **14**:54–64.

KLEIN, G., GIOVANELLA, B., LINDAHL, T., FIALKOW, P., SINGH, S., AND STEHLIN, J., 1974b, Direct evidence for the presence of EBV DNA and nuclear antigen in malignant epithelial cells from patients with poorly differentiated carcinoma of the nasopharynx, *Proc. Natl. Acad. Sci.*, in press.

KOHLHAGE, H., 1964, Differentiation of plaque variants of the herpes simplex virus by gradient centrifugation and column chromatography, *Arch. Ges. Virusforsch.* **14**:348–365 (*Zbl. Bakteriol.* **191**:252–256).

KOHLHAGE, H., AND SCHIEFERSTEIN, G., 1965, Untersuchungen über die genetische stabilität des plaquebildes beim Herpes-simplex-Virus in Zellkulturen (Investigations on the genetic stability of the plaque picture of herpes simplex virus in cell cultures), *Arch. Ges. Virusforsch.* **15**:640–650.

KOHLHAGE, H., AND SIEGERT, R., 1962, Zwei genetische determinierte Varianten eines Herpes-simplex-Stammes, *Arch. Ges. Virusforsch.* **12**:273–286.

KOHN, G., MELLMAN, W. J., MOORHEAD, P. S., LOFTUS, J., AND HENLE, G., 1967, Involvement of C group chromosomes in five Burkitt lymphoma cell lines, *J. Natl. Cancer Inst.* **38**:209–222.

KUFE, D., MAGRATH, I., ZIEGLER, J., AND SPIEGELMAN, S., 1973, Burkitt's tumors contain particles encapsulating RNA instructed DNA polymerase and high molecular weight virus related RNA, *Proc. Natl. Acad. Sci.* **70**:737–741.

LAIBSON, P. R., AND KIBRICK, S., 1969, Recurrence of herpes simplex virus in rabbit eyes: Results of a three-year study, *Invest. Ophthalmol.* **8**:346–350.

LANDO, D., AND RYHINER, M.-L., 1969, Pouvoir infectieux du DNA d'herpesvirus hominis en culture cellulaire, *Compt. Rend. Acad. Sci. Paris* **269**:527–530.

LANDON, J. C., ELLIS, L. B., ZEVE, V. H., AND FABRIGIO, D. P. A., 1968, Herpes-type virus in cultured leukocytes from chimpanzees, *J. Natl. Cancer Inst.* **40**:181–192.

LARSON, C. L., USHIJIMA, R. N., KARIM, R., BAKER, M. B., AND BAKER, R. E., 1972, Herpesvirus hominis type 2 infections in rabbits: Effect of prior immunization with attenuated *Mycobacterium bovis* (BCG) cells, *Infect. Immun.* **6**:465–468.

LEE, L. F., KIEFF, E. D., BACHENHEIMER, S. L., ROIZMAN, B., SPEAR, P. G., BURMESTER, B. R., AND NAZERIAN, K., 1971, Size and composition of Marek's disease virus DNA, *J. Virol.* **7**:289–294.

LEIBOLD, W., FLANAGAN, T. D., MENEZES, J., AND KLEIN, G., 1974, Induction of Epstein–Barr virus (EBV)-associated nuclear antigen (EBNA) during *in vitro* transformation of human lymphoid cells, *J. Natl. Cancer Inst.*, in press.

LERNER, A. M., BAILEY, E. J., AND NOLAN, D. C., 1970, Complement-requiring neutralizing antibodies in herpesvirus hominis encephalitis, *J. Immunol.* **104**:607–615.

LEVIN, A. G., FRIBERG, S., JR., AND KLEIN, E., 1969, Xenotransplantation of a Burkitt lymphoma culture line with surface immunoglobulin specificity, *Nature (Lond.)* **222**:997–998.

LEVINE, P. H., ABLASHI, D. V., BERARD, C. W., CARBONE, P. P., WAGGONER, D. E., AND MALAN, L., 1971, Elevated antibody titers to Epstein–Barr virus in Hodgkin's disease, *Cancer* **27**:416–421.

LEVINE, P. H., O'CONOR, G. T., AND BERARD, C. W., 1972, Antibodies to Epstein–Barr virus (EBV) in American patients with Burkitt's lymphoma, *Cancer* **30**:610–615.

LEVY, J. A., AND HENLE, L., Indirect immunofluorescence test with sera from African children and cultured Burkitt lymphoma cells, *J. Bacteriol.* **92**:275–276.

LINDAHL, T., KLEIN, G., REEDMAN, B., JOHANSSON, B., AND SINGH, S., 1974, Relationship between EBV DNA and EBNA in Burkitt lymphoma biopsies and other lymphoproliferative malignancies, *Int. J. Cancer* **13**:764–772.

LIPMAN, M., ANDREWS, L., AND MILLER, G., 1974, Direct visualization of enveloped herpes-like virus from throat washing with leukocyte transforming activity, in: *Abstracts of the Annual Meeting of the American Society for Microbiology* (H. Godder, ed.), American Society for Microbiology, Washington, D.C.

LODMELL, D. L., NIWA, A., HAYASHI, K., AND NOTKINS, A. L., 1973, Prevention of cell-to-cell spread of herpes simplex virus by leukocytes, *J. Exp. Med.* **137**:706–720.

313

HERPES
SIMPLEX AND
EPSTEIN–BARR
VIRUSES IN
HUMAN CELLS
AND TISSUES:
A STUDY IN
CONTRASTS

LOGAN, W. S., TINDALL, J. P., AND ELSON, M. L., 1971, Chronic cutaneous herpes simplex, *Arch. Dermatol.* **103**:606–614.

LONDON, W. T., CATALANO, L. W., NAHMIAS, A. J., FUCILLO, D. A., AND SEVER, J. L., 1971, Genital herpesvirus type 2 infection of monkeys, *Obstet. Gynecol.* **37**:501–509.

LOWRY, S. A., MELNICK, J. L., AND RAWLS, W. E., 1971, Investigation of plaque formation in chick embryo cells as a biological marker for distinguishing herpesvirus type 2 from type 1, *J. Gen. Virol.* **10**:1–19.

LUDWIG, H. O., 1972, Untersuchungen am genetischen Material von Herpesviren. I. Biophysikalisch-chemische Charakterisierung von Herpesvirus-Desoxyribonucleinsauren, *Med. Microbiol. Immunol.* **157**:186–211.

LUDWIG, H. O., BISWAL, N., AND BENYESH-MELNICK, M., 1971, Characterization of DNA isolated from metaphase chromosomes of cells containing Epstein–Barr virus, *Biochim. Biophys. Acta* **232**:261–270.

LUDWIG, H. O., BISWAL, N., AND BENYESH-MELNICK, M., 1972, Studies on the relatedness of herpesviruses through DNA–DNA hybridization, *Virology* **49**:95–101.

LUSE, S. A., AND SMITH, M. G., 1959, Electron microscope studies of cells infected with the salivary gland viruses, *Ann. N.Y. Acad. Sci.* **81**:133–144.

MANOLOV, G., AND MANOLOVA, Y., 1972, Marker band in one chromosome 14 from Burkitt lymphomas, *Nature (Lond.)* **237**:33–34.

MARTIN, E. M., 1967, Marital and cortal factors in cervical cancer, *Am. J. Pub. Health* **57**:803–814.

MAURER, B. A., GLICK, J. L., AND MINOWADA, J., 1970, DNA synthesis in EB virus–containing Burkitt lymphoma cultures during a temperature cycling procedure, *Proc. Soc. Exp. Biol. Med.* **133**:1026–1030.

MAYYASI, S., SCHIDLOVSKY, G., BULFERRE, L., AND BUSCHEK, F., 1967, Coating reaction of herpes type virus isolated from malignant tissues with an antibody present in sera, *Cancer Res.* **27**:2020–2023.

MENEZES, J., LEIBOLD, W., AND KLEIN, G., 1974, Biological differences between different Epstein–Barr virus (EBV) strains with regard to lymphocyte transforming ability, in press.

MILLER, G., LISCO, H., KOHN, H. I., AND STITT, D., 1971, Establishment of cell lines from normal adult human blood leukocytes by exposure to Epstein–Barr virus and neutralization by human sera with Epstein–Barr virus antibody, *Proc. Soc. Exp. Biol. Med.* **137**:1459–1465.

MILLER, G., NIEDERMAN, J. C., AND STITT, D. A., 1972a, Infectious mononucleosis: Appearance of neutralizing antibody to Epstein–Barr virus measured by inhibition of formation of lymphoblastoid cell lines, *J. Infect. Dis.* **125**:403–406.

MILLER, G., SHOPE, T., LISCO, H., STITT, D., AND LIPMAN, M., 1972b, Epstein–Barr virus: Transformation, cytopathic changes, and viral antigens in squirrel monkey and marmoset leukocytes, *Proc. Natl. Acad. Sci.* **69**:383–387.

MILLER, G., NIEDERMAN, J. C., AND ANDREWS, L., 1973, Prolonged oropharyngeal excretion of EB virus following infectious mononucleosis, *New Engl. J. Med.* **288**:229–232.

MILLER, G., ROBINSON, J., HESTON, L., AND LIPMAN, M., 1974, Differences between laboratory strains of Epstein–Barr virus based on immortalization, abortive infection and interference, *Proc. Natl. Acad. Sci.* **71**:4006–4010.

MILLER, M. H., STITT, D., AND MILLER, G., 1970, Epstein–Barr viral antigen in single cell clones of two human leukocytic lines, *J. Virol.* **6**:699–701.

MOORE, G. E., AND MINOWADA, J., 1973, B and T lymphoid cell lines, *New Engl. J. Med.* **288**:106.

MOORE, G. E., GRACE, J. T., JR., CITRON, P., GERNER, R., AND BURNS, A., 1966, Leukocyte cultures of patients with leukemia and lymphomas, *N.Y. State Med. J.* **66**:2757–2764.

MORGAN, C., ROSE, H. M., AND MEDNIS, B., 1968, Electron microscopy of herpes simplex virus. I. Entry, *J. Virol.* **2**:507–516.

MORI, R., TASAKI, T., AND KIMURA, G., 1967, Depression of acquired resistance against herpes simplex virus in neonatally thymectomized mice, *Arch. Ges. Virusforsch.* **21**:459–462.

MORRIS, V. L., WAGNER, E. K., AND ROIZMAN, B., 1970, RNA synthesis in cells infected with herpes simplex virus. III. Absence of virus-specified arginyl- and seryl-tRNA in infected HEp-2 cells, *J. Mol. Biol.* **52**:247–263.

MORSE, D., AND POPE, J., 1972, Assay of the infectivity of EBV by transformation of human leukocytes in vitro, *J. Gen. Virol.* **17**:233–236.

MUIR, C. S., 1972, Nasopharyngeal carcinoma in non-Chinese populations, in: *Oncogenesis and Herpesvirus* (P. M. Biggs, G. de Thé, and L. N. Payne, eds.), pp. 367–371, International Agency for Research on Cancer, Lyon.

MULLER, S. A., HERRMANN, E. C. JR., AND WINKELMANN, R. K., 1972, Herpes simplex infections in hematologic malignancies, *Am. J. Med.* **52:**102–114.

MUNK, K., AND DARAI, G., 1973, Human embryonic lung cells transformed by herpes simplex virus, *Cancer Res.* **33:**1535–1538.

MUNK, K., AND SAUER, G., 1964, Relationship between cell DNA metabolism and nucleocytoplasmic alterations in herpes virus–infected cells, *Virology* **22:**153–154.

MUNYON, W., KRAISELBURD, E., DAVIS, D., AND MANN, J., 1971, Transfer of thymidine kinase to thymidine kinaseless L cells by infection with ultraviolet-irradiated herpes simplex virus, *J. Virol.* **7:**813–820.

MUNYON, W., KRAISELBURD, E., DAVIS, D., ZEIGEL, R., BUCHSBAUM, R., AND PAOLETTI, E., 1972*a*, Biochemical transformation of L-cells with ultraviolet irradiated herpes simplex virus, *Fed. Proc.* **31:**1669–1672.

MUNYON, W., BUCHSBAUM, R., PAOLETTI, E., MANN, J., KRAISELBURD, E., AND DAVIS, D., 1972*b*, Electrophoresis of thymidine kinase activity synthesized by cells transformed by herpes simplex virus, *Virology* **49:**683–689.

NADKARNI, J. S., NADKARNI, J. J., CLIFFORD, P., MANOLOV, G., FENJO, E. M., AND KLEIN, E., 1969, Characteristics of new cell lines derived from Burkitt lymphomas, *Cancer* **23:**64–79.

NADKARNI, J. S., NADKARNI, J. J., KLEIN, G., HENLE, W., HENLE, G., AND CLIFFORD, P., 1970, EB viral antigens in Burkitt tumor biopsies and early cultures, *Int. J. Cancer* **6:**10–17.

NAHMIAS, A. J., 1970, Disseminated herpes-simplex-virus infections, *New Engl. J. Med.* **282:**684–685.

NAHMIAS, A. J., 1972, Herpesviruses from fish to man—A search for pathobiological unity, *Pathobiol. Ann.* **2:**153–182.

NAHMIAS, A. J., AND ROIZMAN, B., 1973, Infection with herpes simplex virus 1 and 2, *New Engl. J. Med.* **289:**667–674, 719–725, 781–789.

NAHMIAS, A. J., DOWDLE, W. R., NAIB, Z. M., JOSEY, W. E., AND LUCE, C. F., Genital infection with herpesvirus hominis types 1 and 2 in children, *Pediatrics* **42:**659–666.

NAHMIAS, A. J., DOWDLE, W. R., KRAMER, J. H., LUCE, C. F., AND MANSOUR, S. C., 1969*a*, Antibodies to herpesvirus hominis types 1 and 2 in the rabbit, *J. Immunol.* **102:**956–962.

NAHMIAS, A. J., HIRSCH, M. S., KRAMER, J. H., AND MURPHY, F. A., 1969*b*, Effect of antithymocyte serum on herpesvirus hominis (type 1) infection in adult mice, *Proc. Soc. Exp. Biol. Med.* **132:**696–698.

NAHMIAS, A. J., JOSEY, W. E., NAIB, Z. M., LUCE, C., AND DUFFEY, C., 1970*a*, Antibodies to herpesvirus hominis types 1 and 2 in humans. I. Patients with genital herpetic infections, *Am. J. Epidemiol.* **91:**539–546.

NAHMIAS, A. J., JOSEY, W. E., NAIB, Z. M., LUCE, C., AND GUEST, B., 1970*b*, Antibodies to herpesvirus hominis types 1 and 2 in humans. II. Women with cervical cancer, *Am. J. Epidemiol.* **91:**547.

NAHMIAS, A. J., DEL BUONO, I., PIPKIN, J., HUTTON, R., AND WICKLIFFE, C., 1971, Rapid identification and typing of herpes simplex virus types 1 and 2 by a direct immunofluorescence technique, *Appl. Microbiol.* **22:**455–458.

NAHMIAS, A. J., NAIB, Z. M., JOSEY, W. E., FRANKLIN, E., AND JENKINS, R., 1973, Prospective studies of the association of genital herpes simplex infection and cervical anaplasia, *Cancer Res.* **33:**1491–1497.

NAIB, Z. M., NAHMIAS, A. J., JOSEY, W. E., AND KRAMER, J. H., 1969, Genital herpetic infection, *Cancer* **23:**940–946.

NIEDERMAN, J. C., MCCOLLUM, R. W., HENLE, G., AND HENLE, W., 1968, Infectious mononucleosis—Clinical manifestations in relation to EB virus antibodies, *J. Am. Med. Assoc.* **203:**205–209.

NIEDERMAN, J. C., EVANS, A. S., SUBRAHMANYAN, L., AND MCCOLLUM, R. W., 1970, Prevalence, incidence and persistence of EB virus antibody in young adults, *New Engl. J. Med.* **282:**361–365.

NII, S., 1971*a*, Electron microscopic observations on FL cells infected with herpes simplex virus. I. Viral forms, *Biken J.* **14:**177–190.

NII, S., 1971*b*, Electron microscopic observations on FL cells infected with herpes simplex virus. II. Envelopment, *Biken J.* **14:**325–348.

NII, S., AND KAMAHORA, J., 1961, Cytopathic changes induced by herpes simplex virus, *Biken J.* **4:**255–270.

NII, S., AND KAMAHORA, J., 1963, High frequency appearance of amitotic nuclear divisions in PS cells induced by herpes simplex virus, *Biken J.* **6:**33–36.

NII, S., MORGAN, C., AND ROSE, H. M., 1968*a*, Electron microscopy of herpes simplex virus. II. Sequence of development, *J. Virol.* **2:**517–536.

315

HERPES
SIMPLEX AND
EPSTEIN–BARR
VIRUSES IN
HUMAN CELLS
AND TISSUES:
A STUDY IN
CONTRASTS

NII, S., MORGAN, C., ROSE, H. M., AND HSU, K. C., 1968b, Electron microscopy of herpes simplex virus. IV. Studies with ferritin-conjugated antibodies, *J. Virol.* **2:**1172–1184.

NILSSON, K., 1971, High frequency establishment of human immunoglobulin-producing lymphoblastoid lines from normal and malignant lymphoid tissue and peripheral blood, *Int. J. Cancer* **8:**432–442.

NILSSON, K., KLEIN, G., HENLE, W., AND HENLE, G., 1971, The establishment of lymphoblastoid lines from adult and fetal human lymphoid tissue and its dependence on EBV, *Int. J. Cancer* **8:**443–450.

NILSSON, K., KLEIN, G., HENLE, G., AND HENLE, W., 1972, The role of EBV in the establishment of lymphoblastoid cell line from adult and foetal lymphoid tissue, *IARC Monogr.* **2:**285–290.

NONOYAMA, M., AND PAGANO, J. S., 1971, Detection of Epstein–Barr viral genome in nonproductive cells, *Nature New Biol* **233:**103–106.

NONOYAMA, M., AND PAGANO, J. S., 1972a, Replication of viral deoxyribonucleic acid and breakdown of cellular deoxyribonucleic acid in Epstein–Barr virus infection, *J. Virol.* **9:**714–716.

NONOYAMA, M., AND PAGANO, J., 1972b, Separation of Epstein–Barr virus DNA from large chromosomal DNA in non–virus producing cells, *Nature New Biol.* **238:**169–171.

NONOYAMA, M., AND PAGANO, J. S., 1973, Homology between Epstein–Barr virus DNA and viral DNA from Burkitt's lymphoma and nasopharyngeal carcinoma determined by DNA–DNA reassociation kinetics, *Nature (Lond.)* **242:**44–47.

NONOYAMA, M., HUANG, C. H., PAGANO, J. S., KLEIN, G., AND SINGH, S., 1973, DNA of Epstein–Barr virus detected in tissue of Burkitt's lymphoma and nasopharyngeal carcinoma, *Proc. Natl. Acad. Sci.* **70:**3265–3268.

NOTKINS, A. K., 1971, Infectious virus–antibody complexes: Interaction with anti-immunoglobulins. complement and rheumatoid factor, *J. Exp. Med. Suppl.* **134:**41–51.

O'CONNOR, G. T., AND RABSON, A. S., 1965, Herpes-like particles in an American lymphoma: Preliminary note, *J. Natl. Cancer Inst.* **35:**899–903.

OETTGEN, H. F., AOKI, T., AND GEERING, G., 1967, Definition of an antigenic system associated with Burkitt's lymphoma, *Cancer Res.,* **27:**2532–2534.

OLD, L. J., BOYSE, E. A., OETTGEN, H. F., DE HARVEN, E., GEERING, G., WILLIAMSON, B., AND CLIFFORD, P., 1966, Precipitating antibody in human serum to an antigen present in cultured Burkitt's lymphoma cells, *Proc. Natl. Acad. Sci.* **56:**1699–1704.

O'NEILL, F. J., AND RAPP, F., 1971a, Synergistic effect of herpes simplex virus and cytosine arabinoside on human chromosomes, *J. Virol.* **7:**692–695.

O'NEILL, F. J., AND RAPP, F., 1971b, Early events required for induction of chromosome abnormalities in human cells by herpes simplex virus, *Virology* **44:**544–553.

PAGANO, J. S., 1974, The EBV genome and its interactions with human lymphoblastoid cells and chromosomes, in: *Viruses, Evolution, and Cancer* (K. Marmarosch and E. Kurstak, eds.), Academic Press, New York.

PAGANO, J. S., HUANG, C. H., AND LEVINE, P., 1973, No EB viral DNA in American Burkitt's lymphoma, *New Engl. J. Med.* **289:**1395–1399.

PAINE, T. F., 1964, Latent herpes simplex infection in man. *Bacteriol. Rev.* **28:**472–479.

PARK, J. H., AND BARON, S., 1968, Herpetic keratoconjunctivitis: Therapy with synthetic double-stranded RNA, *Science* **162:**811–813.

PATRIZI, G., MIDDELKAMP, J. N., AND REED, C. A., 1968, Fine structure of herpes simplex virus hepatoadrenal necrosis in newborn, *Am. J. Clin. Pathol.* **49:**325–341.

PATTENGALE, P. K., SMITH, R. W., AND GERBER, P., 1973, Selective transformation of B lymphocytes by E.B. virus, *Lancet* **2:**93–94.

PEARSON, G., DEWEY, F., KLEIN, G., HENLE, G., AND HENLE, W., 1970a, Correlation between antibodies of Epstein–Barr virus (EBV)–induced membrane antigens and neutralization of EBV infectivity, *J. Natl. Cancer Inst.* **45:**989–995.

PEARSON, G., DEWEY, F., KLEIN, G., HENLE, G., AND HENLE, W., 1970b, Relation between neutralization of Epstein–Barr virus and antibodies to cell membrane antigens induced by the virus, *J. Natl. Cancer Inst.* **45:**989–995.

PEREIRA, M. S., BLAKE, J. M., AND MACRAE, A. D., 1969, EB virus antibody at different ages, *Brit. Med. J.* **4:**526–527.

PEREIRA, M. S., FIELD, A. M., BLAKE, J. M., RODGERS, F. G., BAILEY, L. A., AND DAVIES, J. R., 1972, Evidence for oral excretion of EB virus in infectious mononucleosis, *Lancet* **1:**710–712.

PETTERSSON, U., AND SAMBROOK, J., 1973, Amount of viral DNA in the genome of cells transformed by adenovirus type 2, *J. Mol. Biol.* **73:**125–130.

PFEFFERKORN, E. R., BURGE, B., AND COADY, H. M., 1966, Characteristics of the photoreactivation of pseudorabies virus, *J. Bacteriol.* **92**:856–861.

PLUMMER, G., 1964, Serological comparison of the herpes viruses, *Brit. J. Exp. Pathol.* **45**:135–141.

PLUMMER, G., AND MASTERSON, J. G. C., 1970, Herpes simplex virus and cancer of the cervix, *Am. J. Obstet. Gynecol.* **3**:81–84.

PLUMMER, G., HOLLINGSWORTH, D. C., AND PHUANGSEB, A., 1970, Chronic infections by herpes simplex viruses and by the horse and cat herpesviruses, *Infect. Immun.* **1**:351–355.

POPE, J. H., 1967, Establishment of cell lines from peripheral leukocytes in infectious mononucleosis, *Nature (Lond.)* **216**:810–811.

POPE, J. H., HORNE, M. K., AND SCOTT, W., 1968a, Transformation of foetal human leukocytes *in vitro* by filtrates of a human leukaemic cell tine containing herpes-like virus, *Int. J. Cancer* **3**:857–866.

POPE, J. H., ACHONG, B., AND EPSTEIN, M., 1968b, Cultivation and pure structure of virus bearing lymphoblasts from 2nd N. G. Burkitt lymphoma establishment, *Int. J. Cancer* **3**:171–182.

POPE, J. H., HORNE, M. K., AND SCOTT, W., 1969a, Identification of the filterable leukocyte-transforming factor QIMRL-WIL cells as herpes-like virus, *Int. J. Cancer* **4**:255–260.

POPE, J. H., HORNE, M. K., AND WETTERS, E. J., 1969b, Significance of a complement-fixing antigen associated with herpes-like virus and detected in the Raji cell line, *Nature (Lond.)* **222**: 186–187.

PORTER, D. D., WIMBERLY, I., AND BENYESH-MELNICK, M., 1969, Prevalence of antibodies to EB virus and other herpesviruses, *J. Am. Med. Assoc.* **208**:1675–1679.

PRIDEN, M., AND LILIENFELD, A. M., 1971, Carcinoma of the cervix in Jewish women in Israel 1960–1969, an epidemiological study, *Israel J. Med. Sci.* **7**:1465–1470.

PRITCHETT, R., HAYWARD, D., AND KIEFF, E., 1974, DNA of EBV. I. Comparative studies of the DNA of EBV from HR1 and B95-8 cells: Size, structure and relatedness, *J. Virol.,* **15**:(in press, March 1975).

PULVERTAFT, R. J. V., 1964, Cytology of Burkitt's tumor (African lymphoma), *Lancet* **1**:238–240.

RABSON, A., O'CONNOR, G., BARON, S., WHANG, J., AND LEGALLAIS, F., 1966, Morphologic, cytogenetic and virologic studies *in vitro* of a malignant lymphoma from an African child, *Int. J. Cancer* **1**:89–106.

RAFFERTY, K. A., JR., 1964, Kidney tumors of the leopard frog: A review, *Cancer Res.* **24**:169–185.

RAKUSANOVA, T., BEN-PORAT, T., HIMENO, M., AND KAPLAN, A. S., 1971, Early functions of the genome of herpesvirus. I. Characterization of the RNA synthesized in cycloheximide-treated, infected cells, *Virology* **46**:877–889.

RAKUSANOVA, T., BEN-PORAT, T., AND KAPLAN, A. S., 1972, Effect of herpesvirus infection on the synthesis of cell-specific RNA, *Virology* **49**:537–548.

RAPP, F., AND DUFF, R., 1972a, Transformation of hamster cells after infection by inactivated herpes simplex virus type 2, in: *Oncogenesis and Herpesviruses* (P. M. Biggs, G. de Thé, and L. N. Payne, eds.), pp. 447–450, International Agency for Research on Cancer, Lyon.

RAPP, F., AND DUFF, R., 1972b, *In vitro* cell transformation by herpesviruses, *Fed. Proc.* **21**:1660–1668.

RAPP, F., AND DUFF, R., 1973, Transformation of hamster embryo fibroblasts by herpes simplex viruses type 1 and 2, *Cancer Res.* **33**:1527–1534.

RAPP, F., CONNER, R., GLASER, R., AND DUFF, R., 1972, Absence of leukosis virus markers in hamster cells transformed by herpes simplex virus type 2, *J. Virol.* **9**:1059–1063.

RAPP, F., LI, J., AND JERKOFSKY, M., 1973, Transformation of mammalian cells by DNA-containing viruses following photodynamic inactivation, *Virology* **55**:339–346.

RAWLS, W. E., 1973, *Herpes Simplex Virus in Herpesviruses* (A. S. Kaplan, ed.), pp. 291–325, Academic Press, New York.

RAWLS, W. E., TOMPKINS, W. A. F., AND MELNICK, J. L., 1969, The association of herpesvirus type 2 and carcinoma of the uterine cervix, *Am. J. Epidemiol.* **89**:547–554.

RAWLS, W. E., IWAMOTO, K., ADAM, E., MELNICK, J. L., AND GREEN, G. H., 1970, Herpes virus type 2 antibodies and carcinoma of the cervix, *Lancet* **2**:1142–1143.

RAWLS, W. E., ADAM, E., AND MELNICK, J. L., 1973, An analysis of seroepidemiological studies of herpesvirus type L and carcinoma of the cervix, *Cancer Res.* **33**:1477–1482.

REEDMAN, B. M., AND KLEIN, G., 1973, Cellular localization of an Epstein–Barr virus (EBV)–associated complement-fixing antigen in producer and nonproducer lymphoblastoid cell lines, *Int. J. Cancer* **11**:499–520.

REISSIG, M., AND KAPLAN, A. S., 1960, The induction of amitotic nuclear division by pseudorabies virus multiplying in single rabbit kidney cells, *Virology* **11**:1–11.

317

HERPES
SIMPLEX AND
EPSTEIN–BARR
VIRUSES IN
HUMAN CELLS
AND TISSUES:
A STUDY IN
CONTRASTS

ROANE, P. R., JR., AND ROIZMAN, B., 1964a, Requirement for continuous protein synthesis for the development of resistance to UV light in HEp-2 cells infected with herpes simplex virus, *Biochim. Biophys. Acta* **91**:168–170.

ROANE, P. R., JR., AND ROIZMAN, B., 1964b, Studies of the determinant antigens of viable cells. II. Demonstration of altered antigenic reactivity of HEp-2 cells infected with herpes simplex virus, *Virology* **22**:1–8.

ROCCHI, G., HEWETSON, J., AND HENLE, W., 1973, Specific neutralizing antibodies in EBV associated diseases, *Int. J. Cancer* **11**:637–647.

ROGERS, H. W., SCOTT, L. V., AND PATNODE, R. A., 1972, Sensitization of guinea pigs to herpes simplex virus, *J. Immunol.* **109**:801–806.

ROIZMAN, B., 1962a, Polykaryocytosis induced by viruses, *Proc. Natl. Acad. Sci.* **48**:228–234.

ROIZMAN, B., 1962b, Polykaryocytosis, *Cold Spring Harbor Symp. Quant. Biol.* **27**:327–342.

ROIZMAN, B., 1963, The programming of herpes virus multiplication in doubly-infected and in puromycin-treated cells, *Proc. Natl. Acad. Sci.* **49**:165–171.

ROIZMAN, B., 1965, An inquiry into the mechanisms of recurrent herpes infections of man, in: *Perspectives in Virology* Vol. IV (M. Pollard, ed.), pp. 283–304, Hoeber, New York.

ROIZMAN, B., 1969, The herpesviruses—A biochemical definition of the group, in: *Current Topics in Microbiology and Immunology*, Vol. 49, pp. 1–79, Springer, Heidelberg.

ROIZMAN, B., 1971a, Herpesvirus, man and cancer—Or the persistence of the viruses of love, in: *Of Microbes and Life* (J. Monod and E. Borek, eds.), pp. 189–214, Columbia University, New York.

ROIZMAN, B., 1971b, Herpesviruses, membranes and the social behavior of infected cells, in: *Proceedings of the Third International Symposium on Applied and Medical Virology*, Fort Lauderdale, Fla., pp. 37–72, Warren Green Pub., St. Louis.

ROIZMAN, B., 1972, Biochemical features of herpesvirus infected cells particularly as they relate to their potential oncogenicity, in: *Oncogenesis and Herpesviruses* (P. M. Biggs, G. de Thé, and L. N. Payne, eds.), pp. 1–17, International Agency for Research on Cancer, Lyon.

ROIZMAN, B., AND AURELIAN, L., 1965, Abortive infection of canine cells by herpes simplex virus. I. Characterization of viral progeny from cooperative infection with mutant differing in ability to multiply in canine cells, *J. Mol. Biol.* **11**:528–538.

ROIZMAN, B., AND FURLONG, D., 1974, The replication of herpesviruses, in: *Comprehensive Virology*, Vol. 3 (H. Fraenkel Conrat and R. R. Wagner, eds.), pp. 229–403, Plenum Press, New York.

ROIZMAN, B., AND ROANE, P. R., JR., 1961a, A physical difference between two strains of herpes simplex virus apparent on sedimentation in cesium chloride, *Virology* **15**:75–79.

ROIZMAN, B., AND ROANE, P. R., JR., 1961b, Studies of the determinant antigens of viable cells. I. A method, and its application in tissue culture studies, for enumeration of killed cells, based on the failure of virus multiplication following injury by cytotoxic antibody and complement, *J. Immunol.* **87**:714–727.

ROIZMAN, B., AND ROANE, P. R., JR., 1963, Demonstration of a surface difference between virions of two strains of herpes simplex virus, *Virology* **19**:198–204.

ROIZMAN, B., AND ROANE, P. R., JR., 1964, The multiplication of herpes simplex virus. II. The relation between protein synthesis and the duplication of viral DNA in infected HEp-2 cells, *Virology* **22**:262–269.

ROIZMAN, B., AND SPEAR, P. G., 1971, Herpesvirus antigens on cell membranes detected by centrifugation of membrane–antibody complexes, *Science* **171**:298–300.

ROIZMAN, B., AND SPEAR, P. G., 1973, Herpesviruses, in: *Ultrastructure of Animal Viruses and Bacteriophages: An Atlas* (A. J. Dalton and F. Haguenau, eds.), pp. 83–107, Academic Press, New York.

ROIZMAN, B., AND SPRING, S. B., 1967, Alteration in immunologic specificity of cells infected with cytolytic viruses, in: *Proceedings of the Conference on Cross-Reacting Antigens and Neoantigens* (J. J. Trentin, ed.), pp. 85–96, Williams and Wilkins, Baltimore.

ROIZMAN, B., BORMAN, G. S., AND KAMALI-ROUSTA, M., 1965, Macromolecular synthesis in cells infected with herpes simplex virus, *Nature (Lond.)* **206**:1374–1375.

ROIZMAN, B., SPRING, S. B., AND ROANE, P. R., JR., 1967, Cellular compartmentalization of herpesvirus antigens during viral replication, *J. Virol.* **1**:181–192.

ROIZMAN, B., BACHENHEIMER, L., WAGNER, E. K., AND SAVAGE, T., 1970, Synthesis and transport of RNA in herpesvirus-infected mammalian cells, *Cold Spring Harbor Symp. Quant. Biol.* **35**: 753–771.

ROIZMAN, B., SPEAR, P. G., AND KIEFF, E. D., 1973, Herpes simplex viruses I and II: A biochemical definition, in: *Perspectives in Virology, Vol. VIII* (M. Pollard, ed.), pp. 129–169, Academic Press, New York.

ROIZMAN, B., KOZAK, M., HONESS, R. W., AND HAYWARD, G. 1974, Regulation of herpesvirus macromolecular synthesis: Evidence for multilevel regulation of herpes simplex 1 RNA and protein synthesis, *Cold Spring Harbor Symp. Quant. Biol.* **39:** in press, April, 1975.

ROIZMAN, B., HAYWARD, G., JACOB, R., WADSWORTH, S., FRENKEL, N., HONESS, R., AND KOZAK, M., 1975, A model for molecular organization and regulation of herpesviruses, in: *Proceedings of a Symposium on Oncogenesis and Herpesviruses* (H. zur Hausen, G. de Thé, and M. Epstein, eds.), International Agency for Research on Cancer, Lyon, in press.

ROSENBERG, G. L., WOHLENBERG, C., NAHMIAS, A. J., AND NOTKINS, A. L., 1972, Differentiation of type 1 and type 2 herpes simplex virus by *in vitro* stimulation of immune lymphocytes, *J. Immunol.* **109:**413–414.

ROSS, L. J. N., WATSON, D. H., AND WILDY, P., 1968, Development and localization of virus-specific antigens during the multiplication of herpes simplex virus in BHK 21 cells, *J. Gen. Virol.* **2:**115–122.

ROSS, L. J. N., CAMERON, K. R., AND WILDY, P., 1972a, Ultraviolet irradiation of herpes simplex virus: Reactivation processes and delay in virus multiplication, *J. Gen. Virol.* **16:**299–311.

ROSS, L. J. N., FRAZIER, J. A., AND BIGGS, P. M., 1972b, An antigen common to some avian and mammalian herpesviruses, in: *Oncogenesis and Herpesvirus* (P. M. Biggs, G. de Thé, and L. N. Payne, eds.), pp. 480–484, International Agency for Research on Cancer, Lyon.

ROTKIN, I. D., 1967, Sexual characteristics of a cervical cancer population, *Am. J. Pub. Health* **57:**815–829.

ROTKIN, I. D., 1973, A comparison review of key epidemiologic studies in cervical cancer related to current searches for transmissible agents, *Cancer Res.* **33:**1353–1367.

ROYSTON, I., AND AURELIAN, L., 1970a, The association of genital herpesvirus with cervical atypia and carcinoma *in situ, Am. J. Epidemiol.* **91:**531–538.

ROYSTON, I., AND AURELIAN, L., 1970b, Immunofluorescent detection of herpesvirus antigens in exfoliated cells from human cervical carcinoma, *Proc. Natl. Acad. Sci.* **67:**204–212.

RUBENSTEIN, D. S., GRAVELL, M., AND DARLINGTON, R., 1972, Protein kinase in enveloped herpes simplex virions, *Virology* **50:**287–290.

SABIN, A. B., 1974, Herpes simplex-genitalis virus nonvirion antigens and their implication in certain human cancers: Unconfirmed, *Proc. Natl. Acad. Sci.* **71:**3248–3252.

SABIN, A. B., AND TARRO, G., 1973, Herpes simplex and herpes genitalis viruses in etiology of some human cancers, *Proc. Natl. Acad. Sci.* **70:**3225–3229.

SAVAGE, T., ROIZMAN, B., AND HEINE, J. W., 1972, The proteins specified by herpes simplex virus. VII. Immunologic specificity of the glycoproteins of subtypes I and II, *J. Gen. Virol.* **17:**31–48.

SAWYER, R., EVANS, A., NIEDERMAN, J., AND MCCOLLUM, R., 1971, Prospective studies of a group of Yale University freshmen. I. Occurrence of infectious mononucleosis, *J. Infect. Dis.* **123:**263–270.

SCHIDLOVSKY, G., AND TOPLIN, I., 1966, Partial purification and electron microscopy of the virus in the EB-3 cell line derived from a Burkitt lymphoma, *Science* **152:**1084–1085.

SCHIEK, W., 1967, Die Massendichte des Herpes simplex-Virus im Casiumchlorid-Wasser-Gradienten: Beziehungen zur Plaquemorphologie auf HeLa-Zellen und sum serologischen Typ, *Z. Immunitat.* **132:**207–217.

SCHIEK, W., AND SCHNEWEISS, K. E., 1968, Beitrag zur Massendichte von Plaque Varianten des Herpesvirus hominis im Caesiumchlorid-Wasser-Gradienten (Density of plaque variants in type herpes simplex virus under cesium chloride–water gradients), *Arch. Ges. Virusforsch.* **23:**280–283.

SCHNEWEISS, K. E., 1962, Der cytopatische Effekt des Herpes simplex Virus, *Zbl. Bakteriol.* **186:**467–485.

SCHNEWEISS, K. E., SOMMERHAUSER, H., AND HUBER, D., 1972, Biologic and immunologic comparison of two plaque variants of herpes simplex virus type 1, *Arch. Ges. Virusforsch.* **38:**338–346.

SCHULTE-HOLTHAUSEN, H., AND ZUR HAUSEN, H., 1970, Partial purification of the Epstein–Barr virus and some properties of its DNA, *Virology* **40:**776–779.

SCHWARTZ, J., AND ROIZMAN, B., 1969a, Similarities and differences in the development of laboratory strains and freshly isolated strains of herpes simplex virus in HEp-2 cells: Electron microscopy, *J. Virol.* **4:**879–889.

SCHWARTZ, J., AND ROIZMAN, B., 1969b, Concerning the egress of herpes simplex virus from infected cells: Electron microscope observations, *Virology* **38:**42–49.

319

HERPES
SIMPLEX AND
EPSTEIN–BARR
VIRUSES IN
HUMAN CELLS
AND TISSUES:
A STUDY IN
CONTRASTS

SCOTT, T. F. MCN., BURGOON, C. F., CORIELL, L. L., AND BLANK, M., 1953, The growth curve of the virus of herpes simplex in rabbit corneal cells grown in tissue culture with parallel observations on the development of the intranuclear inclusion body, *J. Immunol.* **71**:385–396.

SHANMUGARATNAN, K., 1972, The pathology of nasopharyngeal carcinoma, in: *Oncogenesis and Herpesvirus* (P. M. Biggs, G. de Thé, and L. N. Payne, eds.), pp. 239–248, International Agency for Research on Cancer, Lyon.

SHARP, P., PETTERSSON, U., AND SAMBROOK, J., 1974, Viral DNA in transformed cells, *J. Mol. Biol.* **86**:709–725.

SHELDON, P. J., PAPAMICHAEL, M., HEMSTED, E. H., AND HOLBOROW, E. J., 1973, Thymic origin of atypical lymphoid cells in infectious mononucleosis, *Lancet* **2**:1153–1155.

SHELDRICK, P., AND BERTHELOT, N., 1974, Inverted repetitions in the chromosome of herpes simplex virus, *Cold Spring Harbor Symp. Quant. Biol.* **39**: in press.

SHELDRICK, P., LAITHIER, M., LANDO, D., AND RYHINER, M. L., 1973, Infectious DNA from herpes simplex virus: Infectivity of double-stranded and single-stranded molecules, *Proc. Natl. Acad. Sci.* **70**:3621–3625.

SHOPE, T. C., AND MILLER, G., 1973, Epstein–Barr virus: Heterophile responses in squirrel monkeys inoculated with virus-transformed autologous leukocytes, *J. Exp. Med.* **137**:140–147.

SIEGERT, R. S., AND FALKE, D., 1966, Electron microscopic investigation of the development of herpes hominis virus in culture cells, *Arch. Ges. Virusforsch.* **19**:230–249.

SILVERSTEIN, S., BACHENHEIMER, S. L., FRENKEL, N., AND ROIZMAN, B., 1973, The relationship between post transcriptional adenylation of herpesvirus RNA and mRNA abundance (paper No. 8 in the series on RNA synthesis in cells infected with herpes simplex virus), *Proc. Natl. Acad. Sci.* **70**:2101–2104.

SILVESTRE, D., KOWILSKY, F., KLEIN, G., YATH, Y., NEUPORT SAUTES, C., AND LEVY, J., 1971, Relationship between EBV associated membrane antigen on B L cells and the viral envelope demonstrated by immunofunction labelling, *Int. J. Cancer* **8**:222–233.

SKINNER, G. R. B., THOULESS, M. E., AND JORDAN, J. A., 1971, Antibodies to type 1 and type 2 herpesvirus in women with abnormal cervical cytology, *J. Obstet. Gynecol. Brit. Commonw.* **78**:1031–1038.

SMITH, J. D., AND DE HARVEN, E., 1973, Herpes simplex virus and human cytomegalovirus replication in W1-38 cells. I. Sequence of viral replication, *J. Virol.* **12**:919–930.

SMITH, J. W., ADAM, E., MELNICK, J. L., AND RAWLS, W. E., 1972*a*, Use of the ^{51}Cr release test to demonstrate patterns of antibody response in humans to herpesvirus types 1 and 2, *J. Immunol.* **109**:554–564.

SMITH, J. W., LOWRY, S. P., MELNICK, J. L., AND RAWLS, W. E., 1972*b*, Antibodies to surface antigens of herpesvirus type 1 and type 2 infected cells among women with cervical cancer and control women, *Infect. Immun.* **5**:305–310.

SMITH, K. O., 1963, Physical and biological observations on herpes virus, *J. Bacteriol.* **86**:999–1009.

SMITH, K. O., 1964, Relationship between the envelope and infectivity of herpes simplex virus, *Proc. Soc. Exp. Biol. Med.* **115**:814–816.

SPEAR, P. G., AND ROIZMAN, B., 1967, The buoyant density of herpes simplex virus in CsCl solutions, *Nature (Lond.)* **214**:713–714.

SPEAR, P. G., AND ROIZMAN, B., 1970, The proteins specified by herpes simplex virus. IV. The site of glycosylation and accumulation of viral membrane proteins, *Proc. Natl. Acad. Sci.* **66**:730–737.

SPEAR, P. G., AND ROIZMAN, B., 1972, Proteins specified by herpes simplex virus. V. Purification and structural proteins of the herpesvirion, *J. Virol.* **9**:143–159.

SPEAR, P. G., KELLER, J. M., AND ROIZMAN, B., 1970, The proteins specified by herpes simplex virus. II. Viral glycoproteins associated with cellular membranes, *J. Virol.* **5**:123–131.

SPRING, S. B., AND ROIZMAN, B., 1968, Herpes simplex virus products in productive and abortive infection. III. Differentiation of infectious virus derived from nucleus and cytoplasm with respect to stability and size, *J. Virol* **2**:979–985.

SPRING, S. B., ROIZMAN, B., AND SCHWARTZ, J., 1968, Herpes simplex virus products in productive and abortive infection. II. Electron microscopic and immunological evidence for failure of virus envelopment as a cause of abortive infection, *J. Virol.* **2**:384–392.

SPRINGER, G. F., SEIFERT, M. H., ADYE, J. C., AND EYQUEM, A., 1974, Immunization of humans with infectious mononucleosis receptors from mammalian erythrocytes, *Clin. Immunol. Immunopathol.*, in press.

STEEL, C., MCBEATH, S., AND O'RIORDAN, M., 1971, Human lymphoblastoid cell lines. II. Cytogenetic studies, *J. Natl. Cancer Inst.* **47:**1203–1214.

STEIN, S., TODD, P., AND MAHONEY, J., 1970, The arginine requirement for nucleocapsid maturation in herpes simplex development, *Canad. J. Micros.* **16:**851–854.

STERN, H., 1972, Cytomegalovirus and EB virus infections of the liver, *Brit. Med. Bull.* **28:**180–185.

STERTZ, H., LUDWIG, H., AND ROTT, R., 1974, Immunologic and genetic relationship between herpes simplex virus and bovine herpes mammillitis virus, *Intervirology* **2:**1–13.

STEVENS, J. G., AND COOK, M. L., 1971*a*, Latent herpes simplex virus in spinal ganglia of mice, *Science* **173:**843–845.

STEVENS, J. G., AND COOK, M. L., 1971*b*, Restriction of herpes simplex virus by macrophages: An analysis of the cell–virus interaction, *J. Exp. Med.* **133:**19–38.

STEVENS, J. G., AND COOK, M. L., 1972, Latent herpes simplex virus in sensory ganglia, in: *Perspectives in Virology, Vol. VIII* (M. Pollard, ed.), pp. 171–188, Academic Press, New York.

STEVENS, J. G., AND COOK, M. L., 1973, Latent infections induced by herpes simplex virus, *Cancer Res.* **33:**1399–1401.

STEWART, S., LOVELACE, E., WHANG, J., AND NGU, V., 1965, Burkitt tumor, tissue culture, cytogenetic and viral studies, *J. Natl. Can. Inst.* **34:**319–328.

STICH, H. F., HSU, T. C., AND RAPP, F., 1964, Viruses and mammalian chromosomes. I. Localization of chromosome aberrations after infection with herpes simplex virus, *Virology* **22:**439–445.

STOKER, M. G. P., 1959, Growth studies with herpes virus, in: *Ninth Symposium of the Society for Microbiology*, pp. 142–170, Cambridge University Press, Cambridge.

STOKER, M. G. P., AND NEWTON, A. A., 1959, Mitotic inhibitors in HeLa cell and caused by herpes virus, *Ann. N.Y. Acad. Sci.* **81:**129–132.

SUBAK-SHARPE, H., AND HAY, J., 1965, An animal virus with DNA of high guanine + cytosine content which codes for sRNA, *J. Mol. Biol.* **12:**924–928.

SUBAK-SHARPE, H., SHEPHERD, W. M., AND HAY, J., 1966, Studies on sRNA coded by herpes virus, *Cold Spring Harbor Symp. Quant. Biol.* **31:**583–594.

SUGAWARA, K., MIZUNO, F., AND OSATO, T., 1972, Epstein–Barr virus–associated antigens in nonproducing clones of human lymphoblastoid cell lines, *Nature New Biol.* **239:**242–243.

SVEDMYR, A., AND DEMISSIE, A., 1968, Age distribution of antibodies to Burkitt cells, *Acta Pathol. Microbiol. Scand.* **73:**653–654.

SVEDMYR, A., AND DEMISSIE, A., 1971, Complexity of antigen–antibody systems associated with Epstein–Barr virus, *Ann. N.Y. Acad. Sci.* **177:**241–249.

SWANSON, J. L., CRAIGHEAD, J. E., AND REYNOLDS, E. S., 1966, Electron microscopic observations on herpesvirus hominis (herpes simplex virus) encephalitis in man, *Lab. Invest.* **15:**1966–1981.

SYDISKIS, R. J., AND ROIZMAN, B., 1966, Polysomes and protein synthesis in cells infected with a DNA virus, *Science* **153:**76–78.

SYDISKIS, R. J., AND ROIZMAN, B., 1967, The disaggregation of host polyribosomes in productive and abortive infection with herpes simplex virus, *Virology* **32:**678–686.

SYDISKIS, R. J., AND ROIZMAN, B., 1968, The sedimentation profiles of cytoplasmic polyribosomes in mammalian cells productively and abortively infected with herpes simplex virus, *Virology* **34:**562–565.

TANIGUCHI, S., AND YOSHINO, K., 1965, Studies on the neutralization of herpes simplex virus. II. Analysis of complement as the antibody–potentiating factor, *Virology* **26:**54–60.

TARRO, G., AND SABIN, A. B., 1970, Virus specific, labile, nonvirion antigen in herpesvirus-infected cells, *Proc. Natl. Acad. Sci.* **65:**753–760.

TARRO, G., AND SABIN, A. B., 1973, Nonvirion antigens produced by herpes simplex viruses 1 and 2, *Proc. Natl. Acad. Sci.* **70:**1032–1036.

TERNI, M., 1971, Infection with the virus of herpes simplex, the recrudescence of the disease and the problem of latency, *G. Mal. Infet. Parassit.* **28:**433–468.

TEVETHIA, S. S., LOWRY, S., RAWLS, W. E., MELNICK, J. L., AND MCMILLAN, V., 1972, Detection of early cell surface changes in herpes simplex virus infected cells by agglutination with concanavalin A., *J. Gen. Virol.* **15:**93–97.

THOULESS, M. E., 1972, Serological properties of thymidine kinase produced in cells infected with type 1 or type 2 herpesvirus, *J. Gen. Virol.* **17:**307–315.

TOKUMARU, T., 1957, Pseudorabies virus in tissue culture: Differentiation of two distinct strains of virus by cytopathogenic pattern induced, *Proc. Soc. Exp. Biol. Med.* **96:**55–60.

321

HERPES
SIMPLEX AND
EPSTEIN–BARR
VIRUSES IN
HUMAN CELLS
AND TISSUES:
A STUDY IN
CONTRASTS

TOKUMARU, T., 1966, A possible role of γA-immunoglobulin in herpes simplex virus infection in man, *J. Immunol.* **97**:248–259.

TOPLIN, I., AND SCHIDLOVSKY, G., 1966, Partial purification and electron microscopy of virus in the EB-3 cell line derived from a Burkitt lymphoma, *Science* **152**:1084–1085.

UNIVERSITY HEALTH PHYSICIANS AND PHLS, 1971, Infectious mononucleosis and its relationship to EB virus antibody, *Brit. Med. J.* **4**:643–646.

VAHLNE, A. G., AND BLOMBERG, J., 1974, Purification of herpes simplex virus, *J. Gen. Virol.* **22**:297–302.

VAN HOOSIER, G. L., AND MELNICK, J. L., 1961, Neutralizing antibodies in human sera to herpes simiae (B virus), *Texas Rep. Biol. Med.* **19**:376–380.

VANTIS, J. T., AND WILDY, P., 1962, Interaction of herpes virus and HeLa cells: Comparison of cell killing and infective center formation, *Virology* **17**:225–232.

VONKA, V., BENYESH-MELNICK, M., AND MCCOMBS, R., 1970*a*, Antibodies in human sera to soluble and viral antigens found in Burkitt lymphoma and other lymphoblastoid cell lines, *J. Natl. Cancer Inst.* **44**:865–872.

VONKA, V., BENYESH-MELNICK, M., LEWIS, R. T., AND WIMBERLY, I., 1970*b*, Some properties of the soluble (S) antigen of cultured lymphoblastoid cell lines, *Arch. Ges. Virusforsch.* **31**:113–124.

WAGNER, E. K., 1972, Evidence for transcriptional control of the herpes simplex genome in infected human cells, *Virology* **47**:502–506.

WAGNER, E. K., AND ROIZMAN, B., 1969*a*, RNA synthesis in cells infected with herpes simplex virus. I. The patterns of RNA synthesis in productively infected cells, *J. Virol.* **4**:36–46.

WAGNER, E. K., AND ROIZMAN, B., 1969*b*, RNA synthesis in cells infected with herpes simplex virus. II. Evidence that a class of viral mRNA is derived from a high molecular weight precursor synthesized in the nucleus, *Proc. Natl. Acad. Sci.* **64**:626–633.

WAGNER, E. K., ROIZMAN, B., SAVAGE, T., SPEAR, P. G., MIZELL, M., DURR, F. E., AND SYPOWICZ, D., 1970, Characterization of the DNA of herpesviruses associated with Lucké adenocarcinoma of the frog and Burkitt lymphoma of man, *Virology* **42**:257–261.

WAGNER, E. K., TEWARI, K. K., KOLODNES, R., AND WARNER, R. C., 1974, The molecular size of the herpes simplex virus type 1 genome, *Virology* **57**:436–447.

WAHREN, B., CARLENS, E., ESPMARK, A., LUNDBECK, H., LÖFGREN, S., MADAR, E., HENLE, G., AND HENLE, W., 1971, Antibodies to various herpes viruses in sera from patients with sarcoidosis, *J. Natl. Cancer Inst.* **47**:747–756.

WALLIS, C., AND MELNICK, J. L., 1971, Herpesvirus neutralization: The role of complement, *J. Immunol.* **107**:1235–1242.

WALTERS, M. K., AND POPE, J. H., 1971, Studies of the EB virus–related antigens of human leukocyte cell lines, *Int. J. Cancer* **8**:32–40.

WATKINS, J. F., 1964, Adsorption of sensitized sheep erythrocytes to HeLa cells infected with herpes simplex virus, *Nature (Lond.)* **202**:1364–1365.

WATSON, D. H., WILDY, P., AND RUSSELL, W. C., 1964, Quantitative electron microscope studies on the growth of herpes virus using the techniques of negative staining and ultramicrotomy, *Virology* **24**:523–538.

WATSON, D. H., WILDY, P., HARVEY, B. A. M., AND SHEDDEN, W. I. H., 1967, Serological relationship among viruses of the herpes group, *J. Gen. Virol.* **1**:139–141.

WEINBERG, A., AND BECKER, Y., 1969, Studies on EB virus of Burkitt's lymphoblasts, *Virology* **39**:312–321.

WETMUR, J., AND DAVIDSON, N., 1968, Kinetics of renaturation of DNA, *J. Mol. Biol.* **31**:349–370.

WHEELER, C. E., 1964, Biologic comparison of a syncytial and a small giant cell–forming strain of herpes simplex, *J. Immunol.* **93**:749–756.

WILBANKS, G. D., AND CAMPBELL, J. A., 1972, Effect of herpesvirus hominis type 2 on human cervical epithelium: Scanning electron microscopic observations, *Am. J. Obstet. Gynecol.* **112**:924–929.

WILDY, P., 1973, Antigens of herpes simplex virus of oral and genital origin, *Cancer Res.* **33**:1465–1468.

WILDY, P., RUSSELL, W. C., AND HORNE, R. W., 1960, The morphology of herpes virus, *Virology* **12**:204–224.

WILKIE, N. M., 1973, The synthesis and substructure of herpesvirus DNA: The distribution of alkali-labile single strand interruptions in HSV-1 DNA, *J. Gen. Virol.* **21**:453–467.

WILTON, J. M. A., IVANYI, L., AND LEHNER, T., 1972, Cell-mediated immunity in herpesvirus hominis infections, *Brit. Med. J.* **1**:723–726.

WOLF, H., ZUR HAUSEN, H., AND BECKER, V., 1973, EB viral genomes in epithelial nasopharyngeal carcinoma cells, *Nature New Biol.* **244:**245–247.

WRIGHT, D. H., 1972, The pathology of Burkitt's lymphoma, in: *Oncogenesis and Herpesvirus* (P. M. Biggs, G., de Thé, and L. N. Payne, eds.), pp. 217–229, International Agency for Research on Cancer, Lyon.

YAMAGUCHI, J., HINUMA, Y., AND GRACE, J. T., JR., 1967, Structure of virus particles extracted from a Burkitt lymphoma cell line, *J. Virol.* **1:**640–642.

YAMAMOTO, Y., 1966, A re-evaluation of the skin test of herpes simplex virus, *Jap. J. Microbiol.* **10:**67–77.

YOSHINO, K., AND TANIGUCHI, S., 1965, Studies on the neutralization of herpes simplex virus. III. Mechanism of the antibody-potentiating action of complement, *Virology* **26:**61–72.

YOSHINO, K., AND TANIGUCHI, S., 1966, Evaluation of the demonstration of complement-requiring neutralizing antibody as a means for early diagnosis of herpes virus infections, *J. Immunol.* **96:**196–203.

ZAJAC, B. A., AND KOHN, G., 1970, Epstein–Barr virus antigens, marker chromosome, and interferon production in clones derived from cultured Burkitt tumor cells, *J. Natl. Cancer Inst.* **45:**399–406.

ZEMLA, J., COTO, C., AND KAPLAN, A. S., 1967, Correlation between loss of enzymatic activity and of protein from cells infected with pseudorabies virus, *Virology* **31:**736–738.

ZIMMERMAN, J. E., JR., GLASER, R., AND RAPP, F., 1973, Effect of dibutyryl cyclic AMP on the induction of Epstein–Barr virus in hybrid cells, *J. Virol.* **12:**1442–1445.

ZISMAN, B., HIRSCH, M. S., AND ALLISON, A. C., 1970, Selective effects of antimacrophage serum, silica and anti-lymphocyte serum on pathogenesis of herpes virus infection of young adult mice, *J. Immunol.* **104:**1155–1159.

ZUR HAUSEN, H., 1972, EBV in human tumor cells, in: *International Review of Experimental Pathology,* Vol. II (G. Richter and M. Epstein, eds.), pp. 233–258, Academic Press, London.

ZUR HAUSEN, H., AND SCHULTE-HOLTHAUSEN, H., 1970, Presence of EB-virus nucleic acid homology in a "virus-free" line of Burkitt tumor cells, *Nature* (*Lond.*) **227:**245–248.

ZUR HAUSEN, H., AND SCHULTE-HOLTHAUSEN, H., 1972, Detection of Epstein–Barr viral genomes in human tumor cells by nucleic acid hybridization, in: *Oncogenesis and Herpesvirus* (P. M. Biggs, G. de Thé, and L. N. Payne, eds.), pp. 321–325, International Agency for Research on Cancer, Lyon.

ZUR HAUSEN, H., HENLE, W., HUMMELER, K., DIEHL, V., AND HENLE, G., 1967, Comparative study of cultured Burkitt tumor cells by immunofluorescence autoradiography and electronmicroscopy, *J. Virol.* **1:**830–837.

ZUR HAUSEN, H., SCHULTE-HOLTHAUSEN, H., KLEIN, G., HENLE, W., HENLE, G., CLIFFORD, P., AND SANTESSON, L., 1970, EBV DNA in biopsies of Burkitt tumors and anaplastic carcinomas of the nasopharynx, *Nature* (*Lond.*) **228:**1056–1058.

ZUR HAUSEN, H., DIEHL, V., WOLF, H., SCHULTE-HOLTHAUSEN, H., AND SCHNEIDER, U., 1972, Occurrence of Epstein–Barr virus genomes in human lymphoblastoid cell lines, *Nature New Biol.* **237:**189–190.

8

Papilloma–Myxoma Viruses

Yohei Ito

1. Introduction

The two groups of viruses to be discussed in this chapter are apparently dissimilar, although they do share DNA as their essential component. The papilloma viruses belong to the papovavirus group and are included in the medium-sized DNA viruses, while myxoma virus and its allied agents belong to the larger DNA viruses of the pox group. Nevertheless, an acceptable basis for bringing them together may derive from the fact that they both are literally the most "classical" tumor viruses (Shope, 1932, 1933). Two viruses representing these groups, Shope papilloma and myxoma, have played a very important role in setting the stage for the earliest identification of tumor viruses in mammalian species; they were first reported by the pioneering investigator in the field, Richard Shope. The other feature common to them is that the tumors they induce are benign in the sense that the tumor cells rarely metastasize to remote tissues and organs. In many cases, even spontaneous regression is not uncommon. However, myxoma virus as an infectious agent can be lethal to the host.

Accordingly, it is much easier to point out the obvious differences between the viruses of the two groups. One of the most remarkable differences is reflected in their mode of replication and in their mechanism of tumor induction. The papilloma viruses are known to go through a phase of very close interaction with the genetic material of the host cell during its cycle of replication, which is a rather common process for the "genuine" tumor viruses, while the interrelationship of myxoma group viruses and the host cells seems to be much less intimate. The

YOHEI ITO ● Department of Microbiology, Faculty of Medicine, University of Kyoto, Kyoto, Japan.

"masking phenomenon" of the rabbit papilloma is possibly the result of integration of the viral genetic component into that of the host cell. This relationship is consistent throughout the whole system of the Shope papilloma–carcinoma complex and presumably applies to other members of the papilloma virus group. On the other hand, the myxoma group viruses merely utilize a particular area in the cytoplasm close to the nucleus and convert it as a site of replication. This shows up as a conspicuous figure, the inclusion body. When the replication process of the myxoma virus is crippled for some reason or other and the viral particles disappear from the host cells, the tumorous growth also subsides and the neoplastic nature of the tissue fades away.

2. Papilloma Virus Group

2.1. Biological Properties

The papilloma viruses are frequently seen in nature as a "spontaneous" causative agent of warts or superficial benign tumors of skin and mucous membrane. As understood from the unique model of Shope papillomatosis, the virus persists in the proliferating basal cell layer of the skin in the form of free DNA and matures into the complete virion in concert with the differentiation of the epithelial cells. The process takes place as the whole tissue moves upward and outward to eventually form the keratinized layer at the surface of the skin (Noyes and Mellors, 1957). The degenerating cells and cellular debris shed from the surface of the tumor contain a considerable amount of virus and can be accounted for as the source of "natural" infection. These papillomatous growths can be excised and preserved in buffered glycerin and the infectious virus readily extracted from them by differential centrifugation (Beard et al., 1939).

2.2. Classification

The papilloma viruses can be classified into two major groups with respect to the host cell or tissue for which they show affinity: (1) those which infect the skin epithelium (cutaneous type) and (2) those which infect the mucous membrane primarily (mucous type). This classification is shown in Table 1 together with some other properties of the viruses.

The affinity of the papilloma virus for the host cell is known to be rather specific. Rarely does the cutaneous-type virus infect the cells of the mucous membrane and vice versa. When Shope papilloma virus (SPV) is inoculated into the area around the mouth of a rabbit by a line of scarification extending straight from the skin part to the mucosa of the lip, the papilloma appears only in the skin part and never extends further into the lip. The same is true when SPV is injected intravenously into a rabbit. The virus becomes localized at the scarified area of the skin and a papillomatous growth develops. Other organs and tissues remain unaffected.

TABLE 1

Classification of Papilloma Viruses

Type	Name of tumors	Viruses		
		Infectivity	EM particles	Type of nucleic acid
Cutaneous	Verruca vulgaris	+	+	DNA[a]
	Shope rabbit papilloma	+	+	DNA[a]
	Bovine papilloma	+	+	DNA
	Equine papilloma	+	ns[b]	ns
Mucous	Condylomata acuminata	+	+	DNA?
	Multiple largyngeal papilloma	ns	ns	ns
	Rabbit oral papilloma	+	+	ns
	Canine oral papilloma	+	+	DNA

[a] Described as closed circular double-stranded DNA.
[b] Not studied.

2.3. Morphology and Ultrastructure

SPV, a *bona fide* representative of the papilloma virus group, was one of the "classical viruses" obtained in a purified preparation by physical methods (Beard *et al.*, 1939) and was studied extensively long before the electron microscope and refined modern methodology became available to virologists. Yet only recently has its fine structure been studied with respect to modern concepts of virus architecture.

It is well known that the dimensions of the virus particles differ considerably according to the preparatory procedure employed. In air-dried and metal-shadowed preparations, SPV appears as spherical particles with an average diameter of 70 nm (Kahler and Lloyd, 1952), while air-dried and unshadowed preparations give a diameter of only about 45 nm according to early electron microscopic techniques (Beard, 1948a). In PTA negatively stained preparations, however, SPV appears as spherical particles with diameter of 50–60 nm (Chambers *et al.*, 1966). Electron micrographs of SPV and three other papilloma viruses treated in the same fashion are shown on Fig. 1 (Chambers *et al.*, 1966). PTA staining also clearly visualizes the surface structure of the papilloma virions. This led to an attempt to determine the exact number of capsomeres in the virion, which unfortunately has left us in the middle of a controversy. The figure still remains to be decided between 42 and 72 for both SPV and human papilloma virus (HTV) (Williams *et al.*, 1961; Klug and Finch, 1965).

In clear contrast to the complete or intact virion, considerable numbers of hollow or empty particles are often seen under the electron microscope. In addition, a variety of abnormal particles are observed in SPV preparations (Williams *et al.*, 1960). Elongated particles varying from oval to rodshaped or

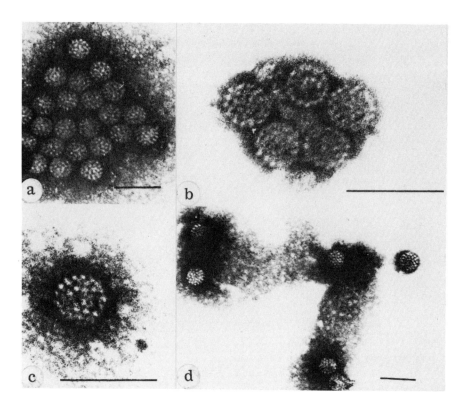

FIGURE 1. Electron micrographs of *papilloma viruses*. (a) Shope papilloma virus, (b) bovine papilloma virus, (c) canine oral papilloma virus, (d) human papilloma virus. All in PTA-negative stain. Each bar represents 100 nm.

filamentous in structure are detectable. These abnormal particles probably lack nucleic acid and infectivity as well, and are presumably the results of misassembly of the subunits of viral structural protein.

The disassembly of the SPV virion occurs, naturally or artificially, by drying and other physical forces, giving rise to discrete capsomeres which appear as short, hollow cylinders approximately 100 Å long (Breedis *et al.*, 1962; Howatson and Crawford, 1963).

2.4. Physical and Chemical Properties

The viral nucleic acid (DNA) is readily extracted from purified SPV by a mild deproteinization procedure employing an agent such as phenol or sodium dodecylsulfate. The SPV DNA extracts thus obtained have been shown to possess infectious and tumorigenic capabilities (Ito, 1960). These biological activities of the SPV DNA exhibit unusual resistance to heat (Ito, 1961). For example, tumorigenicity is unaffected by heating at 100°C for 30 min. Based on this, it has been possible to recover active DNA extracts from once heat-inactivated SPV

TABLE 2

Recovery of Tumorigenic Nucleic Acid Extracts from Heat-Inactivated SPV Preparations

Time of exposure at 70°C (min)	Preparation	Number of tumors/number of inoculation sites	Percent takes	Average incubation period (days)
0	Whole virus	6/6	100	13
0	Viral DNA	11/18	62	19
30	Whole virus	±1/16[a]	0	—
80	Whole virus	0/16	0	—
80	Viral DNA	9/19	56	22
180	Whole virus	0/16	0	—
180	Viral DNA	5/10	50	21
360	Viral DNA	4/18	27	22

[a] A scanty growth after 60 days.

preparations. Some data pertaining to this topic are shown in Table 2. Attempts were also made to link this finding to the tumorigenic potential of the DNA molecules, with little success. The interpretation at present is that it merely reflects the molecular configuration of the viral nucleic acid; i.e., the intact DNA molecule of both SPV and HPV is closed circular and double stranded (Crawford, 1964, 1965). Heating denatures it to the single-stranded state, but renaturation readily takes place upon cooling (Watson and Littlefield, 1960) and its biological activity is probably restored through such mechanism. Papilloma virus DNA samples prepared by the protein film method reveal the unique pattern of "supercoiled" circular molecules (Vinograd et al., 1965). The estimated molecular weights of the papilloma DNAs so far studied are all close to 5×10^6 daltons (Crawford, 1964, 1965; Watson and Littlefield, 1960; Kleinschmidt et al., 1965; Crawford et al., 1966).

The base composition of SPV DNA has been thoroughly studied by Watson and Littlefield (1960). More data were obtained for the other papilloma DNAs by Crawford and Crawford (1963). For SPV DNA, the AT/GC ratio ranged from 1.08 to 1.02 and the (G + C)% from 48 to 49.5 as determined by a variety of methods (Watson and Littlefield, 1960). The (G + C)% values calculated from the buoyant density of the DNAs for HPV, canine papilloma virus, bovine papilloma virus, and SPV were given as 41, 43, 45.5, and 47 respectively (Crawford and Crawford, 1963). It has also been pointed out that these values for the base compositions of the papilloma virus are close to those for the host DNA. The pattern of nearest-neighbor frequency analysis of SPV and HPV DNA gives the same results (Morrison et al., 1967; Subak-Sharpe et al., 1966). These findings suggest that a considerable similarity exists between the base compositions of the papilloma DNAs and the host DNA in both the overall frequency and the distribution of the bases. Whether this finding indicates the possibility of integration of the viral genome in the process of tumorigenesis remains speculative.

The concepts and techniques of nucleic acid hybridization were applied to HPV and SPV to see whether any relatedness exists between the two viral DNAs (Crawford, 1964). No evidence of homology was detectable between these two molecular species. However, similar series of experiments by the same investigator indicated a small degree of homology between rabbit host cell DNA and SPV DNA. These data were interpreted as evidence that a small amount of host cell DNA becomes enclosed in the SPV capsid rather than that true homology exists between virus and host DNAs (Winocour, 1965).

The number of proteins which could be coded for by the amount of DNA contained in the SPV particle is assumed to be approximately 10–15. However, the available data suggest the presence of only one protein in the SPV preparation, probably the structural protein of the viral capsid (Knight, 1950). The amino acid composition of this SPV protein has been studied in detail by Knight and his associates (Knight, 1950; Kass and Knight, 1965).

The presence of lipid among the ingredients of SPV particles has been known for a long time, yet the available information is meager. A rather remote possibility, that it could be a contaminating element of cellular origin, is also not completely excludable. The value of 1.5% is given by Beard (1948b) for lipid content in SPV. The possible participation of such viral lipid in the biological activity of the virus may be excluded by the evidence of ether resistance of SPV (Andrewes and Horstman, 1949).

2.5. Infection, Replication, and Transformation

Again, SPV shall serve as a model for discussion of infection, replication, and transformation. The papilloma viruses mature into infectious virion only in the cells at the superficial horny layer of the skin of their natural host, the cottontail rabbit (Noyes and Mellors, 1957). No other cells, either *in vivo* or *in vitro*, can sustain the replication of the virus. Accordingly, no cytopathic effect of SPV is observable in tissue culture. It is not clear whether this is due to lack of susceptible cell types in the cultures employed in the current studies or to unsuitable cultural conditions, which may be improved in future investigations. There are, however, some reports suggesting that an "abortive" type of infection takes place in the SPV *in vitro* system. In embryonic skin cultures of domestic rabbit infected with SPV, T-antigen-like immunofluorescence was observed in the nuclei of cells 10–30 h after exposure (Yoshida and Ito, 1968). When cottontail rabbit kidney cells are employed, the synthetic process of SPV seems to proceed as far as the production of SPV virion antigen in the nuclei of the cultured cells (Osato and Ito, 1968).

No definite reports are available describing *in vitro* transformation by SPV, although transformation of bovine and murine cells *in vitro* by bovine papilloma virus has been reported (Black *et al.*, 1963; Thomas *et al.*, 1964). Transformed cell foci have been observed in skin–muscle cultures of fetal material exposed to HTV *in vitro* (Noyes, 1965).

Transformation *in vivo* of the target cells of epithelial origin is readily performed by SPV, both spontaneously and experimentally. In fact, tumor induction on the skin of rabbits still is the only way of titrating SPV. The efficiency of this titration method is known to be very low (Bryan and Beard, 1940). A minimum of 10^5 SPV particles is calculated to be necessary to induce a tumor. The tumors thus induced in domestic rabbits ordinarily fail to yield infectious SPV.

The occurrence of a new enzyme, arginase (Rogers, 1959), in SPV-induced papillomas has attracted interest from the point of view that the enzymatic activity could possibly be interpreted as the expression of the introduced SPV genome (Passen and Schultz, 1965). However, controversy exists over whether this is indeed a SPV-induced enzyme (Orth *et al.*, 1967; Satoh *et al.*, 1967). More recently, another enzyme, ornithine transcarbamoylase, also joined the argument (Satoh and Ito, 1968).

Another SPV-induced event is the appearance of surface antigen (Ishimoto and Ito, 1969). This can be demonstrated by immunofluorescence techniques as an annular or semicircular pattern on the surface of unfixed cultured cells derived from cottontail papilloma tissue.

2.6. Virus–Host Relationship

2.6.1. Primary Host: Cottontail Rabbit

As repeatedly stated, the epithelial cells and tissues of the wild cottontail rabbit are the only target cells in which the SPV can replicate. Accordingly, papillomas induced in the animal in the wild are the only source of SPV. If the animal can be successfully tamed to be kept in a cage, infectious SPV will become available by experimental inoculation with either the virus or viral DNA. In the tumors induced by SPV DNA preparations, the presence of complete SPV virion can be shown both by infectivity testing and by electron microscopy (Chambers and Ito, 1964). Such findings point to the fact that all genetic information essential for the synthesis of SPV is indeed contained in the viral DNA.

Even in papillomas induced in the natural host, the heterogeneity in distribution of infectious SPV is of great interest. As already discussed, the infectious and complete virions of SPV are found only in the upper keratinized or horny layers of the neoplasm. One factor which possibly determines the maturation process of SPV is the genetic makeup of the host animals as seen in the difference between cottontails *(Sylvilagus floridanus)* and domestics *(Oryctolagus cuniculus)*. However, the factor(s) which controls the maturation of SPV in cottontail papillomas is obscure. Phenomenologically, it seems as though when the balance of power between the host cell and the viruses harbored in it comes to a certain point, e.g., when deterioration of the epithelial cells begins to take place at the very surface of the skin, the maturation of the viruses also commences. One tempting speculation emerges from the fact that the temperature at the superficial layer of the skin is considerably lower than that in the inner part of the animal's body and that it is possible to restore production of specific SPV antigen in cultured Shope

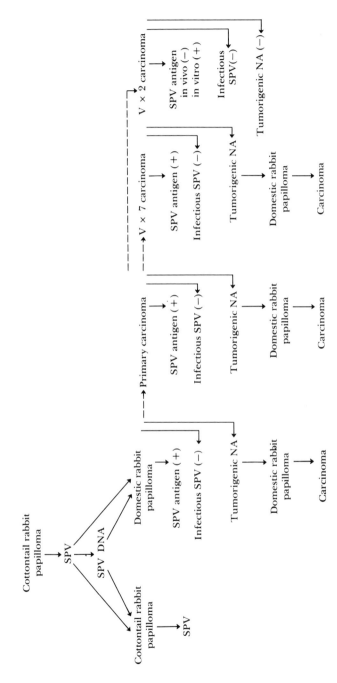

FIGURE 2. Virus, host, and tumor relationship in Shope papilloma–carcinoma complex.

papilloma cells which seemingly have ceased such function by lowering the temperature of cultivation from 37°C to 30°C (Shiratori *et al.*, 1969).

2.6.2. Secondary Host: Domestic Rabbit

Soon after the discovery of SPV, it was revealed that the infectivity of the virus seemingly disappears when the agent is inoculated into an "artificial host," the domestic rabbit. Nevertheless, antibody against SPV remains detectable in the serum of the tumor-bearing animal. Shope proposed the concept of "masking" to explain this unusual phenomenon (Shope, 1962). This was the very first recognition of the peculiar virus–host relationship which is now known to exist in essentially all of the tumor virus systems. The relationship between the virus, the tumor, and the host in the Shope papilloma–carcinoma complex is diagrammed in Fig. 2 (Ito, 1970a). In light of the concepts of modern biology, this merely suggests the persistence of the SPV genome throughout the whole system. Even the very early findings of Shope describing the presence of SPV-neutralizing antibody in the domestic host carrying SPV-induced papilloma point to the fact that the SPV virion capsid antigen is in fact being produced in spite of the lack of infectious viruses in the papillomas. This assumption has been strengthened by a series of experiments demonstrating that biologically active nucleic acid preparations capable of inducing typical papillomas in rabbits could be obtained not only from cottontail papillomas (Ito, 1960) but also from domestic papillomas (Ito and Evans, 1961), primary carcinomas (Ito, 1963), and transplantable V × 7 carcinomas (Ito, 1970a). The only exception was the transplantable V × 2 carcinomas, which failed to yield tumorigenic nucleic acid extracts even after many repeated trials. These data are summarized in Table 3 (Ito, 1970a).

It was also possible to detect the persistence of SPV virion antigen in cultured cells from cottontail and domestic papillomas and from V × 7 and V × 2 carcinomas employing indirect immunofluorescence techniques (Osato and Ito, 1967). SPV antigen was found to be localized in the nuclei and the cytoplasm, sometimes only in the latter. The most interesting fact was the demonstration of

TABLE 3

Relative Efficiency of Tumorigenesis of Various Nucleic Acid Extracts from Shope Papilloma–Carcinoma Complex[a]

Nucleic acid extracts from	Percent positive takes[b]
Partially purified SPV	100
Cottontail papilloma	100
Domestic rabbit	
Papilloma	25
Primary carcinoma	4
V × 7 carcinoma	4
V × 2 carcinoma	0

[a] Tested in domestic rabbits.
[b] Figures given in round numbers.

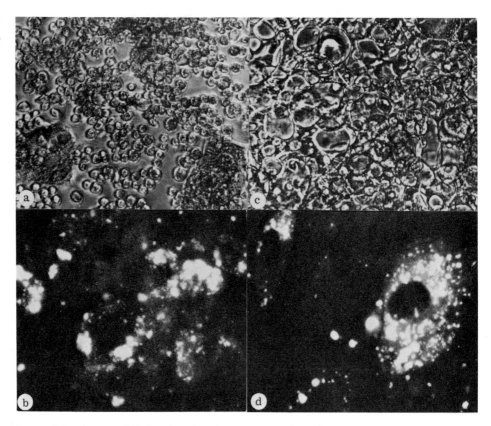

FIGURE 3. Persistence of viral antigen in cultures V × 2 and V × 7 cells. (a,b) V × 2 carcinoma, (c,d) V × 7 carcinoma. Upper: phase-contrast; Lower: immunofluorescence.

SPV antigen in cells cultured from V × 2 carcinomas, which had been thought to have lost the viral antigen during some transfer generation in the past. In Fig. 3, phase-contrast and fluorescence photomicrographs of V × 7 and V × 2 cultured cells are shown in pairs. However, the ratio of immunofluorescence-positive or SPV antigen–harboring cells in V × 2 cultures to that in V × 7 cultures was less than 1/100. From all these findings together, it is plausible to conclude that the SPV genome, carrying the code for SPV virion antigen at least, has persisted in the neoplastic cells of the system well over 20 yr since first being transformed by SPV.

2.6.3. Immunological Aspects

Most if not all animals once affected by a virus of the papilloma group become refractory to reinfection. This is apparently due to the presence of neutralizing antibody produced against the viral antigen, the structural protein of the virion. In the case of SPV, such refractoriness can often be overcome by a very heavy dose of virus inoculum or, more efficiently, by use of viral nucleic acid preparations.

On the other hand, it has been known from the early phase of study of SPV that spontaneous regression sometimes takes place in papillomas induced in domestic rabbits (Kidd, 1938). It was also known that the virus-neutralizing antibodies of

the serum have little effect on the sequence of events (Evans *et al.*, 1962*b*). Although not as yet conclusive, there is considerable evidence indicating that the phenomenon probably is a consequence of a specific immunological reaction against the tumor, as follows (Evans *et al.*, 1962*a*; Evans, 1963; Kreider, 1963): The regression occurs systemically; i.e., multiple tumors in one animal all regress together. In rabbits with both SPV-induced and SPV DNA–induced tumors, regression takes place in all of the tumors regardless of their origin. The regression is observed to occur approximately 5–6 wk after inoculation of SPV or SPV DNA. Those animals in which the papillomas fail to regress during this period seem to carry the tumor almost indefinitely. An example of long-term observation of regression and persistence of SPV-induced papillomas in domestic rabbits is shown in Fig. 4 together with the data on papillomas induced by nucleic acid extracts from V × 7 carcinoma tissues. Although there is more tendency for the nucleic acid–induced tumors to regress compared to the SPV-induced papillomas, the overall pattern is very much the same (Ito, 1970*a*).

The animals in which regression has occurred are refractory to reinfection not only with SPV but also with SPV DNA, while rabbits with persisting papillomas or carcinomas are resistant only to reinfection with SPV. It is possible to induce secondary papillomas in these persistor rabbits with SPV DNA. These secondary tumors persist together with the primary growths and never show any sign of regression. The reason for the refractoriness of the regressor rabbits against reinfection with SPV DNA is not clear (Evans and Ito, 1966).

Spontaneous regression of cutaneous papillomas is also known to occur in humans, cattle, and horses.

2.6.4. Malignant Conversion

Although the papillomas induced both in cottontails and in domestic rabbits by SPV are ordinarily classified as benign growths, they are endowed with definite

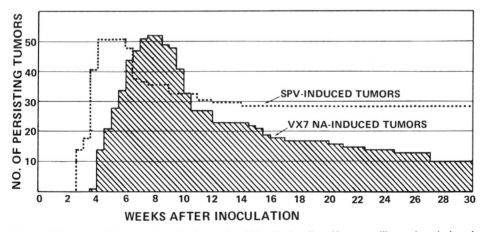

FIGURE 4. Fate of papillomas induced in domestic rabbits. Broken line, Shope papilloma virus–induced tumors; solid line, tumors induced by nucleic acid extracts from V × 7 transplantable carcinomas.

malignant potential. This was recognized soon after the discovery of SPV (Rous and Beard, 1935). If SPV-induced papillomas in domestic rabbits persist over 12 months, approximately 75% of them become converted spontaneously into squamous cell carcinomas (Syverton, 1952; Syverton and Berry, 1935). As a common process for malignancy, these carcinomatous cells metastasize to lungs and other remote organs, causing eventual death of the host animal. Although it has been clearly demonstrated that the SPV genome does persist in the tumor during the whole sequence of events, the most fundamental and interesting question—whether the SPV genome actually plays a role in inducing the carcinoma, or whether it only participates in induction of the papilloma and the subsequent papilloma-to-carcinoma sequence is an independent event—still remains unanswered. However, it might be worth pointing out that when tumors are being induced with nucleic acid extracts from the primary and transplantable V × 7 carcinomas they all first appear as papillomas and never as carcinomas, although some of them go through the papilloma-to-carcinoma sequence later on. It is also known that the combined application of chemical carcinogens directly on the SPV-induced papillomas apparently accelerates this process of conversion (Rous and Friedewald, 1944). This fragmentary evidence seems to favor the latter of the two possibilities.

3. Myxoma Virus Group

3.1. Biological Properties

The myxoma viruses have been included in the poxviruses, a group of large-DNA animal viruses. Although all members of the group are known to possess a capacity to cause cell proliferation to some extent, among them are viruses endowed with more apparent capabilities of inducing tumorous growth in the host they infect. However, infection with these viruses does not result in "true" neoplastic transformation of the cells. In general, the tumors induced are benign. They ordinarily persist in the host for a certain period of time and regress spontaneously, possibly by the involvement of an immune mechanism. The regression coincides with the disappearance of the viruses from the infected cells or tissues. Thus the classical definition of "autonomous growth" in neoplasia does not apply to this virus–host relationship. Although the tumor *per se* is benign, the disease itself proves to be fatal to the host under certain conditions, as is well known in some cases of myxomatosis.

3.2. Classification

If we are to stick to the criterion that myxoma viruses are a sub group within the pox group (Joklik, 1966), only three viruses, i.e., myxoma, Shope fibroma, and squirrel fibroma, come under this heading. If the concept is broadened to

TABLE 4

335

PAPILLOMA–
MYXOMA
VIRUSES

Classification of Oncogenic Poxviruses

Virus (subgroup)[a]	Host (species)	Histology of tumor
Myxoma (myxoma)	Rabbit	
	Oryctolagus	Myxoma
	Sylvilagus	Fibroma
Shope fibroma (myxoma)	Rabbit	
	Oryctolagus	Fibroma
	Sylvilagus	Fibroma[b]
Squirrel fibroma (myxoma)	Squirrel (*Sciurus carolinensis*)	Fibroma
Molluscum contagiosum (Paravaccinia)	Human	Papillomatous growth
Yaba monkey tumor (unclassified)	Monkey	Histiocytoma
	Macaca rhesus	
	Macaca irus	
	Macaca fuscatus	
	Cercopithecus	

[a] Subgroup of the poxvirus (Joklik, 1966).
[b] Long-lasting tumor.

"oncogenic poxviruses," two more primate viruses are to be added to complete the list, as shown in Table 4.

3.3. Morphology and Ultrastructure

Of the viruses of the myxoma subgroup, the Shope fibroma virus has been studied most extensively. Both in shadowed and negatively stained preparations, it appears as a characteristic form of ovoid or brick shape with dimensions of approximately 280 by 240 by 110 nm (Lloyd and Kahler, 1955). With respect to these and other morphological findings, the fibroma virus is indistinguishable from vaccinia virus and others of the same group. The surface structure and inner architecture of these viruses are highly complex (Westwood *et al.*, 1964).

3.4. Physical and Chemical Properties

The essential nucleic acid of viruses of the myxoma group is DNA. Very little information is available on the molecular characteristics of the DNA of myxoma group viruses *per se*, although the general picture probably is close to that of the thoroughly investigated vaccinia virus (Sarov and Becker, 1967), which is the largest viral DNA molecule yet reported, with a weight of about 160×10^6 daltons and with typical double strandedness according to a number of criteria (Joklik, 1962).

Studies on the protein moiety of the poxviruses have also been carried out on vaccinia virus as a model, with refined techniques of polyacrylamide gel electrophoresis (Holowczak and Joklik, 1967) and immunoelectrophoresis (Rodriguez-Burgos *et al.*, 1966), only to result in data just as complex as their ultrastructure. The discovery of the so-called NP antigen (Woodroofe and Fenner, 1962) shared by all poxviruses and definitely present in all members of the myxoma group was more rewarding.

Little is known about the lipid component of poxviruses; however, it might be worth mentioning that both myxoma and fibroma viruses are sensitive to ether (Andrewes and Horstman, 1949), whereas the vaccinia virus is not. The reason for this difference is not clear.

3.5. Infection, Replication, and Tumor Induction

The myxoma, fibroma, and other members of the group all replicate in the cytoplasm (Potz, 1957). The site of virus replication appears as a conspicuous inclusion body. The inclusion body is Feulgen positive (Kato and Cutting, 1959) and is known as the "B type," common in all pox group viruses. Radioautographic studies with ^{3}H-thymidine clearly demonstrate that it is indeed a site of DNA synthesis taking place within the cytoplasm (Kato *et al.*, 1963). Electron microscopic observations also have revealed that the maturation process of the virus occurs inside this inclusion body. Available data suggest that DNA synthesis in the nuclei of cells infected with the fibroma virus is remarkably suppressed. Accordingly, it seems improbable that cells harboring a cluster of replicating viruses can continue to divide and multiply. The process of virus replication is relatively slow and the cytopathic effect is not remarkable. Nevertheless, the infection eventually leads to death of the cell. Kato *et al.* (1967) have proposed a model that the tumorous growth induced by viruses of the myxoma group is composed of two coexisting cycles of events, as outlined in Fig. 5 (Kato *et al.*, 1967). From this model,

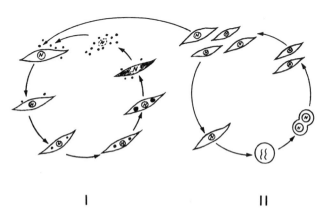

I   II

FIGURE 5. Two coexisting cycles in tumor induction by oncogenic poxviruses.

they have postulated that the major constituents of the tumor are the cells in the

proliferating cycle and not those infected and declining to degeneration.

Both myxoma and fibroma viruses can readily be propagated *in vitro* employing a variety of cell cultures, including rabbit kidney cells and rabbit heart fibroblasts (Chaproniere, 1956). Methods to induce plaques in primary rabbit kidney monolayer cells have been devised which offer a sensitive and accurate method of assay for both myxoma and fibroma viruses (Schwerdt and Schwerdt, 1962; Verna and Eylar, 1962; Woodroofe and Fenner, 1965). It has been also possible to propagate myxoma virus serially on the chorioallantoic membrane of chick embryos (Lush, 1937; Hoffstadt and Pilcher, 1938; Fenner and McIntyre, 1956). As the result of virus infection, small pocks can be observed to develop on the surface of the membrane, which facilitates titration of the virus by counting how many there are. This pock counting is useful as an assay method; however, reproducibility of results is considered to be better in the plaque assay.

A difference in thermoresistance between the two viruses has been pointed out; i.e., propagation of the fibroma virus is suppressed at 40°C, but the myxoma virus still propagates well at this temperature (Kilham, 1959).

As early as in 1936, Shope provided some data suggesting the possible existence of cross-immunity between the myxoma and fibroma viruses (Shope, 1936). The phenomenon known as the "Berry–Dedrick transformation" (Berry and Dedrick, 1936*a,b*) provides more direct evidence that the two viruses are indeed closely related. Heat-inactivated myxoma virus can be revived both *in vivo* and *in vitro* (Kilham, 1957) by mixed culture with live fibroma virus; mechanism is probably a kind of reactivation phenomenon rather than transformation (Avery *et al.*, 1944), which involves exchange of genetic substance between the two entities.

3.6. Virus–Host Relationship

When fibroma virus is inoculated subcutaneously into a rabbit, it ordinarily induces benign fibroma. However, it is known that the pathological reaction varies according to the condition of the host. In the natural host, the cottontail rabbit, the tumor often persists for a long period. When fibroma virus is inoculated into suckling domestic rabbits in excess dose, generalized multiple tumors are induced which eventually result in death of the host (Duran-Reynals, 1940, 1945). If adult rabbits are treated with cortisone, 6-mercaptopurine (Hurst, 1939), and other immunosuppressant drugs prior to virus inoculation, the tumors tend to grow more invasively, last more than 2–6 months, establish generalized fibromatosis, and sometimes even progress to fibrosarcoma. Such an accelerating effect is also observed when the host is pretreated with X-rays (Clemmessen, 1939) or ^{60}Co irradiation (Kato *et al.*, 1966). Thus it seems plausible to conclude that the immunological reactivity of the host is one of the basic factors which controls the progression of infection with fibroma virus.

Myxoma virus induces only a localized lesion in its natural host, *Sylvilagus brasiliensis*. However, it produces a devastating, generalized, and consistently fatal disease in domestic rabbits, *Oryctolagus cuniculus*. Many North American wild cottontail rabbits are relatively resistant to this virus (Gross, 1966). Such a difference in susceptibility could be due to a genetic factor or possibly to acquired immunity in wild rabbits by natural infection with virus of the same group. It has been shown experimentally that infection of domestic rabbits with fibroma virus rapidly induces active immunity to myxoma virus infection (Shope, 1936).

4. References

ANDREWES, C. H., AND HORSTMAN, D. M., 1949, The susceptibility of virus to ethyl ether, *J. Gen. Microbiol.* **3**:290.

AVERY, O. T., MACLEOD, C. M., AND MCCARTY, M., 1944, Studies on the chemical nature of the substance inducing transformation of pneumococcal types: Induction of transformation by a deoxyribonucleic acid fraction isolated from *Pneumococcus* III, *J. Exp. Med.* **79**:137.

BEARD, J. W., 1948a, Review: Purified animal viruses, *J. Immunol.* **58**:49.

BEARD, J. W., 1948b The chemical, physical and morphological properties of animal viruses, *Physiol. Rev.* **28**:349.

BEARD, J. W., BRYAN, W. R., AND WYCKOFF, R. W. G., 1939, Isolation of the rabbit papilloma virus protein, *J. Infect. Dis.* **65**:43.

BERRY, G. P., AND DEDRICK, H. M., 1936a, A method for changing the virus of rabbit fibroma (Shope) into that of infectious myxomatosis (Sanarelli), *J. Bacteriol.* **31**:50.

BERRY, G. P., AND DEDRICK, H. M., 1936b, Further observations on the transformation of the virus of rabbit fibroma (Shope) into that of infectious myxomatosis (Sanarelli), *J. Bateriol.* **32**:356.

BLACK, P. H., HARTLEY, J. W., ROWE, W. P., AND HUEBNER, R. J., 1963, Transformation of bovine tissue culture cells by bovine papilloma virus, *Nature (Lond.)* **199**:1016.

BREEDIS, C., BERWICK, L., AND ANDERSON, T. F., 1962, Fractionation of Shope papilloma virus in cesium chloride density gradients, *Virology* **17**:84.

BRYAN, W. R., AND BEARD, J. W., Correlation of frequency of positive inoculations with inoculation period and concentration of purified papilloma protein, *J. Infect. Dis.* **66**:245.

CHAMBERS, V. C., AND ITO, Y., 1964, Morphology of Shope papilloma virus associated with nucleic acid–induced tumors of cottontail rabbits, *Virology* **23**:434.

CHAMBERS, V. C., ITO, Y., AND EVANS, C. A., 1966, Technique for visualizing papovaviruses in tumors and in tissue cultures, *J. Bacteriol.* **91**:2090.

CHAPRONIERE, D. M., 1956, The effect of myxoma virus on cultures of rabbit tissues, *Virology* **2**:599.

CLEMMESSEN, J., 1939, The influence of roentgen radiation on immunity to Shope fibroma virus, *Am. J. Cancer* **35**:378.

CRAWFORD, L. V., 1964, A study of Shope papilloma virus DNA, *J. Mol. Biol.* **8**:489.

CRAWFORD, L. V., 1965, A study of human papilloma virus DNA, *J. Mol. Biol.* **13**:362.

CRAWFORD, L. V., AND CRAWFORD, E. M., 1963, A comparative study of polyoma and papilloma viruses, *Virology* **21**:258.

CRAWFORD, L. V., FOLLETT, E. A. C., AND CRAWFORD, E. M., 1966, An electron microscopic study of DNA from three tumor viruses, *J. Micros.* **5**:597.

DURAN-REYNALS, F., 1940, Production of degenerative inflammatory or neoplastic effects in the newborn rabbit by the Shope fibroma virus, *Yale J. Biol. Med.* **13**:99.

DURAN-REYNALS, L., 1945, Immunological factors that influence the neoplastic effects of the rabbit fibroma virus, *Cancer Res.* **5**:25.

EVANS, C. A., 1963, Immunological studies of the Shope papilloma–carcinoma complex of rabbits, *Acta Unio. Int. Contra. Cancrum* **19**:110.

EVANS, C. A., WEISER, R. S., AND ITO, Y., 1962a, Antiviral and antitumor immunologic mechanism operative in the Shope papilloma–carcinoma system, *Cold Spring Harbor Symp. Quant. Biol.* **27**:722.

EVANS, C. A., GORMAN, L. R., ITO, Y., AND WEISER, R. S., 1962b, Antitumor immunity in the Shope papilloma–carcinoma complex of rabbits. I. Papilloma regression induced by homologous and autologous tissue vaccines, *J. Natl. Cancer Inst.* **29**:277.

FENNER, F., AND MCINTYRE, G. A., 1956, Infectivity titrations of myxoma virus in the rabbit and the developing chick embryo, *J. Hyg. (Camb.)* **54**:246.

GROSS, L., 1966, *Oncogenic Viruses*, p. 23, Pergamon Press, New York.

HOFFSTADT, R. E., AND PILCHER, K. S., 1938, The use of chorioallantoic membrane of the developing chick embryo as a medium in the study of virus myxomatosum, *J. Bacteriol.* **35**:353.

HOLOWCZAK, J. A., AND JOKLIK, W. K., 1967, Studies on the proteins of vaccinia virus. I. Structural proteins of virions and cores, *Virology* **33**:717.

HOWATSON, A. F., AND CRAWFORD, L. V., 1963, Direct-counting of the capsomers in polyoma and papilloma viruses, *Virology* **21**:1.

HURST, E. W., 1939, The effect of cortisone and of 6-mercaptopurine on the Shope fibroma, *J. Pathol. Bacteriol.* **87**:29.

ISHIMOTO, A., AND ITO, Y., 1969, Specific surface antigen in Shope papilloma cells, *Virology* **39**:595.

ITO, Y., 1960, A tumor-producing factor extracted by phenol from papillomatous tissue (Shope) of cottontail rabbits, *Virology* **12**:596.

ITO, Y., 1961, Heat-resistance of the tumorigenic nucleic acid of Shope papillomatosis, *Proc. Natl. Acad. Sci.* **47**:1897.

ITO, Y., 1963, Studies on subviral tumorigenesis: Carcinoma derived from nucleic acid–induced papillomas of rabbit skin, *Acta Unio. Int. Contra. Cancrum.* **19**:280.

ITO, Y., 1970*a*, Induction of papillomas in rabbits with nucleic acid extracts from V × 7 carcinomas, *Brit. J. Cancer* **26**:16.

ITO, Y., 1970*b*, "Masking" and "unmasking" of Shope papilloma virus–coded functions in transformed rabbit cells, in: *Defectiveness, Rescue and Stimulation on Oncogenic Viruses*, Centre National de la Recherche Scientifique, Paris.

ITO, Y., AND EVANS, C. A., 1961, Induction of tumors in domestic rabbits with nucleic acid preparations from partially purified Shope papilloma virus and from extracts of the papillomas of domestic and cotton tail rabbits, *J. Exp. Med.* **114**:485.

JOKLIK, W. K., 1962, Some properties of poxvirus DNA, *J. Mol. Biol.* **5**:265.

JOKLIK, W. K., 1966, The poxviruses, *Bacteriol. Rev.* **30**:33.

KAHLER, H., AND, LLOYD, B. J., 1952, Electron microscopic study of the Shope Papilloma virus, *J. Natl. Cancer Inst.* **12**:1167.

KASS, S. J., AND KNIGHT, C. A., 1965., Purification and chemical analysis of Shope papilloma virus, *Virology* **27**:273.

KATO, S., AND CUTTING, W., 1959, A study of the inclusion bodies of rabbit myoxma fibroma virus and a consideration of the relationship between all pox virus inclusion bodies, *Stanford Med. Bull.* **17**:34.

KATO, S., TAKAHASHI, M., MIYAMOTO, H., AND KAMAHORA, J., 1963, Shope fibroma and rabbit myoxma viruses. I. Autoradiographic and cytoimmunological study on "B" type inclusions, *Biken J.* **6**:127.

KATO, S., ONO, K., MIYAMOTO, H., AND MANTANI, M., 1966, Virus–host interaction in rabbit fibrosarcoma produced by Shope fibroma virus, *Biken J.* **9**:51.

KATO, S., MIYAMOTO, H., ONO, K., TSURU, K., MANTANI, M., AND TANIGAKI, T., 1967, Virus–host cell interaction in cellular proliferation induced by poxvirus, in: *Second International Symposium for Cellular Chemistry*, Pergamon Press, New York.

KIDD, J. G., 1938, The course of virus-induced rabbit papillomas as determined by virus, cells and host, *J. Exp. Med.* **67**:551.

KILHAM, L., 1957, Transformation of fibroma into myxoma virus in tissue culture, *Proc. Soc. Exp. Biol. Med.* **95**:59.

KILHAM, L., 1959, Relation of thermoresistance among fibroma and myxoma viruses, *Virology* **9**:486.

KLEINSCHMIDT, A. K., KASS, S. J., AND KNIGHT, C. A., Cyclic DNA of Shope papilloma virus, *J. Mol. Biol.* **13**:749.

KLUG, A., AND FINCH, J. T., 1965, Structure of viruses of the papilloma polyoma type. I. Human wart virus, *J. Mol. Biol.* **11**:403.

KNIGHT, C. A., 1950, Amino acids of Shope papilloma virus, *Proc. Soc. Exp. Biol. Med.* **75**:843.

KREIDER, J. W., 1963, Studies on the mechanism responsible for the spontaneous regression of the Shope rabbit papilloma, *Cancer Res.* **23**:1593.

LLOYD, B. J., JR., AND KAHLER, H., 1955, Electron microscopy of rabbit fibroma, *J. Natl. Cancer Inst.* **15**:991.

LUSH, D., 1937, The virus of infectious myxomatosis of rabbits on the chorioallantoic membrane of the developing egg, *Austral. J. Exp. Biol. Med. Sci.* **15**:131.

MORRISON, J. M., KEIR, H. M., SUBAK-SHARPE, H., AND CRAWFORD, L. V., 1967, Nearest neighbor base sequence analysis of the deoxyribonucleic acids of a further three mammalian viruses: Simian virus 40, human papilloma virus and adenovirus type 2, *J. Gen. Virol.* **1:**101.

NOYES, W. F., 1965, Studies on the human wart virus. II. Changes in primary human cell cultures, *Virology* **25:**358.

NOYES, W. F., AND MELLORS, R. C., 1957, Fluorescent antibody detection of the antigens of the Shope papilloma virus in papillomas of the wild and domestic rabbit, *J. Exp. Med.* **106:**555.

ORTH, G., VIELLE, F., AND CHANGEUX, J. P., 1967, On the arginase of the Shope papillomas, *Virology* **31:**729.

OSATO, T., AND ITO, Y., 1967, *In vitro* cultivation and immunofluorescent studies of transplantable carcinoma V × 2 and V × 7, *J. Exp. Med.* **126:**881.

OSATO, T., AND ITO, Y., 1968, Immunofluorescence studies of Shope papilloma virus in cottontail rabbit kidney tissue cultures, *Proc. Soc. Exp. Biol. Med.* **128:**1025.

PASSEN, S., AND SCHULTZ, R. B., 1965, Use of papilloma virus–induced arginase as a biochemical marker *in vitro*, *Virology* **26:**122.

POTZ, L., 1957, Elektronenmikroskopische Untersuchungen der Kaninchenhaut bei infectktioser Myxmatose, *Beitr. Pathol. Anat.* **118:**1.

RODRIGUEZ-BURGOS, A., CHORDI, A., DIAZ, R., AND TORMO, J., 1966, Immunoelectrophoretic analysis of vaccinia virus, *Virology* **30:**569.

ROGERS, S., 1959, Induction of arginase in rabbit epithelium by the Shope papilloma virus, *Nature (Lond.)* **183:**1815.

ROUS, P., AND BEARD, J. W., 1935, The progression to carcinoma of virus-induced rabbit papillomas (Shope), *J. Exp. Med.* **63:**523.

ROUS, P., AND FRIEDEWALD, W. F., 1944, The effect of chemical carcinogens on virus-induced rabbit papillomas, *J. Exp. Med.* **79:**511.

SAROV, I., AND BECKER, Y., 1967, Studies on vaccinia virus DNA, *Virology* **33:**112.

SATOH, P. S., AND ITO, Y., 1968, Ornithine transcarbamoylase in Shope papilloma, *Virology* **35:**335.

SATOH, P. S., YOSHIDA, T. O., AND ITO, Y., 1967, Studies on the arginase activity of Shope papilloma: Possible presence of isozymes, *Virology* **33:**354.

SCHWERDT, P. R., AND SCHWERDT, C. E., 1962, A plaque assay for myxoma virus infectivity, *Proc. Soc. Exp. Biol. Med.* **109:**717.

SHIRATORI, O., OSATO, T., AND ITO, Y., 1969, "Induction" of viral antigen in established cell line (SP-8) derived from Shope virus–induced cutaneous papilloma of rabbits, *Proc. Soc. Exp. Biol. Med.* **130:**115.

SHOPE, R. E., 1932, A transmissible tumor-like condition in rabbits, *J. Exp. Med.* **56:**793.

SHOPE, R. E., 1933, Infectious papillomatosis of rabbits; with a note on the histopathology, *J. Exp. Med.* **58:**607.

SHOPE, R. E., 1936, Infectious fibroma of rabbits. IV. The infection with virus myxomatosum of rabbits recovered from fibroma, *J. Exp. Med.* **63:**43.

SHOPE, R. E., 1962, Are animal tumor viruses always virus-like? (review), *J. Gen. Physiol.* **45:** Suppl. 143.

SUBAK-SHARPE, H., BURK, R. R., CRAWFORD, L. V., MORRISON, J. M., HAY, J., AND KEIR, H. M., 1966, An approach to evolutionary relationships of mammalian DNA viruses through analysis of the pattern of nearest neighbor base sequences, *Cold Spring Harbor Symp. Quant. Biol.* **31:**737.

SYVERTON, J. T., 1952, The pathogenesis of the rabbit papilloma-to-carcinoma sequence, *Ann. N.Y. Acad. Sci.* **54:**1126.

SYVERTON, J. T., AND BERRY, G. P., 1935, Carcinoma in the cottontail rabbit following spontaneous virus papilloma (Shope), *Proc. Soc. Exp. Biol. Med.* **33:**399.

THOMAS, M., BOIRON, M., TANZER, J., LEVY, J. P., AND BERNARD, J., 1964, *In vitro* transformation of mice cells by bovine papilloma virus, *Nature (Lond.)* **202:**709.

VERNA, J. E., AND EYLAR, O. R., 1962, Rabbit fibroma virus plaque assay and *in vitro* studies, *Virology* **16:**266.

VINOGRAD, J., LEOWITZ, J., RADLOFF, R., WATSON, R., AND LAIPIS, P., 1965, The twisted circular form of polyoma viral DNA, *Proc. Natl. Acad. Sci.* **53:**1104.

WATSON, J. D., AND LITTLEFIELD, J. W., 1960, Some properties of DNA from Shope papilloma virus, *J. Mol. Biol.* **2:**161.

WESTWOOD, J. C. N., HARRIS, W. J., ZWARTOUW, H. T., TITMUSS, D. H. J., AND APPLEYARD, G., 1964, Studies on the structure of vaccinia virus, *J. Gen. Microbiol.* **34:**67.

WILLIAMS, M. G., HOWATSON, A. F., AND ALMEIDA, J. D., 1961, Morphological characterization of the viruses of human common wart *(Verruca vulgaris)*, *Nature (Lond.)*, **189**:895.

WILLIAMS, R. C., KASS, S. J., AND KNIGHT, C. A., 1960, Structure of Shope papilloma virus particles, *Virology* **12**:48.

WINOCOUR, E., 1965, Attempts to detect an integrated polyoma genome by nucleic acid hybridization. II. Complementarity between polyoma virus DNA and mouse synthetic RNA, *Virology* **27**:520.

WOODROOFE, G. M., AND FENNER, F., 1962, Serological relationship within the poxgroup: An antigen common to all members of the group, *Virology* **16**:334.

WOODROOFE, G. M., AND FENNER, F., 1965, Viruses of the myxoma–fibroma subgroup of the poxviruses. I. Plaque production in cultured cells, plaque-reduction tests and cross–protection tests in rabbits, *Austral. J. Exp. Biol. Med. Sci.* **43**:123.

YOSHIDA, T. O., AND ITO, Y., 1968, Immunofluorescent study on early virus–cell interaction in Shope papilloma *in vitro* system, *Proc. Soc. Exp. Biol. Med.* **128**:587.

9

Replication and Transformation by Papovaviruses

GEORGE KHOURY AND NORMAN P. SALZMAN

1. General Properties of Papovaviruses

The principal members of the papova group are polyoma virus (Stewart *et al.*, 1957), simian virus 40 (SV40), which is a vacuolating virus of monkeys (Sweet and Hilleman, 1960), and the papilloma viruses (Melnick, 1962). The name for this group of viruses is derived from the first two letters of the names of each of the viruses that were first included in the group, *pa*pilloma, *po*lyoma, *va*cuolating virus (Melnick, 1962). The viruses are 40–57 nm in diameter and, as determined by negative staining, the outer shell has symmetry of the T = 7 icosahedral surface lattice and is composed of 72 morphological subunits (Finch and Klug, 1965; Anderer *et al.*, 1967). The viruses contain no lipids and therefore are resistant to ether. Polyoma and SV40 do not share common antigens, and presently there is no evidence for the existence of homology betweeen their DNAs. The papovaviruses are capable of initiating a lytic cycle of replication or a latent infection. For the papilloma viruses it is difficult to obtain a suitable cell line in which the lytic cycle can be studied; therefore, studies that we will discuss concerning viral replication will deal exclusively with SV40 and polyoma.

In general, studies of the lytic cycle of virus replication of polyoma have been carried out with whole mouse embryo cultures or embryonic mouse kidney

GEORGE KHOURY and NORMAN P. SALZMAN ● Laboratory of Biology of Viruses, National Institutes of Allergy and Infectious Diseases, National Institutes of Health, Bethesda, Maryland.

cultures or with 3T3 cells (a continuous mouse cell line), while hamster cultures have been used for studies of viral transformation. For SV40, primary African green monkey kidney (AGMK) cell cultures or various continuous monkey kidney cell lines, e.g., BSC-1, CV-1, or Vero, have been used to study the lytic cycle, and mouse, hamster, and human cell cultures have been used in studies dealing with transformation.

The papovaviruses contain DNA within the core of the virus particle, which is present as a covalently closed duplex molecule. Each of the papilloma DNAs that have been examined has a molecular weight close to 5×10^6 daltons, which is higher than the molecular weights of SV40 (3.6×10^6) (Tai *et al.*, 1972) and polyoma (3.0×10^6) (Weil and Vinograd, 1963). The DNAs of the papovaviruses are infectious (McCutchan and Pagano, 1968) and are able to transform cells *in vitro* (Crawford *et al.*, 1964; Bourgaux *et al.*, 1965; Aaronson and Todaro, 1969; Aaronson and Martin, 1970). The small size of the viral genomes and their ability to transform cells have made them of great interest as models for studying the mechanism of transformation of a normal to a malignant cell. It seems likely that precise definition of the lytic cycle will be required in order to define the mechanism of cell transformation.

1.1 Initiation of the Replication Cycle—Adsorption, Penetration, and Uncoating of the Virus

We have already mentioned those virus–cell systems that are presently used for studies of viral replication. One reason that a cell is resistant to infection is that there is a block which prevents virus adsorption and/or penetration. The adsorption of polyoma virus occurs in two stages. The first stage of adsorption can be reversed by changing either the ionic conditions or the pH. After the first stage, the virus is irreversibly adsorbed, and the subsequent virus replication cycle is no longer affected by the addition of antiserum. A similar two-stage mechanism of adsorption has been observed for many other animal viruses and bacteriophages. Adsorption of polyoma virus does not occur if the cells have been treated with neuraminidase, which destroys the cell receptors that contain sialic acid (Crawford, 1962; Fried, 1970).

An interesting biological observation which relates to virus adsorption and/or penetration is the frequency of transformation by SV40 of human cell lines derived from individuals with certain metabolic diseases. Cell lines established from skin biopsies of patients with Fanconi's anemia or Down's syndrome can be transformed by SV40 with a much higher frequency than control human skin cultures (Todaro and Martin, 1967; Todaro *et al.*, 1966). However, these differences in transformation frequency are not observed when cells are transformed using SV40 DNA instead of virions (Aaronson and Martin, 1970). Thus the frequency with which SV40 virions can transform cells is determined by cellular differences that affect the rate of adsorption, penetration, or uncoating of the virus. Virion capsid proteins and receptor sites on the cell surface are two of the determinants which define the process of virus adsorption. While a number of chemical studies have provided a partial molecular characterization of the capsid proteins, thus far there are no comparable studies on cell receptor sites.

The changes in cell surfaces that are associated with viral transformation have provided the stimulus for additional studies in this general area. In many cases, cells that are permissive for SV40 replication can also be transformed by SV40. These transformed cells become resistant to superinfection with SV40 virions, but remain susceptible to infection with SV40 DNA (Swetly *et al.*, 1969; Rapp and Trulock, 1970; Shiroki and Shimojo, 1971; Reznikoff *et al.*, 1972). There are, however, transformed cell lines which become either partially or completely resistant to superinfection by SV40 DNA as well as by SV40 virions. One such example is a line of monkey kidney cells which are transformed by a defective virion fraction (a T fraction; Uchida *et al.*, 1968) of SV40. When these cells are reinfected with SV40 DNA, a yield of 10^{-2}–10^{-3} PFU (plaque forming units)/cell is obtained, as compared with a yield of 10 PFU/cell when SV40 DNA is used to infect independently isolated transformed cells (Shiroki and Shimojo, 1971). These results suggest that only one transformed cell in 10^3–10^4 may be permissive, even when a cycle of replication is initiated with viral DNA. Still other transformed lines have been obtained which do not produce any infectious virus after superinfection with either SV40 virions or SV40 DNA (Shiroki and Shimojo, 1971; Butel *et al.*, 1971). The mechanism by which certain transformed clones become resistant to superinfection with either virions or DNA is still unclear. In bacterial systems, there are restriction enzymes which degrade heterologous DNA and which can block a cycle of virus replication (Arber and Linn, 1969; Boyer, 1971). It is possible that viral nucleic acid modification and mammalian restriction enzymes play some role in the determination of susceptibility or resistance of animal cells to infection.

Many of the properties that are used to select for transformed cells depend on changes in the cell surface properties that occur following exposure to oncogenic viruses. Most transformed cells show a loss of contact inhibition; they are able to grow in soft agar and to form colonies in depleted growth medium. These surface properties, as well as the enhanced agglutination of transformed cells with wheat germ agglutinin or concanavalin A, would suggest extensive changes in the cell surface. Therefore, it may not be surprising that transformed cells are resistant to superinfection. However, in another well-characterized transformed cell system only limited surface changes have been demonstrated at the molecular level. Chick embryo fibroblasts (CEF) have been infected with a Rous sarcoma virus which is temperature sensitive (*ts*) in its ability to transform cells. Among the many proteins that can be resolved when isolated plasma membranes of uninfected CEF cells are examined is a polypeptide of about 45,000 mol wt. This polypeptide is present in normal amounts in cells infected with the *ts* virus that are cultivated at the restrictive temperature. It is present in reduced amounts or absent in cells infected with the *ts* mutant virus that are cultivated at the permissive temperature. There are also reduced amounts of the polypeptide in plasma membranes isolated from CEF cells transformed with the wild-type Schmidt Ruppin RSV-A (Wickus and Robbins, 1973). Clearly, there are wide biological differences between the avian tumor viruses and the papovaviruses, and there is no basis for predicting that they will behave in a parallel way. However, it will be interesting to see if there is a class of SV40 transformants in which minimal membrane changes occur and if such transformants are resistant to superinfection with SV40 virions. It is hoped that biochemical studies in these systems will provide more precise data on the role of the cell membrane in virus adsorption and penetration.

Studies to define the events that occur during adsorption, penetration, and uncoating have been carried out using purified radioactive virion preparations. When the process of virus uptake was studied using purified SV40 virus (Hummeler *et al.*, 1970), the most frequently observed mode of entry of virus into the cell was by pinocytosis of single particles. Virus particles were transported through the cytoplasm to the nucleus, where they were observed as early as 1 h after infection. Since virus particles seen at 1 and 2 h post infection (p.i.) were no longer present at 4 h p.i., it is assumed that they were uncoated by this time. When studied with radiolabeled virus, 50% of input virus is adsorbed within 2 h after infection (Ozer and Takemoto, 1969; Barbanti-Brodano *et al.*, 1970). Input viral DNA can be found in the nucleus many hours before any detectable events in the replication cycle are observed.

In these studies, which employ biochemical or cytological procedures to define the fate of the input virus, it is not possible to relate the experimental observations to that small fraction of the particles which are the infectious ones or which are involved in transformation. In general, there are at least 100 physical particles for every particle that causes an infection. In studies with viral DNA, 10,000–100,000 DNA molecules are needed for each infection; to produce one transformant (with a susceptible strain), approximately 10^7 DNA molecules are required. In view of this, biological conclusions which are derived from studies with purified virions must be considered almost speculative in nature.

A temperature-sensitive mutant of SV40, *ts* 101, which at the restrictive temperature cannot induce synthesis of either T or U antigen, can adsorb to and penetrate the cell. This may be useful in defining the very early events in a lytic cycle of virus replication (Robb and Martin, 1972).

1.2. Time Course of Synthesis of Viral Macromolecules

The replication cycle can be considered to occur in two phases. Viral macromolecules either are synthesized early, prior to the time of initiation of viral DNA replication, or are synthesized late, coincident with, or subsequent to viral DNA synthesis. In the early phase, there is synthesis of early mRNA and T and U antigens. In the late phase of replication, both early and late mRNA and capsid proteins are synthesized. When DNA synthesis is blocked by a metabolic inhibitor such as cytosine arabinoside or 5-fluorodeoxyuridine, the early events occur but viral DNA and capsid proteins are not synthesized. Both SV40 and polyoma show a lag phase of 6–8 h after virus infection before the initial events in virus replication are detected. Factors that determine the length of this lag phase have not been defined. In a lytic cycle of replication, the synthesis of early mRNA can be detected as early as 6 h p.i., and T-antigen synthesis, which is observed to start at 8–9 h p.i., is next observed. Viral DNA synthesis can be detected at 15–18 h p.i., and at this time one also observes the induction of enzyme synthesis and late viral mRNA; 2 or 3 h later, synthesis of viral capsid proteins is observed. There is considerable asynchrony within an infected population. When the rates of viral RNA, DNA, or protein synthesis are measured using uptake of radioactive precursors, the extent of incorporation reflects the fraction of the population which is carrying out synthesis as well as the true rate of synthesis. As a consequence of the asynchronous induction of the infectious cycle, synthesis of viral macromolecules and infectious virus formation (which is seen by 20 h p.i.) continues for a prolonged period (during the next 40 h).

While the kinetics of macromolecular synthesis depend on the virus stock and the cell line used in a particular study, the sequence of events noted above should be the same when studied during the lytic cycle. With regard to the time of induction of synthesis, this depends on the sensitivity of the detection procedure used; thus there can be considerable uncertainty when the induction of macromolecular synthesis occurs. For example, the detection of viral mRNA at an earlier time than the detection of T antigen is consistent with T antigen being a virus-coded function. Since procedures with different sensitivities are used for the detection of T antigen and early mRNA, however, there remains considerable uncertainty about the exact times of induction of these two processes.

2. DNA Replication

There are two general areas that have been investigated during the replication of papovaviruses. One series of studies has attempted to describe the mechanism of chain growth, i.e., to provide a description of events that occur at the replication fork. The second area of interest concerns the mechanism of semiconservative replication of a covalently closed molecule. Both areas are important in almost all studies of DNA replication. Besides the papovavirus DNAs, a number of DNAs exist as covalently closed structures within cells, and these include the chromosomes of bacteria, several bacterial and animal viruses, mitochondrial DNA, and bacterial plasmids.

2.1. DNA Configurations

A ring form for DNA was first observed for ϕX174 (Fiers and Sinsheimer, 1962). While the circular DNA within this virion is single stranded, during a cycle of virus replication the DNA is converted to a covalently closed duplex molecule (Burton and Sinsheimer, 1963). Soon after this initial observation, it was demonstrated that the DNA of polyoma virus was in the form of a covalently closed circular

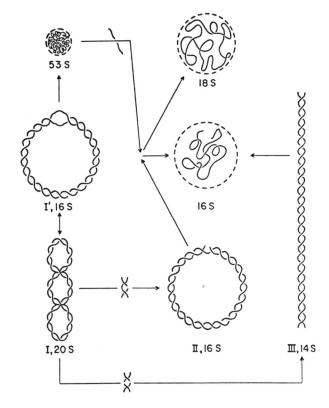

FIGURE 1. Diagram of the several forms of polyoma and SV40 DNA. The dashed circles around the denatured forms indicate the relative hydrodynamic diameters. The sedimentation coefficients were measured in neutral and alkaline NaCl solutions. The twist in I should be right-handed. From Vinograd and Lebowitz (1966).

duplex molecule (Dulbecco and Vogt, 1963; Weil and Vinograd, 1963). Subsequently, SV40, rabbit papilloma, and human papilloma were all shown to contain covalently closed circular DNA (Crawford and Black, 1964; Crawford, 1964, 1965). These interesting and important studies with circular DNA have been reviewed (Vinograd and Lebowitz, 1966).

Two forms of viral DNA are obtained when DNA is extracted from virions. There is DNA I, a covalently closed duplex, and DNA II, a form which can be generated from DNA I by breaking a single phosphodiester bond in either DNA strand. The forms in which papova DNA molecules exist are seen in Fig. 1. DNA I is the predominant type of DNA that is found in virions. DNA III refers to a linear duplex form of DNA which is formed when DNA I or II is cleaved by restriction enzymes. Double-stranded cellular of about 2–3 × 10^6 daltons DNA is also found in varying amounts in purified polyoma preparations, but is found rarely in SV40 preparations. There are wide variations in the amounts of DNA II and cellular DNA present in purified virion preparations. The significance of the DNA II which is obtained from virions is not clear. It can be considered to arise by nicking of DNA I during the extraction procedure. The amount of DNA II obtained from virions has been observed to change when conditions for the extraction of DNA are varied (Vinograd *et al.*, 1965). However, there are no apparent steric reasons why DNA II could not be encapsidated. In support of this idea is the finding that a cellular DNA does occur in an encapsidated form. DNA II has been shown to be an intermediate during SV40 DNA replication (Fareed *et al.*, 1973*b*). With methods now available for determining if the nick in DNA II occurs at a specific site in the molecule, it will be possible to determine whether the DNA II present in virion-extracted DNA is synthesized and encapsidated as such or whether it is simply generated from DNA I during preparation of viral DNA.

DNA I forms of polyoma, SV40, and rabbit and human papilloma (Crawford and Black, 1964; Crawford, 1964, 1965) possess common structural features. Each DNA is a covalently closed duplex in which the DNA contains no free ends. Each of these molecules also contains superhelical turns in which the DNA double helix winds on itself. This latter property results from constraints within the DNA molecule which prevent a change in the pitch of the double helix since the molecule contains neither nicks nor free ends. If, at the time DNA I is formed, the pitch of the helix differs from the pitch which the molecule will assume *in vitro*, then this molecule will generate superhelical turns under *in vitro* conditions. A nicked circular duplex moleculer or linear duplex DNA may have a different helical pitch *in vivo* and *in vitro*, but since there are no constraints in the molecule (one strand being free to wind around the other) the molecule will not generate superhelical turns under *in vivo* or *in vitro* conditions. Both polyoma and SV40 DNAs contain a deficiency of about 19 turns in the double helix at the time of formation of DNA I, and they both contain about 19 negative superhelical turns. The presence of superhelical turns in polyoma and SV40 provides the molecule with a decreased intrinsic viscosity (Opschoor *et al.*, 1968), and therefore its rate of sedimentation (20–21S) is more rapid than that of DNA II (16S) during velocity gradient analysis in neutral conditions. All naturally occurring, covalently closed DNAs similarly contain negative superhelical turns, although the superhelix density (the number of superhelical turns per ten base pairs) is somewhat variable among different DNAs. A number of reagents can change the average pitch of the duplex and thus the superhelix density. The binding of intercalative dyes, changes in ionic conditions, or partial alkaline denaturation may all produce these changes (Helinski and Clewell, 1971). It can be seen (Fig. 1) that when DNA I is partially denatured by alkali it loses superhelical turns and assumes a configuration equivalent to DNA II. A similar effect is observed in the presence of critical concentrations of ethidium bromide. When the two strands in DNA I are completely denatured by alkali, a compact structure which sediments rapidly in alkali is obtained.

After denaturation of DNA I at pH values of 12.1–12.6, a rapidly sedimenting DNA (53S) is obtained, but if these DNA preparations are neutralized the process of denaturation is reversible and 21S DNA I is reformed. However, at pH values above 12.6, denaturation is no longer a reversible process (Westphal, 1970;

Salzman *et al.*, 1973*a*). Similar behavior is observed for the replicative form of ϕX174 (Rush and Warner, 1970).

When DNA II is treated with alkali, it gives rise to a linear single strand of DNA (16S) and a single-stranded circle (18S).

2.2 Use of Enzyme and Chemical Probes to Study Papovaviruses

Studies of restriction and modification in bacterial systems (Arber and Linn, 1969; Boyer, 1971) have provided a number of enzymes which have proven extremely powerful reagents for studies with SV40 and polyoma. Those enzymes which have been purified, although not in each case to a homogeneous state, include enzymes from *Hemophilus influenzae* (R · *Hin*) (Smith and Wilcox, 1970), from *Hemophilus* (sp.) *aegypticus* (R · *Hae*) (Middleton *et al.*, 1972), from *Escherichia coli* carrying an R factor (R · *Eco* R$_I$ and R · *Eco* R$_{II}$), and from *Hemophilus parainfluenzae* (R · *Hpa*) (Gromkova and Goodgal, 1972). Subsequent studies with R · *Hin* (Danna *et al.*, 1973) and with R · *Hpa* (Sharp *et al.*, 1973) have revealed that in each case the original isolation procedures had yielded at least two restriction activities which could be further resolved. The enzymes recognize a particular sequence of nucleotides in the DNA molecule, and in this region they cleave both DNA strands. The first cleavage site to be sequenced, R · *Hin* (Kelly and Smith, 1970), possessed a twofold axis of symmetry. Its structure is shown in Fig. 2, as are the structures for the R · *Eco* R$_I$ and R · *Eco* R$_{II}$ cleavage sites, which have also been characterized (Hedgpeth *et al.*, 1972; Bigger *et al.*, 1973; Boyer *et al.*, 1973). They have the same symmetry as first observed for the R · *Hin* cleavage site; however, the R · *Eco* R$_I$ and R · *Eco* R$_{II}$ cleavage products possess single-stranded ends; these molecules can thus be recyclized at low temperatures, and then covalently closed duplex rings can be generated by the sealing action of ligase. It was first reported that the R · *Hin* endonuclease would cleave SV40 into 11 fragments (Danna and Nathans, 1971) and that R · *Hpa* would cleave SV40 into four fragments (Sack and Nathans, 1973). Later it was demonstrated that the single cleavage of SV40 by R · *Eco* R$_I$ occurred at a specific site in the molecule (Morrow and Berg, 1972; Mulder and Delius, 1972; Fareed *et al.*, 1972). Cleavage of SV40 with several restriction enzymes has been used recently (Danna *et al.*, 1973) in a study which

5′ .... GpTpPy ↓ pPupApC .... 3′
3′ .... CpApPup ↑ PypTpG .... 5′
Hemophilus influenza endonuclease

5′ .... A/TpG ↓ pApApTpTpCpT/A .... 3′
3′ .... T/ApCpTpTpApAp ↑ GpA/T .... 5′
E. coli R$_I$ endonuclease

5′ .... N ↓pCpCpApGpGpN′ .... 3′
3′ .... NpGpGpTpCpCp ↑ N .... 5′
E. coli R$_{II}$ endonuclease

FIGURE 2. The recognition sequences of three restriction endonucleases: *H. influenzae* d$_{II}$ (Kelly and Smith, 1970), *E. coli* R$_I$ (Hedgpeth *et al.*, 1972), and *E. coli* R$_{II}$ (Bigger *et al.*, 1973; Boyer *et al.*, 1973). Both the *Eco* · R$_I$ and *Eco* · R$_{II}$ endonucleases produce a staggered cleavage which results in cohesive termini, while the *Hin* d$_{II}$ endonuclease does not. The substrate sites for all three enzymes possess a twofold rotational axis of symmetry.

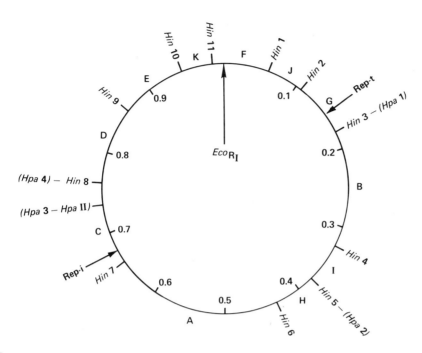

FIGURE 3. A cleavage map of the SV40 genome (Danna and Nathans, 1972; Danna *et al.*, 1973). The R · *Eco* R₁ site (Morrow and Berg, 1972; Mulder and Delius, 1972) is used as a reference for the *Hin* and *Hpa* cleavage sites. Note that the *Hpa* 3 cleavage site appears to be recognized by a unique enzyme, *Hpa* II (Sharp *et al.*, 1973). Therefore, *Hpa* 1, 2, and 4 are the *Hpa* I sites. The positions on the map for initiation (Rep-i) and termination (Rep-t) of DNA replication are indicated (Danna and Nathans, 1972; Fareed *et al.*, 1972).

has defined an impressively detailed cleavage map of the SV40 genome (Fig. 3). In some of the studies described below, which relate to DNA replication and transcription, the usefulness of these enzymes will be illustrated. Clearly, they represent extraordinarily useful reagents, and their use has made possible the rapid progress during the past 4 years in our understanding of the papovaviruses.

There are a number of other methods which have been used to gain information about the anatomy of the viral genome. Several studies have reported denaturation maps for both polyoma (Bourguignon, 1968; Follett and Crawford, 1968) and SV40 (Yoshiike *et al.*, 1972; Mulder and Delius, 1972). Those regions rich in adenine and thymine are the first to become denatured, and the denaturation map gives some idea of the clustering of nucleotides within the molecule. The combined action of restriction enzymes and determination of both base composition and purine and pyrimidine tracts in various fragments will be an alternative method to obtain similar data in a more precise manner.

The T4 gene-32 protein binds to supercoiled SV40 DNA I but not to SV40 DNA II (Mulder and Delius, 1972; Morrow and Berg, 1972). The site(s) at which the gene-32 protein binds to SV40 DNA I is in a region corresponding to 0.44–0.48 SV40 map unit from the *Eco* · R₁ cleavage site (Morrow and Berg, 1973).

This is the same region which is preferentially denatured at alkaline pH values (Mulder and Delius, 1972).

The finding that supercoiled molecules have unpaired bases is based on the binding of formaldehyde to the replicative form of ϕX174 and to PM2 (Dean and Lebowitz, 1971). It is estimated that 3–4% of the bases in ϕX174-RF can bind methylmercury and are therefore in an unpaired state (Beerman and Lebowitz, 1973). Single-strand regions in covalently closed molecules can be cleaved by the single-strand-specific nuclease from *Neurospora crassa,* which converts the super-coiled molecule to the relaxed form (Kato *et al.,* 1973), or by S_1 nuclease of *Aspergillus oryzae,* which produces unit-length, linear, duplex molecules from supercoiled SV40 DNA (Beard *et al.,* 1973). In this latter case, cleavage occurs predominantly at 0.45 and 0.55 SV40 map unit, the same regions at which denaturation and gene-32 protein binding occurs.

The reagent N-cyclohexyl-N'-β-(4-ethylmorpholinium)ethylcarbodiimide (CMEC) reacts preferentially with single-stranded DNA and it has the advantage, as compared to formaldehyde, that a stable reaction product is obtained. The product of the reaction, SV40 I–(CMEC), has an $s_{w,20}$ of 22.5S, which is higher than that of SV40 DNA I (21S), and it also shows a small decrease in buoyant density. When ^{14}C-CMEC is reacted with ^{3}H-SV40 DNA I, the reaction product can be cleaved by the restriction endonuclease R · *Hin* d, and the bound ^{14}C-CMEC is found associated with only three of the 11 cleavage fragments, namely fragments A, B, and G. The degree of single strandedness in these three fragments is estimated to be 7%, 4%, and 2.8%, respectively. When either SV40 DNA I or SV40 DNA I–(CMEC) is cleaved by the single-strand-specific nuclease of *N. crassa,* the population of fragments that is obtained is consistent with cleavage at three sites at approximately 0.2, 0.45, and 0.55 genome length from the *Eco* R_1 cleavage site. This is in agreement with the ^{14}C-CMEC binding data (M. Chen, J. Lebowitz, M. Garon, and N. Salzman, unpublished results).

2.3. Structure of Replicating Molecules

A number of procedures have facilitated studies of SV40 and polyoma DNA replication. The method in which cells are lysed by the addition of SDS, and high molecular weight DNA is separated from low molecular weight DNA by selective salt extraction, is of particular value (Hirt, 1967). In general, cellular DNA is precipitated, and SV40 DNA and intermediates involved in SV40 DNA replication are found in the low molecular weight (LMW) supernatant fluid. The absence of the large amounts of cellular DNA greatly facilitates subsequent sedimentation and electron microscopic analyses. A second important technical advantage in studies with papovaviruses derives from the unique properties of covalently closed, duplex molecules which enable them to be separated from nicked molecules in either alkaline or neutral velocity gradients or by isopycnic centrifugation in the presence of ethidium bromide.

To determine if polyoma DNA replication occurred by a semiconservative mechanism, infected mouse kidney cell cultures were labeled with ^{3}H-thymidine for 20 min at 24 or 36 h p.i. to generate a pool of ^{3}H-labeled LL (light, light) DNA I ($d = 1.709$). These cells were then incubated in the presence of ^{14}C-BUdR and FUdR for an additional 2 h. The presence of hybrid HL (heavy, light; $d = 1.753$) and HH ($d = 1.795$) polyoma DNA I and DNA II containing ^{3}H-thymidine was observed. This HL and HH polyoma DNA was encapsidated. These data show that polyoma DNA replication proceeds by a semiconservative mechanism (Hirt, 1969).

Intermediates in polyoma DNA replication were seen after short (3.5- to 5-min) pulses (Bourgaux *et al.*, 1969). These intermediates seemed to sediment like DNA I in neutral velocity gradients, but they banded in cesium chloride–ethidium bromide (CsCl-EtBr) like DNA II, and they were designated DNA II*. When DNA II* was sedimented in an alkaline gradient, the labeled, newly synthesized DNA sedimented at a rate equal to or slower than that of intact single polyoma DNA strands (16S). These data are consistent with replicating polyoma DNA possessing a Cairn's-type structure (Cairns, 1963). They are not consistent with a rolling-circle model for polyoma DNA replication (Gilbert and Dressler, 1968), which has been reported to be the mechanism by which ϕX174 replicates. One prediction of the rolling-circle model is the presence of a covalent link between parental DNA and one strand of newly synthesized DNA. This would require that a fraction of the newly synthesized DNA sediment more rapidly than 16S, the length of an intact single strand, and no newly synthesized DNA has been observed with these properties.

A more accurate description of replicating molecules was provided in studies of SV40 DNA replication in primary African green monkey kidney cells (Levine *et al.*, 1970). In this system, synthesis of SV40 DNA I is observed to start at 15 h p.i., and a maximum rate of synthesis is observed at 30 h p.i. DNA synthesis continues until 70 h p.i. Since the cells have been infected at a rather high input multiplicity (25–100 PFU/cell), the extended time of synthesis is not a consequence of the failure to rapidly infect each cell. There is asynchrony within the population as to when macromolecular synthesis commences. This study showed clearly that isotope is first incorporated (after a 2.5-min pulse) into replicating molecules which sediment in neutral sucrose gradients with a mean S value of 25–26S. Newly synthesized DNA I is not detected until the labeling time has been extended to 10 min, and by pulse-chase experiments these 25S replicating forms can be shown to be precursors of DNA I. The structures of replicating molecules appear in the electron microscope as Cairn's type structures, with two branch points, three branches, and no free ends, findings similar to those previously observed for polyoma (Hirt, 1969). It was subsequently shown (Sebring *et al.*, 1971) that while these structures are replicating forms of SV40 DNA, only a small fraction of the replicative molecules are seen to have this configuration. Most of the replicating molecules (80–90%) have a structure in which there are two branch points, three branches, and no free ends. In addition, one branch contains superhelical turns (Fig. 4). From length measurements of replicative molecules it is clear that the two branches, L1 and L2, are of equal length and correspond to the replicated portion of the molecule. Superhelical turns are contained in the unreplicated part of the

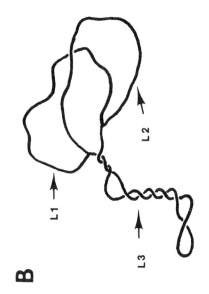

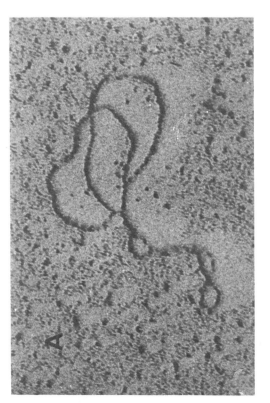

FIGURE 4. A twisted SV40 replicating DNA molecule. (A) Electron micrograph obtained by modification of the technique described by Davis *et al.* (1971). The hypophase was distilled water and the DNA was contrasted by shadowing from one direction with 80% platinum–20% paladium. In some regions the individual strands which comprise the superhelical branch can be seen. Magnification is 1.5×10^{5}. (B) An interpretive drawing of the molecule. The branches of the molecule measured are indicated. The two branches that were not superhelical were designated L1 and L2. The superhelical branch was designated L3. From Sebring *et al.* (1971).

molecule. The reason these structures contain superhelical turns is that the parental template strands are covalently closed. While the replicative intermediates contain covalently closed structures, during the replication cycle nicks must be introduced into the parental strands. This is discussed more fully below.

Since the superhelical turns are contained in the unreplicated part of the molecule, it follows that as replication proceeds the size of the unreplicated region will decrease and the total number of superhelical turns in the replicative intermediates will decrease. This feature of replicative intermediates provides a simple way of sorting molecules as a function of the extent of replication. Covalently closed molecules bind less ethidium bromide than the corresponding nicked DNA II structures, and consequently the two can be easily separated by isopycnic banding in CsCl-EtBr (Bauer and Vinograd, 1968). The DNA II, which binds more dye, bands at a lower density. It is clear that young replicating molecules which contain almost the same number of superhelical turns as DNA I will band close to the position of DNA I. As the DNA molecules progress through a replicative cycle, the number of superhelical turns decreases. This results in a gradual shift in the position at which they band to a lower density, so that almost fully replicated molecules band with DNA II. Once they give rise to progeny DNA I molecules, they then band at the position of DNA I. The isopycnic banding of DNA I, DNA II, and replicating molecules is seen in Fig. 5. DNA I and II band

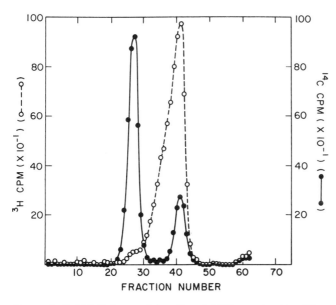

FIGURE 5. CsCl-EtBr isopycnic banding of DNA contained in a Hirt supernatant fluid. At 30 h after infection with SV40, an African green monkey kidney cell monolayer was pulsed for 2 min with medium containing 50 μCi of ^{3}H-thymidine/ml. The Hirt supernatant fluid was prepared and dialyzed. A sample of this fluid and purified ^{14}C-SV40 DNA marker were centrifuged to equilibrium in a CsCl-EtBr gradient (volume, 6 ml; CsCl density, 1.564; ethidium bromide, 200 μg/ml). Fractions were collected directly into scintillation vials and counted. From Sebring et al. (1971).

sharply and are well resolved, while replicative intermediates band heterogeneously in the region from DNA I to DNA II. For most studies involving electron microscopy of replicating molecules, that region between DNA I and DNA II is most readily studied since this fraction will be richest in replicative intermediates. In contrast, regions close to DNA I will be obscured by the large amount of DNA I that is an end product of replication and therefore accumulates in great quantities, while in the region where DNA II bands, even trace contamination with cellular DNA and DNA II will make the examination of mature replicating molecules more difficult. As was observed for polyoma (Bourgaux et al., 1969), all of the newly synthesized SV40 DNA in replicative intermediates is also released by alkaline treatment (Sebring et al., 1971; Jaenisch et al., 1971). The evidence which established that replicative intermediate molecules are effectively separated by CsCl-EtBr was obtained by alkaline sedimentation of replicative intermediates which had banded at different densities. It can be seen that the size of the newly synthesized DNA strands released by alkaline treatment is that predicted if molecules band at progressively lower densities as they go through the replication cycle (Fig. 6). In this experiment, molecules were obtained that had, on the average, completed 23, 36, 57, and 85% of the replication cycle. Since there is a unique site for the initiation of replication (see below), the strands of DNA released by alkali correspond to particular regions of the viral genome. By electron microscopic examination of the replicating molecules in the presence of ethidium bromide, it has been shown that the sense of the superhelix in replicating molecules was the same as that of SV40 DNA I. Replicating DNA molecules of differing extents of replication were also analyzed by sedimentation in varying concentrations of ethidium bromide. It was observed that the superhelix density of the unreplicated portion of replicating molecules was greater than that of DNA I and that it increased as the degree of replication increased. In contrast to the increase in superhelix density that was related to the extent of replication, all replicating molecules contained a rather constant number (two to five) of additional superhelical turns per molecule, irrespective of the extent of replication. This suggests that a region (or regions) of about 20–50 nucleotides may exist in a denatured state in replicating molecules, presumably at the replicating forks of the molecules (Sebring et al., 1974).

Recent studies have shown that replicative intermediates are found in association with a nuclear membrane fraction, and are released from the membranes when replication is complete (LeBlanc and Singer, 1974).

The structure of replicating molecules is shown schematically in Fig. 7. Certain features possessed by replicating molecules that are shared commonly by polyoma and SV40 are the following:

1. The parental strands of the replicative intermediates exist in a covalently closed form (Sebring et al., 1971; Jaenisch et al., 1971; Bourgaux and Bourgaux-Ramoisy, 1972a).
2. The dissociation of newly synthesized strands from parental strands establishes the absence of a covalent linkage between them, and also the absence of a covalent linkage between the two newly synthesized strands.

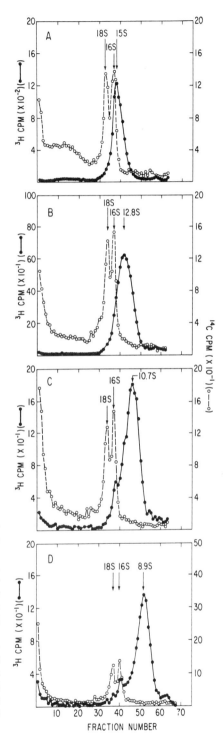

FIGURE 6. Velocity sedimentation in alkaline sucrose of molecules taken from CsCl-EtBr densities of (A) 1.548, (B) 1.555, (C) 1.562, and (D) 1.570. Each fraction was extracted three times with CsCl-saturated isopropanol to remove the ethidium bromide, dialyzed against 0.01 M tris–0.01 M EDTA (pH 7.2) buffer, and concentrated. A sample was layered onto an 11.6-ml 10–30% alkaline sucrose gradient and sedimented at 10°C for 13 h at 40,000 rpm in a SW41 rotor. Fractions were collected directly into scintillation vials, neutralized by the addition of two drops of glacial acetic acid, and counted. Sedimentation is from right to left. The ^{14}C cpm reflect not only the small amount of ^{14}C present in the double-labeled sample but also a purified ^{14}C-SV40 DNA that was added to each gradient as a marker. From Sebring et al. (1971).

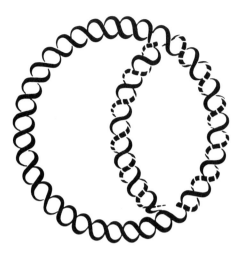

FIGURE 7. Diagram of replicating SV40 DNA. The salient features of the molecule are that (1) both parental DNA strands (solid lines) are covalently closed, and (2) the two newly synthesized DNA strands (broken lines) are neither covalently linked to the parental DNA nor linked together. From Sebring *et al.* (1971).

3. There are single-stranded regions at each of the two replicating forks. This was suggested by the binding of replicative intermediates to benzoylated naphthoylated DEAE-cellulose and their subsequent elution by caffeine (Levine *et al.*, 1970). These binding properties depend on the presence of single-stranded DNA regions (Kiger and Sinsheimer, 1969). More direct evidence has been obtained by demonstrating the susceptivity of replicative intermediates to cleavage by a single-strand-specific nuclease from *N. crassa* which generates, as one product of digestion, ring-shaped structures with tails (Bourgaux and Bourgaux-Ramoisy, 1972*a*).

2.4. Site of Initiation and Direction of DNA Replication

Two separate experimental approaches have been used to demonstrate that DNA synthesis is initiated at a specific site. The first depends on the cleavage of replicating SV40 molecules or newly synthesized SV40 DNA by the bacterial restriction endonuclease from *H. influenzae*. This enzyme preparation cleaves SV40 and yields 11 fragments, which can be resolved by polyacrylamide gels; they range in size from 6.5×10^5 to 7.4×10^4 daltons (Danna and Nathans, 1971). If there is a preferred site for DNA initiation, then in molecules labeled for a period slightly longer than the time required to complete one round of DNA replication the fragment which corresponds to the DNA initiation site will be most highly labeled in the replicative intermediates. However, when the pulse time is shorter than that required for a round of replication and newly synthesized DNA I is examined, the region where termination occurs will be preferentially labeled. Based on the rates of labeling, it was concluded that replication of SV40 DNA starts in *Hin* fragment C and terminates in *Hin* fragment G (see Fig. 3) (Danna and Nathans, 1972).

A preferred initiation site for SV40 DNA replication was also demonstrated in experiments based on the reassociation rates of the strands of replicating molecules. When the rate of duplex formation of strands of newly synthesized DNA, isolated from molecules which had undergone different extents of replication, was studied, the time required to effect 50% renaturation increased at a rate proportional to the increase in the length of the newly synthesized strands. These results are those predicted if there is a specific site for initiation of DNA synthesis (Thoren *et al.*, 1972).

In order to determine if DNA replication, which was initiated at a unique site, proceeds unidirectionally or bidirectionally SV40 replicative intermediates were cleaved with R · *Eco* R$_1$ (Fareed *et al.*, 1972). The structures that are predicted, depending on the mode of DNA replication, are shown in Fig 8. After cleavage, linear structures containing one bubble will be generated. If replication is unidirectional, all molecules, regardless of their extent of replication, will have one branch, L1, of constant length. With bidirectional replication, both L1 and L4 will decrease as replication proceeds. In the case of bidirectional replication, if each replication fork moves at the same rate the lengths of both L1 and L4 will decrease at the same rate as replication proceeds.

The structures that were observed demonstrated that DNA synthesis proceeds bidirectionally, and that the two replication forks move at the same rate. This study also located the R · *Eco* R$_1$ cleavage site at 0.33 (or 0.67) genome length from the initiation site for DNA replication. A parallel study has been carried out with polyoma DNA in which the R · *Eco* R$_1$ endonuclease also introduces a single break.

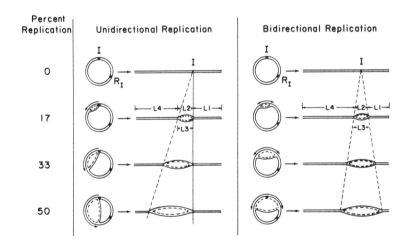

FIGURE 8. Unreplicated SV40 molecules or molecules which have replicated to different extents are schematically represented, as are the molecules which are obtained after cleavage with the R · *Eco* R$_1$ endonuclease. The solid lines represent the parental strands and the broken lines are the newly synthesized strands. I is the site at which DNA replication is initiated. Molecules are cleaved by the R · *Eco* R$_1$ endonuclease at site R$_1$. The arrow indicates the direction of replication. It can be seen that during unidirectional replication the length of one branch remains constant while the second branch decreases in length. Since the R · *Eco* R$_1$ cleavage site is 17% of the genome length from the termination site of DNA synthesis, it is the short arm L1 which would remain constant during unidirectional replication. During bidirectional replication, both L1 and L4 decrease in length as replication proceeds. From Salzman *et al.* (1973a).

Bidirectional replication from a unique origin was also observed (Crawford *et al.*, 1973). When the distribution of ^{3}H-thymidine within R · *Hin*-produced fragments of newly completed SV40 DNA I molecules was measured, a similar conclusion was reached, i.e., that DNA replication proceeds in a bidirectional manner (Danna and Nathans, 1972).

2.5. Mechanism of Chain Growth

When SV40-infected cells are pulsed for short time periods (15 s to 1 min) and replicating molecules are isolated in neutral sucrose gradients, subsequent examination in alkaline sucrose gradients demonstrates two populations of newly synthesized DNA strands. One population consists of growing SV40 DNA chains ranging from 6S to almost 16S, while the second consists of a discrete peak sedimenting at 4S. These 4S fragments, which correspond to DNA chains of 50,000 daltons, are present in molecules at all stages of replication; by pulse-chase experiments, it is seen that these short fragments are precursors of growing SV40 chains. Thus a discontinuous mechanism of synthesis of DNA, as first proposed by Okazaki *et al.* (1968) for bacterial DNA, is also observed for this small circular genome (Fareed and Salzman, 1972). A similar discontinuous mechanism of synthesis for polyoma DNA is observed during *in vitro* incubation with nuclei from infected cells. In addition, the presence of RNA which is covalently linked at the 5′-end of the 4S fragments has been observed during these *in vitro* studies (Magnusson *et al.*, 1973).

It is likely that attachment of the 4S fragments to growing chains requires the action of a DNA polymerase which may be different from that which carries out the synthesis of the 4S fragment. The basis for this theory emerges from three separate studies (Salzman and Thoren, 1973; Magnusson, 1973; Laipis and Levine, 1973). For both SV40 and polyoma, under conditions where DNA synthesis is first inhibited by FUdR and then restarted by the addition of thymidine, or where DNA synthesis is partially blocked by hydroxyurea, there is an accumulation of 4S fragments, both free and within replicating molecules. These 4S fragments in replicative intermediates cannot be joined *in vitro* to growing chains by the action of ligase, but the combined action of T4 DNA polymerase and ligase does effect a joining to growing chains (Laipis and Levine, 1973). The synthesis of 4S DNA fragments, together with the failure to continue chain elongation, suggests that two polymerase activities are involved in this process. Since the RNA which has been found joined to growing chains is excised prior to the incorporation of the 4S fragment into the growing chain, one can speculate that gaps between the 4S fragment and the growing chain are located at the site where RNA previously existed. The presence of enzymes in eukaryotic cells which excise RNA from RNA–DNA hybrids has been described (Keller and Crouch, 1972), and it is possible that such an enzyme removes the RNA primer from the 4S DNA fragments.

When 4S fragments are isolated from replicating molecules and then allowed to reanneal, 70–90% are converted to a double-stranded form (Fareed *et al.*, 1973*a*).

Similarly, when 4S fragments are isolated from hydroxyurea-treated polyoma-infected cells, a lower but still significant percentage of the 4S DNA is converted to a double-stranded form (Magnusson, 1973). These are the results that are expected only if both strands, at each of the replication forks, are made in a discontinuous manner.

In contrast to these findings are results obtained under certain *in vitro* conditions where a significant fraction of the radioactivity is always contained in growing chains, suggesting that chain growth in the 5′ to 3′ direction occurs in a continuous way (Francke and Hunter, 1974; Qasba, 1974). These results are not necessarily inconsistent with discontinuous synthesis of both chains. It may be that growth of the 4S fragment in the 3′ to 5′ direction cannot be initiated until growth of the complementary 4S fragment that has been synthesized in the 5′ to 3′ direction has been completed. Under these circumstances, it is easy to imagine preferential ligation of 4S fragments formed in the 5′ to 3′ direction.

Based on our present understanding of SV40, the following series of events can be specified:

1. DNA synthesis is initiated at a specific site located 0.67 genome length from the R · *Eco* R₁ cleavage site.
2. Replication then proceeds bidirectionally with an equal rate of chain growth at each of the replication forks.
3. Chain growth occurs by a discontinuous mechanism in which 4S DNA fragments are first synthesized. A fraction of the 4S fragments are covalently linked to RNA. The RNA must be removed rapidly since the association of 4S DNA with RNA can be demonstrated during *in vitro* studies or *in vivo* only when DNA synthesis has been modified by metabolic inhibitors.
4. Each of the chains at each of the replication forks is made in a discontinuous manner.
5. There is a gap between the 4S fragment and the growing chain. It seems likely that an enzyme other than the one which synthesizes the 4S DNA is involved in filling in the gap.
6. The newly synthesized fragment is joined to the growing chain by a covalent link which is probably formed by ligase, an enzyme present in animal cells (Sambrook and Shatkin, 1969).

While these facts seem quite likely, based on present experimental evidence, it may also be worthwhile to mention some general areas of DNA replication which are not at all understood. While there is a specific site for initiation of DNA synthesis, there is no evidence as to the precise mechanism of DNA initiation. Is nicking involved as the first step in DNA replication? If initiation involves an RNA polymerase which recognizes and transcribes a region that serves as an RNA primer to which DNA is linked, why is this region recognized preferentially compared with the other sites where RNA synthesis presumably occurs? When 4S DNA fragments are linked to an RNA primer, any one of four deoxynucleotides can lie adjacent to the terminal ribonucleotide (Magnusson *et al.*, 1973). What are the signals, then, within the DNA which determine initiation of RNA synthesis and termination of 4S DNA synthesis? It should also be noted that there has been only a partial characterization of the enzymes involved in DNA replication in mammalian cells and a large number of questions about the detailed mechanism of chain growth still remain unanswered. Temperature-sensitive mutants of SV40 have been isolated which are able to carry out chain elongation at the restrictive temperature but fail to initiate new rounds of DNA synthesis (Tegtmeyer, 1972). These mutants should be of value in defining the mechanism of initiation. Furthermore, the virus mutants which fail to initiate new rounds of DNA replication are also unable to transform cells at the restricted temperatures and this makes their characterization of considerable interest.

2.6. Termination of DNA Synthesis

Kinetic analysis of the time course of formation of replicative intermediates, as well as of DNAs I and II, suggests that DNA II is the first product to arise by segregation of parental strands (Fareed *et al.*, 1973*b*). The properties of this DNA II, which can only be observed after short pulses with ^{3}H-thymidine, are distinct from those of a pool of DNA II seen after extended periods (1–3 h) of labeling. The latter arises by endonucleolytic cleavage of DNA I and the nick is randomly located. In contrast, precursor DNA II (pDNA II) contains all of the newly synthesized DNA in the discontinuous (16S) strand. It can also be shown by cleavage with *Eco* · R$_I$ endonuclease that the nick in the newly synthesized strand is located 0.5 genome length from the initiation site for DNA replication (Fareed *et al.*, 1973*b*). This is the expected site for termination since replication has been shown to be bidirectional and both of the two replication forks were observed to move at the same rate (Fareed *et al.*, 1972).

2.7. Mechanism for Effecting Semiconservative Replication of Covalently Closed Duplex DNA

For each covalently closed duplex DNA molecule, the topological winding number is fixed; it can be changed only by introducing a break into one of the two strands, allowing unwinding to occur, and then sealing the break. The topological winding number is related to the superhelix winding number by the relationship

$$\tau = \alpha - \beta$$

where the topological winding number, α, is the number of revolutions made by one strand about the duplex axis when the axis is constrained to lie in a plane; the duplex winding number, β, is the number of revolutions made by one strand about the duplex axis in the unconstrained molecule; and the superhelix winding number, τ, is the number of revolutions made by the duplex about the superhelix axis (Vinograd *et al.*, 1968). During DNA replication, unwinding of the parental strands must occur and there will be a decrease in α, the topological winding number. After displacement of the newly synthesized strands from these replicative intermediate structures, the parental molecule will have the potential to form a Watson–Crick base-paired structure in which the value β is the same as in DNA I. Since α decreases as a result of replication, it is clear that these structures will have an increased number of negative superhelical turns, which can be quantitated experimentally.

Parental DNA strands have been obtained from replicating molecules after dissociation of the newly synthesized strands by treatment at pH 12.2. When examined by alkaline velocity gradient analysis or isopycnic banding in CsCl-EtBr, they provide direct experimental confirmation that the topological winding number of the parental template strands does progressively decrease as replication proceeds (Salzman *et al.*, 1973*b*; Bourgaux and Bourgaux-Ramoisy, 1972*a*).

A DNA-untwisting enzyme has been found in mammalian cells. This activity breaks one parental strand, allows the DNA strands to unwind, and then restores the covalently closed structure (Champoux and Dulbecco, 1972). A similar type of enzymatic activity has been obtained from bacterial cells and has been extensively purified (Wang, 1971). Such an enzyme is a good candidate to carry out the unwinding that must occur as DNA replication proceeds.

2.8. SV40 DNA Synthesis in Heterokaryons of SV40-Transformed Cells and Cells Permissive for SV40

Induction of extremely low levels of virus has been noted after treatment of SV40-transformed cells with chemical agents (Rothschild and Black, 1970). In general, however, a cell line which is transformed by SV40 cannot be induced to synthesize infectious virus after treatment with agents that cause induction of lysogenic bacteria. A finding of great interest and importance was that by cocultivation of an SV40-transformed mouse line with monkey kidney cells, which are permissive for SV40 replication, there was "activation" of the integrated genome and synthesis of infectious virus (Gerber, 1966). The amount of virus that is rescued is higher when the two cell lines, the susceptible and the transformed, are treated with inactivated Sendai virus in order to enhance the extent of cell fusion (Gerber, 1966; Koprowski *et al.*, 1967; Watkins and Dulbecco, 1967; Burns and Black, 1968; Dubbs *et al.*, 1967). It is difficult to use this system for biochemical studies since only a fraction of the cells can be induced to synthesize virus, even after fusion with inactivated Sendai virus. The time of appearance of infectious SV40 DNA is about the same after cell fusion as it is during a lytic cycle. Thus viral DNA synthesis was detected 19 h after fusion (Kit *et al.*, 1968). When cell fusion was carried out between a transformed mouse and a transformed human cell line, infectious virus was rescued. By using plaque mutants it was shown that only that virus which had been used to transform the mouse cell line was released and no SV40 virus was released from the transformed human line.

SV40-transformed hamster cells have been fused with susceptible CV-1 cells, and nuclei were isolated from the heterokaryons. The nuclei from the two cell species could be separated by sucrose gradient analysis. Virus was first found in the transformed nucleus (40 h) and later (68–72 h) was found associated with both nuclei (Wever *et al.*, 1970). Additional studies with this system may provide some interesting insight into factors which determine a permissive state for DNA synthesis and virus replication starting with an integrated viral genome.

2.9. SV40 DNA-Containing Cellular DNA Sequences

A field of current interest has been the characterization of covalently closed SV40 DNA molecules in which a fraction of the viral genome has been deleted and/or in which there is an insertion of cellular sequences. The first suggestion that cellular DNA is present in SV40 was the finding that SV40 DNA I was able to hybridize to an appreciable extent with DNA from BSC-1 cells (Aloni *et al.*, 1969). However, when the hybridization reaction between SV40 DNA I and cellular DNA was studied in various laboratories, there were considerable quantitative differences in the degree of hybridization. At that time, the reasons for these differences were not understood. It was finally shown that incorporation of cellular DNA into covalently closed molecules occurred when virus was passaged at a high input multiplicity. Infection of BSC-1 cells with a plaque-purified virus at either low or high multiplicities, or with low multiplicities of a virus pool that was not plaque purified, yielded virions which did not hybridize with cellular DNA. However, infection with high inputs of non-plaque-purified virus yielded viral DNA that hybridized to cellular DNA as well as to viral DNA. Similar results were obtained after multiple passages at high input multiplicities of plaque-purified SV40 (Lavi and Winocour, 1972). At the same time that these homology studies of high- and low-passage SV40 were reported, SV40 DNA was obtained from progeny virus that was purified after infection of BSC-1 cells with either high or low virus input multiplicities (Tai *et al.*, 1972). The DNA I was converted to DNA II, which was denatured and then reannealed. Using formamide-spreading of the DNA to prepare the grids, both single- and double-stranded DNA could be distinguished. The low-input-multiplicity DNA was of uniform size (1.7 µm) while the high-input DNA showed considerable size heterogeneity, and a significant fraction of the molecules were smaller than 1.7 µm. Similarly, the heteroduplexes from low-input-multiplicity DNA gave evidence for only a very low level of DNA deletions (2.5%). In contrast, high-input-multiplicity DNA contained 13% deletions (seen as single-stranded loops) and 7–12% substitutions (which are seen as a region where two single strands of DNA replace the duplex structure). The conclusion from both of the above studies is that under conditions of high input multiplicity there is recombination between viral and cellular DNA, and one consequence is the incorporation of host DNA sequences into covalently closed SV40 DNA molecules. This may involve the integration of the viral DNA into the cell genome and its subsequent excision. The findings cited above are clearly related to earlier studies where it was first reported that at high input multiplicities a population of defective particles was formed and that these contained covalently closed DNA molecules smaller than SV40 DNA I (Yoshiike and Furano, 1969). A

consequence of the insertion of cellular DNA and deletion of viral sequences is the
production of particles which are noninfectious. It is only under conditions where
cells are coinfected with a defective and nondefective virus particle that the
defective virus particle can replicate, presumably as a result of complementation.
While defective particles are unable to replicate, they can support a partial cycle of
virus replication (Yoshiike, 1968*a,b*). The loss of infectivity which is a result of a
loss of a random segment of the viral genome suggests that the entire viral genome
is required for infectivity, and this agrees with UV and X-ray inactivation studies
(Basilico and DiMayorca, 1965; Benjamin, 1965). In these studies, infectivity was
lost with one-hit kinetics; i.e., a single break anywhere in the virus genome
inactivated the virus.

These studies of alterations in the viral genome are important for a number of
reasons. It is clear, for example, that stock virus pools must be prepared at low
input multiplicities. The significance of early studies with purified viral DNA that
involved nucleic acid homology, nearest-neighbor analysis, etc., in which the
purity of the viral DNA was not known, is questionable.

The answers to questions of whether the covalent insertion of cellular DNA into
SV40 DNA I is biologically significant and whether this insertion occurs at a
specific site in the host cell genome are unknown. In an attempt to answer the
latter question, the progeny SV40 DNA molecules from a set of serial passages
were examined by digestion with R · *Hin* endonuclease (Rozenblatt *et al.*, 1973).
The cleavage fragments were then examined in hybridization experiments in an
attempt to analyze the incorporated cellular DNA sequences. The results of this
study showed that independent series of passages produced different defective
progeny viral DNA. It will, of course, be necessary to examine other serial-passage
populations in order to determine if there is a consistent pattern either in the
incorporated host cell sequences or in the deleted viral sequences. The defective
virus particles containing host DNA sequences are presumed to have been formed
by integration and excision, and they are then replicated at a rate which assures
their presence at significant levels in the final virus preparation. However, there
exist no data at present to support the hypothesis that integration and excision
seen at high input multiplicities are related to integration which occurs when cells
are transformed with polyoma or SV40. Future studies with the high-passage viral
DNA may provide information not only about the mechanisms of integration and
excision but also about the types of molecules which replicate rapidly in defective
populations. In one recent study, it was observed that after multiple passages at
high input multiplicities, certain DNA sequences which include the initiation site
for DNA replication are selectively preserved (Brockman *et al.*, 1973). In another
group of studies (Fareed *et al.*, 1974; Khoury *et al.*, 1974*a*), viral DNA was
generated in which a single DNA molecule contained three regions corresponding to the site for the initiation of DNA replication. Detectable levels of substituted
particles do not arise after infection with low input multiplicities. However, under
these conditions high virus titers are finally achieved. This suggests that integration and excision may not be necessary events during the lytic cycle.

2.10. *Role of Proteins in DNA Replication*

Several groups have studied the effect of an inhibition of protein synthesis on SV40 or polyoma DNA replication. These various studies differed in the time after infection when the inhibitor (cycloheximide) was added and in the length of the pulse time (1–4 h) for labeling newly synthesized DNA. It is difficult to study the fate of intermediates in replication in cases where such long periods of labeling have been used since the time for one round of viral DNA replication is 10–25 min (Danna and Nathans, 1972; Fareed *et al.*, 1973*b*). It is clear, however, in each of these studies, that the presence of cyclohexamide resulted in a decrease in the rate of viral DNA synthesis (Branton *et al.*, 1970; Branton and Sheinin, 1973; Kit and Nakajima, 1971; Kang *et al.*, 1971). These observations are consistent with a requirement for a protein to initiate DNA synthesis. What is not clear is whether a second protein is needed in the conversion of mature replicating molecules to pDNA II or in the conversion of pDNA II to DNA I. The various studies do not agree on this point. Initiation of viral DNA synthesis does not occur when polyoma replication is carried out in an *in vitro* system (Winnacker *et al.*, 1972). However, chain elongation and synthesis of DNA I can occur in this system. Studies in *in vitro* systems may provide the means to determine the role of proteins in virus maturation.

The role of a virus-coded protein for initiation of DNA synthesis has been demonstrated using temperature-sensitive mutants which are blocked in viral DNA synthesis (Tegtmeyer, 1972). These mutants fail to initiate new rounds of replication but can, at the restrictive temperature, continue the process of chain elongation and termination of DNA molecules. Thus a virus-coded protein is apparently required to initiate viral DNA synthesis. If there is a second protein that is required for chain termination, it is likely to be a cellular protein and may also be involved in cellular DNA synthesis.

When cells are exposed to puromycin (Bourgaux and Bourgaux-Ramoisy, 1972*b*), an inhibition of polyoma DNA replication is observed. There is a reduced rate of synthesis of covalently closed DNA molecules in the presence of the inhibitor, and, in addition, these molecules do not seem to contain superhelical turns as judged by the fact that they band at a slightly higher density than DNA I in CsCl-EtBr. This suggests that specific proteins affect the configuration of DNA, perhaps by complexing with them during replication.

3. *Transcription of SV40 and Polyoma DNA*

Synthesis of virus-specific RNA during the lytic cycle of polyoma replication was first demonstrated using a filter hybridization technique (Benjamin, 1966). Polyoma virus RNA was synthesized in very small amounts early after a productive infection of mouse kidney cells, and in significantly greater concentrations (approximately a hundredfold after the onset of polyoma DNA synthesis.

Subsequently it was shown that virus-specific RNA was produced in two phases during the lytic cycle of SV40 (Aloni *et al.*, 1968; Oda and Dulbecco, 1968*b*; Sauer and Kidwai, 1968; Carp *et al.*, 1969). Prior to viral DNA replication (within the first 12 h after infection) "early" SV40 RNA is synthesized. Using competition-hybridization experiments it was shown that the early RNA continues to be produced late in the lytic cycle and represents approximately 30–50% of the total transcribed gene sequences. Furthermore, the fact that late, lytic SV40 RNA could completely compete against the early RNA indicated that all of the early sequences are transcribed late in the cycle. A similar division of the lytic cycle of polyoma virus into early and late phases of transcription has also been reported (Hudson *et al.*, 1970).

In order to determine the extent of transcription of SV40 (Martin and Axelrod, 1969*a*) or polyoma DNA (Martin and Axelrod, 1969*b*), a saturation hybridization technique was employed (see Fig. 9). A known amount of ^{14}C-labeled viral DNA was bound on filters, and increasing amounts of ^{32}P-labeled lytic RNA preparations of known specific activity were hybridized to the DNA until a plateau was reached. From the amount of RNA required to saturate the DNA on each filter it was determined that approximately 50%, or the equivalent of one full strand of the polyoma or SV40 DNA, was bound in a hybrid. Since the total transcription

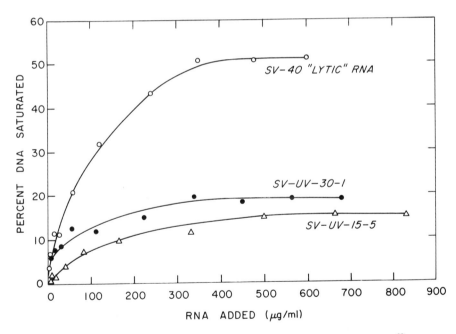

FIGURE 9. A saturation hybridization experiment in which increasing amounts of ^{32}P-labeled lytic (or SV–UV-transformed cell) RNA were hybridized with a fixed amount of ^{14}C-SV40 DNA on filters. Since the specific activities of the RNAs and DNA were known, the percentage of DNA saturated could be determined. The plateau of 50% saturation with SV40 late lytic RNA indicates that the equivalent of one full DNA strand is transcribed during productive infection. Lower values were obtained for the two transformed cell lines examined. From Martin and Axelrod (1969*b*).

product of SV40 or polyoma late in infection is equivalent to one full strand of the genome and the early gene sequences represent about one-half of a strand, the true late gene sequences (those transcribed only after the onset of DNA replication) represent about one-half of the coding capacity of the genome.

3.1. Strand Orientation of Transcription

Because of the similar base composition of the two strands of SV40 DNA, strand separation could not be effected by labeling with a heavy base analogue or by selective binding to polyribonucleotides. In 1970 it was shown that *in vitro* transcription of supercoiled SV40 DNA (DNA I) with *E. coli* DNA-dependent RNA polymerase results in an asymmetrical RNA product which is complementary to only one of the two viral DNA strands (Westphal, 1970). This observation provided a means of separating the viral DNA strands on a preparative scale. In order to achieve this separation, hydroxylapatite chromatography (HA) was employed. This method allows for a rapid and large-scale separation of single-stranded DNA from DNA–RNA (or DNA–DNA) hybrid molecules (Britten and Kohne, 1968). Intact or sheared ^{32}P-labeled SV40 DNA was denatured and allowed to anneal with a great excess of *in vitro* SV40 cRNA (complementary RNA). Since the RNA binds almost exclusively to one DNA strand (the minus, or E, strand), passing the renaturation product over HA with subsequent purification effectively provides a strand separation of SV40 DNA. Once separated, the plus and minus strands of the viral DNA were then used in hybridization studies to determine the strand orientation and extent of transcription of early and late lytic SV40 RNA (Khoury and Martin, 1972; Khoury *et al.*, 1972; Sambrook *et al.*, 1972), as well as that of RNA synthesized in abortively infected (Khoury *et al.*, 1972) or transformed cells (Sambrook *et al.*, 1972; Khoury *et al.*, 1973a; Ozanne *et al.*, 1973). The results of these studies indicated that 30–50% of the minus, or E, strand (the strand which is transcribed *in vitro* with *E. coli* RNA polymerase) is transcribed early in the lytic cycle; in addition, 50–70% of the plus, or L, DNA strand is transcribed late in infection. The extent of transcription and strand orientation for early and late viral mRNA, as determined with the separated strands of SV40, agrees with results of the previous competition-hybridization experiments (Aloni *et al.*, 1968; Oda and Dulbecco, 1968b; Sauer and Kidwai, 1968; Carp *et al.*, 1969). These results are also in agreement with studies in which the early or late RNAs from SV40-infected BSC-l cells were annealed with asymmetrical SV40 cRNA (Lindstrom and Dulbecco, 1972); on the basis of ribonuclease resistance, it was concluded that early lytic RNA was synthesized from approximately 40% of the same DNA strand as is the *in vitro* RNA, whereas late lytic RNA was synthesized from about 60% of the opposite strand.

In SV40-transformed cell lines there is little or no stable RNA transcribed from the plus strand. Transcription of the minus strand (30–80%) appears to be more extensive than in the lytic cycle, and, presumably, the "anti-sense" sequences (those homologous to the late lytic RNA) do not code for functional proteins (see Fig. 10).

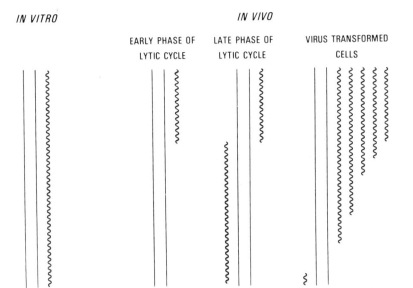

IN VITRO   IN VIVO

EARLY PHASE OF   LATE PHASE OF   VIRUS TRANSFORMED
LYTIC CYCLE   LYTIC CYCLE   CELLS

FIGURE 10. The pattern of transcription of SV40 DNA *in vitro* and *in vivo*. SV40 DNA molecules (=) are represented as linear structures for convenience. The strand orientation and extent of transcription (〰) are based on the abundant, or stable, mRNA species as determined by hybridization experiments described in the text.

On the basis of RNA hybridization to the separated strands of polyoma DNA (Kamen *et al.*, 1974) and RNA–RNA annealing studies similar to those described above (Mueller *et al.*, 1973), it appears that the early and late virus-specific RNAs in the lytic cycle of polyoma are transcribed from opposite DNA strands.

The fact that in the lytic cycle early and late virus-specific RNAs are transcribed from opposite strands of SV40 DNA is especially interesting, and it allows one to propose several novel hypotheses for the control of transcription in lytically infected cells (see below).

The lytic SV40 RNAs studied in the experiments described above (Khoury and Martin, 1972; Lindstrom and Dulbecco, 1972; Khoury *et al.*, 1972; Sambrook *et al.*, 1972) are predominantly the stable or abundant RNA species in the population. In order to determine whether the initial transcription product might be more extensive than the stable species detected above, RNA has been examined after a brief pulse-label of monkey cells with ^{3}H-uridine, 48 h after infection (Aloni, 1972, 1973). These studies suggested that extensive regions of the SV40 genome are transcribed symmetrically. If the brief pulse-label is followed by a 1-h chase or if the 2-min ^{3}H-uridine pulse is extended to 20 min, the labeled RNA exhibits significantly less symmetry. Thus it appears that a substantial portion of the genome is symmetrically transcribed, and, subsequently, specific RNA sequences are rapidly degraded, resulting in the stable transcripts described above. A similar conclusion has been reached in analogous studies with pulse-labeled polyoma RNA (Aloni and Locker, 1973). The important implication of this work is that the control mechanism for selection of stable message occurs at a post-transcriptional level, i.e., the degradation of transcribed nonfunctional regions of RNA. Furthermore, this post-transcriptional control appears to be operative prior to or during transport of mRNA to the cytoplasm, since only the asymmetrical SV40 or polyoma sequences are detected in cytoplasmic RNA (Khoury et al., 1974b, 1975a; Kamen et al., 1974) or on polysomes (Sambrook et al., 1974).

3.2. Control of Late Transcription

A consistent finding in the studies described above is the dependence of transcription of the late gene sequences of SV40 and polyoma on viral DNA synthesis. In the presence of inhibitors of DNA replication, transcription of the late genes does not occur (Carp et al., 1969; Hudson et al., 1970; Sauer, 1971). Current studies have shown that late transcription depends only on the initiation and not the continuation of viral DNA synthesis (Cowan et al., 1973). Cells are infected at the permissive temperature with a temperature-sensitive mutant of SV40, defective in a function necessary for DNA replication. After the initiation of DNA synthesis, the cultures are shifted to the restrictive temperature, effectively terminating viral DNA replication. Nevertheless, subsequent pulses with ^{3}H-uridine demonstrate the continued synthesis of late mRNA. However, the control mechanism which links the transcription of late SV40 and polyoma genes to the initiation of DNA replication is still unclear.

Several possibilities for regulation of late transcription are suggested by existing data. These include the following:

1. The physical state of the viral genome may determine the strand orientation or region of transcription. For example, transcription of late SV40 DNA sequences may occur on replicative intermediates (Girard et al., 1974), thus requiring initiation of viral DNA replication. This hypothesis is based on kinetic data which suggest that transcription of the late viral genes occurs on templates which build up in infected cells in direct relationship to viral DNA replication.

2. Alternatively, virion-associated histones which are associated with infecting SV40 or polyoma DNA may prevent late transcription (Huang et al., 1972b). As these core proteins are removed during DNA replication, late transcription may occur. It is also possible that newly synthesized viral DNA, prior to the addition of core protein, may act as a late transcriptional template.

3. The specificity of the RNA polymerase may be the controlling factor. Since there appears to be no virion-associated RNA polymerase, the early virus-specific RNA is almost certainly synthesized by a host enzyme. This enzyme may be specific for the minus (early) SV40 or polyoma DNA strand. The early viral gene products may provide or induce a new polymerase capable of late transcription. A model system in which the switch from early to late transcription is effected by a "late" RNA polymerase coded for by the early viral genes is the lytic cycle of bacteriophage T7 in E. coli (Chamberlain et al., 1970; Summers and Siegal, 1970).

4. Evidence has been cited for extensive symmetrical transcription of the SV40 genome late in the lytic cycle with subsequent degradation of the RNA sequences which are not translated (Aloni, 1972, 1973). It is conceivable that there is extensive transcription early in the lytic cycle and that the late RNA sequences are efficiently degraded prior to the onset of DNA replication.

While the above hypotheses are highly speculative, each, at least in part, can be tested with techniques presently available. Since the absence of both DNA synthesis and late RNA are hallmarks of SV40- and polyoma-transformed cells, it is hoped that a better understanding of controls which are operative in the lytic cycle will provide an insight into the mechanism of cell transformation.

3.3. Size of the Papovavirus-Specific RNA

Several recent studies have been concerned with the size and potential processing of SV40- and poloyma-specific RNA, synthesized in productively infected cells. Perhaps the most surprising result of these investigations was the detection of intranuclear SV40-specific (Tonegawa et al., 1970; Martin, 1970; Jaenisch, 1972; Rozenblatt and Winocour, 1972) or polyoma-specific (Acheson et al., 1971) RNA molecules which were considerably larger than a unit length of the genome. It seems unlikely that these molecules are simply artifacts due to aggregation since the sizing technique employed in several of these studies was centrifugation in dimethylsulfoxide, a compound which removes secondary structure and aggregation. These large, intranuclear, virus-specific molecules could arise from multiple rounds of transcription of viral DNA. In certain investigations, however, it was shown that nonviral sequences are transcribed in tandem with the SV40 RNA (Jaenisch, 1972; Rozenblatt and Winocour, 1972), suggesting the possibility of transcription from integrated viral genomes.

High molecular weight RNA (HMW RNA) obtained late in the lytic cycle has been hybridized to SV40 DNA on filters (Jaenisch, 1972). The presence of RNA tails which remained susceptible to RNase after the hybridization to SV40 DNA filters is consistent with the idea that these tails contain nonviral sequences, presumably host specific, which are covalently linked to the virus-specific RNA. In a more extensive analysis, it was shown that HMW RNA from a lytic infection which binds specifically to SV40 DNA filters could be eluted and hybridized to host cell DNA filters (Rozenblatt and Winocour, 1972). It is unlikely that the host RNA sequences were transcribed from host DNA incorporated into the virions since the SV40 inoculum was produced by low multiplicity passage, a procedure which selects against host incorporation. Since present evidence points to integration of some viral DNA molecules into host DNA in the lytic cycles of SV40 (Hirai and Defendi, 1972) and polyoma (Babiuk and Hudson, 1972; Ralph and Colter, 1972), the most likely explanation of covalently linked host and viral RNA sequences is that they result from linked transcription of integrated viral DNA and adjacent cellular DNA.

On the other hand, the presence of host-specific sequences in HMW virus-specific RNA in polyoma-infected mouse kidney cells was not observed (Acheson *et al.*, 1971). In this study it was concluded that the HMW virus-specific RNA may represent viral sequences transcribed in tandem or viral RNA linked to unique host RNA sequences which would not be detected by the usual hybridization techniques. Whether these hybrid or nonhybrid HMW RNA molecules have any function in the lytic cycle (as well as whether integration serves any necessary function in a productive infection) is still in question. In other systems, however, most or all of the HMW nuclear RNA never gets to the cytoplasm, which suggests processing or at least selection of the virus-specific RNA which is eventually translated.

3.4. Cytoplasmic Viral RNA

RNA species that are found in the cytoplasm (and presumably on the polysomes) of SV40-infected cells (Weinberg *et al.*, 1972*a*) have been investigated using a formamide hybridization procedure to isolate intact virus-specific RNA. Similar studies have been carried out for cytoplasmic and polysomal polyoma RNA (Buetti, 1974). Prior to viral DNA replication, one can detect a 19S virus-specific moiety; a similar species is found in mouse cells abortively infected with SV40 (May *et al.*, 1973). Subsequent to DNA replication, there are both a 19S and a 16S peak of SV40- or polyoma-specific RNA. While evidence suggests that the 19S and 16S RNAs differ in base compositions as well as in T1 ribonuclease fingerprints (Warnaar and de Mol, 1973), there exist as yet no data which exclude the possibility that part of the 16S peak results from cleavage of a 19S precursor or that a distinct 19S species is synthesized late. In fact, there is preliminary evidence for a distinct 19S late RNA molecule (G. Khoury and B. Carter, unpublished results; Weinberg *et al.*, 1974).

In several studies, it has been demonstrated that a fraction of the SV40 RNA molecules both in the nucleus and in the cytoplasm contain terminal regions of poly(A) about 150–200 nucleotides in length (Weinberg *et al.*, 1972*b*; Aloni, 1973). A number of the observations mentioned above suggested some form of post-transcriptional processing of the SV40 RNA between synthesis in the nucleus and transport to the cytoplasm. If this processing occurs after the addition of the poly(A) sequences, it probably occurs from the 5′-end of the molecules, since it has been shown that the poly(A) is located at the 3′-terminus of mRNA molecules.

3.5. Concentration of Virus-Specific RNA

Extremely small amounts of SV40- and polyoma-specific RNA are synthesized early in the lytic cycle; present estimates suggest that only 0.001–0.01% of the total cell RNA is virus specific prior to SV40 DNA replication. After the onset of viral DNA replication, this fraction increases to 0.1–1% of the total cell RNA (Benjamin, 1966; Khoury and Martin, 1972; Sambrook *et al.*, 1972), in agreement with data which suggested that there is a forty- to fifty-fold increase in the amount of virus-specific RNA late after productive infection (Aloni *et al.*, 1968; Carp *et al.*, 1969). The increase in SV40-specific RNA which occurs after the initiation of viral DNA synthesis includes a commensurate stimulation in the production of early SV40 sequences; this early SV40 RNA appears to account for 20–40% of the total late virus-specific RNA (Martin and Khoury, 1973) yet only 1–5% of the cytoplasmic late virus-specific RNA. Since infection by SV40 (unlike adenovirus) stimulates the production of host cell RNA (Oda and Dulbecco, 1968a), the virus-specific sequences, even late in the lytic cycle, represent a small fraction of the total cellular RNA. For this reason, studies requiring the isolation and purification of virus-specific RNA have proven difficult. Recently, several methods have been developed for the selection of messenger RNA.

3.6. Selection of Viral mRNA

3.6.1. Hybridization and Elution

As noted above, SV40 mRNA can be purified by hybridization of infected cellular RNA to SV40 DNA on filters, with subsequent elution of the bound RNA (Weinberg *et al.*, 1972a). In order to prevent fragmentation of the RNA, annealing is carried out at 37°C in the presence of 50% formamide. Two disadvantages of this technique are a relatively low efficiency of recovery and the introduction of some breaks in the RNA in spite of the precautions taken. The procedure, however, does allow the isolation of a relatively pure virus-specific RNA. This method is currently being used in several laboratories to obtain virus-specific mRNA for translation studies.

3.6.2. Selection of RNA Sequences on the Basis of Poly(A) Tracts

A number of studies have now shown that almost all mammalian cell and animal virus messenger RNAs contain poly(A)-rich regions, about 150–250 nucleotides in length. These tracts are covalently linked to the 3'-ends of the RNA molecules after the message has been synthesized. The poly(A) region contained in SV40 mRNA is not coded for by the viral genome (Weinberg *et al.*, 1972b). Several techniques have been developed for the isolation of mRNA based on specific binding of the poly(A)-rich regions. These methods include preferential selection of mRNA binding to oligo(dT)-cellulose columns (Gilham, 1964), to poly(U) which has been fixed on nitrocellulose filters (Sheldon *et al.*, 1972), or simply to nitrocellulose filters in the presence of high salt (Lee *et al.*, 1971). The separation of mRNA from total cell RNA by any of these methods is relatively simple; the techniques are efficient and provide large quantities of message. Such procedures, however, do not provide for a separation of virus-specific from host-specific messages. Furthermore, transcriptional products which either do not contain poly(A) tracts or have lost them due to breakage or degradation are excluded from these selection procedures.

3.6.3. Immunoprecipitation

The technique of immunoprecipitation relies on the fact that nascent polypeptides, being synthesized on polysomes, can react with specific antibodies (see Palacios and Schinke, 1973). After precipitation of the antigen–antibody complexes, one can isolate and purify the particular mRNA which codes for the precipitated antigen. This procedure has recently been used to obtain the mRNA coding for a mouse immunoglobulin L chain (Schechter, 1973). The mRNA isolated by this procedure retained its biological activity and was translated in a cell-free system forming recognizable L-chain precursors. While this technique requires the use of relatively pure antibodies, it promises to provide specific mRNA species which should prove invaluable both for sequencing experiments and for *in vitro* transitional studies.

3.7. Mapping of Transcriptional Sites on the SV40 Genome

Although previous studies had determined the proportions and strand orientation of SV40 transcription early and late in the lytic cycle, none of the experiments localized these gene sequences on the genome. In order to locate the topographical positions of the early and late gene sequences, the 11 specific fragments of SV40 DNA generated by the restriction endonuclease isolated from *H. influenzae* (R · Hin d) have been used (Khoury et al., 1973b, 1974b). The order of these fragments, which vary in size from 4% to 22.5% of the length of SV40, has been determined (Danna and Nathans, 1971; Danna et al., 1973), as has their relationship to other restriction endonuclease sites (Fig. 3). By reacting unlabeled RNA from SV40-infected monkey cells with the separated strands of the 11 ^{32}P-labeled R · Hin fragments, the early and late gene sequences were localized. Stable species of RNA were complementary to the minus (E) strands of the contiguous fragments A, H, I, and B. The late SV40 RNA is transcribed predominantly from the plus (L) strands of fragments C, D, E, K, F, J, and G, which also form a continuous set on the physical map (Fig. 11). The findings of these experiments were in agreement with previous results which suggested that the early gene sequences are localized on one-half of the minus strand, while the

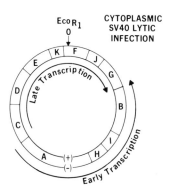

FIGURE 11. Diagram of SV40 transcription in productively infected cells. Arrows indicate the template strand and direction of transcription early and late in the lytic cycle. From Khoury et al. (1973b).

late gene sequences occupy the other one-half of the plus strand (Khoury *et al.*, 1973*b*, 1974*b*; Sambrook *et al.*, 1973).

In this same study, it was found that some of the late lytic SV40 RNA reacted partially with the plus strands of fragments H and I (Khoury *et al.*, 1973*b*), which are located on the physical map in the middle of the early-gene late. This result may reflect an incomplete post-transcriptional degradation of RNA complementary to the plus strands of these fragments.

Initially, the genome appears to be symmetrically transcribed and subsequently portions of each RNA strand are degraded. Since the plus (or late) strand is transcribed at a much higher frequency during the late stages of the lytic cycle, the "anti-early" sequences present in the nuclear component of total cellular RNA lead to an overestimate of the late template (Khoury *et al.*, 1975*a*).

3.8. Direction of SV40 DNA Transcription

It appears to be a general rule that transcription of DNA proceeds in a 5' to 3' direction with respect to the synthesis of the messenger RNA molecule, or 3' to 5' along the DNA template strand. Since the strands of DNA in a duplex molecule have an antiparallel orientation, and since early and late SV40 messages are transcribed from opposite DNA strands (Lindstrom and Dulbecco, 1972; Khoury *et al.*, 1972; Sambrook *et al.*, 1972), it seems clear that the transcription of the early and late SV40 sequences occurs in opposite directions. There are several prerequisites for determining the direction of SV40 transcription:

1. It is necessary to obtain a unique population of linear molecules.
2. One must be able to distinguish the 3'- and 5'-ends of each DNA strand.
3. The strand which codes for the early SV40 RNA must be distinguished from the strand which codes for the late message.

A diagram of the experimental approach used to determine the direction of SV40 transcriptions is shown in Fig. 12. ^{32}P-SV40 DNA I was first cleaved with the R · *Eco* R$_1$ endonuclease to obtain unique, full-length linear molecules. Since the R$_1$ enzymes cleaves within fragment F (Danna *et al.*, 1973), these molecules have the map order F$_1$-J-G-B-I-H-A-C-D-E-K-F$_2$ (see Fig. 11; letters refer to the fragments produced by the R · *Hin* endonuclease as mentioned above). In the next step, the linear molecules were digested with *E. coli* exonuclease III, which removes the 3'-halves of each strand, leaving 5'-"half-molecules." The individual minus and plus 5'-"half-strands" were next separated by annealing with SV40 cRNA. It was then determined which 5'-"half-strand" (plus or minus) contained fragment-J and fragment-G sequences and which contained fragment-K and fragment-E sequences by annealing each "half-strand" with denatured ^{14}C-labeled fragment J, G, K, or E. (The sequences corresponding to these four fragments are nearest to sequence F, which is present at each end of the R$_1$ linear molecules, Fig. 12.) The results indicated that fragments E and K hybridized preferentially with the *plus*

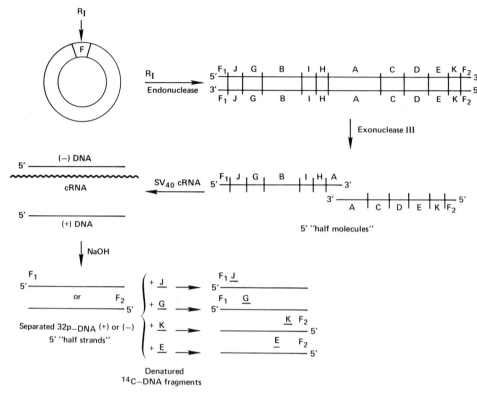

FIGURE 12. Scheme for defining the direction of transcription in SV40-infected cells. This method is based on a determination of the 5'→3' orientation of SV40 DNA strands. See the text for a description of each step. F_1 and F_2 are the parts of fragment F resulting from cleavage by the R_I restriction enzyme, cRNA is SV40 complementary RNA. From Khoury *et al.* (1973*b*).

5'-"half-strand," while fragments G and J hybridized preferentially with the *minus* 5'-"half-strand" of SV40 DNA. Since the minus strand is the template for "early" SV40 RNA, one can conclude that the orientation of the "early" DNA template strand is 5'-F-J-G-B-I-H-A-...-3', i.e., 3' to 5' counterclockwise on the cleavage map shown in Fig. 11, and the orientation of the plus strand ("late" template strand) is 5'-F-K-E-D-C-A-...-3', i.e., 3' to 5' clockwise on the cleavage map. Therefore, transcription of early genes proceeds from A to B *counterclockwise* on the minus DNA strand and transcription of late genes proceeds from A to B in a *clockwise* direction on the plus DNA strand (see Fig. 11). Similar results have been obtained by Sambrook *et al.* (1973) using an analogous procedure.

3.9. In Vitro Studies of Transcription

While much is known about the quantitative aspects of transcription of the SV40 and polyoma genomes, the factors which control transcription are still poorly understood. This is in large part related to the difficulty of studying biochemical events which occur against the complex background of cell-specific functions.

Although it has been shown that transcription of SV40 with the *E. coli* RNA polymerase differs from transcription of the virus *in vivo*, it is possible that the study of viral transcription in cell-free systems will permit investigators to control many of the factors which at present make the study of *in vivo* systems so complex.

The number and location of promoter sites for the *in vitro* transcription of SV40 DNA have been the subject of several recent investigations. It is clear that the results of such studies depend on the form of the DNA template, the enzyme, and the conditions used for *in vitro* transcription.

Both the strand orientation and the efficiency of transcription with the *E. coli* RNA polymerase depend on the form of SV40 DNA employed in the reaction mixture. When supercoiled SV40 DNA (DNA I) is used as a template, the RNA product is highly asymmetrical, heterogeneous in size, and representative of the entire minus (early) DNA strand (Westphal, 1970, 1971; Fried and Sokol, 1972). When the cyclic-coil or nicked form of SV40 DNA (DNA II) is transcribed, a considerable fraction of the RNA is symmetrical, as demonstrated by its ability to self-anneal (Westphal, 1970).

In order to evaluate the relative *in vitro* transcriptional rates of SV40 DNA components I and II, *E. coli* RNA polymerase was allowed to associate with each template and then incubated with a substrate solution containing rifampicin (the drug was added to prevent reinitiation). The kinetics of synthesis of RNA, as determined by the incorporation of ^{3}H-ribonucleotides under conditions of enzyme excess, indicated that the efficiency of transcription of the supercoiled SV40 DNA was significantly greater than that of the component-II DNA template (Westphal, 1971).

Estimates of the rate of *in vitro* RNA synthesis of SV40 component I range from 37 nucleotides per second (Westphal, 1971) to 5 nucleotides per second (Fried and Sokol, 1972), perhaps dependent on the reaction conditions. Most studies agree, however, that the RNA product is asymmetrical and contains some molecules greater in length than unit SV40 (Westphal, 1970; Fried and Sokol, 1972; Delius *et al.*, 1973). This latter finding suggests that the transcriptional complex can, at times, pass its initiation site, which in turn may indicate the absence or lack of recognition of a termination site. There is, however, little evidence at present to suggest multiple rounds of transcription *in vivo*.

The number of polymerase-binding sites on a viral DNA molecule is inversely proportional to the salt concentration (Crawford *et al.*, 1965; Pettijohn and Kamiya, 1967). *E. coli* DNA-dependent RNA polymerase binds to several sites on the SV40 molecule (Herzberg and Winocour, 1970; Delius *et al.*, 1973). Based on an electron microscopic study, it was concluded that these sites are not clustered (Delius *et al.*, 1973). However, when similar experiments were performed using linear SV40 DNA produced with the R · *Eco* R₁ endonuclease, there appeared to be one preferred promoter, in addition to several weaker initiation sites (Westphal *et al.*, 1973). This preferred promoter was localized at a position 0.16 unit from the R · *Eco* R₁ cleavage site, and transcription proceeded toward the short arm of the linear molecule. When transcription of SV40 DNA by *E. coli* RNA polymerase was investigated at reduced temperatures with RNA sequencing studies (Zain *et al.*,

1973), a strong *in vitro* promoter site was found 0.16 unit clockwise from the SV40 R · *Eco* R₁ site. Since transcription on the minus DNA strand (the strand which is transcribed by the *E. coli* polymerase) occurs in a counterclockwise direction (see Fig. 11), *in vitro* transcription almost certainly progresses from the strong promoter toward the R · *Eco* R₁ site. These results are in good agreement with those obtained by electron microscopy as described above (Westphal *et al.*, 1973). The strong promoter for the *E. coli* RNA polymerase does not coincide with that predicted for early RNA synthesized *in vivo* (Khoury *et al.*, 1973*b*; Sambrook *et al.*, 1973). As has been pointed out, however, if lytic messenger RNA represents the product of post-transcriptional degradation, the transcriptional promoters and terminators cannot be definitely localized to the ends of the final product.

Much less is known about the transcription of polyoma DNA with *E. coli* RNA polymerase. It appears, however, that a considerable fraction of the RNA product is symmetrical unless the template has been prepared from a high-multiplicity viral stock (D. Lindstrom, personal communication) or unless the cRNA is synthesized at a particular KCl concentration (Kamen *et al.*, 1974). By using polyoma-specific RNA prepared on such a template with preincubation of the RNA to remove symmetrical regions, it is possible to obtain an RNA which will permit strand separation and transcriptional analysis. The transcriptional map of polyoma appears to be quite similar to that of SV40 (Kamen *et al.*, 1974).

3.10. Applications of in Vitro Virus-Specific RNA

In addition to providing insight into the mechanism of transcription, the *in vitro* product obtained from transcription of SV40 DNA with the *E. coli* DNA-dependent RNA polymerase has proven to be a valuable reagent for a number of other studies.

1. The radiolabeled *in vitro* RNA has been used as a molecular probe in studies designed to determine the number of copies of the viral genome in transformed cells (Westphal and Dulbecco, 1968; Levine *et al.*, 1970) and to establish the integration of the viral DNA within the host DNA of transformed cell lines (Sambrook *et al.*, 1968). It has also been used to determine the transcriptional pattern of the lytic cycles of SV40 (Lindstrom and Dulbecco, 1972), as well as the pattern of transcription from the chromatin of SV40-transformed cells (Astrin, 1973).

2. Since the RNA obtained from transcription of DNA I with the *E. coli* RNA polymerase is essentially asymmetrical, it has been a valuable tool for separating the strands of SV40 DNA (Westphal, 1970; Khoury and Martin, 1972; Sambrook *et al.*, 1972). These separated DNA strands have subsequently been used as probes to determine the transcriptional pattern in lytically infected cells (Khoury *et al.*, 1972; Sambrook *et al.*, 1972), in transformed cells (Sambrook *et al.*, 1972; Khoury *et al.*, 1973*a*; Ozanne *et al.*, 1973), or from the chromatin of transformed cells (Shih *et al.*, 1973). The

separated SV40 DNA strands have also been used to map specific viral deletion mutants (Khoury *et al.*, 1974*a*).

3. The RNA transcribed from unique segments of SV40 DNA has been employed in nucleotide-sequencing studies (Dhar *et al.*, 1973, 1974; Zain *et al.*, 1974; Subramanian *et al.*, 1974).

3.11. Transcription of SV40 DNA by Mammalian Polymerases

The analysis of *in vitro* transcription of viral DNA is directed toward an understanding of the mechanism and control factors which operate *in vivo*. Since *in vivo* transcription of SV40 and polyoma DNA most likely requires a host cell RNA polymerase, it would seem preferable to use mammalian cell polymerases in the *in vitro* studies. Until recently, however, most of our information has been obtained in experiments with the *E. coli* RNA polymerase, primarily because of the difficulty associated with isolating and purifying mammalian enzymes.

It has now been shown that there are two principal DNA-dependent RNA polymerases found in mammalian cells which can be separated by ion-exchange chromatography (Roeder and Rutter, 1969). RNA polymerase I is found in nucleoli and has been associated with the synthesis of ribosomal RNA (Reeder and Roeder, 1972). RNA polymerase II is found in the cell nucleoplasm and is distinguished from polymerase I by its sensitivity to α-amanitin, a toxin extracted from the mushroom *Amanita phalloides* (Stirpe and Fuime, 1967; Roeder and Rutter, 1970).

Using isolated nuclei from SV40-infected cells (since cellular membranes are not uniformly permeable to α-amanitin), transcription of the SV40 sequences was shown to be sensitive to α-amanitin. This evidence suggests that RNA polymerase II is responsible for transcription of viral sequences *in vivo* (Jackson and Sugden, 1972).

While purified DNA-dependent RNA polymerase II from HeLa and KB cells actively transcribes SV40 DNA, the enzymes appear to prefer a single-stranded to a double-stranded DNA template (Sugden and Keller, 1973). The significance of that finding and its relationship to the specificity and activity of mammalian cell RNA polymerase II *in vivo* remain to be determined.

4. The Proteins of SV40 and Polyoma

A number of virus-specific antigens which are synthesized early after infection have been superficially characterized; these are probably proteins and may be products of viral and/or cellular genes. The most fully characterized of the papovavirus proteins are the structural proteins which are synthesized late in the lytic cycle. In addition, during the lytic cycle there is a general stimulation of synthetic enzymes which are probably coded for by the host cell.

4.1. Early Antigens

The early antigens of SV40 and polyoma are synthesized prior to viral DNA replication and also appear in cells transformed by these viruses. These antigens have been detected primarily by immunological methods, and past attempts to purify the early antigens have met with only partial success (Kit *et al.*, 1967; Lazarus *et al.*, 1967; Potter *et al.*, 1969; Del Villano and Defendi, 1973). Nevertheless, several lines of experimentation lead to the conclusion that the early papovavirus antigens are virus specific and, perhaps, virus coded:

1. When cells from different species are infected (Rapp *et al.*, 1964a; Hoggan *et al.*, 1965) or transformed by SV40 or polyoma (Black and Rowe, 1963; Black *et al.*, 1963; Sabin *et al.*, 1964; Rapp *et al.*, 1964c; Habel, 1965; Habel *et al.*, 1965), antigens are synthesized which appear to be immunologically identical.

2. UV irradiation of SV40 (Carp and Gilden, 1965) and polyoma (Benjamin, 1965; Basilico and DiMayorca, 1965; Latarjet *et al.*, 1967) sequentially inhibits the ability of the virus to produce infectious progeny, late antigens, and early antigens. Temperature-sensitive (*ts*) mutants of polyoma virus which are defective at an early stage (prior to DNA replication) either fail to make T antigen or make reduced amounts of it (Oxman *et al.*, 1972). Similarly, early *ts* mutants of SV40 (Tegtmeyer, 1972) also appear to be incapable of making the normal T antigen, although a somewhat altered product with similar antigenicity is detected (R. Tegtmeyer, personal communication; M. Osborn and K. Weber, personal communication).

3. In the SV40 lytic cycle, the synthesis of early SV40 RNA (Oxman and Levin, 1971) and T antigen (Oxman *et al.*, 1967) is inhibited when cultures are treated with interferon. Interferon is considered to be a specific inhibitor of viral protein synthesis, but it does not block cellular protein synthesis. Neither viral RNA nor T antigen is sensitive to inhibitors of DNA synthesis (Gilden *et al.*, 1965; Melnick and Rapp, 1965; Butel and Rapp, 1965), which indicates that they are independent of viral DNA replication. Both, however, are inhibited in the presence of actinomycin D, an agent which blocks viral transcription.

While these experiments appear to make a strong case for the virus-specific nature of early papovavirus antigens, they do not prove that the antigens are virus coded. Such proof will probably require the *in vitro* synthesis of defined viral proteins. Ideally, such experiments would be performed in a coupled system with transcription of the viral DNA and translation of the newly synthesized message. Since transcription of the SV40 and polyoma genomes by *E. coli* RNA polymerase results in a product which differs considerably from stable lytic RNA (see Section 3), future studies may require better characterization of transcriptional intermediates and mammalian RNA polymerases. Until then, preliminary experiments will probably rely on the translation of purified *in vivo* viral mRNA. These experiments are now in progress in a number of laboratories and should provide important answers concerning the nature of viral-coded products.

4.1.1. T Antigen

The best characterized of the early antigens are the SV40 and polyoma T ("tumor") antigens. They were first detected by a complement-fixation (CF) method (Black *et al.*, 1963; Takemoto and Habel, 1965) and are localized in the cell nucleus using immunofluorescence (IF) techniques (Pope and Rowe, 1964; Rapp *et al.*, 1964*a*; Gilden *et al.*, 1965). Antibodies for the detection of T antigen are present in sera from animals bearing SV40 or polyoma tumors. The T antigen can be detected as early as 10–18 h after infection (Rapp *et al.*, 1964*a*; Hoggan *et al.*, 1965) and persists throughout the lytic cycle. The time of appearance of SV40 T antigen and its rate of accumulation have been shown to depend in part on the line of cells infected and the temperature of incubation (Kitahara and Melnick, 1965; Khoury, 1970).

T antigen is heat labile and is sensitive to trypsin, but not to DNase (Gilden *et al.*, 1965). SV40 T antigen does not cross-react with the polyoma T antigen; however, it does share immunological properties with antigens induced by some of the recently discovered papovaviruses isolated from human sources (Takemoto and Mullarkey, 1973).

The synthesis of T antigen is not affected by inhibitors of DNA replication (Gilden *et al.*, 1965; Melnick and Rapp, 1965; Butel and Rapp, 1965), but its synthesis is inhibited by actinomycin D and interferon (Oxman *et al.*, 1967) and by cycloheximide (Gilden and Carp, 1966), thus suggesting that *de novo* transcription and subsequent translation of this message are required for T-antigen production. The presence of T antigen has served as one of the important criteria for determining whether cells are infected or transformed by SV40 or polyoma. Yet, it is still not known whether this antigen has a function in the lytic cycle. Some preliminary data suggest that an altered T antigen may be made at the restrictive temperature, by an early SV40 *ts* mutant (M. Osborn and K. Weber, personal communication). Since this mutant is blocked in SV40 DNA synthesis (Tegtmeyer, 1972), one interpretation would be that T antigen is in some way required for viral DNA synthesis.

One of the major problems in determining the function of T antigen has been an inability to adequately purify this antigen. However, a number of investigators have recently made considerable progress toward that goal (P. Tegtmeyer; D. Livingston; M. Osborn and K. Weber; and R. Carrol—personal communications) and it appears the T antigen may be a DNA-binding protein. A considerable amount of data concerning the structure and function of T antigen should be forthcoming in the next few years, and we may hope that this will result in a fuller understanding of the mechanisms responsible for lytic infection and transformation.

4.1.2. U Antigen

The U antigen has been detected by CF and IF methods in SV40- infected and -transformed cells (Lewis and Rowe, 1971). Like T antigen, the U antigen reacts with serum from SV40-tumor-bearing hamsters. Unlike T antigen, however, U antigen is found at the nuclear membrane and is heat stable (Lewis and Rowe, 1971). While most antisera for T antigen contain anti-U antibodies, there are some batches of anti-T sera which do not. Furthermore, there is a hybrid deletion mutant of adenovirus and SV40 (Ad2$^+$ND$_1$; see Section 7.4) which induces U antigen but not T antigen, thus suggesting that the two antigens differ, at least in part. Nothing is known about the structure or function of this antigen.

4.1.3. Tumor-Specific Transplantation Antigen (TSTA)

The polyoma (Habel, 1961; Sjogren et al., 1961) and SV40 (Habel and Eddy, 1963; Khera et al., 1963; Koch and Sabin, 1963; Defendi, 1963) TSTAs have been studied primarily in transformed cells and have been demonstrated by in vivo immunological methods such as transplantation rejection. In these tests, animals immunized with cells containing the TSTA become resistant to a subsequent challenge with transplantable SV40- or polyoma-transformed cells or tumor cells. TSTA appears to be localized at the cell surface. Newborn hamsters inoculated with membranes from SV40 tumor cells develop a tolerance to immunization as adults against SV40 tumor transplantation (Tevethia and Rapp, 1965). Furthermore, adult animals can be protected against transplantable tumors by immunization with membranes from SV40 tumor cells (Coggin et al., 1969). In more recent studies, TSTA has been shown to be synthesized during the lytic cycle. The ability to block its production with inhibitors of DNA-dependent RNA synthesis and inhibitors of protein synthesis suggests that TSTA appears as a virus-induced protein during productive infection (Girardi and Defendi, 1970). Whether it is virus coded is not known. The antigen has not been purified and its physical and chemical structures are unknown.

4.2. Induction of Host Cell Proteins

The synthesis of a number of enzymes, as well as host cell DNA and RNA synthesis, is stimulated after infection of permissive cells by SV40 and polyoma. Most of the enzymes have a function in DNA-synthetic pathways. The relationship between the early viral antigens and many of the induced enzymes is not clear, but the latter often resemble host enzymes in their properties. It is obvious that a genome of the size of SV40 or polyoma could not code for all of these proteins. Therefore, most, if not all, are presumed to be host enzymes, stimulated by viral infection (Basilico et al., 1969). A more complete discussion of the induction of cellular nucleic acids or enzymes can be found in a number of comprehensive reviews (Kit et al., 1966; Kit, 1967, 1968).

4.3. Virion-Associated Endonucleases

An endonuclease capable of introducing a single-strand endonucleolytic cleavage in the host genome has been found associated with purified polyoma (Cuzin et al., 1971) and SV40 virions (Kaplan et al., 1972; Kidwell et al., 1972). Since a productive infection can be established with viral DNA alone (Crawford *et al.*, 1964), these enzymes, in a virus-associated form, are not essential to the lytic cycle. If the endonuclease could be shown to be virus specific or site specific, however, the implications with respect to an integration function either in lytic or transforming cell interactions would be extremely important.

There is considerable uncertainty at present about whether the SV40-associated enzyme is virus specific; it is not unlikely that association of the endonuclease with the virion can occur as a result of the extraction procedure.

The endonuclease associated with SV40 virions is still present when virus preparations from both early and late temperature-sensitive mutants are grown at permissive temperatures and then incubated at the restrictive temperature for 1–2 h. This suggests that the *ts* functions are not required for the presence or activity of the enzyme (Kidwell *et al.*, 1972). Furthermore, the data at present do not suggest specificity with respect to the site of cleavage in the SV40 DNA, and prolonged incubation of SV40 DNA in the presence of the endonuclease leads to extensive digestion.

On the other hand, the endonuclease from polyoma virus is not associated with the early *ts* mutant, *TsA* (Cuzin *et al.*, 1970). Furthermore, this enzyme appears to introduce a specific break into the polyoma genome (F. Cuzin, A. Parodi, D. Blangy, O. Croissant, and P. Rouget, unpublished results). Determination of the source and activity of these virion-associated endonucleases will, of course, require further investigation.

4.4. Structural Proteins of SV40 and Polyoma

Late in the lytic cycle of SV40 and polyoma, subsequent to viral DNA replication, a new intranuclear antigen (V antigen) can be detected by immunofluorescent staining (Mayor *et al.*, 1962). This antigen reacts specifically with hyperimmune antisera against intact virions and almost certainly represents the viral coat protein(s). Since it is likely that the capsid protein is synthesized in the cytoplasm, its presence in the nucleus is probably the result of a rapid transport of synthesized coat protein to the nucleus for viral assembly. It is possible, however, that V antiserum is specific for assembled coat protein(s) which may be present only in cell nuclei. Whether the anti-V antisera are directed against one or more proteins is not known.

Since the capsid proteins of polyoma and SV40 can be obtained in large quantities and are relatively stable, they have been well characterized (Fine *et al.*, 1968; Girard *et al.*, 1970; Barban and Goor, 1971; Estes *et al.*, 1971; Hirt and Gesteland, 1971; Roblin *et al.*, 1971; Huang *et al.*, 1972a; Frearson and Crawford, 1972; Friedmann and David, 1972) (see Table 1). In the case of SV40, the major capsid polypeptide (VP1) has been shown by SDS-polyacrylamide gel electrophoresis to have a molecular weight between 43,000 and 45,000 and to constitute more than 75% of the total protein. Two other viral structural proteins (VP2, VP3) with molecular weights of approximately 30,000–38,000 and

TABLE 1

The Proteins of SV40 and Polyoma

Protein	Mol wt × 10⁻³	Predicted origin
VP1	43–48[a]	Viral capsid
VP2	30–38	Viral capsid
VP3	20–23	?
VP4	14–16	Host cell histone (F3)[b]
VP5	12–14	Host cell histone (F2b)
VP6	12–13	Host cell histone (F2a2)
VP7	10–12	Host cell histone (F2a1)

[a] In addition, some studies of polyoma proteins have demonstrated the presence of a larger polypeptide (mol wt 86,000) which is thought to be a dimer of VP1 (e.g., see Friedmann, 1974).
[b] The correspondence between the small viral polypeptides and particular host cell histones is based on studies by Lake *et al.* (1973), B. Hirt (personal communication), and D. Pett and M. K. Estes (personal communication).

20,000–23,000 daltons, respectively, have also been described which are present in smaller amounts than the major polypeptide; VP2 appears to be a capsid while the location of VP3 within the virion is uncertain.

The major capsid proteins of polyoma are similar in size to those of SV40 (VPI, 45,000–50,000; VP2, 30,000–35,000; and VP3, 20,000–25,000). In addition, there is a large polypeptide (P1) of approximately 80,000 daltons (Friedmann, 1974), which is thought to be a dimer of VP1. Peptide mapping of the tryptic digests of polyoma structural proteins suggests that some may share common polypeptide sequences and might have arisen by cleavage of a common precursor (Friedmann, 1974). Alternatively, the proteins may have been translated from overlapping segments of a common mRNA molecule. There appears to be no similarity in the peptide maps of the respective tryptic digests of polyoma and SV40 proteins, suggesting that the coat proteins of the two viruses are significantly different.

SDS-polyacrylamide gels have also been used to compare the proteins synthesized in SV40-infected monkey cells with those present in mock-infected cells. Among the new proteins detected in virus-infected cells were two corresponding in mobility to the major and minor capsid proteins (Fischer and Sauer, 1972; Ozer, 1972; Anderson and Gesteland, 1972; Walter *et al.*, 1972). A tryptic digest of the larger protein resulted in a peptide map quite similar to that obtained from the major SV40 capsid protein (Anderson and Gesteland, 1972). The capsid proteins are virus specific, and they are probably coded for by the late region of the viral genomes.

While viral DNA is itself infectious (Crawford *et al.*, 1964), the capsid proteins appear to provide a valuable if not essential function in the reproduction of these viruses. Infection of cells with intact virions is clearly much more efficient than infection with DNA. This may be related to an increased efficiency of absorption and/or penetration in the presence of the coat protein. It is also possible that the capsid protein protects the viral DNA from cellular nucleases.

The amino acid composition of the capsid proteins has been determined for both SV40 (Schlumberger *et al.*, 1968; Greenaway and LeVine, 1973) and polyoma virus (Murakami *et al.*, 1968). By use of an isoelectric focusing technique, differences are seen in the capsid proteins of a large-plaque SV40 strain as compared to small- or minute-plaque virus (Barban, 1973). Various plaque mutants also differ in their host cell restriction, temperature sensitivity, oncogenicity, and antigenicity (Takemoto *et al.*, 1966; Takemoto and Martin, 1970). Which of these properties, if any, is related to the differences in structural polypeptides remains to be determined. Differences in the polypeptides of polyoma plaque mutants have also been reported (Murakami *et al.*, 1968; Thorne *et al.*, 1968). While two large-plaque strains of polyoma have similar amino acid compositions, both appear to differ from a small-plaque polyoma strain (Murakami *et al.*, 1968).

Recent studies have shown that all of the SV40 structural proteins are phosphoproteins (Tan and Sokol, 1972) and that the phosphate groups are linked only to serine residues (Tan and Sokol, 1973). The significance of this finding with relationship to the structure or function of the virion polypeptides is still unknown.

4.5. *Internal Proteins*

A group of low molecular weight proteins (10,000–16,000 daltons; Table 1) have been found associated with the nucleic acid cores of both SV40 (Girard *et al.*, 1970; Barban and Goor, 1971; Estes *et al.*, 1971; Hirt and Gesteland, 1971; Huang *et al.*, 1972*a*; Frearson and Crawford, 1972) and polyoma (Roblin *et al.*, 1971; Frearson and Crawford, 1972; B. Hirt, unpublished results) virions. These polypeptides remain associated with the viral nucleic acid after mild alkaline treatment of intact virions (Estes *et al.*, 1971), and they are not found in empty viral capsids (Frearson and Crawford, 1972). Using SDS-polyacrylamide gel electrophoresis, three low molecular weight basic proteins are observed. But with tris-acetate–SDS-polyacrylamide gel electrophoresis it appears that at least four proteins are associated with SV40 cores (Lake *et al.*, 1973; Fig. 13). A considerable amount of data has been accumulated which strongly suggest that these basic polypeptides are derived from the host cell histones:

1. When permissive cells are labeled with ^{3}H-lysine prior to polyoma infection, a greater amount of label appears in the core proteins of progeny virions than in the viral capsid proteins (Frearson and Crawford, 1972).
2. The mobility of the SV40 basic polypeptides on tris-acetate–SDS-polyacrylamide gels corresponds directly to that of the evolutionarily conserved histones F3, F2b, F2a2, and F2a1 (Lake *et al.*, 1973; see Fig. 13). Similar results for SV40 proteins VP4–6 have been found in an independent study using similar methods (D. Pett and M. Estes, in preparation). Furthermore, the peptide maps of the core proteins of both polyoma and SV40

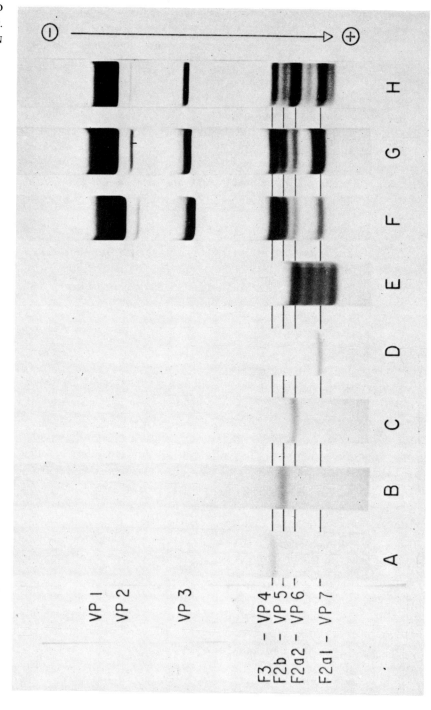

FIGURE 13. A comparison of various calf thymus and Vero cell histone fractions with SV40 structural proteins by 13% tris-acetate–SDS-polyacrylamide gel electrophoresis. (A) Calf thymus F3, (B) Vero cell F3, (C) calf thymus F2b, (D) calf thymus F2a2, (E) Vero cell histone fraction F2a contaminated with cleavage products of Vero F3, (F) SV40 complete, (G) SV40 plus calf thymus F2a1. (H) SV40 plus Vero cell fraction F2a as in (E). From Lake *et al.* (1973).

correspond to those of the basic proteins of the cell lines which support their permissive cycles, mouse and monkey kidney cultures (B. Hirt, unpublished results).

3. Histones are rich in two basic amino acids, arginine and lysine, but are deficient in tryptophan. When polyoma-infected mouse cells were labeled with ^{14}C-arginine and ^{3}H-tryptophan, both isotopes were found in the capsid protein of progeny virions, but only the ^{14}C-arginine was incorporated into a core polypeptide (Roblin *et al.*, 1971).

It has been suggested that although the small internal proteins of polyoma and SV40 may be host derived, it is unlikely that they are histones, on the basis of their higher tryptophan content (Greenaway and LeVine, 1973). This report is in disagreement with the findings previously mentioned. Considering all of the data presently available, it seems most likely that the core polypeptides of SV40 and polyoma are derived from the histones of the host cell.

While the relative proportions of the core proteins are the same in both whole virions and nuclear cores, there is clearly a predominance of VP4 (histone F3) in SV40 virions as compared to the concentration in host Vero cells (Lake *et al.*, 1973). This finding suggests a nonrandom incorporation of core proteins into virions and may be related to the histone's function. However, what role the core proteins perform in the virion is not known. On the basis of *in vitro* transcription studies with SV40 (Huang *et al.*, 1972*b*), it has been suggested that the histone-like proteins may have a regulatory function in the transcription of the genome. The kinetics and extent of transcription of an SV40 DNA template were compared with those of a deoxynucleoprotein template; the latter contained SV40 core proteins. Using the DNA-dependent RNA polymerase from either *E. coli* or a mammalian source, the rate of transcription of the SV40 deoxynucleoprotein complex (DNP I) was shown to be less than that of SV40 DNA I. Furthermore, competition-hybridization experiments showed that the extent of transcription of DNP I was less than that of SV40 DNA I. One interpretation of these data is that the core polypeptides exert a specific control over the transcription of the SV40 genome. It is conceivable that these histones also limit the gene sequences transcribed early after lytic infection.

4.6. SV40 Helper Function for Adenovirus Replication in Monkey Cells

While monkey kidney cells are semipermissive for the replication of adenoviruses, the ability of these viruses to replicate in such cells is greatly enhanced by coinfection with SV40 (Rabson *et al.*, 1964; O'Conor *et al.*, 1965). Whether or not this function relies on the presence of virus-coded protein is not known. It is known, however, that synthesis of new protein(s) is required since pretreatment of cells with cycloheximide prevents the enhancement of adenovirus reproduction (Friedman *et al.*, 1970). Coinfection with the nondefective (ND) adenovirus 2–SV40 hybrid virus [Ad2^{+}ND$_1$] can provide the helper function for adenovirus replication (A. Lewis *et al.*, in preparation). This hybrid virus contains only enough SV40 DNA (approximately 18% of the SV40 genome) to code for the SV40 U antigen (Lewis and Rowe, 1971); thus one might speculate that if the helper function is virus coded it might be provided by (or depend on) the SV40 U antigen.

A number of temperature-sensitive mutants of SV40 (including mutants in both early and late functions) were able to aid the replication of adenoviruses in monkey cells at the restrictive temperature (Jerkofsky and Rapp, 1973). This evidence suggests that the helper function is induced very early in the lytic cycle. In the same study it was shown that the SV40 helper function was ineffective in a particular continuous line of BSC-1 monkey kidney cells. This cell line is unique in that it fails to show an induction of host cell DNA synthesis after infection with SV40. Since the stimulation of host cell DNA synthesis is an event which occurs very early after SV40 infection of most monkey kidney cell lines, and does not occur in these BSC-1 cells, it is possible that the helper function for adenovirus replication is directly linked to the factor responsible for the stimulation of host cell DNA synthesis. Such a conclusion is supported by the demonstration that a clone of BSC-1 cells in which SV40 infection does stimulate host cell DNA synthesis would permit complementation of adenovirus replication by SV40 (Jerkofsky and Rapp, 1973). Kimura (1974) has found that one of his early SV40 mutants does not enhance adenovirus reproduction in monkey cells, thus confirming the need for an early SV40 function. Whether this SV40 mutant induces host cell DNA synthesis remains to be determined.

The nature of the helper function is not understood, but it has been shown that in the absence of coinfection with SV40, adenovirus 2 induces the synthesis of both early and late adenovirus RNA (Fox and Baum, 1972). Furthermore, this RNA is polyadenylated and transported to the cytoplasm. While some investigators have detected the presence of adenovirus proteins after abortive infection of monkey cells by adenoviruses alone (Friedman et al., 1970; Henry et al., 1971; Baum et al., 1972), they are clearly present in decreased quantities unless cells are coinfected with SV40. The block in adenovirus replication and the site of the SV40-related helper function may therefore reside at the level of the interaction of adenovirus mRNA with polyribosomes (Hashimoto et al., 1973; Fox and Baum, 1974), the translation of the message, or the processing of the polypeptides. In any case, the block seems to occur at a post-transcriptional level. This conclusion is further supported by the finding of equivalent amounts of polysome-associated adenovirus-specific RNA in enhanced and unenhanced infections. Furthermore, both populations of mRNA are translated in vitro with equal efficiency (L. Eron, H. Westphal, and G. Khoury, in preparation).

5. Cell Transformation by SV40 and Polyoma

Polyoma virus is able to produce tumors in newborn mice (Stewart et al., 1957) and SV40 will produce tumors in newborn hamsters (Eddy et al., 1962; Ashkenazi and Melnick, 1963; Black and Rowe, 1964). However, neither virus, has been implicated as the causative agent of a spontaneously occurring malignancy in its natural hosts. Since SV40 and polyoma can produce tumors *in vivo* and can transform tissue culture cells *in vitro*, they have been studied intensively during the past 15 years in the belief that they are valid models for defining the role of viral and cellular genes in establishing and maintaining a transformed state. This belief would also presume that tumor induction or cell transformation is analogous to naturally occurring malignant transformations. The small size of the viral genome and the ability to define the virus–cell interactions using biochemical and biophysical methods make it possible to describe some events with precision at the molecular level. There is no doubt that the simplicity of the virus and the distinct advantages in using cloned populations of cultured cells rather than animals are responsible for the rapid progress that has been made. The paucity of knowledge on the mechanisms of growth regulation in normal cells is an enormous barrier that has to be overcome before there can be a broader understanding of changes in cellular regulatory processes that occur after interaction with an oncogenic virus.

When permissive cells are exposed to polyoma virus or SV40, there may be a lytic response in which the cell is killed and virus replication occurs. In a nonpermissive cell, the virus will fail to replicate, but will transform a fraction of the cell population. Although SV40 produces tumors only in hamsters *in vivo*, it can transform mouse (Black and Rowe, 1963), rat (Diderholm *et al.*, 1966), rabbit (Black and Rowe, 1963), monkey (Fernandes and Moorhead, 1965), and human cells (Shein and Enders, 1962; Koprowski *et al.*, 1962) under *in vitro* conditions. Following exposure of human cells to SV40, replication of virus and transformation are both observed, and thus these cells are termed "semipermissive."

When a cell population which is nonpermissive for replication is exposed to SV40 or polyoma virus, a number of new phenotypic properties are acquired in a fraction of the exposed cell population; these properties are permanently retained by a small fraction of progeny cells and are transmitted in a stable way in cloned cell populations.

5.1. Properties of Transformed Cells

5.1.1. Growth and Metabolic Changes

When primary cells from a normal tissue are trypsinized and grown in tissue culture medium containing nutrients and serum factors, they will divide until confluency is reached. It appears that "signals" mediated by the proximity of normal cells to each other result, in contact inhibition of cell movement (Abercrombie and Heaysman, 1954) and division (Dulbecco, 1970). The addition of fresh serum at his point results in some additional growth. After several cell passages, however, the growth potential declines, and unless some type of spontaneous, chemical-induced, or viral-induced "transformation" occurs the culture will not persist. In response to inoculation with polyoma or SV40, a wide variety of cells will undergo a series of changes collectively referred to as transformation (see reviews, Enders, 1965; Sambrook, 1972). The growth potential and rate are markedly increased. In addition, cells lose their capacity for growth in an orderly array, and they no longer remain contact inhibited. Transformed cells form randomly oriented, dense colonies, and confluent monolayers often contain more than 10 times as many cells as their normal counterparts. An increased production of lactic acid has been related not only to the rate of growth but also to a shift in the cellular metabolism towards anaerobic glycolysis. The transformed cells frequently differ in morphology from the cells from which they were derived.

The increased growth potential of transformed cells is also demonstrated by their ability to grow under stringent conditions, and this allows for the selection of transformants. Examples of these selective conditions include the ability of transformed cells to grow in soft agar or methylcellulose (Macpherson and Montagnier, 1964), on monolayers of normal cells (Temin and Rubin, 1958), or in a medium which is deficient in serum or growth factors (Smith et al., 1971). Even more impressive than the vigorous growth of the transformed cells is the fact that they no longer are constrained to a finite lifetime in tissue culture; under the proper growth conditions, they will persist and can be passaged indefinitely.

It is generally believed that only a fraction of the cell population is transformed, even when the cells are exposed to very high levels of virus. Using mouse 3T3 cells, 40% of the cells are transformed when exposed to 10^4 TCID/cell (Todaro and Green, 1966b). With polyoma, 5–10% of the BHK cells are transformed at high input multiplicities (Macpherson and Montagnier, 1964; Williams and Till, 1964). The failure to transform the entire cell population cannot be explained on the basis of genetic heterogeneity of the cell population, since cloned cells have been used in some studies; neither can it be due to the fact that cells can be transformed only if they are in a particular part of the cell cycle (Basilico and Marin, 1966). In the studies cited above, cells were scored as transformants using a single criterion, i.e., if they grew in soft agar or if they gave rise to fusiform colonies. Recently 3T3 cells that had been exposed to SV40 (2000 PFU/cell) were selected at random. When they were scored on the basis of a single criterion, fusiform colony formation, 10% of the population appeared to be transformed. In contrast, the randomly selected population had altered genetic properties. In addition to cells which finally were scored as "normal transformants," 40% of the cells studied had acquired the ability to grow in low concentrations of calf serum but were T-antigen negative. It was concluded that the ability to grow in medium containing low serum concentrations is the primary effect when nonpermissive cells are exposed to SV40 infection (Risser and Pollack, 1974).

In human cell lines, which show a wide difference in the frequency of transformation, there is a direct relationship between the transformation frequency and the fraction of SV40 T-antigen-producing cells. However, in all of the human cell lines there seems to be a fixed probability (1 in 250) that T-antigen-positive cells can give rise to a cell transformant (Aaronson and Todaro, 1968). These results would suggest that the initial expression of T antigen is a necessary but not sufficient condition for cells which finally give rise to transformants. It would be interesting to know if the transient expression of T antigen is a necessary event in those cells which acquire the ability to grow in low serum concentrations but which eventually become T-antigen negative.

5.1.2. Chromosomal Changes

In parallel with the morphological and growth changes, a number of chromosomal modifications have been documented. Sequential chromosomal aberrations are abundant and include chromosomal breakage, the appearance of dicentric rings and other abnormal forms, and a general tendency toward heteroploidy (often a hypotetraploid number). The problem in evaluating many of these cytogenetic changes is in deciding whether they represent the cause or the effect of transformation. Most karyotypic analyses have been performed long after the transformation event, and it is clear that there is a progression of chromosomal changes which continue long after the detection of the transformed phenotype by other methods. It is possible that the heritable changes associated with viral transformation may affect the chromosomes, especially in light of the association between viral transformation and integration of the viral genome. But so far there has been little information from karyological analysis which could offer an explanation for the alterations associated with transformed cells. The techniques previously applied for chromosome analysis were not sensitive enough to describe the important changes. Recent progress, however, promises to eliminate some of these problems. It is hoped that some of our newer tools, such as restriction enzymes, will help us to localize the site and function of transforming agents even more precisely.

5.1.3. Cell Surface Changes

As was mentioned above, a basic property of "normal" cells in tissue culture is their apparent recognition of and respect for the boundaries of adjacent cells. It is at the cell membrane where these contacts are made; therefore, it would seem reasonable to investigate the membranes of normal and transformed cells in hopes of finding differences which could be related to a loss of contact inhibition. A number of investigators have been able to demonstrate quantitative differences in the chemical composition of membranes from transformed cells and their untransformed counterparts. The technique of membrane staining with ruthenium red followed by visualization with electron microscopy has also been used in an attempt to distinguish normal and transformed cell membranes (Vorbrodt and Koprowski, 1969). These studies have demonstrated increased undulation and microvilli formation on the free surface of S40-transformed cells, changes not seen in "normal" cells. The function of these structures is unknown.

Of more immediate interest are a number of studies which point to a functional difference between the surfaces of normal and transformed cells. One of the properties of transformed cells which has recently received much attention is their agglutinability by concanavalin A and wheat germ agglutinin. These compounds are in the category of lectins, glycoproteins which are frequently obtained from plant sources and have an affinity for binding to the carbohydrate groups on cell surfaces (see Tooze, 1973, for a discussion of the properties of these compounds).

Of particular interest is the fact that these compounds preferentially agglutinate transformed cells (Burger, 1969; Pollack and Burger, 1969; Inbar and Sachs, 1969). However, if "normal" cells are treated for a limited time with proteolytic enzymes, they demonstrate enhanced agglutinability. Studies with lectins suggest that the surface structure of the transformed cell which is responsible for increased agglutination is virus induced, but not virus specific, since exposure to virus or a proteolytic enzyme appears to uncover the same binding sites (Burger, 1969; Inbar and Sachs, 1969). A virus function may be responsible for exposure of the lectin binding site, since cells transformed by an early polyoma temperature-sensitive mutant (ts-3) showed a much lower level of agglutination when grown at the nonpermissive temperature as compared with the permissive temperature. Furthermore, there is a particular group of host range polyoma virus mutants which neither induce cell transformation nor increase the agglutinability of cells infected by them (Benjamin and Burger, 1970).

To make the picture even more complex, several careful investigations employing radiolabeled lectins have clearly demonstrated that there are an equal number of binding sites on normal, trypsin-treated, and transformed cells (Cline and Livingstone, 1971; Ozanne and Sambrook, 1971b). While there are some investigators who still feel that a substantial difference exists in the number of binding sites on normal and transformed cells, it now seems that a difference in the distribution of binding sites in the two cell types may be responsible for the differential agglutination. Thus it is possible that transformation or trypsinization leads to a clustering of binding sites, which in turn is responsible for the increased agglutination reaction. These studies, as well as others relating to membrane function, appear to have reached a level where a better understanding of membrane biochemistry is required for further progress.

5.1.4. Antigenic Changes

The early antigens, which appear in the lytic cycle prior to DNA replication (T antigen and, in the case of SV40, U antigen), are found in all cells transformed by the papovaviruses. The tumor-specific transplantation antigen (TSTA), which is found during the lytic infection, is also present in transformed cells. This antigen is present on the cell surface and has been detected only by in vivo experiments involving the establishment of immunity to tumor transplantation. The properties of these antigens have already been discussed in some detail (see Section 4.1). Experiments to develop an in vitro test for TSTA have employed the serum from an immunized hamster responding to a challenge with transformed cells (Tevethia and Rapp, 1965). By use of this antiserum in both cytotoxicity and indirect immunofluorescence tests, it is possible to demonstrate the presence of an antigen on the surface of transformed cells. Other investigators using similar techniques confirmed the presence of an S antigen(s) in SV40-transformed cells. It was at first thought that the S antigen might be identical to TSTA. Considerable

doubt resulted from the study of a series of transformed hamster cell lines, some
clones of which contained the S but not the T antigen (Diamandopoulos *et al.*, 1968). In further studies it was found that these S^+T^- lines contained no detectable SV40-specific DNA or RNA (Levine *et al.*, 1970) and could not induce immunity to transplantation of other SV40-transformed cells (Tevethia *et al.*, 1968). Thus it seems clear that at least this S antigen is different from the SV40 TSTA and is not virus specific. Nevertheless, the presence of S antigen in SV40-transformed cells, but not in normal cells or cells transformed by other viruses, suggests that it may be virus induced. A possible clue to the identity of the S antigen was provided by the demonstration that sera from pregnant hamsters would react with it (Duff and Rapp, 1970). This study was based on the assumption that S antigen may in fact represent a fetal antigen which is derepressed by the virus in the transformed cell. However, other studies suggest that certain S antigen(s) may be unique in each transformed line and may, at times, exist in a cryptic form (Collins and Black, 1973*a,b*).

How the S antigen relates to the sites for lectin binding is not known. It should be mentioned, however, that the S antigen may be virus specific, whereas increased agglutinability by lectins resulted from viral, chemical, or even spontaneous transformation. Therefore, unless the S antigen is just one of many lectin binding sites, the two may well be unrelated (see also review by Butel *et al.*, 1972).

5.2. Detection of the Viral Genome in Transformed Cells

In all stably transformed cells there is evidence for the persistence of at least part of the viral genome. A number of procedures have been used to demonstrate the presence of viral DNA. The first of these employed *E. coli* DNA-dependent RNA polymerase to synthesize radioactive RNA, complementary to DNA I. This radioactive probe was then hybridized with transformed cellular DNA which had been immobilized on a nitrocellulose filter. The amount of bound RNA was compared to the amount which annealed with DNA from nontransformed cells (background) and, in order to calibrate the reaction, with known quantities of SV40 DNA that were immobilized on filters. The initial estimates of the number of integrated viral genomes (5–60 SV40 DNA equivalents per cell) appear to have been high (Westphal and Dulbecco, 1968), and more recent studies have given values closer to 1–10 viral genome equivalents per cell (Levine *et al.*, 1970). A second method uses as a probe viral DNA, which can be labeled either *in vivo* with $^{32}PO_4$ or ^3H-thymidine, or *in vitro* using DNA polymerase I, ^{32}P- or ^3H-deoxyribonucleotides, and unlabeled SV40 DNA II. When this DNA is denatured and reannealed, the rate of duplex formation is a function of the DNA concentration. If the DNA concentration of the probe is doubled, the time required to effect 50% reannealing is reduced by one-half. High concentrations of cellular DNA from control cells have only a slight accelerating effect on the rate at which the probe (the labeled DNA) reanneals. However, transformed cell DNA does accelerate the rate of reassociation of the probe, and the extent of enhancement in the rate of renaturation can be related to the number of viral genome equivalents in the transformed cell DNA. With this procedure it has been calculated that various transformed cell lines contain 1–3 genome equivalents (Gelb et al., 1971; Ozanne et al., 1973). One interesting modification of this procedure has been the use of probes generated by restriction enzymes which correspond to specific fractions of the viral genome (Sharp et al., 1974; Botchan et al., 1974). By use of this procedure, it can be demonstrated that certain parts of the adenovirus genome may not be present in transformed cell lines but that other specific regions are present in all of the transformed lines. Another recent procedure employs radioactive strand-separated SV40 DNA as a probe (Khoury et al., 1974b). The concentration of cellular DNA which is required to convert 50% of the single-stranded probe to a duplex form is determined, and this gives a quantitative measure of the gene equivalents in the cell. In this system the probe cannot self-anneal, so reannealing with DNA from transformed cells can be carried out for extended time periods, allowing the use of less cellular DNA even when examining viral genomes present in a low copy number. The results obtained using this method are in agreement with those of Gelb et al. (1971).

5.3. State of the Viral DNA Within Transformed Cells

It is now generally assumed that viral DNA in transformed cells is integrated within the cell genome. However, this assumption is based on the few cases where it has been convincingly demonstrated that the viral sequences in transformed cells are covalently linked to high molecular weight cellular DNA. Viral DNA sequences have also been demonstrated in chromosomes isolated from transformed cells (Sambrook et al., 1968; Hirai and Defendi, 1971). When chromosomes were isolated from transformed Chinese hamster cells and transferred to permissive BSC-1 cells, there was a low but consistent activation of T antigen and infectious virus (Shani et al., 1974). These findings also support the presence of SV40 in an integrated state and provide an alternative procedure for determining the site of integration.

Studies with mouse–SV40-transformed human cell hybrids suggest that integration of the viral DNA occurs at a specific site in the cell genome. The expression of T antigen has been scored in these hybrid cells where there is a selective loss of the human chromosomes. The human chromosome C7 was present in all hybrid clones positive for T antigen. Hybrid cells that contain the C7 chromosome and are T-antigen positive give rise, after fusion with CV-1 cells, to V-antigen-positive fused cells (Croce et al., 1973). Based on this finding, it is likely that SV40 is integrated into this chromosome. It will be interesting to have direct evidence for the number of viral gene equivalents in these hybrid cells.

The data on the conditions that are necessary to effect integration are somewhat unclear, and very limited. Current studies with ts mutants provide clear evidence that mutants defective in the early function(s) are unable to transform cells at the restrictive temperature. If SV40 is added to nonpermissive CH cells, in which virus does not replicate but in which transformation does occur, SV40 DNA is found linked to high molecular weight cellular DNA. This linkage is observed even when inhibitors which block DNA replication are present (Hirai and Defendi, 1971). Since there is integration of viral DNA into the cell genome during a lytic cycle, it is unclear whether this integration in the nonpermissive CH cells provides a meaningful insight into those events which produce a stably transformed cell. Cell growth and cell division are necessary to effect transformation. When contact-inhibited 3T3 cells are infected with SV40, the frequency in the number of transformed cells decreases as a function of time prior to cell division (Todaro and Green, 1966a).

The sites of integration which are observed when cells are first transformed may differ from the integration sites in stably transformed cell lines. By study of the reassociation of restriction enzyme fragments of SV40 DNA, the properties of a stably transformed line have been analyzed (Botchan *et al.*, 1974). The effect of the cellular DNA from SVT2 cells (an SV40-transformed mouse cell line) on the rate of reassociation of four Endo R · *Hpa* I + R · *Eco* R$_1$ SV40 fragments (see Fig. 3) has been measured. It was concluded that at least a single copy of the entire viral genome was present, but that an early part of the genome was present six times. Since transformation can be effected by a single virus particle, this would suggest that extensive rearrangements have occurred either during or subsequent to the establishment of the stably transformed cell line. Again, it is unclear whether this rearrangement is a necessary condition for the maintenance of transformation. The application of reassociation kinetic methodology to a number of transformed lines, at different times during their development, will be of great interest.

5.4. Transcription in Transformed Cells

While it is still conceivable that following integration the papovavirus genomes play no further role in the maintenance of transformation, most investigators would prefer to believe in the active contribution of a viral coded function. There is some evidence from studies with temperature-sensitive mutants of polyoma and SV40 that this is the case (see Section 6). In addition, we have no evidence that there are any papovavirus-transformed cell lines in which virus-specific RNA is not synthesized. A considerable effort has been devoted to characterizing virus-specific RNA in transformed cells in the hope that this information might give some clue to the possible gene(s) involved in a putative maintenance function.

5.5. Patterns of Transcription

The results of these studies evolved in parallel with the various hybridization techniques used for analysis of virus-specific RNA and are best evaluated chronologically (see also Tooze, 1973).

5.5.1. Filter Hybridization

As mentioned previously, Benjamin was the first to detect polyoma virus-specific ^{3}H-labeled RNA on filters containing immobilized polyoma virus DNA (Benjamin, 1966). This technique was essentially that described by Gillespie and Spiegelman (1965).

5.5.2. Competition Filter Hybridization

A number of investigators subsequently employed a modification of the filter hybridization procedure to compare the gene sequences transcribed in lytically infected cells with those from transformed cells (Aloni et al., 1968; Oda and Dulbecco, 1968b; Sauer and Kidwai, 1968). Saturating amounts of a radiolabeled RNA were annealed to a fixed amount of viral DNA on a filter. A second filter with the same amount of DNA was first incubated with a saturating amount of unlabeled "competitor RNA"; subsequently, saturating amounts of the first radiolabeled RNA were added to this second filter. The decrease in radioactivity on the second filter was a reflection of the common sequences (competition) shared with the unlabeled RNA. With this technique, there was general agreement that RNA from transformed cells could compete with 30–50% of late virus-specific lytic RNA and most if not all of the early viral RNA.

5.5.3. Saturation Filter Hybridization

In the saturation filter hybridization technique, devised by Martin and Axelrod (1969a,b; see Section 3), a known amount of ^{14}C-radiolabeled DNA was bound on filters. To these filters, increasing amounts of ^{32}P-labeled transformed cell RNA of known specific activity were added. The RNA/DNA ratio at saturation was therefore an indication of the extent of transcription. In a series of SV40-transformed cell lines, it was shown that the equivalent of 50–100% of a strand of SV40 DNA was transcribed. The finding of transformed lines with transcription levels of greater than 50% of a strand equivalent is in contrast with the results of competition-hybridization studies.

5.5.4. Solution Hybridization

Separation of the strands of SV40 DNA (Khoury et al., 1972; Sambrook et al., 1972) and polyoma DNA (Kamen et al., 1974) eliminated the need for immobilization of DNA on filters to prevent DNA–DNA renaturation, and thus some of the problems inherent in filter hybridization experiments could be circumvented. Background hybridization levels were reduced essentially to zero, allowing for a more detailed evaluation of low levels of hybridization, but more importantly the template function of the viral DNA strands could be evaluated separately. Hybridization experiments with transformed cell RNAs and the separated strands of SV40 DNA were performed by the groups which had used this technique to describe the pattern of transcription in the lytic cycle (Sambrook et al., 1972; Khoury et al., 1973a; Ozanne et al., 1973). Their results are in rather good agreement with each other and with the recent analysis of RNA from polyoma-transformed cells (Kamen *et al.*, 1974). Most transformed cell lines contain RNA complementary only to the minus (early) strand of viral DNA, and the extent of this transcription for that strand varies from about 40 to 80%. A few transformed cell lines appear to contain RNA homologous to small regions of the plus (late) strand, and these RNA sequences are present at low concentrations.

In liquid-phase *summation hybridization experiments*, saturating amounts of early RNA and/or RNA of a particular transformed cell were incubated with the separated strands of SV40 DNA. The extent of annealing with the minus (early) strand was the same whether or not early lytic RNA was added to the transformed cell RNA (Khoury *et al.*, 1973*a*). This result showed that each of the transformed cell RNAs contained a full complement of early RNA.

The presence of early SV40 RNA in transformed cell lines has been confirmed by mapping experiments using the separated strands of restriction enzyme fragments of SV40 and polyoma DNA (Khoury *et al.*, 1973; Sambrook *et al.*, 1973; Kamen *et al.*, 1974). In addition, the "anti-late" sequences in various transformed cell lines have been localized to the 5' RNA end of the early region (Khoury *et al.*, 1974*c*; B. Ozanne *et al.*, personal communication). In a kinetic analysis, it has been shown that these "anti-late" sequences are present in considerably lower concentrations than the true early RNA sequences (Khoury *et al.*, 1975*b*). In summary, the mapping experiments with transformed cell RNAs confirm and extend the models for expression of integrated DNA which have previously been proposed (Sambrook *et al.*, 1972; Khoury *et al.*, 1973*a*; Ozanne *et al.*, 1973). Integration of SV40 DNA into the host cell genome almost certainly occurs with a cleavage in the late-gene region of the virus. Two models for the mechanism of transcription then seem possible, and both make use of the fact that transcription of the DNA strand expressed in transformed cells (minus strand) proceeds in a counterclockwise direction (Khoury *et al.*, 1973*b*; Sambrook *et al.*, 1973). In model A, most rounds of transcription recognize the early viral promoter (P_E) and terminator (T_E). Occasionally, transcription is initiated within the host genome and continues through the viral genes to the viral terminator T_E. This latter event is responsible for the low levels of transcription of anti-late RNA sequences and would provide some indication (based on which anti-late sequences are present) about the site of cleavage within the viral genome. Alternatively, extensive regions of one or both DNA strands may be transcribed, as is the case during the lytic cycle (model B, Fig. 14). Subsequent degradation of all but the early viral sequences would lead to their abundance. Incomplete degradation of the anti-late RNA might result in its detection at a lower concentration, and the localization of these sequences to the 5' RNA side of the early region may indicate that a putative processing enzyme proceeds in that direction. If model B is correct, the integration site in the viral DNA may be anywhere within the late gene region. Since the evaluations of transcription in transformed cells have thus far employed total cellular RNA, we do not yet know if the anti-late RNA sequences are present in the cytoplasm of transformed cells. If they are not, the analogy to transcription and processing in the lytic system might lead one to favor a model similar to B.

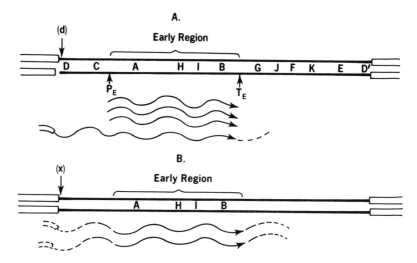

FIGURE 14. Two models for the transcription of SV40 DNA in transformed cell lines. See the text for a description of each model. ▭, Host cell DNA; ——, viral DNA; P_E and T_E, putative promoter and terminator for transcription of the early viral genes; ——, abundant viral RNA sequences; ---, scarce RNA sequences; A–K, *Hin* fragments of SV40 DNA; (d), a specific cleavage site (in *Hin* D) for integration of viral into host cell DNA; (x), a random cleavage site (in the late SV40 genes) for integration. From Khoury *et al.* (1975*b*).

5.6. Concentration and Size of Virus-Specific RNA

A number of investigators have obtained estimates for the fraction of transformed cellular RNA which is SV40 or polyoma specific (Benjamin, 1965). Values appear to range from 0.001 to 0.04%, and, considering the relative scarcity of virus-specific sequences as well as the variety of techniques employed, these results are in quite good agreement (see review by Winocour, 1969). As has been pointed out previously, it is this paucity of virus-specific RNA which has limited the analysis of transcription in transformed cells. Fortunately, the use of highly radiolabeled DNA probes, hybridization techniques with little or no background levels, and methods for concentrating mRNA (see Section 3) should provide a successful approach to this analysis.

The size of RNA in SV40-transformed cells has been studied in several laboratories (Tonegawa *et al.*, 1970; Martin, 1970; Wall and Darnell, 1971; Weinberg *et al.*, 1974). There is general agreement that some of the virus-specific RNA molecules in SV40-transformed cells are larger than a single strand of DNA (i.e., greater than 1.6×10^6 daltons). For the most part, these sequences are localized in the nucleus and are not found in cytoplasm. Although this suggests a precursor–product relationship, none has yet been established. Since it is known that SV40 and polyoma DNAs are integrated within the transformed cellular DNA, a plausible explanation for these large RNA molecules would be the cotranscription of host and viral gene sequences, analogous to the mechanism proposed for the transcription of integrated SV40 and polyoma DNA during the lytic cycle (see Section 3.3). This explanation would fit with either model of Fig. 14 and the data from mapping studies which led to its proposal. In fact, there is evidence that these large virus-specific RNA molecules can be selected on SV40 DNA-containing filters, eluted, and reannealed to filters containing host cellular DNA (Wall and Darnell, 1971). This would suggest that the host and viral RNA sequences are contained within the same RNA molecules. This study would also suggest that viral sequences are adjacent to a repetitive fraction of host RNA sequences, since the conditions of annealing to the host cell DNA filters would select almost exclusively for reiterated RNA. Such a result might appear to be in contrast to the finding of Gelb and Martin (1973), who showed by renaturation kinetics that the S40 genome was primarily adjacent to unique cellular sequences in transformed cell lines. However, Gelb and Martin did detect some association between SV40 and reiterated host DNA, and it may be this set of sequences that was detected by Wall and Darnell.

When RNA from a number of SV40-transformed cell lines was first selected on the basis of poly(A)-associated tracts and then subjected to acrylamide gel electrophoresis, the major species of virus-specific RNA was found to migrate between 18S and 28S (Weinberg *et al.*, 194). This appears to be somewhat larger than 19S early species found by these same authors. Whether the larger size reflects the presence of the 5' RNA "anti-late" sequences described above remains to be determined.

5.7. Properties of "Untransformed Revertants" Selected from Transformed Cell Cultures

Studies with temperature-sensitive mutants suggest that a viral gene is involved in establishing and maintaining the transformed state. One approach to analyzing its role is to isolate revertant cells which have regained the phenotype of untransformed cells. When these revertants are selected based on reversion of one cell property, one can then test to see which other properties of transformed cells also revert and try to establish what obligatory linkages exist between the various transformed cell properties.

All of the procedures that are used to select revertants employ conditions where preferential killing of transformed cells can be effected. When confluent transformed cell cultures are maintained in medium containing bromodeoxyuridine or 5-fluorodeoxyuridine, transformed cells continue to synthesize DNA and as a consequence are killed. Cell revertants which fail to grow in confluent cultures can be recovered and these revertants will have regained a number of properties of untransformed cells (Pollack *et al.*, 1968). Similarly, revertants can be selected from transformed cell populations using methylcellulose or soft agar to effect selective growth. Transformed cells which can grow in semisolid medium will incorporate the base analogue 5-bromodeoxyuridine, and these cells are killed by exposing the culture to blue light (Wyke, 1971), thus allowing the selection of revertants which are unable to grow in this medium. Isolation of revertants and selective killing of transformed cells have also been carried out with nucleic acid analogues in medium containing 1% serum, where revertants are unable to grow and therefore survive (Vogel and Pollack, 1973). Other investigators have employed concanavalin A, which will preferentially kill transformed cells (Ozanne and Sambrook, 1971a; Culp and Black, 1972; Wollman and Sachs, 1972). Preferential survival of revertant cells contained in a transformed cell population has been demonstrated when cells are plated on monolayers that have been fixed with glutaraldehyde (Rabinowitz and Sachs, 1968) or when the cells are plated at very low cell concentrations (Rabinowitz and Sachs, 1969). There is no obvious biological reason why these latter two methods should select for revertants. In fact, the cells which are selected by these procedures seem to differ from revertant cells selected by the other procedures that result in the killing of growing transformed cells. The procedures that employ glutaraldehyde-fixed monolayers and plating at high dilutions yield a 200-fold higher number of cell revertants (2%) compared to the 0.01% frequency of reversion obtained by the alternative procedures described above. Furthermore, the frequency of reversion of the phenotypically normal cells to the transformed phenotype is very high with these procedures.

The properties of revertants are listed in Table 2. There seem to be a number of common properties shared by the revertants. As might be expected from the way

TABLE 2

Characteristics of Revertant Cell Lines Isolated from SV40-Transformed 3T3 Cells[a]

	Saturation density[b]	Serum requirement[c]	Anchorage requirement[d]
Line			
3T3	Normal	Normal	Normal
SV101	Transformed	Transformed	Transformed
Density revertants selected with			
FUdR	Normal	Transformed	Normal
BUdR	Normal	Transformed	Normal
Colchicine	Normal	Normal	Normal
Concanavalin A revertants			
	Normal	Transformed	Normal
Serum revertants selected in			
1% calf serum	Normal	Normal	Normal
Aγ-depleted calf serum	Normal	Normal	Transformed

[a] We are grateful to Dr. Robert Pollack, who provided some of these data prior to publication.
[b] Normal cells have saturation densities less than 15×10^4 cells/cm^2 in 10% calf serum.
[c] Assayed by growth in 1% calf serum. Normal cells have doubling times greater than 80 h; transformed cells double in 35 h or less.
[d] Assayed by ability to form a colony in Methocel. Normal cells do not form colonies in Methocel; transformed cells do.

in which they are selected, the cells have a more normal phenotype; that is, they grow with a more ordered cell orientation, achieve lower saturation cell densities, fail to grow in soft agar, and are not agglutinated by plant lectins. Yet with few exceptions (Martin and Macpherson, 1969) the cells would be classified as transformed cells according to biochemical criteria. They contain quantities of viral RNA and DNA that are similar to those contained in the transformants from which they arose. They are T-antigen positive and infectious virus can be rescued by cell fusion. There may be specific chromosome losses or gains which can be related to transformation and reversion (Hitotsumachi *et al.*, 1971). In most of the selection procedures, cell revertants obtained from confluent monolayers or from soft agar still behave as transformants with regard to their ability to grow in medium containing 1% serum. Revertants selected after preferential killing of transformed cells that grew in 1% serum had properties that were the same as those of other revertants except that they required 10% serum for growth (Vogel and Pollack, 1973).

The findings with revertant cells provide some insight into the process of transformation. Since revertants contain the viral genome, and since infectious virus can be rescued by cell fusion, the presence of the complete viral genome within the cell is not sufficient to produce a transformed cell. At this time we don't know if there are several separate classes of transformants which are phenotypically equivalent but which differ depending on the procedure used for their selection. While there is some evidence for a specific integration site of the viral genome in transformed cells, it is not clear whether a meaningful relationship exists between the number of viral genome equivalents present in the transformed lines and the properties of the transformed and/or revertant cells selected from these populations. It is known that primary cells, which have a limited lifetime in culture, become capable of infinite survival after transformation. Perhaps there is some connection between this fact and the observation that in almost every case revertants still retain the viral genome.

When revertants are selected from transformed cell populations by procedures that depend on cell properties initially used to select the transformants, revertants always differ significantly from the originally untransformed cells. As we have already noted, in a biochemical sense the revertants are still similar to transformed cells. Phenotypically, the cells, while similar to untransformed cells, achieve somewhat higher densities at confluency than the parental untransformed cells, and in the confluent monolayers there is still some continued DNA synthesis. The revertant cells at confluency do not consistently accumulate in the G_1 phase as do normal cells (R. Pollack, personal communication). The study of revertants of transformed cells demonstrates clearly that certain phenotypic properties are regulated in a number of independent ways.

A number of phenotypic changes can be effected in transformed cells in a reversible way using cyclic AMP and/or its derivatives. These morphological changes are noted within a few hours and the effects are reversible. Pastan and Johnson (1974) have reviewed the relationship of cyclic AMP to transformation in some detail.

5.8. *Transformation of Cells with Viral DNA Fragments*

A useful procedure has recently been devised for demonstrating the biological activity of viral DNA. When viral DNA is coprecipitated with calcium phosphate, there is an effective uptake of the precipitated DNA by cells (Graham and van der Eb, 1973). This technique has proven effective in assaying the infectivity of adenovirus DNA types 1 and 5, and SV40 DNA. When adenovirus DNA is fragmented, infectivity is lost, but the DNA fragments can effect transformation of rat cells as efficiently as intact DNA (Graham *et al.*, 1974). DNA fragments as small as 1×10^6 daltons are capable of transformation, and studies with DNA fragments generated by restriction enzymes demonstrate that this transforming activity resides in a specific portion of the viral genome. Similar studies with SV40 suggest that in this virus, too, transformation can be effected by that fraction of the viral genome which codes for the early viral function(s) (F. L. Graham and A. J. van der Eb, personal communication).

6. *Genetic Approach to SV40 and Polyoma*

It would appear from the discussion in previous sections that the interaction between papovaviruses and their host cells is quite complex. Yet the SV40 and polyoma virus genomes are small, with a coding capacity for three to seven proteins. By isolating and studying the properties of conditionally lethal mutants, it was hoped that particular biological properties could be directly related to the function of specific viral proteins and that these functions, in turn, could be mapped on the viral genome. This approach has been particularly successful in the last 4 years, largely through the efforts of several investigators who have isolated and characterized large numbers of temperature-sensitive (*ts*) mutants.

6.1. *SV40 ts Mutants*

At this time, more than 150 SV40 *ts* mutants have been isolated and partially characterized (Tegtmeyer *et al.*, 1970; Kit *et al.*, 1968; Tegtmeyer and Ozer, 1971; Robb and Martin, 1972; Kimura and Dulbecco, 1972, 1973; Chou and Martin, 1974; Dubbs *et al.*, 1974). These mutants can be organized into five classes on the basis of physiological function and/or their behavior in complementation assays.

6.1.1. *Group A*

The *ts* mutants of complementation group A appear to be defective in an early viral function. At the nonpermissive temperature, they are able to infect cells and synthesize early virus-specific RNA (Cowan *et al.*, 1973; R. Saral, G. Khoury, J. Chou, and R. Martin, unpublished results), but T antigen appears to be abnormal (P. Tegtmeyer, and M. Osborn and K. Weber, personal communications).

Furthermore, the group A mutants are able to induce neither host cell (J. Chou and R. Martin, personal communication) nor SV40 (Tegtmeyer, 1972) DNA synthesis. If, however, a cycle of viral DNA synthesis is initiated at the permissive temperature and the cells are then shifted to the nonpermissive temperature, that cycle of DNA synthesis is completed (Tegtmeyer, 1972) and late virus-specific RNA synthesis continues (Cowan et al., 1973; Girard et al., 1974). Group A mutants are able to transform a variety of cells at the permissive temperature but do not transform these cells at the nonpermissive temperature. Of particular interest is the recent finding with cells that have been transformed by group A ts mutants at the permissive temperature. When these transformed cells are shifted to the restrictive temperature, certain transformed phenotypic properties may revert (R. Tegtmeyer; R. Martin, J. Chou, J. Avila, and R. Saral; J. Butel, J. S. Brugge, and C. A. Noonan; M. Osborn and K. Weber—personal communications).

The mutants of group A are not thermolabile, and infection under nonpermissive conditions does not result in the production of detectable structural proteins (Tegtmeyer and Ozer, 1971; Chou and Martin, personal communication). Finally, in elegant marker rescue experiments, Lai and Nathans (1974) showed that these group A mutants map in Hin fragments H and I, which are located in the middle of the early SV40 region (see Fig. 12). Whether there are one or more subgroups within group A is still a matter of speculation. However, the recent findings of Kimura (1974) suggest there may be at least two subgroups. His results show that a particular group A mutant could not assist the replication of adenovirus in monkey cells (see Section 4.6). These results are in contrast to those of Jerkofsky and Rapp (1973), who found an early SV40 mutant which did provide the helper function at the nonpermissive temperature. One possible explanation for these results would be the presence of two distinct early subgroups. Whether the difference in these early mutants relates to their ability to induce host cell DNA synthesis is presently under investigation.

In summary, then, it seems likely that group A mutants represent a defect in the early SV40 gene region which codes for an early viral protein(s). The early region now appears to represent 45–50% of the genome (see Section 3.7) and therefore could code for a protein as large as T-antigen. At any rate, the early function(s) appears to directly or indirectly induce the synthesis of host cell DNA, viral DNA, and, in turn, late viral mRNA. A candidate protein would most likely be a DNA-binding protein, and such properties have recently been ascribed to T antigen (R. Carrol, D. Livingston, personal communications). This protein might be a polymerase, an unwinding protein, and/or an endonuclease, and considerable effort is presently being devoted to its purification and characterization.

6.1.2. Groups B, C, and BC

SV40 ts mutants of groups B and C (complementing) and BC (noncomplementing) are thermolabile and induce the synthesis of an altered V antigen or capsid protein (Tegtmeyer et al., 1970; Tegtmeyer and Ozer, 1971; Kimura and

Dulbecco, 1972; Dubbs *et al.*, 1974; Chou and Martin, 1974). Since they have been shown by marker rescue experiments (Lai and Nathans, 1974) to map in a relatively circumscribed late region of the genome corresponding to *Hin* fragments F, J, and G (see Fig. 12), it is thought that they might all contain a defect in the major capsid protein, VP1. As might be expected, the early viral functions appear normally in cells infected with these mutants and cells can be transformed at the nonpermissive temperature by them.

6.1.3. Group D

Mutants of group D proved difficult to study because of their "leakiness" at the nonpermissive temperature. Nevertheless, extensive studies with these mutants, and in particular *ts* 101, have shown that this group is essentially noncomplementing. While infection with viral DNA leads to a normal lytic cycle and the production of temperature-sensitive progeny, viral infection is itself blocked at a very early stage (Robb and Martin, 1972; Chou *et al.*. 1974; Chou and Martin, 1974). The virus is adsorbed, but there is no subsequent synthesis of early SV40 mRNA (R. Saral, G Khoury, J. Chou, and R. Martin, unpublished results), early viral proteins, or viral DNA. In addition, the "D function" is necessary only very early in the lytic cycle, since infection of cells at the permissive temperature followed by a shift to the restrictive temperature after 10–20 h results in no reduction in the rate of viral DNA synthesis. From consideration of all these properties, it seems most likely that the D mutants are blocked at the restrictive temperature in some stage of uncoating. Thus one might conclude that the D protein is structural (either a capsid- or, perhaps more likely, a core-associated protein), and the removal of this protein is necessary for expression of the viral genome. Nathans and Lai have mapped D mutants in *Hin* fragment E (Fig. 12) which, as might be expected, is located in the late region of the viral genome.

6.2. Polyoma ts Mutants

As was the case for SV40, a number of temperature-sensitive mutants of polyoma have been isolated from viral stocks treated with chemical mutagens (Fried, 1965; DiMayorca *et al.*, 1969; Eckhart, 1969).

These mutants can be classified into four or five groups on the basis of physiological or complementation experiments. In most respects, the groups of polyoma mutants are analogous to those of SV40 and will be discussed only briefly.

6.2.1. Groups I and IV

The polyoma mutants of groups I and IV are late mutants, analogous to the group B and C SV40 *ts* mutants. At the nonpermissive temperature, early functions appear to be normal but there are detectable defects in the synthesis of structural proteins as demonstrated either by the absence of V antigen in infected cells or by heat liability of the mutant virion capsids. Group I and IV mutants will complement each other at restrictive temperatures.

6.2.2. Groups II and III

Groups II and III are early mutants and are in many respects analogous to the SV40 group A mutants. They are unable to synthesize viral DNA at nonpermissive temperatures, and at least group II mutants are defective in the function necessary for establishment of transformation. It is not yet certain that group III mutants can transform at the restrictive temperature (the only characteristic which separates them from group II mutants) or whether this phenomenon is simply a result of multiplicity-dependent leakiness (Eckhart, 1969; Oxman *et al.*, 1972).

At the present time, it appears that the group II function is not necessary for maintenance of the transformed state; BHK-21 cells transformed at the permissive temperature by a group II mutant (*ts-a*) do not appear to lose their phenotypic characteristics of transformation when shifted to the restrictive temperature (Fried, 1965; Eckhart, 1969; DiMayorca *et al.*, 1969). This property is extremely important; it suggests that once transformation has been initiated, the continued synthesis of the viral function which was necessary for initiation of transformation is no longer required. In the light of recent contrasting data which suggest that the early SV40 function may be necessary for maintenance of the transformed state, these early polyoma mutants deserve further examination.

6.2.3. Group V

Mutant *ts-3* is representative of polyoma group V and has certain properties which resemble those of the SV40 D mutants. Virions are not able to induce host cell DNA synthesis or early viral functions at the nonpermissive temperature (Dulbecco and Eckhart, 1970), yet viral DNA is fully infectious under these same conditions (Eckhart, unpublished results). On the other hand, BHK cells transformed by *ts-3* at the permissive temperature lose certain of their transformed characteristics (morphology, wheat germ agglutinin sites, and topoinhibition) (Eckhart *et al.*, 1971) when shifted to the nonpermissive temperature, while other properties of the transformed phenotype (e.g., ability to grow in soft agar) are retained. These temperature-sensitive characteristics of transformation are somewhat analogous to the properties of SV40 group A mutants. It is possible, therefore, that *ts-3* is a double mutant, and with recent advances in mapping of the polyoma genome and the application of marker rescue studies to animal virus systems this question should be answered in the near future.

In summary, temperature-sensitive mutants of SV40 and polyoma have been of tremendous value in the investigation of the viral contribution to virus–cell interactions. There is no doubt that they will continue to be useful in approaching many of the still unanswered questions related to the lytic cycle and cell transformation.

GEORGE
KHOURY AND
NORMAN P.
SALZMAN

7. Other Properties of Papovaviruses

7.1. Induction of Cellular Processes in Infected Cells

As previously described, the lytic infection of either polyoma or SV40 is accompanied by the stimulation of a number of cellular processes; there is the induction of synthesis of cellular DNA (Dulbecco et al., 1965; Hatanaka and Dulbecco, 1966; Ritzi and Levine, 1969) and mitochondrial DNA (Levine, 1971), certain enzymes (Kit, 1967), cellular RNA (Oda and Dulbecco, 1968a), and histones (Shimono and Kaplan, 1969; Hancock and Weil, 1969; Winocour and Robbins, 1970; Rovera et al., 1972). These phenomena are related to the exposure of cells to virus, and, in general, higher levels of induction are seen after infection at higher input multiplicities (Basilico et al., 1966). While these effects are the consequence of exposure to the virus, it is difficult to assess their importance in relation to virus replication. There is some implication in discussion of the induction of cellular processes which results from virus infection that viral gene products are acting in some immediate way as regulators of these processes. For example, it has been proposed that the induction of cellular DNA synthesis by SV40 is an in vitro process parallel to the process of malignant cell transformation that occurs in vivo. However, the very broad stimulation of cellular processes results from the exposure of cells to a virus which codes for only six to ten proteins.

The induction of cellular DNA synthesis is seen following infection with either SV40 or polyoma virus in almost every cell line that has been examined. These cell cultures in which induction of cellular DNA is observed have been held in a contact-inhibited state for several days prior to infection. The cells are presumed to be arrested in the G_1 phase, a phase which is normally characterized as a brief period (of approximately 4–12 h duration) following mitosis and prior to the initiation of DNA synthesis. There has not yet been an adequate characterization of the changes that occur in a cell population which has been kept in a nondividing state for several days prior to infection. It is most likely that these cells may differ markedly from G_1 cells even though both share certain common properties (e.g., a diploid DNA content and the absence of DNA synthesis). In a growing cell population, virus infection does not change the orderly progression of cells through the cycle; i.e., cells which are in different parts of the cell cycle when they are infected are not brought into synchrony in a single phase of the cycle (Ben-Porat and Kaplan, 1967). When growing cells are infected, it has been shown that some biosynthetic event occurs during late G_1 or early S phase which is required for virus replication (Pages et al., 1973; Thorne, 1973).

Given these two facts, (1) that events which are required for virus replication can occur only during G_1 or S phase, and (2) that virus infection per se is not sufficient to change the phase of the cell cycle, it would seem likely that a necessary consequence of infection of a resting cell population is that it affects the cell like a mitogenic agent. This is likely to be a precondition for virus replication, since after resting cells are stimulated to divide they will move through the cell cycle and allow biosynthetic events to occur which are required for virus replication and which are

coupled to particular parts of the cell cycle. The general induction of cellular
processes would then be a reflection of cell growth and division. There are
significant differences between resting cell cultures in which cellular processes are
induced as a consequence of infection and uninfected growing cells. Some of these
differences may be a consequence of the extended time that cultured cells were
held in a contact-inhibited state prior to infection.

7.2. Pseudovirions

Fragmented cellular DNA can be encapsidated within a virus protein coat, giving rise to pseudovirions, which are noninfectious, virus-like particles that contain linear duplex fragments of cellular DNA. It is only cellular DNA that has replicated during the infectious cycle which breaks down to material of about the same molecular weight as viral DNA (Ben-Porat and Kaplan, 1967). In contrast with polyoma, where pseudovirions are commonly found after infection of primary or continuous mouse kidney cell cultures (Michel *et al.*, 1967), SV40 pseudovirions are observed only rarely and not in any consistent or predictable manner (Trilling and Axelrod, 1970, 1972). Three different types of monkey kidney cultures have been compared to determine the conditions in which pseudovirion formation occurs. When these three cell lines were examined following SV40 infection, there was a 13–23% breakdown of prelabeled cellular DNA of primary African green monkey kidney cell cultures within 96 h p.i.; for CV-1 cells there was a 1–2% breakdown, and there was no breakdown of prelabeled BSC-1 cellular DNA (Ritzi and Levine, 1969). These results parallel other studies in the same laboratory which showed that pseudovirions were obtained after infection of primary AGMK cells but not in virus stocks prepared in CV-1 or BSC-1 cells (Levine and Teresky, 1970). While this would suggest that cleavage of cellular DNA is a precondition for pseudovirion formation, it has not been established that cleavage alone is sufficient for pseudovirion production. Treatment of polyoma-infected mouse embryo cells with phleomycin also enhances the incorporation of host cell DNA into virions (Iwata and Consigli, 1971). The three requirements for pseudovirion formation are (1) conditions which permit cellular DNA replication, (2) breakdown of this cellular DNA, and (3) encapsidation of the DNA within a virus protein coat. It has also been suggested that the relative pool sizes of polyoma DNA and degraded cellular DNA at the time of virus assembly may determine the relative proportion of polyoma virions and pseudovirions (Yelton and Aposhian, 1972).

7.3. Nucleoprotein Complexes

The association of proteins with viral nucleic acid in nucleoprotein complexes may occur for a number of reasons. These complexes may be intermediates in the process of uncoating of the virus particle; they may represent the association of enzymes with DNA during replication of viral DNA or during transcription; or

TABLE 3

Properties of the Nondefective Ad 2–SV40 Hybrid Viruses

Virus	Host[a] range	SV40 antigens[b]					Size of integrated SV40 DNA segment[c] (SV40 units)	Size of adenovirus DNA deletion[d] (Ad units)	Extent of SV40 transcription[e] (SV40 units)
		T	U	TSTA	V				
Ad2[+]ND$_1$	AGMK/HEK	–	+	–	–		0.18	0.054	0.17
Ad2[+]ND$_2$	AGMK/HEK	–	+	+	–		0.32	0.061	0.32
Ad2[+]ND$_3$	HEK	–	–	–	–		0.06	0.053	0.07
Ad2[+]ND$_4$	AGMK/HEK	+	+	+	–		0.43	0.045	0.45
Ad2[+]ND$_5$	HEK	–	–	–	–		0.28	0.071	0.26

[a] Lewis *et al.* (1973). AGMK, African green monkey kidney cells; HEK, human embryonic kidney cells.
[b] Lewis *et al.* (1973).
[c] Estimates of integrated SV40 DNA segment (fraction of the SV40 genome), based on electron microscopic heteroduplex mapping experiments (Kelly and Lewis, 1973).
[d] Estimates of the deleted adenovirus DNA segment of each hybrid (fraction of the adenovirus genome), based on electron microscopic heteroduplex mapping experiments (Kelly and Lewis, 1973).
[e] Determined in RNA–DNA hybridization experiments with the separated strands of SV40 DNA (Khoury *et al.*, 1973c).

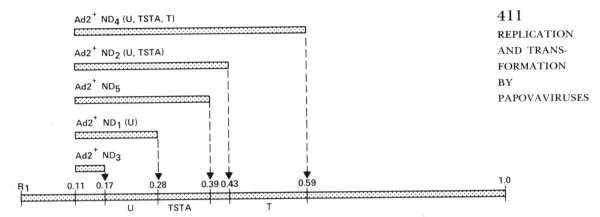

FIGURE 15. Map positions of the SV40 DNA segments incorporated in the five Ad 2–SV40 nondefective hybrid viruses. The SV40-specific antigens induced after infection by certain of these viruses (T, U, or TSTA) are indicated. Note that the SV40 molecule is represented as linear for convenience, with the *Eco·R₁* restriction enzyme cleavage site at 0 map units. From Lewis and Rowe (1973).

SV40-specific RNA is synthesized during the lytic cycle of each of the nondefective hybrid viruses (Levine *et al.*, 1973; Khoury *et al.*, 1973c) and, as was the case for the SV40 DNA segments of these viruses, the specific RNAs have been shown by competition-hybridization experiments to be subsets of each other (Levine *et al.*, 1973; Table 3).

In subsequent studies with the separated strands of SV40 DNA, it was shown that transcription in all of the nondefective hybrid viruses is limited to the minus (or early) DNA strand. Under saturating conditions, it was further demonstrated that the SV40 segment in each of the hybrids is transcribed in its entirety (Khoury *et al.*, 1973c). It had previously been shown that Ad2⁺ND₁ (as well as the other nondefective hybrids) contains both early and late SV40 gene sequences (Patch *et al.*, 1972, 1974). Since the early and late SV40 messages are transcribed from opposite strands of the SV40 DNA, the extent and strand orientation of transcription in the nondefective hybrid viral lytic infections indicate that there is no synthesis of stable late SV40 mRNA, and that stable "anti-late" SV40 RNA sequences are synthesized (Khoury *et al.*, 1973c). More recent data confirm the presence of these "anti-late" transcripts and suggest that they are present in lower concentrations than the true early SV40-specific RNA sequences. Whether this result reflects processing of the initial transcript is not yet known.

Since the direction of RNA synthesis on the minus (early) strand of SV40 DNA has been determined (Khoury *et al.*, 1973b; see Fig. 11), the direction of transcription of the SV40 sequences from the nondefective adenovirus–SV40 hybrids is known. It is clear that this transcription proceeds from the uncommon toward the common end of the SV40 segments (see Figs. 11 and 15). If transcription were to begin in the SV40 portion of the genomes, this would require a different promoter in each of the SV40 segments of the five nondefective hybrid viruses. Thus it was suggested that transcription is initiated at a promoter in the adenovirus portion of the hybrid, proximal to the early SV40 region (Khoury et al., 1973c). This prediction would also suggest that hybrid-adenovirus message is synthesized with adenovirus sequences on the 5'-end of the molecule. Adenovirus–SV40 hybrid mRNA has been detected by filter hybridization techniques (Oxman et al.,, 1974). Although the orientation of the adenovirus and SV40 sequences has not yet been determined, it has been concluded that the hybrid promoter is in adenovirus DNA, since transcription from the hybrid viral DNA is resistant to interferon. In contrast, SV40 transcription (and/or translation) is quite sensitive to interferon (Oxman et al., 1967).

The prototype of these hybrid viruses, $Ad2^+ND_1$, which contains 18% of the SV40 genome (see Table 3), does not induce the SV40 T antigen but does code for the SV40 U antigen. In addition to the U antigen, $Ad2^+ND_2$ (containing 32% of the SV40 genome) codes for the SV40 transplantation antigen (TSTA), while $Ad2^+ND_4$, which contains the largest SV40 segment (48%), codes for U, TSTA, and T antigens.

An analysis of the antigen-inducing ability of the hybrids and the location of the SV40 segments of each on the parental SV40 genome allows one to construct a map of the early SV40 antigens (see Fig 15). The U antigen would be located at the common end of the hybrids, and between 0.11 and 0.28 unit. Similarly, TSTA and T antigens would be associated with 0.28–0.39 and 0.39–0.48 unit, respectively. It should be pointed out, however, that although the SV40 segments of the nondefective hybrid viruses have been carefully mapped, the early "gene" regions associated with these segments have been located only by inference. Furthermore, the three regions of the SV40 genome described above are only large enough to code for proteins of 15,000–25,000 daltons; the early SV40 antigens, on the other hand, may be considerably larger (see above). In spite of these reservations, the map positions of the early SV40 antigens as determined from the adeno–SV40 nondefective hybrid viruses, early ts mutants, and the early transcriptional region of the genome localized by hybridization experiments (Section 3, Fig. 11) are in good agreement.

Two of the nondefective hybrid viruses, $Ad2^+ND_3$ and $Ad2^+ND_5$, induce no known SV40 antigens (Lewis et al., 1973; Table 3). Yet infection by each of these viruses results in the synthesis of SV40-specific RNA, which represents a complete transcript of the incorporated SV40 DNA segment (Khoury et al., 1973c). Perhaps the SV40 gene sequences in $Ad2^+ND_3$ are too small (7% of SV40) to induce any SV40 antigens. Furthermore, most of the SV40-specific RNA transcribed from this hybrid is "anti-late" message (Patch et al., 1974). On the other hand, $Ad2^+ND_5$ contains almost as much SV40 DNA as $Ad2^+ND_2$ (Kelly and Lewis, 1973), a hybrid which induces two of the three SV40 early antigens (Lewis et al., 1973). There appears to be no inhibition of the transcription of $Ad2^+ND_5$; mRNA is synthesized (Levine et al., 1973; Khoury et al., 1973c), transported to the cytoplasm, and is found on polyribosomes (C. S. Crumpacker, M. J. Levin, and A. M. Lewis, unpublished results). Whether there is a block in the initiation of translation or a frame shift resulting in the translation of a nonsense protein is unclear. In addition, it remains to be determined if the fact that $Ad2^+ND_5$ contains the largest adenoviral DNA deletion among the nondefective hybrids relates to the lack of induction of early SV40 antigens.

ACKNOWLEDGMENT

We thank Marilyn Thoren for her help in preparing this manuscript.

8. References

AARONSON, S. A., AND MARTIN, M. A., 1970, Transformation of human cells with different forms of SV40 DNA, *Virology* **42**:848.

AARONSON, S. A., AND TODARO, G. J., 1968, SV40 T antigen induction and transformation in human fibroblast cell strains, *Virology* **36**:254.

AARONSON, S. A., AND TODARO, G. J., 1969, Human diploid cell transformation by DNA extracted from the tumor virus SV40, *Science* **166**:390.

ABERCROMBIE, M., AND HEAYSMAN, J. E. M., 1954, Observations on the social behavior of cells in tissue culture, *Exp. Cell Res.* **6**:293.

ACHESON, N. H., BUETTI, E., SCHERRER, K., AND WEIL, R., 1971, Transcription of the polyoma virus genome: Synthesis and cleavage of giant late polyoma-specific RNA, *Proc. Natl. Acad. Sci.* **68**:2231.

ALONI, Y., 1972, Extensive symmetrical transcription of simian virus 40 DNA in virus-yielding cells, *Proc. Natl. Acad. Sci.* **69**:2024.

ALONI, Y., 1973, Poly A and symmetrical transcription of SV40 DNA, *Nature New Biol.* **243**:2.

ALONI, Y., AND LOCKER, H., 1973, Symmetrical *in vivo* transcription of polyoma DNA and the separation of self-complementary viral and cell DNA, *Virology* **54**:495.

ALONI, Y., WINOCOUR, E., AND SACHS, L., 1968, Characterization of the simian virus 40-specific RNA in virus-yielding and -transformed cells, *J. Mol. Biol.* **31**:415.

ALONI, Y., WINOCOUR, E., SACHS, L., AND TORTEN, J., 1969, Hybridization between SV40 DNA and cellular DNA's, *J. Mol. Biol.* **44**:333.

ANDERER, F. A., SCHLÜMBERGER, H. D., KOCH, M. A., FRANK, H., AND EGGERS, H. J., 1967, Structure of simian virus 40. II. Symmetry and components of the virus particle, *Virology* **32**:511.

ANDERSON, C. W., AND GESTELAND, R. F., 1972, Pattern of protein synthesis in monkey cells infected by simian virus 40, *J. Virol.* **9**:758.

ARBER, W., AND LINN, S., 1969, DNA modification and restriction, in: *Annual Review of Biochemistry*, pp. 467–500, Annual Reviews, Palo Alto, Calif.

ASHKENAZI, A., AND MELNICK, J. L., 1963, Tumorigenicity of simian papovavirus SV40 and of virus-transformed cells, *J. Natl. Cancer Inst.* **30**:1227.

ASTRIN, S. M., 1973, *In vitro* transcription of simian virus 40 sequences in SV3T3 chromatin, *Proc. Natl. Acad. Sci.* **70**:2304.

BABIUK, L. A., AND HUDSON, J. B., 1972, Integration of polyoma virus DNA into mammalian genomes, *Biochem. Biophys. Res. Commun.* **47**:111.

BARBAN, S., 1973, Electrophoretic differences in the capsid proteins of simian virus 40 plaque mutants, *J. Virol.* **11**:971.

BARBAN, S., AND GOOR, R. S., 1971, Structural proteins of simian virus 40, *J. Virol.* **7**:198.

BARBANTI-BRODANO, G., SWETLY, P., AND KOPROWSKI, H., 1970, Early events in the infection of permissive cells with simian virus 40: Adsorption, penetration, and uncoating, *J. Virol.* **6**:78.

BASILICO, C., AND DIMAYORCA, G., 1965, Radiation target size of the lytic and the transforming ability of polyoma virus, *Proc. Natl. Acad. Sci.* **54**:125.

BASILICO, C., AND MARIN, G., 1966, Susceptibility of cells in different steps of the mitotic cycle to transformation by polyoma virus, *Virology* **28**:429.

BASILICO, C., MARIN, G., and DIMAYORCA, G., 1966, Requirement for the intregrity of the viral genome for the induction of host DNA synthesis by polyoma virus, *Proc. Natl. Acad. Sci* **56**:208.

BASILICO, C., MATSUYA, Y., AND GREEN, M. H., 1969, Origin of the thymidine kinase induced by polyoma virus in productively infected cells, *J. Virol.* **3:**140.

BAUER, W., AND VINOGRAD, J., 1968, The interaction of closed circular DNA with intercalative dyes. I. The superhelix density of SV40 DNA in the presence and absence of dye, *J. Mol. Biol.* **33:**141.

BAUM, S. G., HORWITZ, M. S., AND MAIZEL, J. V., JR., 1972, Studies of the mechanism of enhancement of human adenovirus infection in monkey cells by simian virus 40, *J. Virol.* **10:**211.

BEARD, P., MORROW, J. F., AND BERG, P., 1973, Cleavage of circular superhelical SV40 DNA to a linear duplex by S_1 nuclease, *J. Virol.* **12:**1303.

BEERMAN, T. A., AND LEBOWITZ, J., 1973, Further analysis of the altered secondary structure of superhelical DNA: Sensitivity of methylmercuric hydroxide, a chemical probe for unpaired bases, *J. Mol. Biol.* **79:**451.

BENJAMIN, T. L., 1965, Relative target sizes for the inactivation of the transforming and reproductive abilities of polyoma virus, *Proc. Natl. Acad. Sci.* **54:**121.

BENJAMIN, T. L., 1966, Virus-specific RNA in cells productively infected or transformed by polyoma virus, *J. Mol. Biol.* **16:**359.

BENJAMIN, T. L., AND BRUGER, M. M., 1970, Absence of a cell membrane alteration function in non-transforming mutants of polyoma virus, *Proc. Natl. Acad. Sci.* **67:**929.

BEN-PORAT, T., AND KAPLAN, A. S., 1967, Correlation between replication and degradation of cellular DNA in polyoma virus–infected cells, *Virology,* **32:**457.

BEN-PORAT, T., COTO, C., AND KAPLAN, A. S., 1966, Unstable DNA synthesized by polyoma virus infected cells, *Virology* **30:**74.

BIGGER, C., MURRAY, K., AND MURRAY, N. E., 1973, Recognition sequence of a restriction enzyme, *Nature New Biol.* **244:**7.

BLACK, P. H., AND ROWE, W. P., 1964, Viral studies of SV40 tumorigenesis in hamsters, *J. Natl. Cancer Inst.* **32:**253.

BLACK, P. H., AND ROWE, W. P., 1963, SV40-induced proliferation of tissue culture cells of rabbit, mouse and porcine origin, *Proc. Soc. Exp. Biol. Med.* **114:**721.

BLACK, P. H., ROWE, W. P., TURNER, H. C., AND HUEBNER, R. J., 1963, A specific complement-fixing antigen present in SV40 tumor and transformed cells, *Proc. Natl. Acad. Sci.* **50:**1148.

BOTCHAN, M., OZANNE, B., SUDGEN, B., SHARP, P. A., AND SAMBROOK, J., 1974, Viral DNA in transformed cells. III. The amounts of different regions of the SV40 genome present in a line of transformed mouse cells, *Proc. Natl. Acad. Sci.* **71:**4183.

BOURGAUX, P., AND BOURGAUX-RAMOISY, D., 1972a, Unwinding of replicating polyoma virus DNA, *J. Mol. Biol.* **70:**399.

BOURGAUX, P., AND BOURGAUX-RAMOISY, D., 1972b, Is a specific protein responsible for the supercoiling of polyoma DNA? *Nature (Lond.)* **235:**105.

BOURGAUX, P., BOURGAUX-RAMOISY, D., AND STOKER, M., 1965, Further studies on transformation by DNA from polyoma virus, *Virology* **25:**364.

BOURGAUX, P., BOURGAUX-RAMOISY, D., AND DULBECCO, R., 1969, The replication of ring-shaped DNA of polyoma virus. I. Identification of the replicative intermediate, *Proc. Natl. Acad. Sci.* **64:**701.

BOURGUIGNON, M. F., 1968, A denaturation map of polyoma virus DNA, *Biochim. Biophys. Acta.* **166:**242.

BOYER, H. W., 1971, DNA restriction and modification mechanisms in bacteria, in: *Annual Review of Microbiology,* pp. 153–176, Annual Reviews, Palo Alto, Calif.

BOYER, H. W., CHOW, L. T., DUGAICZYK, A., HEDGPETH, J., AND GOODMAN, H. M., 1973, DNA substrate site for the Eco_{RII} restriction endonuclease and modification methylase, *Nature New Biol.* **244:**172.

BRANTON, P. E., AND SHEININ, R., 1973, Studies on the replication of polyoma DNA: Physicochemical properties of viral DNA synthesized when protein synthesis is inhibited, *Can. J. Biochem.* **51:**305.

BRANTON, P. E., CHEEVERS, W. P. AND SHEININ, R., 1970, The effect of cycloheximide on DNA synthesis in cells productively-infected with polyoma virus, *Virology* **42:**979.

BRITTEN, R. J., AND KOHNE, D. E., 1968, Repeated sequences in DNA, *Science* **161:**529.

BROCKMAN, W. W., LEE, T. N. H., AND NATHANS, D., 1973, The evolution of new species of viral DNA during serial passage of simian virus 40 at high multiplicity, *Virology* **54:**384.

BUETTI, E., 1974, Characterization of late polyoma mRNA, *J. Virol.* **14:**249.

BURGER, M. M., 1969, A difference in the architecture of the surface membrane of normal and virally transformed cells, *Proc. Natl. Acad. Sci.* **62:**994.

BURNS, W. H., AND BLACK, P. H., 1968, Analysis of simian virus 40 induced transformation of hamster kidney tissue *in vitro.* V. Variability of virus recovery from cell clones inducible with mitomycin C and cell fusion, *J. Virol.* **2:**606.

BURTON, A., AND SINSHEIMER, R. L., 1963, Process of infection with φX174: Effect of exonucleases on the replicative form, *Science* **142**:962.

BUTEL, J. S., AND RAPP, F., 1965, The effect of arabinofuranosylcytosine on the growth cycle of simian virus 40, *Virology* **27**:490.

BUTEL, J. S., GUENTZEL, M. J., AND RAPP, F., 1969, Variants of defective simian papovavirus 40 (PARA) characterized by cytoplasmic localization of simian papovavirus 40 tumor antigen, *J. Virol.* **4**:632.

BUTEL, J. S., RICHARDSON, L. S., AND MELNICK, J. L., 1971, Variation in properties of SV40-transformed simian cell lines detected by superinfection with SV40 and human adenoviruses, *Virology* **46**:844.

BUTEL, J. S., TEVETHIA, S. S., AND MELNICK, J. L., 1972, Oncogenicity and cell transformation by papovavirus SV40: The role of the viral genome, *Advan. Cancer Res.* **15**:1.

CAIRNS, J., 1963, The chromosome of *Escherichia coli, Cold Spring Harbor Symp. Quant. Biol.* **28**:43.

CARP, R. I., AND GILDEN, R. V., 1965, The inactivation of simian virus 40 infectivity and antigen-inducing capacity by ultraviolet light, *Virology* **27**:639.

CARP, R. I., SAUER, G., AND SOKOL, F., 1969, The effect of actinomycin D on the transcription and replication of simian virus 40 deoxyribonucleic acid, *Virology* **37**:214.

CHAMBERLIN, M., MCGRATH, J., AND WASKELL, L., 1970, New RNA polymerase from *Escherichia coli* infected with bacteriophage T7, *Nature (Lond.)* **228**:227.

CHAMPOUX, J. J., AND DULBECCO, R., 1972, An activity from mammalian cells that untwists superhelical DNA—A possible swivel for DNA replication. *Proc. Natl. Acad. Sci.* **69**:143.

CHOU, J. Y., AND MARTIN, R. G., 1974, Complementation analysis of SV40 mutants, *J. Virol.* **13**:1101.

CHOU, J. Y., AVILA, J., AND MARTIN, R. G., 1974, Viral DNA synthesis in cells infected by temperature sensitive mutants of SV40, *J. Virol.* **14**:116.

CLINE, M. J., AND LIVINGSTONE, D. C., 1971, Binding of ³H-concanavalin A by normal and transformed cells, *Nature New Biol.* **232**:155.

COGGIN, J. H., ELROD, L. H., AMBROSE, K. R., AND ANDERSON, N. G., 1969, Induction of tumor-specific transplantation immunity in hamster with cell fractions from adenovirus and SV40 tumor cells, *Proc. Soc. Exp. Biol. Med.* **132**:328.

COLLINS, J. J., AND BLACK, P. H., 1973a, Analysis of surface antigens on simian virus 40 transformed cells. I. Unique antigenicity of simian virus 40 transformed outbred hamster kidney cell lines, *J. Natl. Cancer Inst.* **51**:95.

COLLINS, J. J., AND BLACK, P. H., 1973b, Analysis of surface antigens on simian virus 40 transformed cells. II. Exposure of simian virus 40 induced antigens on transformed rabbit kidney and inbred hamster kidney cells by phospholipase C, *J. Natl. Cancer Inst.* **51**:115.

COWAN, K., TEGTMEYER, P., AND ANTHONY, D. D., 1973, Relationship of replication and transcription of simian virus 40 DNA, *Proc. Natl. Acad. Sci.* **70**:1927.

CRAWFORD, L. V., 1962, The adsorption of polyoma virus, *Virology* **18**:177.

CRAWFORD, L. V., 1964, A study of Shope papilloma virus DNA, *J. Mol. Biol.* **8**:489.

CRAWFORD, L. V., 1965, A study of human papilloma virus DNA, *J. Mol. Biol.* **13**:362.

CRAWFORD, L. V., AND BLACK, P. H., 1964, The nucleic acid of simian virus 40, *Virology* **24**:388.

CRAWFORD, L., DULBECCO, R., FRIED, M., MONTAGNEIR, L., AND STOKER, M., 1964, Cell transformation by different forms of polyoma virus DNA, *Proc. Natl. Acad. Sci.* **52**:148.

CRAWFORD, L. V., CRAWFORD, E. M., RICHARDSON, J. P., AND SLAYTER, H. S., 1965, The binding of RNA polymerase to polyoma and papilloma DNA, *J. Mol. Biol.* **14**:593.

CRAWFORD, L. V., SYRETT, C., AND WILDE, A., 1973, The replication of polyoma virus, *J. Gen. Virol.* **21**:515.

CROCE, C. M., GIRARDI, A. J., AND KOPROWSKI, H., 1973, Assignment of the T-antigen gene of simian virus 40 to human chromosome C-7, *Proc. Natl. Acad. Sci.* **70**:3617.

CULP, L. A., AND BLACK, P. H., 1972, Contact inhibited revertant cell lines isolated from simian virus 40 transformed cells, *J. Virol.* **9**:611.

CUZIN, F., VOGT, M., DIECKMANN, M., AND BERG, P., 1970, Induction of virus multiplication in 3T3 cells transformed by a thermosensitive mutant of polyoma virus. II. Formation of oligomeric polyoma DNA molecules, *J. Mol. Biol.* **47**:317.

CUZIN, F., BLANGY, D., AND ROUGET, P., 1971. Activité endonucleastique de preparation purifié du virus polyome, *Compt. Rend. Acad. Sci.* **273**:2650.

DANNA, K., AND NATHANS, D., 1971, Specific cleavage of simian virus 40 DNA by restriction endonuclease of *Hemophilus influenza, Proc. Natl. Acad. Sci.* **68**:2913.

DANNA, K. J., AND NATHANS, D., 1972, Bidirectional replication of simian virus 40 DNA, *Proc. Natl. Acad. Sci.* **69**:3097.

DANNA, K. J., SACK, G. H., JR., AND NATHANS, D., 1973, Studies of simian virus 40 DNA. VII. A cleavage map of the SV40 genome, *J. Mol. Biol.* **78**:363.

DAVIS, R., SIMON, M., AND DAVIDSON, N., 1971, Electron microscope heteroduplex methods for mapping regions of base sequence homology in nucleic acids, in: *Methods in Enzymology* (L. Grossman and K. Moldave, eds.), pp. 413–428, Academic Press, New York.

DEAN, W. W., AND LEBOWITZ, J., 1971, Partial alteration of secondary structure in native superhelical DNA, *Nature New Biol.* **231**:5.

DEFENDI, V., 1963, Effect of SV40 virus immunization on growth of transplantable SV40 and polyoma virus tumors in hamsters, *Proc. Soc. Biol. Med.* **113**:12.

DELIUS, H., WESTPHAL, H., AND AXELROD, N., 1973, Length measurements of RNA synthesized *in vitro* by *E. coli* polymerase, *J. Mol. Biol.* **74**:677.

DEL VILLANO, B. C., AND DEFENDI, V., 1973, Characterization of the SV40 T antigen, *Virology* **51**:34.

DHAR, R., ZAIN, S., WEISSMAN, S. M., PAN, J., AND SUBRAMANIAN, K., 1973, Nucleotide sequences of RNA transcribed in infected cells and by *E. coli* polymerase from a segment of simian virus 40 DNA, *Proc. Natl. Acad. Sci.* **71**:371.

DHAR, R., WEISMANN, S. M., ZAIN, B. S., PAN, J., AND LEWIS, A. M., 1974, II. The sequence of the early strand, *Nucleic Acid Res.* **1**:595.

DIAMANDOPOULOS, G. T., TEVETHIA, S. S., RAPP, F., AND ENDERS, J. F., 1968, Development of S and T antigens and oncogenicity in hamster embryonic cell lines exposed to SV40, *Virology* **34**:331.

DIDERHOLM, H., BERG, R., AND WESSLÉN, T., 1966, Transformation of rat and guinea pig cells *in vitro* by SV40, and the transplantability of the transformed cells, *Int. J. Cancer* **1**:139.

DIMAYORCA, G., CALLENDER, J., MARIN, G., AND GIORDANO, R., 1969, Temperature-sensitive mutants of polyoma virus, *Virology* **38**:126.

DUBBS, D. R.. KIT, S., DETORRES, R. A., AND ANKEN, M., 1967, Virogenic properties of bromodeoxy-uridine-sensitive and bromodeoxyuridine-resistant simian virus 40 transformed mouse kidney cells, *J. Virol* **1**:968.

DUBBS, D. R., RACHMELER, M., AND KIT, S., 1974, Recombination between temperature sensitive mutants of SV40, *Virology* **57**:161.

DUFF, R., AND RAPP, F., 1970, Reaction of serum from pregnant hamsters with surface of cells transformed by SV40, *J. Immunol.* **105**:521.

DULBECCO, R., 1970, Topoinhibition and serum requirement of transformed and untransformed cells, *Nature (Lond.)* **227**:802.

DULBECCO, R., AND ECKHART, W., 1970, Temperature dependent properties of cells transformed by a thermosensitive mutant of polyoma virus, *Proc. Natl. Acad. Sci.* **67**:1775.

DULBECCO, R., AND VOGT, M., 1963, Evidence for a ring structure of polyoma virus DNA, *Proc. Natl. Acad. Sci.* **50**:236.

DULBECCO, R., HARTWELL, L. H., AND VOGT, M., 1965, Induction of cellular DNA synthesis by polyoma virus, *Proc. Natl. Acad. Sci.* **53**:403.

ECKHART, W., 1969, Complementation and transformation by temperature-sensitive mutants of polyoma virus, *Virology* **38**:120.

ECKHART, W., DULBECCO, R., AND BURGER, M., 1971, Temperature dependent surface changes in cells infected or transformed by a thermosensitive mutant of polyoma virus, *Proc. Natl. Acad. Sci.* **68**:283.

EDDY, B. E., BORMAN, G. S., GRUBBS, G. E., AND YOUNG, R. D., 1962, Identification of the oncogenic substance in rhesus monkey cell cultures as simian virus 40, *Virology* **17**:65.

ENDERS, J. F., 1965, Cell transformation by viruses as illustrated by the response of human and hamster renal cells to simian virus 40, *Harvey Lect.* **59**:113.

ESTES, M. K., HUANG, E.-S., AND PAGANO, J. S., 1971, Structural polypeptides of simian virus 40, *J. Virol.* **7**:635.

FAREED, G. C., AND SALZMAN, N. P., 1972, Intermediate in SV40 DNA chain growth, *Nature New Biol.* **238**:274.

FAREED, G. C., GARON, C. F., AND SALZMAN, N. P., 1972, Origin and direction of simian virus 40 deoxyribonucleic acid replication, *J. Virol.* **10**:484.

FAREED, G. C., KHOURY, G., AND SALZMAN, N. P., 1973a, Self-annealing of 4 S strands from replicating simian virus 40 DNA, *J. Mol. Biol.* **77**:457.

FAREED, G. C., MCKERLIE, M. L., AND SALZMAN, N. P., 1973b, Characterization of simian virus 40 DNA component II during viral DNA replication, *J. Mol. Biol.* **74**:95.

FAREED, G. C., BYRNE, J. C., AND MARTIN, M. A., 1974, Triplication of a unique genetic segment in an SV40-like virus of human origin and evolution of new viral genomes. *J. Mol. Biol.* **86**:275.

FERNANDES, M., AND MOOREHEAD, P., 1965, Transformation of African green monkey kidney cultures infected with simian vacuolating virus (SV40), *Texas Rep. Biol. Med.* **23**:242.

FIERS, W., AND SINSHEIMER, R. L., 1962, The structure of the DNA of bacteriophage φX174, *J. Mol. Biol.* **5**:408.

FINCH, J. T., AND KLUG, A., 1965, The structures of viruses of the papilloma-polyoma type. III. Structure of rabbit papilloma virus, *J. Mol. Biol.* **13**:1.

FINE, R., MASS, M., AND MURAKAMI, W. T., 1968, Protein composition of polyoma virus, *J. Mol. Biol.* **36**:167.

FISCHER, H., AND SAUER, G., 1972, Identification of virus-induced proteins in cells productively infected with simian virus 40, *J. Virol.* **9**:1.

FOLLETT, E. A. C., AND CRAWFORD, L. V., 1968, Electron microscope study of the denaturation of polyoma virus DNA, *J. Mol. Biol.* **34**:565.

FOX, R. I., AND BAUM, S. G., 1972, Synthesis of viral ribonucleic acid during restricted adenovirus infection, *J. Virol.* **10**:220.

FOX, R. I., AND BAUM, S. G., 1974, Post-transcriptional block to adenovirus replication in nonpermissive monkey cell, *Virology* **60**:45.

FRANCKE, B., AND HUNTER, T., 1974, *In vitro* polyoma DNA synthesis: Discontinuous chain growth, *J. Mol. Biol.* **83**:99.

FREARSON, D. M., AND CRAWFORD, L. V., 1972, Polyoma virus basic proteins, *J. Gen. Virol.* **14**:141.

FRIED, A. H., AND SOKOL, F., 1972, Synthesis *in vitro* by bacterial RNA polymerase of simian virus 40 specific RNA: Multiple transcription of the DNA template into a continuous polyribonucleotide, *J. Gen. Virol* **17**:69.

FRIED, M., 1965, Isolation of temperature-sensitive mutants of polyoma virus, *Virology* **25**:669.

FRIED, M., 1970, Characterization of a temperature-sensitive mutant of polyoma virus, *Virology* **40**:605.

FREIDMAN, M. P., LYONS, M. J., AND GINSBERG, H. S., 1970, Biochemical consequences of type 2 adenovirus and simian virus 40 double infections of African green monkey kidney cells, *J. Virol.* **5**:586.

FRIEDMANN, T., 1974, Novel genetic economy of polyoma virus: Capsid proteins are cleavage products of same viral gene, *Proc. Natl. Acad. Sci.* **71**:257.

FRIEDMANN, T., AND DAVID, D., 1972, Structural roles of polyoma virus proteins, *J. Virol.* **10**:776.

GELB, L. D., KOHNE, D. E., AND MARTIN, M. A., 1971, Quantitation of simian virus 40 sequences in African green monkey, mouse and virus transformed cell genomes, *J. Mol. Biol.* **57**:129.

GELB, L. D., AND MARTIN, M. A., 1973, Simian virus 40 DNA integration within the genome of virus transformed mammalian cells, *Virology* **51**:351.

GERBER, P., 1966, Studies on the transfer of subviral infectivity from SV40-induced hamster tumor cells to indicator cells, *Virology* **28**:501.

GILBERT, W., AND DRESSLER, D., 1968, DNA replication: The rolling circle model, *Cold Spring Harbor Symp. Quant. Biol.* **33**:473.

GILDEN, R. V., AND CARP, R. I., 1966, Effects of cycloheximide and puromycin on synthesis of simian virus 40 T antigen in green monkey kidney cells, *J. Bacteriol.* **91**:1295.

GILDEN, R. V., CARP, R. I., TAGUCHI, F., AND DEFENDI, V., 1965, The nature and localization of the SV40 induced complement-fixing antigen, *Proc. Natl. Acad. Sci.* **53**:684.

GILHAM, P. T., 1964, The synthesis of polynucleotide celluloses and their use in the fractionation of polynucleotides, *J. Am. Chem. Soc.* **86**:4982.

GILLESPIE, D., AND SPIEGELMAN, S., 1965, A quantitative assay for DNA–RNA hybrids with DNA immobilized on a membrane, *J. Mol. Biol.* **12**:829.

GIRARD, M., MARTY, L., AND SUAREZ, F., 1970, Capsid proteins of simian virus 40, *Biochem. Biophys. Res. Commun.* **40**:97.

GIRARD, M., MARTY, L., AND MANTEUIL, S., 1974, Viral DNA–RNA hybrids in simian virus 40 infected cells: The simian virus 40 transcriptional intermediates, *Proc. Natl. Acad. Sci.* **71**:1267.

GIRARDI, A. J., AND DEFENDI, V., 1970, Induction of SV40 transplantation antigen (TrAg) during the lytic cycle, *Virology* **42**:688.

GOLDSTEIN, D. A., HALL, M. R., AND MEINKE, W., 1973, Properties of nucleoprotein complexes containing replicating polyoma DNA, *J. Virol.* **12**:887.

GRAHAM, F. L., AND VAN DER EB, A. J., 1973, A new technique for the assay of infectivity of human adenovirus 5 DNA, *Virology* **52**:456.

GRAHAM, F. L., VAN DER EB, A. J., AND HEYNEKER, H. L., 1974, Size and location of the transforming region in human adenovirus type 5 DNA, *Nature (Lond.)* **251**:687.

GREEN, M. H., MILLER, H. I., AND HENDLER, S., 1971, Isolation of a polyoma nucleoprotein complex from infected mouse cell cultures, *Proc. Natl. Acad. Sci.* **68:**1032.

GREENAWAY, P. J., AND LEVINE, D., 1973, Amino acid compositions of simian virus 40 structural proteins, *Biochem. Biophys. Res. Commun.* **52:**1221.

GROMKOVA, R., AND GOODGAL, S. H., 1972, Action of *Haemophilus* endodeoxyribonuclease on biologically active deoxyribonucleic acid, *J. Bacteriol.* **109:**987.

HAAS, M., VOGT, M., AND DULBECCO, R., 1972, Loss of simian virus 40 DNA–RNA hybrids from nitrocellulose membranes: Implications for the study of virus–host DNA interactions, *Proc. Natl. Acad. Sci.* **69:**2160.

HABEL, K., 1961, Resistance of polyoma virus immune animals to transplanted polyoma tumors, *Proc. Soc. Exp. Biol. Med.* **106:**722.

HABEL, K., 1965, Specific complement-fixing antigens in polyoma tumors and transformed cells, *Virology* **25:**55.

HABEL, K., AND EDDY, B. E., 1963, Specificity of resistance to tumor challenge of polyoma and SV40 virus immune hamsters, *Proc. Soc. Exp. Biol. Med.* **113:**1.

HABEL, K., JENSEN, J., PAGANO, J., AND KOPROWSKI, H., 1965, Specific complement-fixing tumor antigen in SV40-transformed human cells, *Proc. Soc. Exp. Biol. Med.* **118:**4.

HALL, M. R., MEINKE, W., AND GOLDSTEIN, D. A., 1973, Nucleoprotein complexes containing replicating simian virus 40 DNA: Comparison with polyoma nucleoprotein complexes, *J. Virol.* **12:**901.

HANCOCK, R., AND WEIL, R., 1969, Biochemical evidence for induction by polyoma virus of replication of the chromosomes of mouse kidney cells, *Proc. Natl. Acad. Sci.* **63:**1144.

HARTLEY, J. W., HUEBNER, R. J., AND ROWE, W. P., 1956, Serial propagation of adenoviruses (APC) in monkey kidney tissue cultures, *Proc. Soc. Exp. Biol. Med.* **92:**667.

HASHIMOTO, K., NAKAJIMA, K., ODA, K., AND SHIMOJO, H., 1973, Complementation of translational defect for growth of human adenovirus type 2 in simian cells by an SV40 induced factor, *J. Mol. Biol.* **81:**207.

HATANAKA, M., AND DULBECCO, R., 1966, Induction of DNA synthesis by SV40, *Proc. Natl. Acad. Sci.* **56:**736.

HEDGPETH, J., GOODMAN, H. M., AND BOYER, H. W., 1972, DNA nucleotide sequence restricted by the R1 endonuclease, *Proc. Natl. Acad. Sci.* **69:**3448.

HELINSKI, D. R., AND CLEWELL, D. B., 1971, Circular DNA, in: *Annual Review of Biochemistry*, pp. 899–942, Annual Reviews, Palo Alto, Calif.

HENRY, C. J., SLIFKIN, M., AND MERKOW, L., 1971, Mechanism of host cell restriction in African green monkey kidney cells abortively infected with human adenovirus type 2, *Nature New Biol.* **233:**39.

HERZBERG, M., AND WINOCOUR, E., 1970, Simian virus 40 deoxyribonucleic acid transcription *in vitro*: Binding and transcription patterns with a mammalian ribonucleic acid polymerase. *J. Virol.* **6:**667.

HIRAI, K., AND DEFENDI, V., 1971, Homology between SV40 DNA and DNA of normal and SV40-transformed Chinese hamster cells, *Biochem. Biophys. Res. Commun.* **42:**714.

HIRAI, K., AND DEFENDI, V., 1972, Integration of SV40 DNA into the DNA of permissive monkey cells, *J. Virol.* **9:**705.

HIRT, B., 1967, Selective extraction of polyoma DNA from infected mouse cell cultures, *J. Mol. Biol.* **26:**265.

HIRT, B., 1969, Replicating molecules of polyoma DNA *J. Mol. Biol.* **40:**141.

HIRT, B., AND GESTELAND, R. F., 1971, Characterization of SV40 and polyoma virus, *Lepetit Colloq. Biol. Med.* **2:**98.

HITOTSUMACHI, S., RABINOWITZ, Z., AND SACHS, L., 1971, Chromosomal control of reversion in transformed cells, *Nature (Lond.)* **231:**511.

HOGGAN, M. D., ROWE, W. P., BLACK, P. H., AND HEUBNER, R. J., 1965, Production of "tumor-specific" antigens by oncogenic viruses during acute cytolytic infections, *Proc. Natl. Acad. Sci.* **52:**12.

HÖLZEL, F., AND SOKOL, F., 1974, Integration of progeny simian virus 40 DNA into the host cell genome, *J. Mol. Biol.* **84:**423.

HUANG, E.-S., ESTES, M., AND PAGANO, J., 1972a, Structure and function of the polypeptides in simian virus 40. I. Existence of subviral deoxynucleoprotein complexes, *J. Virol.* **9:**923.

HUANG, E.-S., NONOYANA, M., AND PAGANO, J. S., 1972b, Structure and function of the polypeptides in simian virus 40. II. Transcription of subviral deoxynucleoprotein complexes *in vitro*, *J. Virol.* **9:**930.

HUDSON, J., GOLDSTEIN, D., AND WEIL, R., 1970, A study on the transcription of the polyoma viral genome, *Proc. Natl. Acad. Sci.* **65:**226.

HUEBNER, R. J., CHANOCK, R. M., RUBIN, B. A., AND CASEY, M. J., 1964, Induction by adenovirus type 7 of tumors in hamsters having the antigenic characteristics of SV40 virus, *Proc. Natl. Acad. Sci.* **52**:1333.

HUMMELER, K., TOMASSINI, N., AND SOKOL, F., 1970, Morphological aspects of the uptake of simian virus 40 by permissive cells, *J. Virol.* **6**:87.

INBAR, M., AND SACHS, L., 1969, Interaction of the carbohydrate-binding protein concanavalin A with normal and transformed cells, *Proc. Natl. Acad. Sci.* **63**:1418.

IWATA, A., AND CONSIGLI, R. A., 1971, Effect of phleomycin on polyoma virus synthesis in mouse embryo cells, *J. Virol.* **7**:29.

JACKSON, A. H., AND SUGDEN, B., 1972, Inhibition by α-amanitin of simian virus 40 specific ribonucleic acid synthesis in nuclei of infected monkey cells, *J. Virol*, **10**:1086.

JAENISCH, R., 1972, Evidence for SV40-specific RNA-containing virus and host-specific sequences, *Nature New Biol.* **235**:46.

JAENISCH, R., MAYER, A., AND LEVINE, A. J., 1971, Replicating SV40 molecules containing closed circular template DNA strands, *Nature (Lond.)* **233**:72.

JERKOFSKY, M., AND RAPP, F., 1973, Host cell DNA synthesis as a possible factor in the enhancement of replication of human adenoviruses in simian cells by SV40, *Virology* **51**:466.

KAMEN, R., LINDSTROM, D. M., SHURE, H., AND OLD, R., 1974, Transcription of polyoma virus DNA, *Cold Spring Harbor Symp. Quant. Biol.* **39**:187.

KANG, H. S., ESHBACH, T. B., WHITE, D. A., AND LEVINE, A. J., 1971, Deoxyribonucleic acid replication in simian virus 40 infected cells. IV. Two different requirements for protein synthesis during simian virus 40 deoxyribonucleic acid replication, *J. Virol.* **7**:112.

KAPLAN, J. C., WILBERT, S. M., AND BLACK, P. H., 1972, Endonuclease activity associated with purified simian virus 40 virions, *J. Virol.* **9**:800.

KATO, A. C., BARTOCK, K., FRASER, M. J., AND DENHARDT, D. T., 1973, Sensitivity of superhelical DNA to a single-strand specific endonuclease, *Biochim. Biophys. Acta* **308**:68.

KELLER, W., AND CROUCH, R., 1972. Degradation of DNA-RNA hybrids by ribonuclease H and DNA polymerases of cellular and viral origin, *Proc. Natl. Acad. Sci.* **69**:3360.

KELLY, T. J., JR., AND LEWIS, A. M., 1973, Use of nondefective adenovirus–simian virus 40 hybrids for mapping the simian virus 40 genome, *J. Virol.* **12**:643.

KELLY, T. J., JR., AND ROSE, J. A., 1971, Simian virus 40 integration site in an adenovirus 7–SV40 hybrid DNA molecule, *Proc. Natl. Acad. Sci.* **68**:1037.

KELLY, T. J., JR., AND SMITH, H. O., 1970, A restriction enzyme from *Hemophilus influenza.* II. Base sequence of the recognition site, *J. Mol. Biol.* **51**:393.

KHERA, K. S., ASHKENAZI, A., RAPP, F., AND MELNICK, J. L., 1963, Immunity in hamsters to cells transformed *in vitro* and *in vivo* by SV40: Tests for antigenic relationships among the papovaviruses, *J. Immunol.* **91**:604.

KHOURY, G., 1970, An investigation of the properties of SV40-transformed human cells, Harvard Medical School thesis.

KHOURY, G., AND MARTIN, M. A., 1972, Comparison of SV40 DNA transcription *in vivo* and *in vitro.* *Nature New Biol.* **238**:4.

KHOURY, G., BYRNE, J. C., AND MARTIN, M. A., 1972, Pattern of simian virus 40 DNA transcription after acute infection of permissive and non-permissive cells, *Proc. Natl. Acad. Sci.* **69**:1925.

KHOURY, G., BYRNE, J. C., TAKEMOTO, K. K., AND MARTIN, M. A., 1973a, Patterns of simian virus 40 deoxyribonucleic acid transcription. II. In transformed cells, *J. Virol.* **11**:54.

KHOURY, G., MARTIN, M. A., LEE, T. N. H., DANNA, K. J., AND NATHANS, D., 1973b, A map of simian virus 40 transcription sites expressed in productively infected cells, *J. Mol. Biol.* **78**:377.

KHOURY, G., LEWIS, A. M., OXMAN, M. N., AND LEVINE, A. S., 1973c, Strand orientation of SV40 transcription in cells infected by the nondefective adenovirus 2–SV40 hybrid viruses, *Nature New Biol.* **246**:202.

KHOURY, G., FAREED, G. C., BERRY, K., MARTIN, M. A., LEE, T. N. H., AND NATHANS, D., 1974a, Characterization of a rearrangement in viral DNA: Mapping of the circular SV40-like DNA containing a triplication of a specific one-third of the viral genome, *J. Mol. Biol.* **87**:289.

KHOURY, G., HOWLEY, P., BROWN, M., AND MARTIN, M., 1974b, The detection and quantitation of SV40 nucleic acid sequences using single-stranded DNA probes, *Cold. Spring Harbor Symp. Quant. Biol.* **39**:147.

KHOURY, G., HOWLEY, P., NATHANS, D., AND MARTIN, M., 1975a, Post-transcriptional selection of SV40-specific RNA, *J. Virol.* **15**:433.

KHOURY, G., MARTIN, M. A., LEE, T. N. H., AND NATHANS, D., 1975*b*, A transcriptional map of the SV40 genome, *Virology* **63**:263.

KIDWELL, W. R., SARAL, R., MARTIN, R. G., AMD OZER, H. L., 1972, Characterization of an endonuclease associated with simian virus 40 virions, *J. Virol.* **10**:410.

KIGER, J. A., JR., AND SINSHEIMER, R. L., 1969, Vegetative lambda DNA. IV. Fractionation of replicating lambda DNA on benzoylated-naphthoylated DEAE cellulose, *J. Mol. Biol.* **40**:467.

KIMURA, G., 1974, Genetic evidence for SV40 gene function in enhancement of human adenovirus in similar cells, *Nature (Lond.)* **248**:590.

KIMURA, G., AND DULBECCO, R., 1972, Isolation and characterization of temperature-sensitive mutants of SV40, *Virology* **49**:394.

KIMURA, G., AND DULBECCO, R., 1973, A temperature-sensitive mutant of SV40 affecting transforming ability, *Virology* **52**:529.

KIT, S., 1967, Enzyme inductions in cell cultures during productive and abortive infections by papovavirus SV40, in: *The Molecular Biology of Viruses* (J. S. Colter and W. Paranchyeh, eds.), pp. 495–525, Academic Press, New York.

KIT, S., 1968, Viral-induced enzymes and viral carcinogenesis, *Advan. Cancer Res.* **11**:73.

KIT, S., AND NALAJIMA, K., 1971, Analysis of the molecular forms of simian virus 40 deoxyribonucleic acid synthesized in cycloheximide treated cell cultures, *J. Virol.* **7**:87.

KIT, S., DUBBS, D. R., AND FREARSON, P. M., 1966, Enzymes of nucleic acid metabolism in cells infected with polyoma virus, *Cancer Res.* **26**:638.

KIT, S., MELNICK, J. L., ANKEN, M., DUBBS, D. R., deTORRES, R. A., AND KITAHARA, T., 1967, Non-identity of some simian virus 40 induced enzymes with tumor antigen, *J. Virol.* **1**:684.

KIT, S., KURIMURA, T., SALVI, M. L., AND DUBBS, D. R., 1968, Activation of infectious SV40 DNA synthesis in transformed cells, *Proc. Natl. Acad. Sci.* **60**:1239.

KITAHARA, T., AND MELNICK, J. L., 1965, Thermal separation of the synthesis of papovavirus SV40 tumor and virus antigen, *Proc. Soc. Exp. Biol. Med.* **120**:709.

KOCH, M. A., AND SABIN, A. B., 1963, Specificity of virus induced resistance to transplantation of polyoma and SV40 tumors in adult hamsters, *Proc. Soc. Exp. Biol. Med.* **113**:4.

KOPROWSKI, H., PONTÉN, J. A., JENSEN, F., RAUDIN, R. G., MOORHEAD, P., AND SAKSELA, E., 1962, Transformation of cultures of human tissue infected with simian virus 40, *J. Cell. Comp. Physiol.* **59**:281.

KOPROWSKI, H., JENSEN, F. C., AND STEPLEWSKI, Z., 1967, Activation of production of infectious tumor virus SV40 in heterokaryon cultures, *Proc. Natl. Acad. Sci.* **58**:127.

LAI, C. J., AND NATHANS, D., 1974, Mapping temperature-sensitive mutants of simian virus 40: Rescue of mutants by fragments of viral DNA, *Virology* **60**:466.

LAIPIS, P., and LEVINE, A. J., 1973, Deoxyribonucleic acid replication in SV40 infected cells. IX. The inhibition of a gap filling step during discontinuous synthesis of SV40 DNA, *Virology* **56**:580.

LAKE, R. S., BARBAN, S., and SALZMAN, N. P., 1973, Resolutions and identification of the core deoxynucleoproteins of the simian virus 40, *Biochem. Biophys. Res. Commun.* **54**:640.

LATARJET, R., CRAMER, R., and MONTAGNIER, L., 1967, Inactivation by UV-, X-, and α-radiations of the infecting and transforming capacities of polyoma virus, *Virology* **33**:104.

LAVI, S., AND WINOCOUR, E., 1972, Acquisition of sequences homologous to host deoxyribonucleic acid by closed circular simian virus 40 deoxyribonucleic acid, *J. Virol.* **9**:309.

LAZARUS, H. M., SPORN, M. B., SMITH, J. M., AND HENDERSON, W. R., 1967, Purification of T antigen from nuclei of simian virus 40 induced hamster tumors, *J. Virol.* **5**:1093.

LeBLANC, D. J., AND SINGER, M. F., 1974, Localization of replicating DNA of simian virus 40 in monkey kidney cells, *Proc. Natl. Acad. Sci.* **71**:2236.

LEBOWITZ, P., AND KHOURY, G., 1974, The simian virus 40 DNA segment of the adenovirus 7-SV40 hybrid, E46⁺, and its transcription during permissive infection of monkey kidney cells, *J. Virol.* **15**: in press.

LEE, Y., MENDECKI, J., AND BRAWERMAN, G., 1971, A polynucleotide segment rich in adenylic acid in the rapidly labeled polyribosomal RNA component of mouse sarcoma 180 ascites cells, *Proc. Natl. Acad. Sci.* **68**:1331.

LEVIN, M. J., CRUMPACKER, C. S., LEWIS, A. M., OXMAN, M. N., HENRY, P. H., AND ROWE, W. P., 1971, Studies of nondefective adenovirus 2–simian virus 40 hybrid viruses. II. Relationship of adenovirus 2 deoxyribonucleic acid and simian virus 40 deoxyribonucleic acid in the Ad2⁺ND₁ genome, *J. Virol.* **7**:343.

LEVINE, A. J., 1971, Induction of mitochondrial DNA synthesis in monkey cells infected by SV40 and (or) treated with calf serum, *Proc. Natl. Acad. Sci.* **68:**717.

LEVINE, A. J., AND TERESKY, A. K., 1970, Deoxyribonucleic acid replication in simian virus 40 infected cells. II. Detection and characterization of simian virus 40 pseudovirions, *J. Virol.* **5:**451.

LEVINE, A. J., KANG, H. S., AND BILLHEIMER, F., 1970, DNA replication in SV40 infected cells. I. Analysis of replicating SV40 DNA, *J. Mol. Biol.* **50:**549.

LEVINE, A. S., OXMAN, M. N., HENRY, P. N., LEVIN, M. J., DIAMANDOPOULOS, G. T., AND ENDERS, J. F., 1970, Virus-specific deoxyribonucleic acid in simian virus 40 exposed hamster cells: Correlation with S and T antigens, *J. Virol.* **6:**199.

LEVINE, A. S., LEVIN, M. J., OXMAN, M. N., AND LEWIS, A. M., 1973. Studies of nondefective adenovirus 2–simian virus 40 hybrid viruses. VII. Characterization of the simian virus 40 RNA species induced by five nondefective hybrid viruses. *J. Virol.* **11:**672.

LEWIS, A. M., AND ROWE, W. P., 1971, Studies on nondefective adenovirus–simian virus 40 hybrid viruses, *J. Virol.* **7:**189.

LEWIS, A. M., LEVIN, M. J., WEISE, W. H., CRUMPACKER, C. S., AND HENRY, P. H., 1969, A nondefective (competent) adenovirus–SV40 hybrid isolated from the AD2–SV40 hybrid population, *Proc. Natl. Acad. Sci.* **63:**1128.

LEWIS, A. M., LEVINE, A. S., CRUMPACKER, C. S., LEVIN, M. J., SAMAHA, R. J., AND HENRY, P. H., 1973, Studies of nondefective adenovirus 2–simian virus 40 hybrid viruses. V. Isolation of five hybrids which differ in their simian virus 40 specific biological properties, *J. Virol.* **11:**655.

LINDSTROM, D. M., AND DULBECCO, R., 1972, Strand orientation of simian virus 40 transcription in productivity infected cells, *Proc. Natl. Acad. Sci.* **69:**1517.

MACPHERSON, I., AND MONTAGNIER, L., 1964, Agar suspension culture for the selective assay of cells transformed by polyoma virus, *Virology* **23:**291.

MAGNUSSON, G., 1973, Hydroxyurea-induced accumulation of short fragments during polyoma DNA replication. I. Characterization of fragments, *J. Virol* **12:**600.

MAGNUSSON, G., PIGIET, V., WINNACKER, E. L., ABRAMS, R., AND REICHARD, P., 1973, RNA-linked short DNA fragments during polyoma replication, *Proc. Natl. Acad. Sci.* **70:**412.

MANTEUIL, S., PAGES, J., STEHELIN, D., AND GIRARD, M., 1973, Replication of simian virus 40 deoxyriboncleic acid: Analysis of the one-step growth cycle, *J. Virol.* **11:**98.

MARIN, G., AND MACPHERSON, I., 1969, Reversion in polyoma transformed cells: Retransformation, induced antigens and tumorigenicity, *J. Virol.* **3:**146.

MARTIN, M. A., 1970, Characteristics of SV40 DNA transcription during lytic infection, abortive infection, and in transformed mouse cells, *Cold Spring Harbor Symp. Quant. Biol.* **35:**833.

MARTIN, M. A., AND AXELROD, D., 1969a, SV40 gene activity during lytic infection and in a series of SV40 transformed mouse cells, *Proc. Natl. Acad. Sci.* **64:**1203.

MARTIN, M. A., AND AXELROD, D., 1969b, Polyoma virus gene activity during lytic infection and in transformed animal cells, *Science* **164:**68.

MARTIN, M. A., AND KHOURY, G., 1973, Transcription of SV40 DNA in lytically infected and transformed cells, in: *Virus Research* (C. F. Fox and W. S. Robinson, eds.), pp. 33–50, Academic Press, New York.

MAY, E., MAY, P., AND WEIL, R., 1973, "Early" virus-specific RNA may contain information necessary for chromosome replication and mitosis induced by simian virus 40, *Proc. Natl. Acad. Sci.* **70:**1658.

MAYOR, H. D., STINEBAUGH, S. E., JAMISON, R. M., JORDAN, L. E., AND MELNICK, J. L., 1962, Immunofluorescent, cytochemical, and microcytological studies on the growth of the simian vacuolating virus (SV40) in tissue culture, *Exp. Mol. Pathol.* **1:**397.

McCUTCHAN, J. H., AND PAGANO, J. S., 1968, Enhancement of the infectivity of simian virus 40 deoxyribonucleic acid with diethylamino-ethyldextran, *J. Natl. Cancer Inst.* **41:**351.

MELNICK, J. L., 1962, Papova virus group, *Science* **135:**1128.

MELNICK, J. L., AND RAPP, F., 1965, The use of antiviral compounds in analyzing the sequential steps in the replication of SV40 papovavirus, *Ann. N.Y. Acad. Sci.* **130:**291.

MICHEL, M. R., HIRT, B., AND WEIL, R., 1967, Mouse cellular DNA enclosed in polyoma viral capsids (pseudovirions), *Proc. Natl. Acad. Sci.* **58:**1381.

MIDDLETON, J. H., EDGELL, M. H., AND HUTCHISON, C. A., III, 1972, Specific fragmentation of ϕX174 deoxyribonucleic acid produced by a restriction enzyme from *Haemophilus aegypticus* endonuclease 2, *J. Virol.* **10:**42.

MORROW, J. F., AND BERG, P., 1972, Cleavage of simian virus 40 DNA at a unique site by a bacterial restriction enzyme, *Proc. Natl. Acad. Sci.* **69:**3365.

MORROW, J. F., AND BERG, P., 1973, The location of the T4 gene 32 protein binding site on SV40 DNA, *J. Virol.* **12**:1631.

MORROW, J. F., BERG, P., KELLY, T. J., JR., AND LEWIS, A. M., 1973, Mapping of simian virus 40 early functions on the viral chromosome, *J. Virol.* **12**:653.

MULDER, C., AND DELIUS, H., 1972, Specificity of the break produced by restricting endonuclease R_1 in simian virus 40 DNA, as revealed by partial denaturation mapping, *Proc. Natl. Acad. Sci.* **69**:3215.

MUELLER, N., ZEMLA, J., AND BRANDNER, G., 1973, Strand switch during *in vitro* polyoma transcription, *FEBS (Fed. Eur. Biochem. Soc.)* **31**:222.

MURAKAMI, W. T., FINE, R., HARRINGTON, M. R., AND BEN SASSAN, Z., 1968, Properties and amino acid composition of polyoma virus purified by zonal ultracentrifugation, *J. Mol. Biol.* **36**:153.

O'CONOR, G. T., RABSON, A. S., MALMGREN, R. A., BEREZESKY, I. K., AND PAUL, F. J., 1965, Morphologic observations of green monkey kidney cells after single and double infection with adenovirus 12 and simian virus 40, *J. Natl. Cancer Inst.* **34**:679.

ODA, K., AND DULBECCO, R., 1968a, Induction of cellular mRNA synthesis in BSC-1 cells infected by SV40, *Virology* **35**:439.

ODA, K., AND DULBECCO, R., 1968b, Regulation of transcription of the SV40 DNA in productively infected and in transformed cells, *Proc. Natl. Acad. Sci.* **60**:525.

OKAZAKI, R., OKAZAKI, T., SAKABE, K., SUGIMOTO, K., AND SUGINO, A., 1968, Mechanism of DNA chain growth, I. Possible discontinuity and unusual secondary structure of newly synthesized chains, *Proc. Natl. Acad. Sci.* **59**:598.

OPSCHOOR, A., POUWELS, P. H., KNIJNENBURG, C. M., AND ATEN, J. B. T., 1968, Viscosity and sedimentation of circular native deoxyribonucleic acid, *J. Mol. Biol.* **37**:13.

OXMAN, M. N., AND LEVIN, M. J., 1971, Interferon and transcription of early virus-specific RNA in cells infected with simian virus 40, *Proc. Natl. Acad. Sci.* **68**:299.

OXMAN, M.,N., ROWE, W. P., AND BLACK, P. H., 1967, Differential effects of interferon on SV 40 and adenovirus T antigen formation in cells infected with SV40 virus, adenovirus, and adenovirus–SV40 hybrid virus, *Proc. Natl. Acad. Sci.* **57**:941.

OXMAN, M. N., TAKEMOTO, K. K., AND ECKHART, W., 1972, Polyoma T antigen synthesis by temperature-sensitive mutants of polyoma virus, *Virology* **49**:675.

OXMAN, M. N., LEVIN, M. J., AND LEWIS, A. M., 1974, Control of SV40 gene expression in adenovirus–SV40 hybrid viruses: The synthesis of hybrid adenovirus 2–SV40 RNA molecules in cells infected with a nondefective adenovirus 2–SV40 hybrid virus, *J. Virol.* **13**:322.

OZANNE, B., AND SAMBROOK, J., 1971a, Isolation of lines of cells resistant to agglutination by concanavalin A from 3T3 cells transformed by SV40, *Lepetit Colloq. Biol. Med.* **2**:248.

OZANNE, B., AND SAMBROOK, J., 1971b, Binding of radioactivity labelled concanavalin A and wheat germ agglutinin to normal and virus-transformed cells. *Nature New Biol. (Lond.)* **232**:156.

OZANNE, B., VOGEL, A., SHARP, P., KELLER, W., AND SAMBROOK, J., 1972, Transcription of SV40 DNA sequences in different cell lines, *Lepetit Coloq. Biol. Med.* **4**:176.

OZANNE, B., SHARP, P. A. , AND SAMBROOK, J., 1973, Transcription of simian virus 40. II. Hybridization of RNA extracted from different lines of transformed cells to the separated strands of simian virus 40 DNA, *J. Virol.* **12**:90.

OZER, H. L., 1972, Synthesis and assembly of simian virus 40. I. Differential synthesis of intact virions and empty shells, *J. Virol.* **9**:41.

OZER, H., AND TAKEMOTO, K. K., 1969, Site of host restriction of simian virus 40 mutants in an established African green monkey kidney cell line, *J. Virol.* **4**:408.

OZER, H. L., AND TEGTMEYER, P., 1972, Synthesis and assembly of simian virus 40. II. Synthesis of the major capsid protein and its incorporation into viral particles, *J. Virol.* **9**:52.

PAGES, J., MANTEUIL, S., STEHELIN, D., FISZMAN, M., MARX, M., AND GIRARD, M., 1973, Relationship between replication of simian virus 40 DNA and specific events of the host cell cycle, *J. Virol,* **12**:99.

PALACIOS, R., AND SCHINKE, R.´T., 1973, Identification and isolation of ovalbumin-synthesizing polysomes, *J. Biol. Chem.* **248**:1424.

PASTAN, I., AND JOHNSON, G. S., 1974, Cyclic AMP and the transformation of fibroblasts, in: *Advances in Cancer Research* (G. Klein, S. Weinhouse, and A. Haddow, eds.), pp. 303–329, Academic Press, New York.

PATCH, C. T., LEWIS, A. M., AND LEVINE, A. S., 1972, Evidence for a transcription-control region of simian virus 40 in the adenovirus 2–simian virus 40 hybrid, $Ad2^+ND_1$, *Proc. Natl. Acad. Sci.* **69**:3375.

PETTIJOHN, D., AND KAMIYA, T., 1967, interaction of RNA polymerase with polyoma DNA, *J. Mol. Biol.* **29**:275.

POLLACK, R. E., AND BURGER, M. M., 1969, Surface-specific characteristics of a contact-inhibited cell line containing the SV40 viral genome, *Proc. Natl. Acad. Sci.* **62**:1074.

POLLACK, R. E., GREEN, H., AND TODARO, G. J., 1968, Growth control in cultured cells: Selection of sublines with increased sensitivity to contact inhibition and decreased tumor producing ability, *Proc. Natl. Acad. Sci.* **60**:126.

POPE, J. H., AND ROWE, W. P., 1964, Detection of a specific antigen in SV40 transformed cells by immunofluorescence, *J. Exp., Med.* **120**:121.

POTTER, C. W., MCLAUGHLIN, B. C., AND OXFORD, J. S., 1969, Simian virus 40 induced T and tumor antigens, *J. Virol.* **4**:574.

QASBA, P. K., 1974, Synthesis of simian virus 40 DNA in isolated nuclei, *Proc. Natl. Acad. Sci.* **71**:1045.

RABINOWITZ, Z., AND SACHS, L., 1968, Reversion of properties in cells transformed by polyoma virus, *Nature (Lond.)* **220**:1203.

RABINOWITZ, Z., AND SACHS, L., 1969, The formation of variants with a reversion of properties of transformed cells. II. *In vitro* formation of variants from polyoma-transformed cells, *Virology* **38**:343.

RABSON, A. S., O'CONOR, G. T., BEREZESKY, I. K., AND PAUL, F. J., 1964, Enhancement of adenovirus growth in African green monkey kidney cell cultures by SV40, *Proc. Soc. Exp. Biol. Med.* **116**:187.

RALPH, R. K., AND COLTER, J. S., 1972, Evidence for the integration of polyoma virus DNA in a lytic system, *Virology* **48**:49.

RAPP, F., AND TRULOCK, S. C., 1970, Susceptibility to superinfection of simian cells transformed by SV40, *Virology* **40**:961.

RAPP, F., KITAHARA, T., BUTEL, J. S., AND MELNICK, J. L., 1964a, Synthesis of SV40 tumor antigen during replication of simian papovavirus (SV40), *Proc. Natl. Acad. Sci.* **52**:1138.

RAPP, F., MELNICK, J. L., BUTEL, J. S., AND KITAHARA, T., 1964b, The incorporation of SV40 genetic material into adenovirus 7 as measured by intranuclear synthesis of SV40 tumor antigen, *Proc. Natl. Acad. Sci.* **52**:1348.

RAPP, F., BUTEL, J. S., AND MELNICK, J. L., 1964c, Virus induced intranuclear antigen in cells transformed by papovavirus SV40, *Proc. Soc, Exp. Biol. Med.* **116**:1131.

REEDER, R. H., AND ROEDER, R. G., 1972, Ribosomal RNA synthesis in isolated nuclei, *J. Mol. Biol.*. **67**:433.

REICH, P. R., BLACK, P. H., AND WEISSMAN, S. M., 1966, Nucleic acid homology studies of SV40 virus–transformed and normal hamster cells, *Proc. Natl. Acad. Sci.* **56**:78.

REZNIKOFF, C., TEGTMEYER, P., DOHAN, C., JR., AND ENDERS, J. F., 1972, Isolation of AGMK cells partially resistant to SV40: Identification of the resistant step, *Proc. Soc. Exp. Biol. Med.* **141**:740.

RISSER, R., AND POLLACK, R., 1974, A non-selective analysis of SV40 transformation of mouse 3T3 cells, *Virology* **59**:477.

RITZI, E., AND LEVINE, A. J., 1969, Deoxyribonucleic acid replication in simian virus 40 infected cells. III. Comparison of simian virus 40 lytic infection in three different monkey kidney cell lines, *J. Virol.* **5**:686.

ROBB, J. A., AND MARTIN, R. G., 1972, Genetic analysis of simian virus 40, III. Characterization of a temperature-sensitive mutant blocked at an early stage of productive infection in monkey cells, *J. Virol.* **9**:956.

ROBLIN, R., HARLE, E., AND DULBECCO, R., 1971, Polyoma virus proteins. I Multiple virion components, *Virology* **45**:555.

ROEDER, R. G., AND RUTTER, W. J., 1969, Multiple forms of DNA-dependent RNA polymerase in eukaryotic organisms, *Nature (Lond.)* **224**:234.

ROEDER, R. G., AND RUTTER, W. J., 1970, Specific nucleolar and nucleoplasmic polymerases, *Proc. Natl. Acad. Sci.* **65**:675.

ROTHSCHILD, H., AND BLACK, P. H., 1970, Analysis of SV40 induced transformation of hamster kidney tissue *in vitro*. VII. Induction of SV40 virus from transformed hamster cell clones by various agents, *Virology* **42**:251.

ROVERA, G., BASERGA, R., AND DEFENDI, V., 1972, Early increase in nuclear acidic protein synthesis after SV40 infection, *Nature New Biol.* **237**:240.

ROWE, W. P., AND BAUM, S. G., 1964, Evidence for a possible genetic hybrid between adenovirus type 7 and SV40 viruses, *Proc. Natl. Acad. Sci.* **52**:1340.

ROWE, W. P., AND BAUM, S. G., 1965, Studies of adenovirus–SV40 hybrid viruses. II. Defectiveness of the hybrid particles, *J. Exp. Med.* **122**:955.

ROZENBLATT, S., AND WINOCOUR, E., 1972, Covalently linked cell and SV40-specific sequences in an RNA from productivity infected cells, *Virology* **50**:558.

ROZENBLATT, S., LAVI, S., SINGER, M. F., AND WINOCOUR, E., 1973, Acquisition of sequences homologous to host DNA by closed circular simian virus 40 DNA. III. Host sequences, *J. Virol.* **12**:501.

RUSH, M. G., AND WARNER, R. C., 1970, Alkali denaturation of covalently closed circular duplex deoxyribonucleic acid, *J. Biol. Chem.* **245**:2704.

SABIN, A. B., SHEIN, H. M., KOCH, M. A., AND ENDERS, J. F., 1964, Specific complement-fixing tumor antigens in human cells morphologically transformed by SV40 virus, *Proc. Natl. Acad. Sci.* **52**:1316.

SACK, G. H., AND NATHANS, D., 1973, Studies of SV40 DNA. VI. Cleavage of SV40 DNA by restriction endonuclease from *Hemophilus parainfluenza*, *Virology* **51**:517.

SALZMAN, N. P., AND THOREN, M. M., 1973, Inhibition in the joining of DNA intermediates to growing simian virus 40 chains, *J. Virol.* **11**:721.

SALZMAN, N. P., FAREED, G. C., SEBRING, E. D., AND THOREN, M. M., 1973*a*, The mechanism of replication of SV40 DNA, in: *Virus Research* (C. F. Fox and W. S. Robinson, eds.), pp. 71–87, Academic Press, New York.

SALZMAN, N. P., SEBRING, E. D., AND RADONOVICH, M., 1973*b*, Unwinding of parental strands during simian virus 40 DNA replication, *J. Virol.* **12**:669.

SAMBROOK, J., 1972, Transformation by polyoma virus and simian virus 40, *Advan. Cancer Res.* **16**:141–180.

SAMBROOK, J., AND SHATKIN, A. J., 1969, Polynucleotide ligase activity in cells infected with simian virus 40, polyoma virus, or vaccinia virus, *J. Virol.* **4**:719.

SAMBROOK, J. F., WESTPHAL, H., SRINIVASAN, P. R., AND DULBECCO, R., 1968, The integrated state of viral DNA in SV40-transformed cells, *Proc. Natl. Acad. Sci.* **60**:1288.

SAMBROOK, J., SHARP, P. A., AND KELLER, W., 1972, Transcription of simian virus 40. I. Separation of the strands of SV40 DNA and hybridization of the separated strands to RNA extracted from lytically infected and transformed cells, *J. Mol. Biol.* **70**:57.

SAMBROOK, J., SUGDEN, B., KELLER, W., AND SARP, P. A., 1973, Transcription of simian virus 40. III. Mapping of "early" and "late" species of RNA, *Proc. Natl. Acad. Sci.* **70**:3711.

SAUER, G., 1971, Apparent differences in transcriptional control in cells productively infected and transformed by SV40, *Nature New Biol.* **231**:135.

SAUER, G., AND KIDWAI, J. R., 1968, The transcription of the SV40 genome in productively infected and transformed cells, *Proc. Natl. Acad. Sci.* **61**:1256.

SCHECHTER, I., 1973, Biologically and chemically pure mRNA coding for a mouse immunoglobin L-chain prepared with the aid of antibodies and immobilized oligothymidine, *Proc. Natl. Acad. Sci.* **70**:2256.

SCHLUMBERGER, H. D., ANDERER, F. A., AND KOCH, M. A., 1968, Structure of the simian virus 40. IV. The polypeptide chains of the virus particle, *Virology* **36**:42.

SEBRING, E. D., KELLY, T. J., JR., THOREN, M. M., AND SALZMAN, N. P., 1971, Structure of replicating simian virus 40 deoxyribonucleic acid molecules, *J. Virol.* **8**:478.

SEEBECK, T., AND WEIL, R., 1974, Polyoma viral DNA replicated as a nucleoprotein complex in close association with the host cell chromatin, *J. Virol.* **13**:567.

SHANI, M., HUBERMAN, E., ALONI, Y., AND SACHS, L., 1974, Activation of simian virus 40 by transfer of isolated chromosomes from transformed cells, *Virology* **61**:303.

SHARP, P. A., SUGDEN, B., AND SAMBROOK, J., 1973, Detection of two restriction endonuclease activities in *Haemophilus parainfluenzae* using analytical agarose–ethidium bromide electrophoresis, *Biochemistry* **12**:3055.

SHARP, P. A., PETTERSSON, U., AND SAMBROOK, J., 1974, Viral DNA in transformed cells. I. A study of the sequences of adenovirus Z DNA in a line of transformed rat cells using specific fragments of the viral genome, *J. Mol. Biol.* **86**:709.

SHEIN, H. M., AND ENDERS, J. F., 1962, Transformation induced by simian virus 40 in human renal cell cultures. I. Morphology and growth characteristics, *Proc. Natl. Acad. Sci.* **48**:1164.

SHELDON, R., JURALE, C., AND KATES, J., 1972, Detection of polyadenylic acid sequences in viral and eukaryotic RNA, *Proc. Natl. Acad. Sci.* **69**:417.

SHIH, T. Y., KHOURY, G., AND MARTIN, M. A., 1973, *In vitro* transcription of the viral specific sequences present in the chromatin of SV40 transformed cells, *Proc. Natl. Acad. Sci.* **70**:3506.

SHIMONO, H., AND KAPLAN, A. S., 1969, Correlation between the synthesis of DNA and histones in polyoma virus infected mouse embryo cells, *Virology* **37**:690.

SHIROKI, K., AND SHIMOJO, H., 1971, Transformation of green monkey kidney cells by SV40 genome: The establishment of transformed cell lines and the replication of human adenoviruses and SV40 in transformed cells, *Virology* **45**:163.

SJOGREN, H. O., HELLSTROM, I., AND KLEIN, G., 1961, Transplantation of polyoma virus induced tumors in mice, *Cancer Res.* **21**:329.

SMITH, H. S., SHER, C. D., AND TODARA, G. J., 1971, Induction of cell division in medium lacking serum growth factor by SV40, *Virology* **44**:359.

SMITH, H. O., AND WILCOX, K., 1970, A restriction enzyme from *Hemophilus influenza.* I. Purification and general properties, *J. Mol. Biol.* **51**:379.

STEWART, S. E., EDDY, B. E., GOCHENOUR, A. M., BORGESE, N. G., AND GRUBBS, G. E., 1957, The inductions of neoplasms with a substance released from mouse tumors by tissue culture, *Virology* **3**:380.

STIRPE, F., AND FIUME, L., 1967, Studies on the pathogenesis of liver necrosis by α-amanitin: Effect of α-amanitin on ribonucleic acid synthesis and on ribonucleic acid polymerase in mouse liver nuclei, *Biochem. J.* **105**:779.

SUBRAMANIAN, K. N., PAN, J., ZAIN, B. S., AND WEISMANN, S. M., 1924, The mapping and ordering of fragments of SV40 DNA produced by restriction endonucleases, *Nucleic Acid Res.* **1**:727.

SUGDEN, B., AND KELLER, W., 1973, Mammalian deoxyribonucleic acid–dependent ribonucleic acid polymerases I. Purification and properties of an α-amanitin-sensitive ribonucleic acid polymerase and stimulatory factors from HeLa and KB cells, *J. Biol. Chem.* **248**:3777.

SUMMERS, W. C., AND SIEGAL, R. B., 1970, Transcription of late phage RNA by T7 RNA polymerase. *Nature (Lond.)* **228**:1160.

SWEET, B. H., AND HILLEMAN, M. R., 1960, The vacuolating virus, SV40, *Proc. Soc. Exp. Biol. Med.* **105**:420.

SWETLY, P., BARBANTI-BRODANO, G., KNOWLES, B., AND KOPROWSKI, H., 1969, Response of simian virus 40 transformed cell lines to superinfection with simian virus 40 and its deoxyribonucleic acid, *J. Virol.* **4**:348.

TAI, H. T., SMITH, C. A., SHARP, P. A., AND VINOGRAD, J., 1972, Sequence heterogeneity in closed simian virus 40 deoxyribonucleic acid, *J. Virol.* **9**:317.

TAKEMOTO, K. K., AND HABEL, K., 1965, Hamster ascitic fluids containing complement-fixing antibody against virus induced tumor antigens, *Proc. Soc. Exp. Biol. Med.* **120**:124.

TAKEMOTO, K. K., AND MARTIN, M. A., 1970, SV40 thermosensitive mutant: Synthesis of viral DNA and virus induced proteins at nonpermissive temperatures, *Virology* **42**:938.

TAKEMOTO, K. K., AND MULLARKEY, M. F., 1973, Human papovavirus, BK strain: Biological studies including antigenic relationship to simian virus 40, *J. Virol.* **12**:625.

TAKEMOTO, K. K., KIRSCHSTEIN, R. L., AND HABEL, K., 1966, Mutants of simian virus 40 differing in plaque size, oncogenicity, and heat sensitivity, *J. Bacteriol.* **92**:990.

TAN, K. B., AND SOKOL, F., 1972, Structural proteins of simian virus 40: Phosphoproteins, *J. Virol.* **10**:985.

TAN, K. B., AND SOKOL, F., 1973, Phosphorylation of simian virus 40 proteins in a cell-free system, *J. Virol.* **12**:676.

TEGTMEYER, P., 1972, Simian virus 40 deoxyribonucleic acid synthesis: The viral replicon, *J. Virol.* **10**:591.

TEGTMEYER, P., AND OZER, H. L., 1971, Temperature sensitive mutants of SV40: Infection of permissive cells, *J. Virol.* **8**:516.

TEGTMEYER, P., DOHAN, C., JR., AND REYNIKOFF, C., 1970, Inactivating and mutagenic effects of nitrosoguanidine on SV40, *Proc. Natl. Acad. Sci.* **66**:745.

TEMIN, H. M., AND RUBIN, H., 1958, Characteristics of an assay for Rous sarcoma virus and Rous sarcoma cells in tissue culture, *Virology* **6**:669.

TEVETHIA, S. S., AND RAPP, F., 1965, Demonstration of new surface antigens in cells transformed by papovavirus SV40 by cytotoxic tests, *Proc. Soc. Exp. Biol. Med.* **120**:455.

TEVETHIA, S. S., DIAMANDAPOULOS, G. T., RAPP, F., AND ENDERS, J. F., 1968, Lack of relationship between virus specific surface and transplantation antigens in hamster cells transformed by simian papovavirus SV40, *J. Immunol.* **101**:1192.

THOREN, M. M., SEBRING, E. D., AND SALZMAN, N. P., 1972, Specific initiation site for simian virus 40 deoxyribonucleic acid replication, *J. Virol.* **10**:462.

THORNE, H. V., 1973, Cyclic variation in susceptibility of Balb-C 3T3 cells to polyoma virus, *J. Gen. Virol.* **18**:163.

THORNE, H. V., EVANS, J., AND WARDEN, D., 1968, Detection of biologically defective molecules in component I of polyoma virus DNA, *Nature (Lond.)* **219**:728.

TODARO, G. J., AND GREEN, H., 1966a, Cell growth and the initiation of transformation by SV40, *Proc. Natl. Acad. Sci.* **55**:302.

TODARO, G. J., AND GREEN, H., 1966b, High frequency of SV40 transformation of mouse cell line 3T3, *Virology* **28**:756.

TODARO, G. J., AND MARTIN, G. M., 1967, Increased susceptibility of Down's syndrome fibroblasts to transformation by SV40, *Proc. Soc. Exp. Biol. Med.* **124**:1232.

TODARO, G. J., GREEN, H., AND SWIFT, M. R., 1966, Susceptibility of human diploid fibroblast strains to transformation by SV40 virus, *Science* **153**:1252.

TONEGAWA, S., WALTER, G., BERNARDINI, A. AND DULBECCO, R., 1970, Transcription of the SV40 genome in transformed cells and during lytic infection, *Cold Spring Harbor Symp. Quant. Biol.* **35**:833.

TOOZE, J., 1973, Interaction of cell surfaces with lectins, in: *The Molecular Biology of Tumour Viruses* (J. Tooze, ed.), pp. 224–253, Cold Spring Harbor Laboratory, Cold Spring Harbor, N.Y.

TRILLING, D. M., AND AXELROD, D., 1970, Encapsidation of free host DNA by simian virus 40: A simian virus 40 pseudovirus, *Science* **168**:268.

TRILLING, D., AND AXELROD, D., 1972, Analysis of the three components of simian virus 40: Pseudo-, mature, and defective viruses, *Virology* **47**:360.

UCHIDA, S., YOSHIIKE, K., WATANABE, S., AND FURANO, A., 1968, Antigen-forming defective viruses of simian virus 40, *Virology* **34**:1.

VINOGRAD, J., AND LEBOWITZ, J., 1966, Physical and topological properties of circular DNA, *J. Gen. Physiol.* **49**:103.

VINOGRAD, J., LEBOWITZ, J., RADLOFF, R., WATSON, R., AND LAIPIS, P., 1965, The twisted circular form of polyoma viral DNA, *Proc. Natl. Acad. Sci.* **53**:1104.

VINOGRAD, J., LEBOWITZ, J., AND WATSON, R., 1968, Early and late helix-coil transitions in closed circular DNA: The number of superhelical turns in polyoma DNA, *J. Mol. Biol.* **33**:173.

VOGEL, A., AND POLLACK, R., 1973, Isolation and characterization of revertant cell lines. IV. Direct selection of serum-revertant sublines of SV40 transformed 3T3 mouse cells, *J. Cell Physiol.* **82**:189.

VORBRODT. A., AND KOPROWSKI, H., 1969. Ruthenium red stained coat of normal and simian virus 40 transformed cells, *J. Natl. Cancer Inst.* **43**:1241.

WALL, R., AND DARNELL, J. E., 1971, Presence of cell and virus specific sequences in the same molecules of nuclear RNA from virus transformed cells, *Nature New Biol.* **232**:73.

WALTER, G., ROBLIN, R., AND DULBECCO, R., 1972, Protein synthesis in simian virus 40 infected monkey cells, *Proc. Natl. Acad. Sci.* **69**:921.

WANG, J. C., 1971, Interaction between DNA and an *Escherichia coli* protein ω, *J. Mol. Biol.* **55**:523.

WARNAAR, S. O., AND DEMOL, A. W., 1973, Characterization of two simian virus 40 specific RNA molecules from infected BSC-1 cells, *J. Virol.* **12**:124.

WATKINS, J. F., AND DULBECCO, R., 1967, Production of SV40 virus in heterokaryons of transformed and susceptible cells, *Proc. Natl. Acad. Sci.* **58**:1396.

WEIL, R., AND VINOGRAD, J., 1963, The cyclic helix and cyclic coil forms of polyoma viral DNA, *Proc. Natl. Acad. Sci.* **50**:730.

WEINBERG, R. A., WARNAAR, S. O., AND WINOCOUR, E., 1972a, Isolation and characterization of simian virus 40 ribonucleic acid, *J. Virol.* **10**:193.

WEINBERG, R. A., BEN-ISHAI, Z., AND NEWBOLD, J. E., 1972b, Poly A associated with SV40 messenger RNA, *Nature New Biol.* **238**:111.

WEINBERG, R. A., BEN-ISHAI, Z., AND NEWBOLD, J. E., 1974, SV40 transcription in productively infected and transformed cells, *J. Virol.* **13**:1263.

WESTPHAL, H., 1970, SV40 DNA strand selection by *Escherichia coli* RNA polymerase, *J. Mol. Biol.* **50**:407.

WESTPHAL, H., 1971, Transcription of superhelical and relaxed circular SV40 DNA by *E. coli* RNA polymerase in the presence of rifampicin, *Lepetit Colloq. Biol. Med.* **2**:77.

WESTPHAL, H., AND DULBECCO, R., 1968, Viral DNA in polyoma and SV40 transformed lines, *Proc. Natl. Acad. Sci.* **59**:1158.

WESTPHAL, H., DELIUS, H. AND MULDER, C., 1973, Visualization of SV40 *in vitro* transcription complexes, *Lepetit Colloq. Biol. Med.* **4**:183.

WEVER, G. H., KIT, S., AND DUBBS, D. R., 1970, Initial site of synthesis of virus during rescue of simian virus 40 from heterokaryons of simian virus 40 transformed and susceptible cells, *J. Virol.* **5**:578.

WHITE, M., AND EASON, R., 1971, Nucleoprotein complexes in simian virus 40 infected cells, *J. Virol.* **8**:363.

WICKUS, G. G., AND ROBBINS, P. W., 1973, Plasma membrane proteins of normal and Rous sarcoma virus transformed chick embryo fibroblasts, *Nature New Biol.* **245:**65.

WILLIAMS, J. F., AND TILL, J. E., 1964, Transformation of rat embryo cells in culture by polyoma virus, *Virology* **24:**505.

WINNACKER, E. L., MAGNUSSON, G., AND REICHARD, P., 1972, Replication of polyoma DNA in isolated nuclei. I. Characterization of the system from mouse fibroblast 3T6 cells, *J. Mol. Biol.* **72:**523.

WINOCOUR, E., 1965, Attempts to detect an integrated polyoma genome by nucleic acid hybridization. I. "Reconstruction" experiments and complementarity tests between synthetic polyoma RNA and polyoma tumor DNA, *Virology* **25:**276.

WINOCOUR, E., 1969, The investigation of oncogenic viral genomes in transformed cells by nucleic acid hybridization, *Advan. Virus Res.* **14:**153.

WINOCOUR, E., AND ROBBINS, E., 1970, Histone synthesis in polyoma and SV40-infected cell DNA, *Virology* **40:**307.

WOLLMAN, J., AND SACHS, L., 1972, Mapping of sites on the surface membrane of mammalian cells. II. Relationship of sites for concanavaline A and an ornithine, leucine copolymer, *J. Membr. Biol.* **10:**1.

WYKE, J., 1971, A method of isolating cells incapable of multiplication in suspension culture, *Exp. Cell. Res.* **66:**203.

YELTON, D. B., AND APOSHIAN, H. V., 1972, Polyoma pseudovirions. I. Sequence of events in primary mouse embryo cells leading to pseudovirus production, *J. Virol.* **10:**340.

YOSHIIKE, K., 1968a, Studies on DNA from low-density particles of SV40. I. Heterogeneous defective virions produced by successive undiluted passages, *Virology* **34:**391.

YOSHIIKE, K., 1968b, Studies on DNA from low-density particles of SV40. II. Noninfectious virions associated with a large-plaque variant, *Virology* **34:**402.

YOSHIIKE, K., AND FURANO, A., 1969, Heterogeneous DNA of simian virus 40, *Fed. Proc.* **28:**1899.

YOSHIIKE, K., FURANO, A., AND SUZUKI, K., 1972, Denaturation maps of complete and defective simian virus 40 DNA molecules, *J. Mol. Biol.* **70:**415.

ZAIN, B. S., DHAR, R., WEISSMAN, S. M., LEBOWITZ, P., AND LEWIS, A. M., 1973, Preferred site for initiation of RNA transcription by *Escherichia coli* RNA polymerase within the simian virus 40 DNA segment of the nondefective adenovirus–simian virus 40 hybrid viruses Ad2$^+$ND$_1$ and Ad2$^+$ND$_3$, *J. Virol.* **11:**682.

ZAIN, B. S., WEISSMAN, S. M., DHAR, R., AND PAN, J., 1974, The nucleotide sequence preceding an RNA polymerase initiation site on SV40 DNA I, *Nucleic Acid Res.* **1:**577.

Index